EVIDENCE-BASED CARDIOLOGY

CHRISTOPHER P. CANNON, MD
Associate Professor of Medicine
Harvard Medical School
Brigham and Women's Hospital
Boston, Massachusetts

BENJAMIN A. STEINBERG, MD
Division of Cardiovascular Medicine
Department of Medicine
Duke University Medical Center
Durham, North Carolina

 Wolters Kluwer | Lippincott Williams & Wilkins
Health

Philadelphia · Baltimore · New York · London
Buenos Aires · Hong Kong · Sydney · Tokyo

Acquisitions Editor: Frances DeStefano
Product Manager: Leanne McMillan
Developmental Editor: Franny Murphy
Production Manager: Bridgett Dougherty
Senior Manufacturing Manager: Benjamin Rivera
Marketing Manager: Kimberly Schonberger
Creative Director: Doug Smock
Production Service: MPS Limited, A Macmillan Company

Printed in China

Library of Congress Cataloging-in-Publication Data
Cannon, Christopher P.
Evidence-based cardiology / Christopher P. Cannon, Benjamin A. Steinberg.—3rd ed.
  p. ; cm.
  Rev. ed. of: Evidence-based cardiology / Peter J. Sharis, Christopher P. Cannon. c2003.
  Includes bibliographical references and index.
  ISBN 978-0-7817-6473-5 (alk. paper)
  1. Heart—Diseases—Handbooks, manuals, etc. 2. Evidence-based
medicine—Handbooks, manuals, etc. I. Steinberg, Benjamin A.
II. Sharis, Peter J. Evidence-based cardiology. III. Title.
  [DNLM: 1. Heart Diseases—therapy—Abstracts. 2. Heart Diseases—therapy—Handbooks. 3.
Evidence-Based   Medicine—methods—Abstracts. 4. Evidence-Based   Medicine—methods—
Handbooks. 5. Heart Diseases—diagnosis—Abstracts. 6. Heart Diseases—diagnosis—Handbooks.
7. Randomized Controlled Trials as Topic—Abstracts. 8. Randomized Controlled Trials as Topic—
Handbooks. WG 39 C226e 2011]
  RC669.15.S53 2011
  616.1'2—dc22

2010025909

10 9 8 7 6 5 4 3 2 1

CCS0910

CONTENTS

2. Invasive Procedures and Revascularization 94

CHRISTOPHER P. CANNON AND BENJAMIN A. STEINBERG

PREFACE

Perhaps more than any other field of medicine, advances in cardiology are guided by data from large clinical trials. The number of major trials evaluating pharmacologic agents and diagnostic and therapeutic procedures continues to undergo significant growth. Since the publication of the previous edition of *Evidence-Based Cardiology*, results of hundreds of major trials have been published.

The two primary goals of *Evidence-Based Cardiology* are to (1) systematically summarize the major trials and (2) provide an overview of the field that integrates all the major trials and guidelines, thereby placing the information from the annotated studies in context. The results of major randomized trials in six major topic areas are presented in systematic fashion, including the design, study population, treatment regimen, results and when needed, additional perspective; some older trials and reviews have been eliminated and newer studies have replaced them. We have included selected meta-analyses, major review articles, and on occasion nonrandomized studies on important topics, usually with more abbreviated summaries. Importantly, the chapter overviews preceding the annotated references have been expanded with particular attention to discussing relevant ACC/AHA Practice Guidelines.

Chapter 1 focuses on preventive cardiology, particularly lipid and diet management, but also each of the multiple risk factors for coronary artery disease. There have been many advances included here. Chapter 2 focuses on major revascularization procedures, primarily coronary artery stenting and bypass surgery. New material includes data on drug-eluting stents and other novel devices. Chapters 3 and 4 cover the wealth of data on acute coronary syndromes. New material includes trial data on new antiplatelet and anticoagulant options for ACS, and a wealth of new studies on invasive strategy in STEMI patients. Chapter 5 focuses on the pharmacologic management of heart failure, with expanded information on biventricular pacing for CHF. Chapter 6 has been greatly expanded to include over 50 new trials, both in atrial fibrillation with new medications, novel strategies, and ablation procedures and in ventricular arrhythmias with expanded information on new drugs and implantable cardioverter defibrillators (ICDs).

We wish to acknowledge the coauthors of Chapters 5 and 6 (Justin M. Dunn and Jonathan Walter Dukes), who provided extensive assistance in revising, updating, and expanding these two chapters. We hope that the new edition will be helpful to you in staying up to date on the latest in evidence-based cardiology, and thereby help improve the management of patients.

Christopher P. Cannon, MD and Benjamin A. Steinberg, MD

CONTRIBUTORS

Christopher P. Cannon, MD
Associate Professor of Medicine
Harvard Medical School
Senior Investigator, TIMI Study Group
Cardiovascular Division
Brigham and Women's Hospital
Boston, Massachusetts

Jonathan Walter Dukes, MD
Postdoctoral Fellow in Cardiovascular Medicine
Department of Medicine
Division of Cardiology
University of California
San Francisco, California

Justin M. Dunn, MD, MPH
Cardiology Fellow
Department of Cardiovascular Medicine
Cleveland Clinic
Cleveland, Ohio

Benjamin A. Steinberg, MD
Division of Cardiovascular Medicine
Department of Medicine
Duke University Medical Center
Durham, North Carolina

The authors wish to acknowledge the work of Dr. Peter Sharis who was a coauthor of the previous edition, and as such a contributor to this volume.

CHAPTER 1

Preventive Cardiology: Risk Factors for Coronary Artery Disease and Primary and Secondary Prevention Trials

Christopher P. Cannon and Benjamin A. Steinberg

CHOLESTEROL, LIPIDS, AND DIET

Epidemiology

An estimated 107 million Americans have elevated total cholesterol (TC) levels, and based on the new National Cholesterol Education Program (NCEP) III guidelines, 37 million (one in five adults) are eligible for cholesterol-lowering therapy. A 10% decrease in TC is associated with an approximately 10% to 15% lower coronary heart disease (CHD) mortality rate and an approximately 20% decrease in the risk of myocardial infarction (MI). When TC levels are reduced by lifestyle modification (e.g., diet, exercise) and/or pharmacologic intervention, more benefit is derived in younger individuals, and the full benefits of a sustained decrease are not achieved for at least 5 years. Very low TC levels have been associated with higher mortality rates than those found with normal TC levels; however, this is likely owing to the higher prevalence of cancer in such individuals. Cardiac risk tables have been created to estimate the risk of CHD death at various cholesterol levels and in combination with other major CRFs. The NCEP III guidelines use modified Framingham risk score tables to estimate the 10-year CHD risk (see **Table 1.1**).

Low-density lipoprotein (LDL) has been shown in several studies, including the Framingham Heart Study, Multiple Risk Factor Intervention Trial (MRFIT), and Lipid Research Clinics (LRC) trial, to be a stronger predictor of CHD than TC. In fact, for every 30 mg/dL rise in LDL-C above 40 mg/dL, relative risk for coronary artery disease (CAD) increases by 30% (*Circulation* 2004;110:227). As a result, LDL levels are the primary focus of the NCEP III guidelines and their subsequent update. Of note, recent evidence suggests that C-reactive protein (CRP), a marker of inflammation, can provide additional prognostic information beyond that of LDL (see page 25).

High levels of high-density lipoproteins (HDLs) are associated with a decreased risk of CHD mortality; a 1% lower HDL-C is associated with a 2% to 3% higher CHD risk (17). The NCEP III guidelines now consider a low HDL level as less than 40 mg/dL (vs. less than 35 mg/dL in NCEP II) an indicator of

TABLE 1.1 Estimate of 10-Year Coronary Heart Disease Risk for Men and Women (Framingham Point Scores)

1. Age (yr)

20–34: −9/−7
35–39: −4/−3
40–44: 0/0
45–49: 3/3
50–54: 6/6
55–59: 8/8
60–64: 10/10
65–69: 11/12
70–74: 12/14
75–79: 13/16

2. Total Cholesterol mg/dL	Age 20–39 yr	Age 40–49 yr	Age 50–59 yr	Age 60–69 yr	Age 70–79 yr
<160	0/0	0/0	0/0	0/0	0/0
160–199	4/4	3/3	2/2	1/1	0/1
200–239	7/8	5/6	3/4	1/2	0/1
240–279	9/11	6/8	4/5	2/3	1/2
≥280	11/13	8/10	5/7	3/4	1/2

3. Smoking Status	Age 20–39 yr	Age 40–49 yr	Age 50–59 yr	Age 60–69 yr	Age 70–79 yr
Nonsmoker	0/0	0/0	0/0	0/0	0/0
Smoker	8/9	5/7	3/4	1/2	1/1

4. HDL (mg/dL)

>60: −1/−1
50–59: 0/0
40–49: 1/1
<40: 2

5. Systolic BP mm Hg	If Untreated	If Treated
<120	0/0	0/0
120–129	0/1	1/3

TABLE 1.1 *(Continued)*

130–139	1/2	2/4
140–159	1/3	2/5
≥160	2/4	3/6

Point Total	10-yr Risk (%)	Point Total	10-yr Risk (%)
<0	<1/<1	13	12/2
1	1/<1	14	16/2
2	1/<1	15	20/3
3	1/<1	16	25/4
4	1/<1	17	≥30/5
5	2/<1	18	≥30/6
6	2/<1	19	≥30/8
7	3/<1	20	≥30/11
8	3/<1	21	≥30/14
9	5/1	22	≥30/17
10	6/1	23	≥30/22
11	8/1	24	≥30/27
12	10/1	25	≥30/30

The score for each of the five components should be added together and the total point total used to estimate the 10-year risk of CHD. If the 10-year risk is >20%, this is considered a CHD risk equivalent (see **Table 1.2**). If the risk is 10–20%, then among those with 2+ CHD risk factors, LDL-lowering drug therapy should be initiated at a LDL level ≥130 (vs. ≥160 if 10-yr risk is <10%) (see **Table 1.2**).

CHD, coronary heart disease; LDL, low-density lipoprotein; BP, blood pressure; HDL, high-density lipoprotein.

COMMENT: Framingham score hasn't changed.

increased risk, whereas a level of 60 mg/dL or greater is a negative cardiac risk factor (**Table 1.2**). Furthermore, low HDL is now one of five diagnostic criteria for the metabolic syndrome (see page xx) (*Circulation* 2005;112:2735). Non-HDL cholesterol levels also have been demonstrated to be predictors of cardiovascular disease (CVD) (18), and the new NCEP guidelines now provide non-HDL goals for various risk categories (see **Table 1.2**).

Growing evidence indicates that high triglyceride (TG) levels are a modest independent predictor of increased CHD mortality (57). One analysis of studies with nearly 60,000 participants found that even after adjustment for multiple

TABLE 1.2. ATP III LDL-C Goals and Cutpoints for TLC and Drug Therapy in Different Risk Categories and Proposed Modifications Based on Recent Clinical Trial Evidence

Risk Category	LDL-C Goal	Initiate TLC	Consider Drug Therapy[i]
High risk: CHD[a] or CHD risk equivalents[b]	<100 mg/dL	≥100 mg/dL[h]	≥100 mg/dL[j]
10-year risk >20%	Optional goal: <70 mg/dL[f]		<100 mg/dL: consider drug options[i]
Moderately high risk: 2+ risk factors[c]	<130 mg/dL[g]	≥130 mg/dL[h]	≥130 mg/dL
10-year risk 10% to 20%[d]			100–129 mg/dL; consider drug options[k]
Moderately risk: 2+ risk factors[c] (10-year risk <10%)[d]	<130 mg/dL	≥130 mg/dL	≥160 mg/dL
Lower risk: 0–1 risk factor[e]	<160 mg/dL	≥160 mg/dL	≥190 mg/dL
			160–189 mg/dL: LDL-lowering drug optional

[a]CHD includes history of myocardial infarction, unstable angina, stable angina, coronary artery procedures (angioplasty or bypass surgery), or evidence of clinically significant myocardial ischemia.

[b]CHD risk equivalents include clinical manifestations of noncoronary forms of atherosclerotic disease (PAD, abdominal aortic aneurysm, and carotid artery disease [transient ischemic attacks or stroke of carotid origin or >50% obstruction of a carotid artery]), diabetes, and 2+ risk factors with 10-year risk for hard CHD >20%.

[c]Risk factors include cigarette smoking, hypertension (BP ≥140/90 mm Hg or on antihypertensive medication), low HDL cholesterol (<40 mg/dL), family history of premature CHD (CHD in male first-degree relative <55 years of age; CHD in female first-degree relative <65 years of age), and age (men ≥45 years; women ≥55 years).

[d]Electronic 10-year risk calculators are available at www.nhlbi.nih.gov/guidelines/cholesterol.

TABLE 1.2 (Continued)

[e]Almost all people with zero or 1 risk factor have a 10-year risk <10%, and 10-year risk assessment in people with zero or 1 risk factor is thus not necessary.

[f]Very high risk favors the optional LDL-C goal of <70 mg/dL, and in patients with high triglycerides, non–HDL-C <100 mg/dL.

[g]Optional LDL-C goal <100 mg/dL.

[h]Any person at high risk or moderately high risk who has lifestyle-related risk factors (e.g., obesity, physical inactivity, elevated triglyceride, low HDL-C, or metabolic syndrome) is a candidate for therapeutic lifestyle changes to modify these risk factors regardless of LDL-C level.

[i]When LDL-lowering drug therapy is employed, it is advised that intensity of therapy be sufficient to achieve at least a 30% to 40% reduction in LDL-C levels.

[j]If baseline LDL-C is <100 mg/dL, institution of an LDL-lowering drug is a therapeutic option on the basis of available clinical trial results. If a high-risk person has high triglycerides or low HDL-C, combining a fibrate or nicotinic acid with an LDL-lowering drug can be considered.

[k]For moderately high-risk persons, when LDL-C level is 100 to 129 mg/dL, at baseline or on lifestyle therapy, initiation of an LDL-lowering drug to achieve an LDL-C level <100 mg/dL is a therapeutic option on the basis of available clinical trial results.

From Grundy et al. Implications of recent clinical trials for the National Cholesterol Education Program Adult Treatment Panel III guidelines. *Circulation* 2004;110:227–239.

CRFs, high TG levels are associated with significant 14% and 37% reductions in cardiovascular risk in men and women, respectively. Obesity, physical inactivity, glucose intolerance, hypothyroidism, and the use of β-blockers, estrogen, and diuretics are associated with an increased risk of hypertriglyceridemia. The NCEP guidelines now classify TG levels of less than 150 mg/dL as desirable, 150 to 199 mg/dL as borderline, 200 to 499 mg/dL as high, and 500 mg/dL or greater as very high. Furthermore, hypertriglyceridemia joins low HDL among the five clinical criteria for diagnosis of the metabolic syndrome (see page xx).

Lipoprotein(a) [Lp(a)], which is structurally similar to LDL except for the addition of a single apolipoprotein(a) molecule, is a weak independent risk factor for CHD. Although individual studies have yielded conflicting results (56,57,59,60), a recent meta-analysis of 27 studies with at least 1 year of follow-up data found a 1.6-fold higher risk among those in top third of Lp(a) levels compared with those in the bottom third (59). Additionally, while the Women's Health Study (WHS) did demonstrate elevated cardiovascular risk in women with the highest levels of Lp(a), it also showed that this prognostication ability was significantly attenuated by hormone therapy (*JAMA* 2006;296:1363; *J Am Coll Cardiol* 2008;52:124). Levels are difficult to measure, and various measurement and storage techniques have been used in different studies. Most important, it is difficult to reduce Lp(a) levels significantly with lipid-lowering agents, and the clinical significance of reducing Lp(a) levels is unknown.

National Cholesterol Education Program Guidelines

The NCEP III guidelines recommended that all adults undergo a lipid panel analysis at least once every 5 years, starting at age 20 years (3,14), and now recommend that the initial screening include LDL measurement and TG measurement. Compared with NCEP II, NCEP III had several other changes, including (a) patients with diabetes and other high-risk disorders [peripheral vascular disease (PVD), symptomatic carotid disease, abdominal aortic aneurysm] are considered a CHD equivalent; (b) use of a modified Framingham risk table to identify higher-risk patients; (c) non–HDL-C targets for different risk categories; and (d) recognition of the metabolic syndrome.

NCEP LDL goals are listed in **Table 1.2**; of note, a 10-year CHD risk of more than 20% is considered a CHD risk equivalent. **Table 1.1** provides the modified Framingham point scores that should be used to estimate this 10-year risk. Drug therapy was listed as optional for those with CHD/CHD risk equivalents and an LDL of 100 to 129 mg/dL; however, subsequently published trials, including the Heart Protection Study (HPS) (44) and the Pravastatin or Atorvastatin Evaluation and Infection—Thrombolysis in Myocardial Infarction 22 (PROVE IT-TIMI 22) (46), led to a 2004 update to the NCEP III guidelines (15). The highlight of this update is the proposal that a LDL-C of <70 mg/dL may be a therapeutic option in patients of high or very high risk. They further amended previous guidelines to suggest that in these patients who have LDL-C ^{3}100 mg/dL, LDL-lowering drugs are indicated simultaneously with lifestyle modification (**Table 1.2**).

DIET AND VITAMINS

The nutrient composition of the therapeutic lifestyle changes (TLC) diet includes the following: saturated fat, less than 7% of total calories; total fat, 25% to 35% of calories; fiber, 20 to 30 g/day; and cholesterol, less than 200 mg/day. Fiber has minimal impact on cholesterol, and approximately 25% of compliant patients have no response; the average response is a reduction in TC of only 10% to 15%.

Increased vitamin E intake was associated with less CVD in several epidemiologic studies, including the Nurses Health Study (62). In the Cambridge Heart Antioxidant Study (CHAOS) (61), a randomized study of 2,002 CAD patients, vitamin E supplementation was associated with a significantly lower incidence of cardiovascular death and MI. However, in the Alpha-Tocopherol Beta-Carotene Cancer Prevention (ATBC) trial (63), GISSI Prevention Study (64), and Heart Outcome Prevention Evaluation (HOPE) study, all found no benefit associated with vitamin E supplementation (65). Most recently, the WHS failed to demonstrate any cardiovascular benefit to vitamin E supplementation (66), and a meta-analysis of high-dose supplementation even hinted at increased mortality in those taking vitamin E (67).

Special Diets

1. Fish and omega-3 fatty acid (FA) consumption: In a study of 852 Dutch men, the mortality rate was more than 50% lower among those consuming over 30 g of fish per day (equivalent of one to two dishes per week). In the 2,033 patient, randomized Diet and Reinfarction trial, the group advised to increase omega-3 fatty acid intake via fish consumption or fish oil supplementation had a 29% lower mortality compared to no advice group. In a prospective, nested case-control analysis of Physicians' Health Study participants with 17 years of follow-up, men with baseline long-chain n-3 fatty acid levels in the third and fourth quartiles had significantly reduced risks of sudden death compared with those in first quartile (adjusted RRs, 0.28, 0.19) (75). In the 11,324 patient GISSI-Prevenzione trial, supplementation with 850 mg of omega-3 fatty acid decreased sudden death by 45% and all-cause mortality by 20%, even in those receiving standard therapy [e.g., aspirin (ASA), statins]. Evidence also exists that increased fish intake results in a reduced risk of ischemic stroke (see *JAMA* 2002;288:3130).

   Based on these and other data, the American Heart Association (AHA) recently issued recommendations that persons with documented CHD should consume about 1 g of omega-3 fatty acids per day (76). In those unable to eat sufficient amounts of fish to meet this requirement, it recommends daily supplementation with 1-g fish oil capsules that contain 180 mg of eicosapentaenoic acid and 120 mg of docosahexaenoic acid. In individuals with high TG levels, higher amounts (2 to 4 g/day) should be considered. However, the AHA has pointed out that the research in omega-3 fatty acids is ongoing; notably, a 2006 systematic review of the data on long- and short-chain omega-3 fatty acids failed to identify a benefit in mortality, CVD, or cancer (77).

2. High fiber: Analysis of 21,930 ABTC patients showed the risk of CHD death to be inversely related to fiber intake [highest quintile (34.8 g/day) vs. lowest quintile (16.1 g/day); RR of CHD death, 0.69] (71). A Nurses' Health Study (NHS) analysis also found a significant association between fiber intake and CHD events. A 10-g/day increase in daily fiber intake was associated with a multivariate RR of 0.81 [95% confidence interval (CI), 0.66 to 0.99]. Finally, a recent analysis of 39,876 female health professionals found a 21% nonsignificant reduction of cardiovascular events among those in the highest quintile (26.3 g/day) of fiber intake compared with those in lowest quintile (12.5 g/day) (74).

3. Mediterranean (includes more bread, fruit, and margarine, and less meat, butter, and cream): The randomized 605-patient Lyon Heart Study found a 73% reduction in death and MI at 2.3-year follow-up, and a significant 56% all-cause mortality reduction at 3.8-year follow-up (68). The benefits of this diet appear correlated with increased omega-3 fatty acid intake (see *Am J Cardiol* 2000;85:1239).

Continuing research into the effects of various diets on weight loss and CVD has yielded varied results. However, there have been some clear messages. In the 2005 OmniHeart randomized trial of three diets low in saturated fat, but enhanced with either (a) carbohydrates, (b) protein, or (c) monounsaturated fat (78). While all three diets demonstrated improved blood pressure (BP) and LDL cholesterol compared to baseline, both the diets enriched in protein and the one enriched with monounsaturated fat demonstrated further improvement of such markers. In their 2005 comparison of four "fad" diets (the Atkins, Ornish, WeightWatchers, and Zone diets), Dansinger et al. found that all four could favorably affect weight and cardiometabolic risk factors—provided patients were able to stick with them long enough (79). The bottom line has been that diet *can* affect weight and cardiovascular health—and it is more important to find a diet that the patient can stick with, than to pick and choose the right ingredients.

DRUGS

Bile Resins (e.g., Cholestyramine, Colestipol)

These agents lower lipid levels by binding and blocking the reabsorption of bile acids. They typically decrease LDL cholesterol by 15% to 30%, increase HDL by 3% to 5%, and possibly increase TG levels. Compliance is often problematic because of their poor taste and gastrointestinal (GI) side effects, such as abdominal fullness, bloating, flatulence, and constipation. Numerous drug interactions also are found, and use is associated with an increased risk of gallstones. In the Lipid Research Clinic Coronary Primary Prevention Trial (22), cholestyramine use in 3,806 men with a mean TC of 291 mg/dL and LDL of 215 mg/dL resulted in 17% fewer MIs and a 19% reduction in CHD death and MI over the 7.4-year follow-up period. However, the all-cause mortality rate was not significantly different. The Cholesterol Lowering Atherosclerosis Study (CLAS) (52) was a smaller angiographic study that evaluated the combination of colestipol and niacin in 162 men with prior coronary artery bypass graft (CABG) surgery. Drug treatment resulted in lower TC (26%) and LDL levels (43%), higher HDL levels (37%), a higher atherosclerosis regression rate (16.2% vs. 2.4%), and fewer new lesions in bypass grafts. The Familial Atherosclerosis Treatment Study (FATS) (53) and a National Heart, Lung, and Blood Institute study were angiographic studies that both showed beneficial lipid-lowering effects and better angiographic outcomes in colestipol-treated patients. Thus, while these agents were pivotal in helping to prove the "lipid hypothesis"—that cholesterol was key to cardiovascular events and thus lowering cholesterol levels would improve clinical outcomes—they have largely fallen by the wayside in clinical practice, owing to their side-effect profile, interactions, and the development of more effective and better-tolerated alternatives.

Fibric Acid Derivatives (e.g., Gemfibrozil, Fenofibrate)

These agents (e.g., gemfibrozil, fenofibrate) typically increase HDL levels by 10% to 15%, decrease TGs by 20% to 50%, and have a minimal effect on LDL levels. They are usually well tolerated. The Helsinki Heart Study (23) evaluated the effect of gemfibrozil in 4,081 asymptomatic hypercholesterolemic men. At 5-year follow-up, gemfibrozil use was associated with 34% fewer cardiac events and a 26% lower CHD mortality rate. However, the overall mortality rate was not significantly different because of more deaths due to accidents, violence, and intracranial hemorrhage in the gemfibrozil group. The Veterans Administration HDL Intervention Trial (VA-HIT), which was a secondary prevention trial of 2,531 patients, found that gemfibrozil was associated with a nonsignificant 10% mortality reduction and 20% reduction in the incidence of CAD-related death and MI (37).

The World Health Organization Cooperative Study (21) evaluated clofibrate in 10,627 hypercholesterolemic men. At an average follow-up of 5.3 years, the clofibrate group had 25% fewer nonfatal MIs, but a 47% increase in overall mortality ($p < 0.05$). The Coronary Drug Project found that clofibrate use had no significant effect on all-cause mortality.

In the 10,000-patient Fenofibrate Intervention and Event Lowering in Diabetes (FIELD) trial, those randomized to fenofibrate (vs. placebo) seemed to have improved clinical outcomes over their counterparts (38). Unfortunately, many more patients in the fenofibrate group than the placebo group initiated statin therapy (see below) during the follow-up period, thus clouding the results.

In the latest assessment of fibrates for cardiovascular prevention, investigators from the ACCORD study group added fenofibrate or placebo to the regimens of 5,518 patients with type 2 diabetes already on simvastatin. At 4.7 years, there was no difference in the primary outcome of cardiovascular death, MI, or stroke. However, based on subgroup analyses, the data do not rule out fenofibrate use for hypertriglyceridemia or low HDL.

Cholesterol Absorption Inhibitors

This new class of agents works by inhibiting the intestinal absorption of dietary and biliary cholesterol by blocking the passage across the intestinal wall. Ezetimibe use results in moderate LDL reduction when used as monotherapy (18% in one study; see *Clin Ther* 2001;23:1209). More important, its effects appear additive to those provided by the statins (28,29). In one randomized study of 769 patients not at LDL goal at baseline, 72% taking ezetimibe and a statin achieved LDL goal compared with 19% taking statin alone. Coadministration is well tolerated (30,32,33). Therefore ezetimibe should be considered in patients not at LDL goal with statin monotherapy. However, further research into the *clinical* benefits of ezetimibe added to statins are still ongoing. In a study of 720 patients with familial hypercholesterolemia, the Ezetimibe and Simvastatin in Hypercholesterolemia Enhances Atherosclerosis Regression (ENHANCE) investigators randomized the group to 80 mg of simvastatin plus either 10 mg ezetimibe or placebo (31). They found no significant difference in changes to carotid-artery intima–media thickness, the primary outcome, as a surrogate for improvement in atherosclerotic disease. The ongoing IMPROVE-IT trial, powered to assess ezetimibe's efficacy for prevention of clinical events when added to a statin, should help address whether reduction in LDL with this nonstatin agent leads to a clinical benefit.

3-Hydroxy-3-Methylglutaryl-Coenzyme A Reductase Inhibitors (Statins)

These agents inhibit the rate-limiting step of cholesterol synthesis in the liver and typically decrease LDL by 20% to 60%, increase HDL by 5% to 15%, and decrease TGs by 10% to 20%. Potency (weakest to strongest on milligram-per-milligram basis) may be characterized as follows: fluvastatin, lovastatin, pravastatin, simvastatin, atorvastatin, rosuvastatin.

All these agents except pravastatin are metabolized by the cytochrome P450 system.

Side effects of the statins are uncommon (approximately 1% to 2%) and include mild GI intolerance, increased liver function test values, myositis (rare and usually with concurrent niacin, cyclosporine, gemfibrozil, or erythromycin). It is important to titrate or increase the dose of a specific agent until the NCEP LDL goal as one analysis of approximately 5,000 CAD patients found that only 25% had met the NCEP LDL goal of less than 100 mg/dL.

Several mechanisms of action ("pleiotropism") are proposed by which these agents achieve significant reductions in CHD and overall mortality:

1. Increased luminal diameter: unlikely because most angiographic trials [e.g., CLAS-I, FATS, MARS, CCAIT, SCRIP, MAAS, PLAC-I, REGRESS, LCAS, SCAT, HATS (52,53,55)] demonstrate minimal or no changes.
2. Restoration of endothelium-dependent vasodilatation: a small study found that initiation early after acute coronary syndromes (ACSs) (10.4 ± 0.7 days) rapidly improved endothelial function after 6 weeks of therapy.
3. Inhibition of thrombus formation (see the later section on early statin initiation).
4. Anti-inflammatory effects: statins significantly reduce CRP levels [see Pravastatin Inflammation/CRP Evaluation (PRINCE) results (179)].
5. Decreased cholesterol content in lesions, leading to more stable fibrous cap and other plaque-stabilization effects (see *Circulation* 2001;103:926).

A recent meta-analysis of 59 randomized, controlled trials found that several classes of lipid agents lower cholesterol, but only the statins significantly reduced CHD-related and all-cause mortality [34% and 25% RR reductions (RRRs), respectively] (4). In another meta-analysis of only statin trials (3), statin-treated patients had a 22% lower overall mortality rate, a 28% lower cardiovascular mortality rate, and 29% fewer strokes. Another analysis found that the effect of these agents widens with time [7% lower mortality in the first 2 years (25% by 5 years)].

Additional, in-depth analysis of the PROVE IT-TIMI 22 trial (see below), highlighted many potential pleiotropic phenomena observed specifically in patients with acute coronary syndromes, and frequently independent of the cholesterol-lowering effect (12). These include effects on endothelial activation/function, mitigation of the coagulation cascade, and favorable effects on markers of inflammation.

PRIMARY PREVENTION TRIALS

The West of Scotland Coronary Prevention Study (WOSCOPS) (24) was a randomized, placebo-controlled trial of 6,595 patients with an average TC of 272 mg/dL. At 5 years, the pravastatin group had 29% fewer nonfatal MIs ($p < 0.001$), a 32% lower cardiovascular mortality rate ($p = 0.033$), and a 22% lower overall mortality rate ($p = 0.051$). The Air Force/Texas Coronary Atherosclerosis Prevention Study (AFCAPS/TexCAPS) (25) randomized 9,605 men and post-menopausal women with average TC and LDL levels and below-average HDL levels to lovastatin or placebo. At average follow-up of 5.2 years, the lovastatin group had a 37% reduction ($p < 0.001$) in the risk for acute major coronary events. Only 17% of AFCAPS/TexCAPS patients would be recommended by the NCEP guidelines for drug therapy, suggesting that perhaps the guidelines should be expanded. Finally, the atorvastatin versus placebo arm of the Anglo-Scandinavian Cardiac Outcomes Trial (ASCOT) (10,305 patients) was stopped in October 2002 because the atorvastatin group had a significant 36% reduction in nonfatal MI and fatal CHD compared with those with placebo (1.9% vs. 3.0%, $p = 0.0005$) (30).

More contemporary primary prevention trials include the Collaborative Atorvastatin Diabetes Study (CARDS) (26), which enrolled 2,838 patients with type 2 diabetes mellitus, but no previously documented CVD; they were randomized to either atorvastatin 10 mg daily or placebo. The trial was stopped early, when a 37% relative risk reduction for the primary endpoint of acute coronary syndrome, coronary revascularization, or stroke was demonstrated in the intervention group. Additionally, one of the latest primary prevention trials to open a new door for primary prevention of atherosclerosis is the Justification for the Use of Statins in Prevention: an Intervention Trial Evaluating Rosuvastatin (JUPITER) study (27). The JUPITER investigators randomly assigned nearly 18,000 apparently healthy adults with LDL cholesterol levels of less than 130 mg/dL and high-sensitivity CRP of 2.0 mg/L or higher to rosuvastatin 20 mg daily or placebo. They demonstrated an impressive 44% reduction in cardiovascular events with rosuvastatin versus placebo ($p < 0.00001$), and highlighting another potential risk-stratification step for patients without documented CVD.

Additionally, several primary prevention studies have been done to look at atherosclerotic burden in patients taking statins, using vascular ultrasound (either carotid or coronary intravascular ultrasound) to assess primary endpoints. Both the ASTEROID study (a study to evaluate the effect of rosuvastatin on intravascular ultrasound-derived coronary atheroma burden) (JAMA 2006;295:1556–1565) and the METEOR trial (measuring effects on intima–media thickness: an evaluation of rosuvastatin) (JAMA 2007;297:1344–1353) assessed plaque burdens in patients taking rosuvastatin. Both demonstrated decreased plaque burden in the respective vascular sites, and the ASTEROID trial even demonstrated regression of such disease with the use of high-dose rosuvastatin, indicating that the improvements in cardiovascular events is accompanied by improvements in measured atherosclerosis.

SECONDARY PREVENTION TRIALS

The Scandinavian Simvastatin Survival Study (4S) (34) was a randomized, placebo-controlled trial enrolling 4,444 patients with an elevated TC ($\geq$213 mg/dL) and a history of CAD. At 5.4-year follow-up, the use of simvastatin, 40 mg/day, was associated with a 25% lower TC, a 35% lower LDL, a 42% lower CHD mortality rate, and a highly significant 30% relative reduction in lower overall mortality rate ($p = 0.0003$). Simvastatin patients also underwent 34% fewer coronary revascularization procedures and had fewer fatal and nonfatal cerebrovascular events.

The Cholesterol and Recurrent Events (CARE) trial (35) examined the use of pravastatin (40 mg/day) in patients with normal or mildly elevated TC (<240 mg/dL). At 5 years, pravastatin was associated with 24% fewer cardiac deaths and nonfatal MIs ($p = 0.003$). If the baseline LDL level was less than 125 mg/dL, only diabetic patients had a significant benefit.

The Long-term Intervention with Pravastatin in Ischemic Disease (LIPID) trial (36) enrolled more than 9,000 patients with known CAD and average TC levels (155 to 271 mg/dL). Pravastatin (40 mg/day) was associated with a 24% RRR in CHD mortality ($p < 0.001$), 22% RRR in overall mortality rate ($p < 0.001$), 19% RRR in strokes ($p = 0.048$), and 20% RRR in revascularization procedures ($p < 0.001$). Thus both the LIPID and CARE trials provide compelling data to support aggressive lipid lowering with statins in CAD patients with normal TC levels.

The Post-CABG trial (54) was an angiographic trial of 1,351 patients with one patent saphenous venous coronary bypass graft that showed that aggressive LDL-lowering therapy with lovastatin, 40 to 80 mg/day (and cholestyramine added if necessary), to achieve a target LDL of less than 85 mg/dL was associated with less graft atherosclerotic progression and 29% fewer revascularization procedures ($p = 0.03$). These data suggest that achieving very low LDL levels in post-CABG patients is important.

Two of the largest, contemporary, secondary prevention trials are the TNT (Treating to New Targets) and the IDEAL (Incremental Decrease in End Points Through Aggressive Lipid Lowering) trials (46,47). Both enrolled patients with stable CAD (10,001 in TNT; 8,888 in IDEAL), randomized them to high or standard-dose statins (10 vs. 80 mg atorvastatin in TNT, 20 mg simvastatin vs. 80 mg atorvastatin in IDEAL), and followed them for roughly 5 years for clinical endpoints. The TNT trial resulted in a 2.2% absolute reduction ($p < 0.001$) in the primary event (composite of cardiovascular death, nonfatal MI, resuscitation from cardiac arrest, or any stroke). In the IDEAL trial, patients in the high-dose statin group (atorvastatin 80 mg) did experience fewer events of the primary endpoint (coronary death, nonfatal MI, or cardiac arrest resuscitation), the hazard ratio of 0.89 for the high-dose group did not meet statistical significance ($p = 0.07$). However, when measured based on the endpoints of any number of other, similar trials, including TNT, the IDEAL results prove consistent with the clinical benefit.

To better identify the best secondary prevention strategy, the Clinical Outcomes Utilizing Revascularization and Aggressive Drug Evaluation (COURAGE) trial randomized 2,287 patients with stable CAD to PCI, medical therapy, and aggressive lifestyle modification versus medical therapy and aggressive lifestyle modification alone (see Chapter 3). The primary outcome was a composite endpoint of death or nonfatal MI, over a follow-up period of 4.6 years. This hotly debated trial resulted in no significant difference in clinical endpoints for patients undergoing PCI or medical therapy alone. It reinforced conclusions from many preliminary studies—that revascularization could improve symptoms, but does not seem to prevent clinical events.

Initiation of statin therapy before hospital discharge, in addition to providing probable non–lipid-lowering benefits, results in higher use rates. In the Cardiac Hospitalization Atherosclerosis Management Program (CHAMP) study, statin use increased from 6% to 86% when started in the hospital, and 58% reached their LDL goal (<100 mg/dL) versus 6% (see *Am J Cardiol* 2001;87:219).

COMBINED PRIMARY AND SECONDARY PREVENTION TRIALS

In the HPS (44), which randomized 20,536 patients with CAD, diabetes, or other occlusive arterial disease to simvastatin, 40 mg/day, or placebo, the statin group had a significantly lower all-cause mortality (12.9% vs. 14.7%; $p = 0.003$). Significant benefit also was observed among those with an initial LDL less than 3 mmol (116 mg/dL). These results significantly expand the population that should be targeted for lipid-lowering therapy.

In the PROspective Study of Pravastatin in the Elderly at Risk (PROS-PER) study, 5,804 patients aged 70 to 82 years with vascular disease or risk factors were randomized to pravastatin, 40 mg/day, or placebo, and the pravastatin group had a 24% relative reduction in CHD death. This large study provides strong evidence that the benefits associated with statin therapy extend to older patients.

EARLY STATIN INITIATION TRIALS

Several studies have examined the early initiation of statins after acute coronary events. In the Myocardial Ischemia Reduction with Aggressive Cholesterol Lowering (MIRACL) study (40), 3,086 patients with unstable angina or non–ST elevation MI (UA/NSTEMI) were enrolled, and atorvastatin, 80 mg/day, was found to have a significant 15% relative reduction in the composite primary end point compared with placebo, primarily because of fewer recurrent ischemic events (14.8% vs. 17.4%; $p = 0.048$). This benefit occurred regardless of LDL level or the percentage by which LDL was lowered, suggesting the presence of non–lipid-lowering, pleiotropic effects.

The PROVE IT-TIMI 22 trial randomized 4,162 patients hospitalized for ACS to either 40 mg pravastatin daily ("standard" therapy) versus 80 mg of ator-vastatin daily ("intensive" therapy), with the primary endpoint being a composite of death, MI, rehospitalization for unstable angina, revascularization, or stroke at a mean follow-up of 24 months (46). After 2 years of mean follow-up, 26.3% of patients in the standard therapy group experienced an event versus 22.4% in the intensive therapy, a significant 16% reduction in the hazard ratio in favor of inten-sive therapy in patients hospitalized for ACS ($p = 0.005$). This benefit appeared to emerge within 30 days.

In the "Z" phase of the Aggrastat to Zocor (A to Z) trial, 4,497 patients with acute coronary syndromes were randomized to simvastatin 40 mg daily for 1 month then 80 mg daily ("early high-dose" group) versus placebo for 4 months and then 20 mg simvastatin ("late standard dosing") (47). They were followed for up to 24 months, with a composite primary endpoint of cardiovascular death, nonfatal MI, readmission for ACS, or stroke. Despite a 2.3% absolute risk reduction in the primary endpoint favoring the early high-dose group, this result did not meet statistical signif-icance ($p = 0.14$), though the overall trends in the trial confirmed the findings of other studies, such as PROVE IT-TIMI 22 and TNT. When these two trials are combined with the results from TNT and IDEAL (see *J Am Coll Cardiol* 2006;48:438–445), the evidence for intensive lipid-lowering therapy in patients with CAD is robust.

Raising HDL Cholesterol

NIACIN

Niacin is a B vitamin that inhibits the mobilization of free FAs from peripheral tis-sues, with a resulting decrease in hepatic synthesis of TGs and secretion of very low density lipoproteins (VLDLs). Niacin typically decreases LDL by 10% to 25%, increases HDL by 15% to 35%, decreases TGs by 20% to 50%, and decreases Lp(a). A common side effect is flushing, which is often controllable by daily ASA use. A long-acting formulation of niacin appears to reduce flushing. Other side effects of niacin include hyperglycemia, increased uric acid levels, increased liver function tests, exacerbation of peptic ulcer disease, and rhabdomyolysis (rare). In the Coronary Drug Project (32), a randomized trial enrolling more than 8,000 men with prior MI, the use of niacin, 3 g/day, was associated with a 27% lower nonfatal MI rate at 5-year follow-up and a significant 11% reduction in overall mortality at 15 years. Other trials evaluating the use of niacin in combination with other agents [e.g., CLAS, FATS, HDL-Atherosclerosis Treatment Study (HATS) (52,53,55)] also showed significant favorable changes in lipid levels and reduced rates of CHD mor-tality. However, the flushing associated with niacin has proven to be a significant hurdle for many patients, and attempts at developing combination agents to mitigate that effect have been to no avail.

With low HDL cholesterol demonstrated to be a risk factor for CVD, therapies targeted to raising HDL have been aggressively pursued. One class has been the cholesterol ester transfer protein (CETP) inhibitors, which had been demonstrated to significantly raise HDL levels (though without data on clinical outcomes). The first agent to make it to phase 3 trials, torcetrapib, was unfortunately abandoned when these trials demonstrated increased mortality in the active-treatment arm (see *N Engl J Med* 2007;356:1304–1316; *N Engl J Med* 2007;357:2109–2122). This could be owing to the drug's tendency to increase BP significantly, through mechanisms not well-understood. However, additional agents geared toward HDL remain in development currently with high hopes for additional cardiovascular benefits (see *Lancet* 2007;370:1907–1914; *Eur Heart J* 2010;31:390–393).

SMOKING

Current smoking is associated with an approximately threefold increased risk of MI and an approximately twofold increased risk of CHD-related death (95–100). Smoking in combination with another major cardiac risk factor [e.g., hypertension (HTN), diabetes, hypercholesterolemia] results in an approximately 20-fold increase in death and MI (96). Among those who quit smoking, the risk gradually returns to baseline after several years (97). Passive or second-hand smoke exposure results in an average 20% to 25% increase in CHD mortality (98,100), whereas frequent or heavy exposure can result in a nearly twofold increased risk (99). In fact, several follow-up studies of smoking bans implemented in public areas have identified measurable declines in coronary disease incidence in these areas (101,102, see also *Circulation* 2006;114:1490–1496; *Arch Intern Med* 2008;168:1950–1960). Financial incentives have also been found to be effective in some scenarios, for assistance in smoking cessation (see also *N Engl J Med*. 2009;360:699–709).

Additional pharmacologic therapies to aid in smoking cessation continue to be developed. In addition to the use of well-known antidepressant, bupropion, as a smoking cessation aid, a newer agent, varenicline has proved even more effective (103). An alpha4beta2 nicotinic acetylcholine receptor partial agonist, varenicline is now approved to aid in smoking cessation and many have found it very effective. Importantly, varenicline also appears safe in patients with known CVD (104).

DIABETES

The American Health Association estimates that 15 million individuals in the United States have diagnosed diabetes mellitus and an additional 6 million are undiagnosed in 2005; more than 95% have the non–insulin-dependent variety of diabetes mellitus (NIDDM). Additionally, the organization estimates that as many as 60 million Americans may have prediabetes, a state of glucose intolerance thought to precede the development of diabetes. The significant decline in CHD mortality seen in the general population in recent decades has not occurred in diabetes (81); 77% of U.S. hospital stays for diabetics are attributable to CVD. NIDDM is associated with approximately two- and threefold increased risks of CHD death in men and women, respectively. The risks of death from MI and CHD are as high in diabetics without prior MIs as in nondiabetics with prior MIs (80,82). As a result, guidelines now consider diabetes a CHD risk equivalent and recommend that all diabetics older than 30 years take ASA ($\geq$81 mg daily). Diabetics also have an approximately twofold increased risk of stroke.

Diabetics frequently have other modifiable risk factors, most often HTN and obesity. Addressing these risk factors [e.g., by exercise, dietary modification, or pharmacologic agent(s)] is essential to reducing an individual's cardiac risk. Prior studies have indicated that BP control significantly reduces the incidence of both macrovascular and microvascular (e.g., retinopathy) complications (87); the Joint National Committee (JNC) 7 Guidelines recommend less than 130/80 mm Hg, as do the American Diabetes Association and National Kidney Foundation. However, the recent ACCORD trial found no benefit of targeting a systolic BP <120 as compared with the more standard approach of <140 (88). In particular, angiotensin-converting enzyme (ACE) inhibitors and angiotensin-II–receptor blockers (e.g., losartan, irbesartan) not only lower BP but also protect against the progression of nephropathy [Irbesartan Microalbuminuria Type 2 Diabetes in Hypertensive Patients Study (IRMA II), Reduction of Endpoints in NIDDM with the Angiotensin II Antagonist Losartan Study (RENAAL) Irbesartan in Diabetic Nephropathy Trial (IDNT) (89,90,93).

Intensive glycemic control of individuals with IDDM in the Diabetes Control and Complications Trial (DCCT) resulted in a 34% reduction in LDL levels and a 41% reduction in major cardiovascular and peripheral vascular events (see *N Engl J Med* 1993;329:977). Current American Diabetes Association guidelines (see *Diabetes Care* 2009;32:S13–S61) recommend target goals of LDL cholesterol of less than 100 mg/dL for patients without overt CVD, and less than 70 mg/dL as an option for those with known CVD; of HDL, more than 45 mg/dL; and of TGs, less than 150 mg/dL.

However, the ACCORD (Action to Control Cardiovascular Risk in Diabetes) and ADVANCE (Action in Diabetes and Vascular Disease: Preterax and Diamicron Modified Release Controlled Evaluation) trials tested the hypothesis that strict glycemic control could improve clinical cardiovascular outcomes. ACCORD randomized 10,251 patients with type 2 diabetes to either standard therapy targeting a hemoglobin A1c (HbA1c) of 7% to 7.9% versus intensive therapy, targeting a1c less than 6%. The trial was discontinued prematurely when an excess rate of death was identified in the intensive glycemic control arm after a mean of 3.5 years of follow-up. The ADVANCE trial randomized 11,140 patients with type 2 diabetes to either standard care or intensive glycemic control to a goal a1c of less than 6.5%, and followed for a mean of 5 years for both macrovascular and microvascular cardiovascular outcomes. While the trial met its primary endpoint (a composite of macro- and microvascular events), this was predominantly driven by a decreased incidence of nephropathy, without statistically significant effects on major adverse cardiovascular events (MACE) (death, MI, stroke, heart failure).

In the STENO-2 study, intensive therapy, consisting of behavioral modification and drug therapy, which targeted all the previously mentioned areas (hyperglycemia, HTN, dyslipidemia, microalbuminuria), reduced the risk of cardiovascular and microvascular events by about 50% compared with conventional therapy (94). This small study however emphasizes the benefits of comprehensive risk factor modification in diabetics.

Metabolic Syndrome

This disorder has received increasing attention and is recognized as a major problem in the NCEP III report. The syndrome is defined as the presence of three or more of the following: (a) abdominal obesity (waist circumference more than 40 inches in men and more than 35 inches in women); (b) TGs, 150 mg/dL or more; (c) HDL, less than 40 mg/dL (men) or less than 50 mg/dL (women) (or on pharmacologic treatment for hypertriglyceridemia); (d) systolic BP more than 129 or diastolic BP more than 84 mm Hg (or on pharmacologic treatment for HTN); and (e) fasting glucose more than 99 mg/dL (or on pharmacologic treatment for elevated glucose). In the National Health And Nutrition Examination Survey (NHANES) III survey, the prevalence of the metabolic syndrome was more than 20% (83). A Finnish study found those with the syndrome had a three- to fourfold increased risk of CHD death (84). A recent study found, however, that patients with metabolic syndrome, in the absence of diabetes, did not appear to have an increased risk (85).

HYPERTENSION

Epidemiology

Approximately 70 million Americans have HTN. HTN occurs in the absence of other CRFs in 20%. From ages 30 to 65 years, systolic blood pressure (SBP) and diastolic blood pressure (DBP) increase by approximately 20 and 10 mm Hg, respectively. According to NHANES data in the JNC 7 report, only 59% receive treatment, and only 34% have adequate control (<140/90 mm Hg at the time of the study); nearly one third are unaware of their HTN. A Framingham Heart Study analysis (108) showing the age-adjusted prevalence of stage 2 HTN (SBP ≥ 160 mm Hg or DBP ≥ 100 mm Hg) declined significantly from 1950 to 1989 (men, 18.5% to 9.2%; women, 28.0% to 7.7%); these findings are likely owing to effective pharmacologic treatment of severe HTN. However, another Framingham analysis found that the lifetime risk of developing HTN is 90% or higher (109). The risks of "mild" HTN are not insignificant; for example, isolated systolic HTN (SBP, 140 to 159 mm Hg) is associated with a 50% to 60% higher incidence of cardiovascular death (107); also, the JNC 7 guidelines stress that SBP >140 mm Hg is a more important CVD risk factor than diastolic BP in those older than 50 years (105).

Etiology

Approximately 90% to 95% of cases have no known cause (essential HTN). Secondary causes include renal parenchymal disease (2% to 5%), renovascular HTN (approximately 1%), primary aldosteronism (adrenal adenoma, 60%; bilateral hyperplasia, 40%), Cushing syndrome, pheochromocytoma [10% malignancy, 10% bilateral, 10% familial (multiple endocrine neoplasia type 2; MEN II)], coarctation of aorta, numerous drugs [e.g., glucocorticoids, anabolic steroids, nonsteroidal anti-inflammatory drugs (NSAIDs) (110), alcohol, oral contraceptives, cocaine, cyclosporine, sympathomimetics, tricyclic antidepressants, and amphetamines], hyperparathyroidism, and acromegaly.

Diagnosis, Joint National Committee 7 Classification

Unless BP is markedly elevated, it should be measured on three separate occasions before initiating therapy. The Joint National Committee (JNC 7) classification is as follows (see also **Table 1.3**) (105):

Prehypertension: SBP, 120 to 139 mm Hg; DBP, 80 to 89 mm Hg
Stage I HTN: SBP, 140 to 159 mm Hg; DBP, 90 to 99 mm Hg
Stage II: SBP, $\geq$160 mm Hg; DBP, $\geq$100 mm Hg

Treatment
NONPHARMACOLOGIC

Weight loss has been shown to reduce the need for antihypertensive medication(s). The Dietary Approaches to Stop Hypertension (DASH) diet, which consists of a diet rich in fruits, vegetables, and low-fat dairy products, has been shown to reduce BP significantly in hypertensive patients (135,137). Sodium restriction also appears to have a modest beneficial effect. One meta-analysis of 56 trials showing a 100 mg/day reduction in urinary sodium excretion was associated with a reduction of 3.7 mm Hg in SBP ($p < 0.001$).

A randomized study (PREMIER) demonstrated the benefit of behavioral modification that included weight loss, sodium reduction, increased physical activity, and limited alcohol intake (see *JAMA* 2003;289:2083). Furthermore, data from the LOOK AHEAD trial demonstrated that intensive lifestyle modification in patients with diabetes not only is more effective for weight loss, but can also have significant impact on cardiovascular risk markers, including lipids and BP (138).

PHARMACOLOGIC

The JNC 7 guidelines advocate the use of thiazide diuretics for most patients with uncomplicated HTN, either alone or in combination with drugs from other classes (**Table 1.3**) (105). A meta-analysis of 18 randomized trials enrolling a total of more than 48,000 patients showed that the use of β-blockers and low-dose

TABLE 1.3 JNC 7 Classification and Management of Blood Pressure

BP Classification (SBP and DBP, mm HG)	Initial Drug Therapy[a] Without Compelling Indication	With Compelling Indications[b]
Normal (<120 and <80)		
Prehypertension (140–159 or 80–89)	No drug indicated	Drug(s) for compelling indications
Stage 1 hypertension (140–159 or 90–99)	Thiazide-type diuretics for most; may consider ACE inhibitor, ARB, β-blocker, CCB, or combination	Drug(s) for compelling indications: Other antihypertensive drugs (diuretics, ACE inhibitor, ARB, β-blocker, CCB) as needed
Stage 2 hypertension (≥160 or ≥100)	Two-drug combination for most (usually thiazide-type diuretic and ACE inhibitor or ARB or β-blocker or CCB)	Same as above

ARB, angiotensin-receptor blocker; CCB, calcium channel blocker.

[a]Lifestyle modification is recommended for those with prehypertension and stages 1 or 2 hypertension.

[b]See Table 6 of JNC 7 Guidelines (examples: post-MI: β-blocker, ACE inhibitor, aldosterone antagonist; heart failure: diuretic, β-blocker, ACE inhibitor, ARB, aldosterone antagonist; diabetes: diuretic, β-blocker, ACE inhibitor, ARB, CCB).

(Adapted from JNC 7, Chobanian AV, et al. The seventh report of the Joint National Committee on prevention, detection, evaluation, and treatment of high blood pressure: the JNC 7 report. *JAMA* 2003;289:2560–2571.)

diuretics was associated with fewer strokes (RRs, 0.71, 0.49, and 0.66) and less congestive heart failure (CHF; RRs, 0.58, 0.17, and 0.58). Low-dose diuretics also were associated with less CAD and lower all-cause mortality rates (RR, 0.90; 95% CI, 0.81 to 0.99).

Several studies have now compared diuretics and β-blockers with newer, more expensive ACE inhibitors and calcium-channel blockers [e.g., CAPP (Cantopril Prevention Project), Nordil (Nordic Diltiazem Study), INVEST (International Verapamil SR-Trandolapril Study), STOP-HTN2 (Swedish Trial in

Old Patients with Hypertension-2 Study), CONVINCE (Controlled Onset Verapamil Investigation of Cardiovascular Endpoints Trial)] and found no significant differences in efficacy (118,119,124,130; see *JAMA* 2003;289:2073).

However, the Anglo-Scandinavian Cardiac Outcomes Trial-Blood Pressure Lowering Arm (ASCOT-BPLA) mega-trial compared regiments of amlodipine plus perindopril versus atenolol plus bendroflumethiazide in nearly 20,000 patients. Though the primary endpoint did not meet statistical significance on account of the trial being stopped early, there was a significantly higher rate of death and stroke, individually, favoring the amlodipine arm (125). Additional analyses did not find this effect mitigated by tachycardia in patients (see *J Am Coll Cardiol* 2009; 54:1154–1161).

The most contemporary Avoiding Cardiovascular Events Through Combination Therapy in Patients Living with Systolic Hypertension (ACCOM-PLISH) trial randomized 11,506 patients with HTN and at high-risk for cardiovascular events to either benazepril plus amlodipine or benazepril plus hydrochlorothiazide (126). The primary endpoint was the composite of death from cardiovascular causes, nonfatal MI, nonfatal stroke, hospitalization for angina, resuscitation after sudden cardiac arrest, or coronary revascularization. The trial was stopped prematurely, after a mean follow-up of 36 months, when a significant absolute reduction in the primary endpoint of 2.2% was observed (relative risk 19.6%) favoring the ACE inhibitor and calcium-channel blocker combination.

In order to test the hypothesis of dual renin–angiotensin–aldosterone system blockade, investigators for the ONTARGET trial randomized over 25,000 high-risk patients to either ramipril, telmisartan, or both (127). While there was no benefit to dual therapy for the primary end point of cardiovascular death, MI, stroke, or CHF hospitalization, there was a significant excess of adverse events in the combination-therapy group. Thus, dual ACE-I/ARB therapy is unlikely to provide substantial clinical benefit over one or the other.

The JNC 7 guidelines do provide for the consideration of different agents in specific types of patients or conditions (105). Most important, the use of ACE inhibitors should definitely be considered in individuals with diabetes, CHF with left ventricular (LV) dysfunction, MI complicated by LV dysfunction, chronic kidney disease, prior stroke, and high coronary disease risk. β-Blockers can be utilized in those with heart failure, MI, diabetes, and high CHD risk. Aldosterone antagonists are indicated in those with heart failure or post-MI. Angiotensin-receptor blockers can be utilized in those with diabetes or chronic kidney disease. Elderly patients with isolated systolic HTN may be treated with calcium-channel antagonists (long-acting dihydropyridines) (117). These agents can also be considered in those with high CHD risk or diabetes. In pregnancy, safe agents include labetalol, hydralazine, and methyldopa.

The Antihypertensive and Lipid-Lowering Treatment to Prevent Heart Attack Trial (ALLHAT) enrolled 33,357 participants aged 55 years or older with HTN and at least one other CHD risk factor (131). Patients received the diuretic chlorthalidone, 12.5 to 25 mg/day; amlodipine, 2.5 to 10 mg/day; or lisinopril, 10 to

40 mg/day [the fourth arm (doxazosin) was stopped early because of increased cardiovascular events and CHF hospitalizations)]. At a mean follow-up of 4.9 years, no significant differences were found between the treatment groups in the incidence of fatal CHD or nonfatal MI (overall rate, 8.9%). Certain secondary outcomes actually occurred less often with the chlorthalidone group compared with the amlodipine group (HF) and lisinopril group (combined CVD, stroke, and HF). Although some criticisms of this important study exist (see comments in annotated summary, page xx), the results suggest that in patients in whom cardiovascular events are the greater risk, a thiazide-type diuretic is the preferred first agent.

The second Australian National Blood Pressure Study (ANBP-2) enrolled 6,083 Caucasian elderly subjects. Patients received any ACE inhibitor or diuretic in an open-label fashion. The ACE inhibitor group had a significantly lower incidence of death or any cardiovascular event; this benefit was restricted to men (HR 0.83 vs. HR 1.00 in women). This study is methodologically weaker than ALLHAT, but its results suggest Caucasian men may benefit more from ACE inhibitor therapy.

Isolated systolic HTN, which is more common in elderly patients, also warrants treatment (115); unfortunately, only one fourth of physicians report routinely starting drug treatment in persons older than 70 years with SBP from 140 to 160 mm Hg.

Target Blood Pressure

The Hypertension Optimal Treatment (HOT) study (129) randomized 18,790 patients to target DBP levels of 90 mm Hg or less, 85 mm Hg or less, or 80 mm Hg or less. The incidence of major events did not differ between the three groups. However, the power to detect such a difference was less than planned for two reasons: (a) actual mean BPs were approximately 2 mm Hg apart instead of 5 mm Hg apart; and (b) only 724 major cardiovascular events occurred over a period of 3.8 years versus the projected 1,100 over a period of 2.5 years. Thus the trial was not adequately powered to determine whether a target DBP of approximately 80 mm Hg results in the fewest major events. Nevertheless, significantly fewer cardiovascular events and deaths were found among diabetic patients assigned to a target DBP of 80 mm Hg or less compared with 90 mm Hg or less ($p = 0.005$; $p = 0.016$). In the African American Study of Kidney (AASK) Disease and Hypertension Study, lower BP control (mean, 128/78 mm Hg) was associated with an 18% lower incidence of cardiovascular mortality and hospitalizations compared with higher BP control (mean, 141/85 mm Hg). (See also updated data on blood pressure goals in patients with diabetes, page 16.)

OBESITY

Approximately two in three U.S. adults are overweight or obese, compared with one in four in the early 1960s. There are U.S. guidelines for weight for men and women. Another measure, BMI (weight/body surface area), is often used (desirable,

18.0 to 24.9; overweight, 25 to 30; obese, greater than 30), however its shortcomings have also been identified—it can be difficult to distinguish adipose obesity from lean muscle mass (see *Eur Heart J* 2007;28:2087–2093).

One analysis of multiple large databases found that obesity reduces life expectancy markedly, especially among younger adults (144). More than 280,000 deaths per year are now attributable to obesity, and it will soon surpass smoking as the primary preventable cause of death in the United States.

Data from the NHS show that even modest weight gains over a period of 18 years result in significantly higher risks of CHD death and nonfatal MI; RRs ranged from 1.25 for a 5- to 7.9-kg gain to 2.65 for a 20-kg gain (137). Other studies have shown that a higher waist/hip ratio and greater waist circumference are independent predictors of CHD death and MI (143). In the Framingham Study, variability in weight was associated with increased all-cause and CHD mortality rates.

SEDENTARY LIFESTYLE AND EXERCISE

Favorable effects associated with exercise include weight loss and favorable alter-ation of lipoprotein profiles, especially HDL levels (see *N Engl J Med* 2002;347:1483). Observational studies have shown that individuals with low fitness levels have a 25% to 100% increased mortality risk. One meta-analysis showed a nearly twofold risk of CHD death among individuals in sedentary (vs. active) occupations.

Studies have shown increasing benefit with increasing intensity and frequency of exercise. An analysis of MRFIT subjects showed a 27% lower CAD mortality rate among subjects with moderate versus less-active physical activity (149). Another study found that running (aerobic) was better than lifting weights (typi-cally more anaerobic) (154). However, in a study of endothelium function follow-ing exercise in patients with recent MI, all forms of exercise resulted in favorable changes (aerobic, resistance, resistance plus aerobic). Of note, these changes disap-peared with cessation of training at 1 month (see *Circulation* 2009;119:1601–1608.

Although high-intensity, aerobic exercise appears to be best, doing less is bet-ter than no activity, as evidenced by two studies of middle-aged women and elderly men that found substantial benefits associated with walking (152,213). An NHS analysis of more than 72,000 women found brisk walking (more than 3 hours a week) associated with a 35% reduction in coronary events (153). Walking also reduces body weight and body fat (see *JAMA* 2003;289:323). Contemporary data have even demonstrated that regular exercise, even *without* significant weight loss, still can reduce cardiovascular risk (see *Arch Intern Med* 2008;168:884–890).

Formal exercise testing can provide a more accurate risk assessment. In the Lipid Research Clinics Mortality Follow-up Study, the least-fit quartile on a stan-dard treadmill test had a greater than eightfold risk of CAD mortality compared with the fittest quartile. In another study of 6,213 men, peak exercise capacity was the strongest predictor of death in those with and without CVD [every 1 metabolic equivalent of the task (MET) increase correlated with a 12% improvement in survival].

Other studies have shown that exertion is a trigger of acute MI, with a markedly increased RR of MI (>100 times) in the 1 hour after heavy exertion in those who exercise infrequently (no more than once per week) (150,151). Thus although exercise is protective, the initiation of any exercise program should generally be preceded by evaluation or consultation with a physician and initiated gradually.

NONMODIFIABLE RISK FACTORS

Family History

A family history of disorders appears most important in those otherwise at low risk. One analysis of 45,317 physicians showed that if a parent had an MI before age 70 years, the RRs of cardiac death, percutaneous transluminal coronary angioplasty (PTCA), and revascularization procedures were approximately twofold higher, whereas a study of 21,004 Swedish twins showed that the risk of CHD death was as high as eightfold greater if the other monozygous twin died of CHD before age 55 years (160). A recent cohort analysis of more than 20,000 individuals found that approximately 15% of CHD cases were attributable to family history, independent of other known risk factors (161).

Age

Advancing age is associated with a gradual deterioration in cardiovascular function (e.g., diastolic function, BP regulation) and increasing risks of CHD death (159). The NCEP guidelines consider age of 45 years or older in men and 55 years or older in women a CAD risk factor (**Table 1.2**).

Gender

CAD-related events are more common in men. This gender disparity is largely owing to a later onset of symptomatic CAD in women (approximately 10 years), which is likely related to the protective effects of estrogen.

ALCOHOL

Several observational studies have shown that moderate alcohol consumption (e.g., one to two drinks per day) is associated with a significantly lower rate of CHD and overall mortality (163). A Physicians Health Study (PHS) analysis reported adjusted relative mortality risks of 0.79 and 0.84 in those consuming one and two drinks per day, respectively. Another study of 38,000 male health professionals found consumption of alcohol at least 3 to 4 days per week was associated with a greater than 30% lower rate of MI (165); neither the type of beverage nor the proportion consumed with meals substantially altered this association.

Mechanisms for the benefits of alcohol appear to include increased HDL levels, antiplatelet effects, and improved insulin resistance. Because of the significant health risks associated with more substantial alcohol consumption, many physicians are hesitant to recommend alcohol consumption as a means to reduce cardiovascular risk. AHA Nutrition Committee recommendations acknowledge the data supporting alcohol's protective effects; however, they do not recommended alcohol solely for CVD prevention. Instead, they recommend that the risks and benefits be weighed, and support its consumption at a maximum of two drinks per day for men, one drink daily for women (see *Circulation* 2006;114:82–96).

HORMONAL STATUS AND HORMONAL THERAPY

Estrogen replacement therapy in postmenopausal women results in an approximately 15% to 20% reduction in LDL and 15% to 20% elevation in HDL levels. Significant epidemiologic data suggested that estrogen replacement was associated with significantly lower CHD mortality (168,169). However, breast cancer rates are 10% to 30% higher, and endometrial cancer occurs up to six times more often.

However, in contrast to the epidemiologic data, the first large prospective, randomized trial [Heart and Estrogen/Progestin Replacement Study (HERS)] showed that a combination of estrogen and progestin in 2,763 women with a CHD event in the preceding 6 months did not result in a significant reduction in cardiovascular death and MI [relative hazard (RH), 0.99] (170,172); the hormone group had more events in year 1 but fewer events in years 4 and 5.

The Women's Health Initiative, which randomized 16,608 postmenopausal women to estrogen and progestin or placebo, was terminated early (at 5.2 years of follow-up) (173). The hormone group had significantly higher rates of CHD (hazard ratio, 1.29), breast cancer (HR, 1.26), and stroke (HR, 1.41), whereas a lower incidence of colorectal cancer (HR, 0.63) and hip fractures (HR, 0.66) was seen. Overall mortality rates were similar. Based on these data, the overall risk–benefit profile for estrogen and progestin therapy does not meet the requirements for a clearly safe and efficacious intervention for primary prevention. The estrogen-only arm of this study is still ongoing.

Raloxifene is a selective estrogen modulator used for treatment of osteoporosis. In the Multiple Outcomes of Raloxifene Evaluation (MORE) trial, 7,705 osteoporotic postmenopausal women were randomized to raloxifene, 60 mg/day; raloxifene, 120 mg/day; or placebo (171). At 4-year follow-up, no significant differences were found between the treatment groups in coronary and cerebrovascular events. However, among the 1,035 women with increased cardiovascular risk at baseline, those assigned to raloxifene (either dose) had a significantly lower risk of cardiovascular events compared with placebo (RR, 0.60; 95% CI, 0.38 to 0.95). Confirmation in a trial with evaluation of cardiovascular outcomes as the primary objective was required—the Raloxifene Use for The Heart (RUTH) trial randomized 10,101 postmenopausal women with CAD or multiple risk factors for CHD to 60 mg of raloxifene daily or placebo and followed them for a median of 5.6 years. The trial had two primary outcomes: (1) a composite of death from coronary causes, MI, or hospitalization for ACS, and (2) invasive breast cancer. The results demonstrated no significant difference in coronary events between the two groups, but did reduce the risk of invasive breast cancer.

C-REACTIVE PROTEIN

CRP is an acute-phase reactant produced by the liver in response to interleukin 6 (IL-6). A high-sensitivity assay (hsCRP) has allowed accurate measurement at the low levels (<10 mg/L) that predict CHD risk. Numerous studies have shown that elevated hsCRP levels are strongly associated with an increased risk of cardiovascular events. CRP also may be more than a marker of CHD risk, as some research suggests it impairs endothelial vasoreactivity and promotes atherosclerosis (see *Circulation* 2000;102:1000, 2165).

In nested case-control studies of WHS and Women's Health Initiative participants (183), the highest hsCRP levels were associated with a more than fourfold higher risk of cardiovascular events and twofold increased risk of CHD, respectively; individuals in the highest quartile of hsCRP had increased rates of stroke (RR, 1.9), MI (RR, 2.9), and PVD (RR, 4.1). In the PHS, high levels of CRP were associated with increased risk of MI (adjusted RR, 1.5), and those in the highest quartiles of both CRP and TC had a fivefold higher risk (177). Another study of both PHS and WHS participants found that those in the highest quintiles of CRP *and* TC/HDL had an eight- to ninefold increased risk of major events (see *Circulation* 2001;103:1813).

CRP also has predictive value in those with known CAD. In the CARE study, those in the highest quintile of CRP levels had nearly a twofold increased risk of recurrent events (179). An analysis of prospective European studies of patients with stable and unstable angina found a 45% increase in nonfatal MI and sudden cardiac death (SCD) in those with increased CRP levels. In patients with ACSs, high CRP levels are predictive of worse prognosis (185). In the initial evaluation of such patients, hsCRP measurement provides additional prognostic information to other markers (see *Circulation* 2002;105:1760) and may prove useful in those with normal troponin levels.

A more impressive finding is that hsCRP appears to be an even stronger predictor of first cardiovascular events than is LDL cholesterol. An analysis of the 27,939 WHS participants found that both baseline LDL and hsCRP levels had a strong linear relation with the incidence of cardiovascular events, although the two were minimally correlated ($r = 0.08$) (184). The adjusted RRs of first cardiovascular events according to increasing quintiles of CRP, as compared with women in the lowest quintile, were 1.4, 1.6, 2.0, and 2.3 ($p < 0.001$), compared with corresponding RRs in increasing quintiles of LDL-C of 0.9, 1.1, 1.3, and 1.5 ($p < 0.001$). Because 46% of major events occurred among those with LDL less than 130 mg/dL, CRP may be particularly helpful in identifying patients at high CHD risk among those with low LDL levels.

CRP levels appear to be effectively lowered by statins. The PRINCE trial enrolled 2,884 patients (including 1,182 with known CVD off statins for at least 12 weeks) (181). In the primary prevention cohort, pravastatin reduced hsCRP by 16.9% compared with no change with placebo. In the open-labeled CVD cohort (all received statin therapy), a similar 14.3% reduction in hsCRP was found. An analysis of AFCAPS/TexCAPS participants found that lovastatin decreased CRP levels by 14% during the course of the study ($p < 0.001$). If LDL was less than the median (149 mg/dL) and CRP was greater than the median (1.6 mg/L), lovastatin conferred significant benefit (182). In the CARE study, the statin group had a 17% reduction in hsCRP; in those treated with pravastatin, an hsCRP above the 90th percentile was associated with a 54% reduction in recurrent events compared with 25% if hsCRP was less than 9.9 mg/L. Several studies have shown that statins lower hsCRP within weeks of therapy initiation, an effect independent of their effect on LDL cholesterol (see *Circulation* 2001;103:1191; 2002;106:1447). Prospective studies to evaluate whether CRP lowering by statins reduces major events are now ongoing.

In regard to ASA, a PHS analysis found that its use was most beneficial among men in the highest quartile of hsCRP values [56% reduction in MI vs. 14% (lowest quartile)] (177). Studies specifically examining the impact of aspirin on hsCRP are conflicting (see *J Thromb Thrombol* 2000;9:37; *J Am Coll Cardiol* 2000;37:2036). Thus further studies are required to determine whether initiation of ASA in patients with high CRP levels results in reduced CHD risk.

Lifestyle modification also lowers hsCRP levels. Several studies have shown that weight loss, exercise, smoking cessation, and modest alcohol consumption reduce hsCRP (see *Circulation* 2002;105:564; 2003;107:443). Because elevated hsCRP levels are seen in those with diabetes and the metabolic syndrome (see *Diabetes Care* 2000;23:1835; *Circulation* 2003;107:391), it is likely that aggressive glycemic control will lower hsCRP levels.

In January 2003, the AHA and Centers for Disease Control (CDC) published a Scientific Statement that identified hsCRP as the most promising inflammatory marker because of the robust data base and its strong ability to predict CHD events (see *Circulation* 2003;107:499). In 2004, the CDC/AHA Workshop on Markers of Inflammation and Cardiovascular Disease further outlined a recommended approach to CRP, with recommendations for clinical practice (see *Circulation* 2004;110:e550–e553). These included the use of hsCRP at the discretion of the physician to further direct evaluation and management in persons of intermediate risk for coronary disease[10% to 20% risk of CHD at 10 years (with modified Framingham tables)], or as global assessment of risk in those with known disease. The report specifically discourages use of hsCRP to monitor therapy, guide management of ACS, or determine secondary prevention strategies. If the level is greater than 10 mg/L, investigations for noncardiac causes should be undertaken. It should be noted that few of these recommendations are based on the highest quality of evidence—randomized controlled trials.

More recently, hsCRP rose to even higher prominence—it can now be used to guide pharmacologic lipid-lowering therapy, according to the FDA. Based on data from the JUPITER trial (27), rosuvastatin is indicated in patients who met entry criteria for this trial: those with normal LDL cholesterol, but increased risk of cardiovascular events based on elevated CRP, age, and at least one other CVD risk factor.

OTHER POTENTIAL RISK FACTORS

Homocysteine

Hyperhomocysteinemia appears to be a modest independent risk factor for CHD, CVD, and PVD. Most studies have confirmed that high homocysteine levels are associated with an increased CHD mortality rate (191,198,200); however, other studies have shown no association (170). A meta-analysis found that in prospective studies, a 25% lower homocysteine level was associated with an 11% lower risk of ischemic heart disease (IHD) and 19% lower stroke risk (190); analysis of 5,569 AFCAPS/TexCAPS participants found that higher baseline homocysteine levels were associated with increased risk of future acute coronary events; however, in contrast to findings in this trial for CRP, homocysteine levels did not help to define low-LDL subgroups with different responses to statin therapy (201). Furthermore, homocysteine levels in elderly persons without known CHD predicted cardiovascular mortality better than the Framingham risk score (see *BMJ* 2009;338:a3083).

Two studies reported that folic acid fortification and multivitamin use are associated with lower homocysteine levels (193). However, multiple trials of homocysteine as a therapeutic target, mostly involving B vitamins, have yielded disappointing results—lowering homocysteine does not appear to prevent events. These trials included NORVIT (194), HOPE 2 (195), a VA study of homocysteine lowering (196), and the WENBIT trial (197) (see also *JAMA* 2008;299(17):2027–2036; *JAMA* 2008;300(7):795–804).

Lipoprotein-associated Phospholipase A2

Lipoprotein-associated phospholipase A_2 (Lp-PLA$_2$) is an enzyme produced predominantly by macrophages and monocytes and is also known as platelet-activating factor acetylhydrolase (PAF-AH). Its action is to convert oxidized LDL within the plaque into two inflammatory compounds: free fatty acids and lyso PC (see *Eur Heart J* 2009;30:2930–2938). While its exact involvement in atherosclerosis is not yet clear, its levels were found to correlate closely with future coronary, as well as cerebrovascular events, in observational and case-cohort studies (see *Circulation* 2004;110:1903–1908; *Circulation* 2005;111:570–575). Statistically, these effects were independent of hsCRP and could help predict relatively high-risk individuals who already had low LDL-C. In further analyses of the PROVE IT-TIMI 22 trial, Lp-PLA$_2$ was *not* found to be useful for risk stratification immediately after ACS; however, Lp-PLA$_2$ levels were reduced following statin therapy and to a greater extent in with a higher-dose statin. Increased levels at 30 days following ACS *did* predict recurrent coronary events (203). Additional data from a large collaborative study supports the significant association between CHD and Lp-PLA$_2$ activity and mass, comparable to that of blood pressure or non-HDL cholesterol (see *Lancet* 2010;375:1536–1544).

Infection

Some studies demonstrated an increased risk of CAD in individuals who are seropositive for certain infectious agents. The most robust evidence accumulated to date is for *Chlamydia pneumoniae*. A meta-analysis (performed in 2000) of 15 prospective studies of *C. pneumoniae* immunoglobulin G (IgG) titers, included 3,169 cases, and found a combined OR of CHD of only 1.15 (95% CI, 0.97 to 1.36), suggesting a weak association of *C. pneumoniae* with CHD.

A nested case-control study of PHS subjects and a prospective cohort study of Framingham Heart Study participants found no increased risk of future MI in those with increasing IgG titers to *C. pneumoniae* (see *J Am Coll Cardiol* 2002;40:1408). The Azithromycin in Coronary Artery Disease: Elimination of Myocardial Infection with Chlamydia (ACADEMIC) trial, which treated patients with CAD and elevated *C. pneumoniae* titers with azithromycin, found no difference between the treated and placebo groups in a 3-month composite of four inflammatory markers and clinical outcomes at 6 months.

Among unstable angina and non–Q-wave MI patients, the Clarithromycin in Acute Coronary Syndrome Patients in Finland (CLARIFY) study found that clarithromycin reduced the risk of ischemic cardiovascular events compared with placebo. In contrast, the AZACS trial found no benefit of azithromycin use in 1,400 unstable angina or acute MI patients (see *Lancet* 2003;361:809), and the larger the Weekly Intervention with Zithromax for Atherosclerosis and its Related Disorders (WIZARD) trial (207), which enrolled more than 7,000 post-MI patients with elevated *C. pneumoniae* titers, showed no significant benefit at 2 years of azithromycin versus placebo.

However, in the antibiotic arm of the PROVE IT-TIMI 22 trial, investigators randomized the 4,162 patients presenting with ACS to gatifloxacin or placebo over a mean treatment duration of 2 years (10 days per month of therapy) (208). After 2 years of follow-up there was no significant difference in the rates of the primary endpoint, a composite of death from all causes, MI, documented unstable angina requiring rehospitalization, revascularization (performed at least 30 days after randomization), and stroke. This study, along with the ACES study using azithromycin effectively ended the concept that infection was a modifiable risk factor for recurrent CV events (see *N Engl J Med* 2005;352(16):1637–1645).

Genetic Markers

The PLA1/PLA2 polymorphism of platelet glycoprotein IIIa and the ACE gene have been most extensively studied. Observational studies of the PLA1/PLA2 polymorphism reported an increased risk of cardiac events among those with the PLA2 allele, whereas larger studies have shown no significant relation (212,213). A meta-analysis performed of 40 studies with a total of 9,095 cases and 12,508 controls found the overall OR of CAD for carriers of the *PLA2* allele was 1.10 (95% CI, 1.03 to 1.18), suggesting a significant but weak association (214). In regard to the ACE gene, a meta-analysis of 15 studies found an approximately 25% increased risk of MI among those homozygous for the deletion allele of the ACE gene (211). Additionally, an exciting association between significant CVD risk and alleles at chromosome location 9p21 has been identified. While this research is still in its infancy, this appears to be a least one heritable risk factor that significantly, though with a small effect, impacts risk of MI (216).

ANTIPLATELET DRUGS FOR PRIMARY AND SECONDARY PREVENTION

Aspirin

PRIMARY PREVENTION TRIALS

The PHS found that ASA-treated patients (325 mg every other day) had 44% fewer nonfatal MIs and a nonsignificant 4% reduction in cardiovascular deaths (222). This study was stopped prematurely because of concerns about the high stroke rate (RR, 2.1). A study of 5,139 British physicians found that ASA use (500 mg/day) resulted in a nonsignificant 10% mortality reduction and no effect on the incidence of nonfatal MI. In the Swedish Angina Pectoris Aspirin Trial (SAPAT) (222), which randomized 2,035 patients to ASA, 75 mg/day, or placebo, ASA was associated with a 34% reduction in MI and sudden death, but a nonsignificant increase in major bleeds was seen (1.0% vs. 0.7%).

While the AHA and the U.S. Preventive Services Task Force (USPSTF) had both previously found insufficient evidence to recommend for or against routine ASA prophylaxis in primary prevention, recent data and subsequent guidelines from the USPSTF mark a change from such a stance. One meta-analysis of over 50,000 patients demonstrated a significant reduction of cardiovascular events, predominantly driven by ischemic stroke in women and MI in men, at the cost of increased GI bleeding (221). This finding confirmed earlier data from the WHS (also cited in the latest guidelines), that low-dose aspirin effectively prevented ischemic strokes in women, with no effect on MI (224). It is based on these, and other subgroup analyses, that in their latest guidelines the USPSTF encourages the use of aspirin for primary prevention in men aged 45 to 79 (when the reduction in MI outweighs the risk of bleeding), and women aged 55 to 79 (when the benefit of stroke reduction outweighs the risk of bleeding). They encourage use of the Framingham risk score to establish long-term risk of cardiovascular events, and potential benefit derived from aspirin therapy. The task force found insufficient data to make recommendations for patients 80 years old and greater (see *Ann Intern Med* 2009;150:396–404). However, in the ATT Collaboration, the FRS was useful in identifying patients at very low risk who had very little benefit, whereas patients above a 5% to 10% risk did have a clinical benefit (see *Lancet* 2009; 373:1849–1860). The American Diabetes Association guidelines recommend that all individuals with diabetes older than 40 years should take ASA because of their increased CHD risk (minimum, 81 mg/day; see *Diabetes Care* 2009;32:S13–S61).

SECONDARY PREVENTION TRIALS

In the second Persantine–Aspirin Reinfarction Study (PARIS II) (1,200), the ASA plus persantine group had a 30% lower 1-year mortality rate. An early meta-analysis that includes the PARIS II results found a similar reduction in mortality with ASA use. In a recent observational study of elderly patients, with no contraindications to ASA, ASA use was associated with a 23% lower mortality rate (214); however, only 76% were given this beneficial therapy at hospital discharge.

The Antithrombotic Trialists' Collaboration recent meta-analysis (published in 2002) examined 287 randomized studies with 135,000 patients in comparisons of antiplatelet therapy versus control and 77,000 in comparisons of different antiplatelet regimens (219). Among high-risk patients [e.g., acute MI, acute stroke, previous stroke or transient ischemic attack (TIA), peripheral arterial disease (PAD), atrial fibrillation], antiplatelet therapy reduced the incidence of serious vascular events (nonfatal MI or stroke, vascular death) by approximately one fourth, nonfatal MI by approximately one third, nonfatal stroke by approximately one fourth, and vascular mortality by approximately one sixth (all $p < 0.00001$). In each of the high-risk categories, the absolute benefits outweighed the absolute risks of major extracranial bleeding (Fig. 1.1).

Though preparations are approved at up to 1,300 mg/day, a recent meta-analysis of aspirin trials for the prevention of CVD demonstrated little benefit to doses higher than 75 to 81 mg/day, and an increased risk of hemorrhage, specifically GI bleeding, at higher doses (see *JAMA* 2007;297:2018–2024).

Aspirin resistance is present in 5% to 10% of individuals. In one study, aspirin resistance was associated with a threefold higher risk of death, MI, or stroke compared to aspirin-sensitive patients (see *J Am Coll Cardiol* 2003;41:966). Whether aspirin-resistant individuals receive adequate or enhanced benefit from Clopidogrel requires further study.

Clopidogrel

The Clopidogrel versus Aspirin in Patients at Risk of Ischaemic Events (CAPRIE) trial randomized more than 19,000 patients with a recent MI, ischemic stroke, or PAD to clopidogrel, 75 mg once daily, or ASA, 325 mg once daily (226) (see page xx). Overall, clopidogrel was associated with a significantly lower incidence in the primary composite end point, consisting of ischemic stroke, MI, or vascular death (5.32% vs. 5.83%/year; $p = 0.043$). Another analysis of all enrolled patients showed a statistically significant 19.2% reduction in the MI event rate ($p = 0.008$)

Figure 1.1 • Antithrombotic Trialists' (ATT) Collaboration. Aspirin in the primary and secondary prevention of vascular disease: collaborative meta-analysis of individual participant data from randomised trials. (Reprinted from *The Lancet*, Vol. 373, Antithrombotic Trialists' (ATT) Collaboration, Aspirin in teh primary and secondary prevention of vascular disease: collaborative meta-analysis of individual participant data from randomised trials, 1849–1860, © 2009, with permission from Elsevier.)

(see *Am J Cardiol* 2002;90:760). Based on these data, the use of clopidogrel in all patients with recent MI or stroke or documented PAD appears to result in a reduced risk of subsequent MI, stroke, or CV death. Furthermore, the subsequent results of the CURE, CREDO, COMMIT, and CLARITY-TIMI 28 studies (see Chapters 2 through 4) confirmed the benefits of clopidogrel for secondary prevention in PCI patients, and across the spectrum of ACS.

In those with history of stroke or PAD or at high risk for CHD events, the combination of clopidogrel and ASA was evaluated in the Clopidogrel for High Atherothrombotic Risk and Ischemic Stabilization, Management, and Avoidance (CHARISMA) trial (227). A total of 15, 603 patients either with known CVD (cardiac, cerebrovascular, or peripheral) or with multiple cardiovascular risk factors (CRFs) were enrolled, and randomized to 75 mg of clopidogrel or placebo over a median follow-up period of 28 months. When taken together, the trial failed to meet its primary endpoint, a composite of stroke, MI, or cardiovascular death at 28 months (6.8% in the clopidogrel group vs. 7.3% in the placebo group). However, in the group with known CVD, clopidogrel proved statistically beneficial (6.9% in the clopidogrel group vs. 7.9% in the placebo group), reaffirming the findings of the CAPRIE study (as this was the "CAPRIE-like" cohort).

REFERENCES

General Articles

1. **Stampfer MJ,** et al. Primary prevention of coronary heart disease in women through diet and lifestyle. *N Engl J Med* 2000;343:16–22.

   This analysis examined the 84,129 NHS participants who were free of diagnosed CVD, cancer, and diabetes at baseline. During 14 years of follow-up, 296 CHD deaths and 832 nonfatal MIs occurred. Low-risk subjects (only 3% of cohort) were defined as follows: nonsmokers, BMI less than 25, alcohol consumption at least half a drink per day, moderate-to-vigorous physical activity for average of approximately 30 minutes per day, scored in highest 40% of cohort for consumption of a diet high in cereal fiber, marine n-3 fatty acids, and folate, with a high ratio of polyunsaturated to saturated fat, and low in trans fat and glycemic load. After adjustment for age, family history, presence or absence of diagnosed HTN or diagnosed high cholesterol level, and menopausal status, all factors independently and significantly predicted risk. Low-risk women had an 83% RRR in CHD death or nonfatal MI compared with all the other women.

2. **Pearson TA,** et al. **AHA Guidelines** for primary prevention of cardiovascular disease and stroke: 2002 update: consensus panel guide to comprehensive risk reduction for adult patients without coronary or other atherosclerotic vascular diseases: American Heart Association Science Advisory and Coordinating Committee. *Circulation* 2002;106:388–391.

3. **Smith SC,** et al. AHA/ACC guidelines for secondary prevention for patients with coronary and other atherosclerotic vascular disease: 2006 update, endorsed by the National Heart, Lung, and Blood Institute. *J Am Coll Cardiol* 2006;47:2130–2139.

4. **Bucher HC,** et al. Systematic review of the risk and benefit of different cholesterol-lowering interventions. *Arterioscler Thromb Vasc Biol* 1999;19:187–195.

This analysis of 59 randomized, controlled trials with 85,431 participants included 13 statin trials, 12 fibrate trials, 8 bile resin trials, 8 hormone trials, 2 niacin trials, 3 n-3 fatty acid trials, and 16 dietary intervention studies. Only statins showed a significant reduction in CHD-related mortality (RRR, 0.66; 95% CI, 0.54 to 0.79) and all-cause mortality rates (RRR, 0.75; 95% CI, 0.65 to 0.86). A meta-regression analysis showed that the variability of results across trials was largely explained by the magnitude of cholesterol reduction.

5. **Mosca L,** et al. Evidence-based guidelines for cardiovascular disease prevention in women: 2007 update. *Circulation* 2007;115:1481–1501.
6. **Yusuf S,** et al. Effect of potentially modifiable risk factors associated with myocardial infarction in 52 countries (the INTERHEART study): case-control study. *Lancet* 2004;364:937–952.

This very large international case-control study of acute MI assessed the relationship of smoking, HTN, diabetes, waist-to-hip ration, dietary patterns, physical activity, alcohol consumption, blood lipids, and psychosocial factors to MI incidence. Among many conclusions, was the demonstration that these modifiable risk factors could account for 90% of the risk of MI in these populations.

7. **Bhatt D,** et al. for the REACH Registry Investigators. International prevalence, recognition, and treatment of cardiovascular risk factors in outpatients with atherothrombosis. *JAMA* 2006;295:180–189.
8. **Steg PG,** et al. for the REACH Registry Investigators. One-year cardiovascular event rates in outpatients with atherothrombosis. *JAMA* 2007;297:1197–1206.

The Reduction of Atherothrombosis for Continued Health (REACH) Registry represents a unique look at over 50,000 outpatients with CVD or significant risk factors. These manuscripts examine the contemporary diagnoses and management of such patients, as well as their events rates. The results are stratified by vascular bed of disease (coronary, cerebral, peripheral, or risk factors only), with patients diagnosed with atherothrombosis of multiple vascular beds having escalating 1-year event rates.

9. **Ford ES,** et al. Explaining the decrease in U.S. deaths from coronary disease, 1980–2000. *N Engl J Med* 2007;356:2388–2398.

The authors examine the rates of CVD mortality in the United States among adults ages 25 to 84 from 1980 to 2000, finding a drop from 542.9 to 266.8 deaths per 100,000 population in men and from 263.3 to 134.4 deaths per 100,000 women. They attribute these declines to both improved medical and surgical treatments (primary and secondary preventive therapies for MI, revascularization, treatments for heart failure, and other therapies), as well as a decline in risk factors (reductions in TC, BP, smoking prevalence, and physical inactivity), with both contributing roughly equally to the improvement. Unfortunately, they found part of these gains offset by an increase in population-wide body mass index, boosting cardiovascular mortality.

Lipids, Cholesterol, and Diet

REVIEW ARTICLES AND META-ANALYSES

10. **Baigent C,** et al. Efficacy and safety of cholesterol lowering treatment: prospective meta-analysis of data from 90,056 participants in 14 randomised trials of statins. *Lancet* 2005;366:1267–1278.

This landmark compilation of 14 trials of statins in CVD, both primary and secondary prevention studies, included 90,056 patients, accruing 8,186 deaths, 14,348 major adverse vascular events, and 5,103 new diagnoses of cancer. Analyses were performed *per unit reduction in LDL*, demonstrating impressive 20% reduction in events per mmol/L reduction, with the absolute events rates related to individual patient characteristics.

11. **Cannon CP,** et al. Meta-analysis of cardiovascular outcomes trials comparing intensive versus moderate statin therapy. *J Am Coll Cardiol* 2006;48(3):438–445. [Epub 2006 Jul 12].

    This analyses of the four major trials (PROVE IT-TIMI 22, A to Z, TNT, IDEAL), totaling 27,548 patients over roughly 4 years, demonstrated significant 16% odds reduction in death or MI, 18% reduction in stroke, and a *trend* (though not significant) in reduced cardio-vascular mortality for patients taking high-dose statins as compared with those on standard doses (including various doses of pravastatin, simvastatin, and atorvastatin).

12. **Ray K,** et al. The potential relevance of the multiple lipid-independent (pleiotropic) effects of statins in the management of acute coronary syndromes. *J Am Coll Cardiol* 2005;46:1425–1433.

    The culmination of a journal supplement devoted to the many lessons from the PROVE IT-TIMI 22 trial, this review highlights the evidence for, potential mechanisms of, and clinical consequences of the many biochemical effects of statins (independent of the LDL-lowering capacity) in CVD.

13. **Briel M,** et al. Association between change in high density lipoprotein cholesterol and cardiovascular disease morbidity and mortality: systematic review and meta-regression analysis. *BMJ* 2009;338:b92.

    This meta-analysis of 108 trials of lipid therapy, measuring HDL and clinical outcomes, involved 299,310 patients at risk of CVD. After adjusting of LDL-C levels, they found little variability in outcomes with respect to HDL levels. While reducing LDL-C demonstrated a strong relationship with reduced clinical events, increasing HDL-C levels did not correlate with clinical improvements. Importantly, this analysis do not differentiate among the treatments used to increase HDL-C, and many different interventions were included in the group of studies.

14. **NCEP Guidelines.** Expert panel on detection, evaluation, and treatment of high blood cholesterol in adults: executive summary of the third report of the National Cholesterol Education Program (NCEP) expert panel on detection, evaluation, and treatment of high blood cholesterol in adults (Adult Treatment Panel III). *JAMA* 2001;285:2486–2497.

    The guidelines focus on LDL cholesterol goals and cut points for TLCs and drug therapy (**Table 1.2**). High-risk groups are identified by using a modified Framingham point score (**Tables 1.1** and **1.3**). Attention also is given to TG levels, non-HDL levels, and the metabolic syndrome.

15. **Grundy SM,** et al. Implications of recent clinical trials for the National Cholesterol Education Program Adult Treatment Panel III guidelines. *Circulation* 2004;110:227–239.

    This update to the 2001 guidelines highlighted the recent evidence from high-dose statin trials (namely HPS, ALLHAT, ASCOT-LLA, PROVE IT-TIMI 22), reviewing their implications on clinical practice. Importantly, the panel offered a new optional therapeutic target of LDL <70 mg/dL in the highest-risk patients.

EPIDEMIOLOGY

16. **Martin MJ,** et al. Multiple risk factor intervention trial (**MRFIT**): serum cholesterol, blood pressure and mortality: implications from a cohort of 361,662 men. *Lancet* 1986;2:933–939.

This analysis of 6-year follow-up data showed that cardiovascular mortality correlated with cholesterol levels. Increased cardiovascular mortality risk was seen with TC levels as low as 181 mg/dL. RR was 3.8 for cholesterol levels above the 85th percentile (>253 mg/dL).

17. **Gordon DJ,** et al. High-density lipoprotein cholesterol and cardiovascular disease: four prospective American studies. *Circulation* 1989;79:8–15.

This analysis examined data from the FHS, Lipid Research Clinics Prevalence Mortality Follow-up Study (LRCF) and Coronary Primary Prevention Trial (CPPT), and MRFIT. A 1-mg/dL (0.026 mM) increment in HDL-C was associated with a significant CHD risk decrement of 2% in men (FHS, CPPT, and MRFIT) and 3% in women (FHS). In LRCF, in which only fatal outcomes were documented, a 1-mg/dL increment in HDL-C was associated with significant 3.7% (men) and 4.7% (women) decrements in cardiovascular mortality rates.

18. **Cui Y,** et al. Non-high-density lipoprotein cholesterol level as a predictor of cardiovascular disease mortality. *Arch Intern Med* 2001;161:1413–1419.

This study analyzed data on 2,406 men and 2,056 women aged 40 to 64 years from the Lipid Research Clinics Program Follow-up Study. At follow-up (average, 19 years), baseline levels of HDL-C and non–HDL-C were strong predictors of CVD death in both sexes, whereas LDL-C level was a slightly weaker CVD predictor. Differences of 30 mg/dL in non–HDL-C and LDL-C levels corresponded to increases in CVD risk of 19% and 15%, respectively, in men, and 11% and 8% in women.

19. **Ridker PM,** et al. Non-HDL cholesterol, apolipoproteins A-I and B100, standard lipid measures, lipid ratios, and CRP as risk factors for cardiovascular disease in women. *JAMA* 2005;294(3):326–333.

This analysis of the WHS looked at several lipid markers to identify those with strong prognostic importance: TC, low-density lipoprotein cholesterol (LDL-C), HDL-C, non–HDL-C, apolipoproteins A-I and B100, high-sensitivity CRP, and the ratios of TC to HDL-C, LDL-C to HDL-C, apolipoprotein B100 to apolipoprotein A-I, and apolipoprotein B100 to HDL-C. They concluded that non–HDL-C and the ratio of TC to HDL-C could be equally useful to apolipoprotein fractions, and that hsCRP added prognostic significance to all lipid markers, after controlling for major clinical risk factors.

20. **Michos ED,** et al. Prevalence of low low-density lipoprotein cholesterol with elevated high sensitivity C-reactive protein in the U.S.: implications of the JUPITER (justification for the use of statins in primary prevention: an intervention trial evaluating rosuvastatin) study. *J Am Coll Cardiol* 2009;53:931–935.

Using data from the NHANES, the investigators estimated the number of patients qualifying for statin therapy under up-to-date guidelines, and those who might additionally qualify were the guidelines to be broadened based on the results of the JUPITER study (broadly, patients with LDL <130 mg/dL and hsCRP $\geq$2 mg/L). They estimated an additional 6.5 million American patients would be eligible for statin therapy as primary prevention for CVD.

PRIMARY PREVENTION

21. World Health Organization (**WHO**) Study. Committee of principal investigators: a cooperative trial in the primary prevention of ischemic heart disease using clofibrate. *Br Heart J* 1978;40:1069–1118.

Design: Prospective, randomized, placebo-controlled, multicenter study; average follow-up 5.3 years.
Purpose: To evaluate the effects of clofibrate on cholesterol levels and the incidence of major cardiovascular events.

Population: 10,627 men aged 30 to 59 years with high TC levels (upper one third of distribution).
Treatment: Clofibrate, 1.6 g/day, or placebo.
Results: Clofibrate group had 8% lower TC, and 20% fewer MIs (4.6% vs. 6.2%, $p < 0.05$) and overall IHD events (5.9% vs. 7.4%, $p < 0.05$).

22. Lipid Research Clinics Coronary Primary Prevention Trial (**LRC-CPPT**) results: reduction in incidence of CHD. *JAMA* 1984;251:351–364.

Design: Prospective, randomized, double-blind, placebo-controlled, multicenter study. Primary end point was CHD-related death and nonfatal MI. The average follow-up was 7.4 years.
Purpose: To evaluate the effects of cholestyramine on cholesterol levels and major cardiac events in hypercholesterolemic men at high risk of CHD events.
Population: 3,806 men aged 35 to 59 years with TC greater than 265 mg/dL and LDL greater than 190 mg/dL.
Treatment: Cholestyramine (24 g/day) or placebo.
Results: Cholestyramine use was associated with 9% lower TC and 13% lower LDL-C. Cholestyramine group had a 19% reduction in CHD-related death and MI (8.1% vs. 9.8%, $p < 0.05$).

23. **Frick MH,** et al. **Helsinki Heart Study**: primary-prevention trial with gemfibrozil in middle-aged men with dyslipidemia. *N Engl J Med* 1987;317:1237–1245.

Design: Prospective, randomized, double-blind, placebo-controlled, multicenter study. Primary end point was cardiac death and MI. The follow-up period was 5 years.
Purpose: To investigate the effect of gemfibrozil on the incidence of CHD in asymptomatic middle-aged men at high risk because of elevated lipid levels.
Population: 4,081 men aged 40 to 55 years with a non-HDL cholesterol level of $\geq$200 mg/dL.
Treatment: Gemfibrozil, 600 mg twice daily, or placebo.
Results: Gemfibrozil initially increased HDL levels by more than 10%, followed by a small decline over time. TC and LDL levels were initially decreased by 11% and 10%, respectively, and remained consistent throughout the trial. The gemfibrozil group had 34% fewer cardiac events (7.3 vs. 41.4/1,000; $p < 0.02$); the decline in incidence became evident in the second year; no significant mortality difference was detected between groups (2.19% vs. 2.07%).
Comments: A subsequent subgroup analysis showed that patients with TG greater than 200 mg/dL and an LDL/HDL ratio of more than 5:1 had a 3.8 times higher risk of cardiac events, and that risk was reduced a substantial 71% with gemfibrozil.

24. **Shepherd J,** et al. West of Scotland Coronary Prevention Study Group (WOSCOPS): prevention of coronary heart disease with pravastatin in men with hypercholesterolemia. *N Engl J Med* 1995;333:1301–1307.

Design: Prospective, randomized, double-blind, multicenter trial. Primary end point was death from CHD and nonfatal MI. The average follow-up period was 4.9 years.
Purpose: To evaluate the effectiveness of an HMG-CoA reductase inhibitor in preventing events in men with moderate hypercholesterolemia and no history of MI.
Population: 6,544 men aged 45 to 64 years with TC $\geq$252 mg/dL (mean, 272) and no history of MI.
Treatment: Pravastatin, 40 mg once daily, or placebo.
Results: Pravastatin group had 20% lower TC, 26% lower LDL, 31% fewer coronary events (nonfatal MI, death from CHD; $p < 0.001$), 32% lower cardiovascular mortality ($p = 0.033$), and nearly significant 22% overall mortality reduction ($p = 0.051$). The reduction in coronary events was independent of baseline cholesterol level (as in 4S trial).

25. **Downs JR,** et al. for the Air Force/Texas Coronary Atherosclerosis Prevention Study (AFCAPS/TexCAPS) Research Group. Primary prevention of acute coronary events

with lovastatin in men and women with average cholesterol levels. *JAMA* 1998;279: 1615–1622.

Design: Prospective, randomized, double-blind, multicenter study. Composite primary end point was fatal or nonfatal MI, unstable angina, and SCD. Average follow-up period was 5.2 years.

Purpose: To compare lovastatin with placebo for the prevention of first major coronary events in those without clinically evident atherosclerosis and with average TC and LDL and below-average HDL levels.

Population: 5,608 men aged 45 to 73 years and 997 postmenopausal women aged 55 to 73 years with TC, 180 to 264 mg/dL; LDL, 130 to 190 mg/dL; and HDL, ≥45 mg/dL (men) or = 47 mg/dL (women).

Exclusion Criteria: Diabetes managed with insulin or with HbA1c of 10 or more, and more than 50% ideal weight.

Treatment: Lovastatin, 20 to 40 mg once daily, or placebo.

Results: Lovastatin was associated with an RRR of 37% in first acute major coronary events (3.51% vs. 5.54%; $p < 0.001$). Several secondary end points occurred less frequently in the lovastatin group: (a) MI, RRR of 40% ($p = 0.002$); (b) unstable angina, RRR of 32% ($p = 0.02$); (c) coronary revascularization procedures, RRR of 33% ($p = 0.001$); (d) coronary events, RRR of 25% ($p = 0.006$); and (e) cardiovascular events, RRR of 25% ($p = 0.003$). Lovastatin reduced LDL levels by 25% and increased HDL levels by 6%; no significant differences in adverse events were detected.

Comments: Differences between the two groups appeared after 1 year (23 vs. 40 events).

26. **Colhoun HM,** et al. on behalf of the CARDS investigators. Primary prevention of cardiovascular disease with atorvastatin in type 2 diabetes in the Collaborative Atorvastatin Diabetes Study (CARDS): multicentre randomised placebo-controlled trial. *Lancet* 2004;364:685–696.

Design: Prospective, randomized, double-blind, multicenter study in the UK and Ireland. Composite primary end point was time to first acute CHD event, coronary revascularization, or stroke.

Purpose: To compare atorvastatin (10 mg daily) with placebo for the prevention of first major cardiovascular events in patients those without clinically evident atherosclerosis and with diabetes at risk for CVD.

Population: 2,838 patients aged 40 to 75 with type 2 diabetes, no known CVD, LDL-cholesterol of 4.14 mmol/L or lower, fasting TG of 6.78 mmol/L or less, and at least one of the following: retinopathy, albuminuria, current smoking, or HTN.

Exclusion Criteria: HbA1c of 12% or more, elevated creatinine.

Treatment: Atorvastatin 10 mg daily, or placebo.

Results: The trial was stopped 2 years short of the anticipated duration, at the second interim analysis, median duration of follow-up was 3.9 years. Atorvastatin was associated with an RRR of 37% in the composite primary endpoint ($p = 0.001$). This yielded a number needed to treat 37, to prevent one primary event over 4 years. There was a nonsignificant reduction in death from any cause ($p = 0.059$).

27. **Ridker PM,** et al. for the JUPITER Study Group. Rosuvastatin to prevent vascular events in men and women with elevated C-reactive protein. *N Engl J Med* 2008;359:2195–2207.

Design: Prospective, randomized, double-blind, multicenter study. Composite primary end point of MI, stroke, arterial revascularization, hospitalization for unstable angina, or death from cardiovascular causes.

Purpose: To compare rosuvastatin (20 mg daily) with placebo for the primary prevention of first major cardiovascular events in apparently healthy men and women with LDL at goal (<130 mg/dL), but elevated hsCRP.

Population: 17,802 men (50 years and older) and women (60 years and older), with no known history of CVD, LDL-cholesterol <130 mg/dL, hsCRP ³2 mg/L.

Exclusion Criteria: Previous or current lipid-lowering therapy, patients with underlying systemic inflammatory conditions, patients taking immunosuppressant agents.

Treatment: Rosuvastatin 20 mg daily, or placebo.

Results: The trial was stopped after a median of 1.9 years of follow-up. In the rosuvastatin group, LDL was reduced by 50% and hsCRP by 37%. There was a hazard reduction of 44% for the primary endpoint in the rosuvastatin group (absolute event rates 0.77 and 1.36 per 100 person-years in the rosuvastatin and placebo groups, respectively, $p < 0.00001$). Each component of the primary endpoint demonstrated strong reductions, with the endpoint driven by clinically adverse events: hazard ratios 0.46 for any MI ($p < 0.0002$), 0.52 for any stroke ($p = 0.002$), 0.54 for arterial revascularization ($p < 0.0001$), 0.59 for hospitalization for unstable angina ($p = 0.09$), 0.80 for death from any cause ($p = 0.02$).

Comments: Importantly, this was a study of using hsCRP to identify an additional population that might benefit from statin therapy, *not* a trial of hsCRP as a *therapeutic goal* of statin therapy. The FDA granted an indication for treatment with rosuvastatin for this patient population, based on this study.

28. **Dujovne CA,** et al. Ezetimibe Study Group: efficacy and safety of a potent new selective cholesterol absorption inhibitor, ezetimibe, in patients with primary hypercholesterolemia. *Am J Cardiol* 2002;90:1092–1097.

Design: Prospective, randomized, double-blind, placebo-controlled, multicenter trial. Primary end point was the percentage reduction in direct plasma LDL at 12 weeks.

Purpose: To evaluate the safety and efficacy of the new cholesterol-absorption inhibitor ezetimibe.

Population: 892 patients with primary hypercholesterolemia.

Exclusion Criteria: Included MI, CABG surgery, or PTCA in previous 6 months; CHF (NYHA class III or IV); unstable angina; impaired renal function; hepatobiliary disease.

Treatment: After 2 weeks or more on an NCEP Step I or stricter diet and a 4- to 8-week single-blind placebo lead-in, those with LDL-C 130 to 250 mg/dL and TGs 350 mg/dL or greater were randomized in 3:1 fashion to ezetimibe, 10 mg, or placebo orally each morning for 12 weeks.

Results: Ezetimibe significantly decreased LDL levels by 17%, compared with a 0.4% increase with placebo ($p < 0.01$). The LDL-lowering effect occurred early (2 weeks) and persisted throughout the 12-week treatment period. Ezetimibe also significantly improved calculated LDL, apolipoprotein B, TC, TGs, HDL, and HDL(3) cholesterol ($p < 0.01$). Ezetimibe was well tolerated: compared with placebo, no differences were seen in laboratory parameters, or GI, liver, or muscle side effects.

29. **Davidson MH,** et al. Ezetimibe coadministered with simvastatin in patients with primary hypercholesterolemia *J Am Coll Cardiol* 2002;40:2125–2134.

After dietary stabilization, a 2- to 12-week washout period, and a 4-week, single-blind, placebo lead-in period, 591 patients with baseline LDL 145 to 250 mg/dL and TGs 350 mg/dL or more were randomized to 1 of 10 groups administered daily for 12 consecutive weeks: ezetimibe, 10 mg; simvastatin, 10, 20, 40, or 80 mg; ezetimibe, 10 mg plus simvastatin 10, 20, 40, or 80 mg; or placebo. Ezetimibe plus simvastatin resulted in LDL-C reductions of 44% to 57%, TG reductions of 20% to 28%, and HDL increases of 8% to 11%, depending on the simvastatin dose. Compared with simvastatin alone, ezetimibe and simvastatin significantly improved LDL-C (incremental 13.8% reduction; $p < 0.01$), HDL (2.4% increase; $p = 0.03$), and TG (7.5% reduction; $p < 0.01$). Coadministration of ezetimibe with simvastatin was well tolerated and comparable with that of simvastatin alone.

30. Sever PS, et al. **ASCOT-LLA.** Prevention of coronary and stroke events with atorvastatin in hypertensive patients who have average or lower-than-average cholesterol concentrations

in the Anglo-Scandinavian Cardiac Outcomes Trial-Lipid Lowering Arm (ASCOT-LAA): a multicenter randomized controlled trial. *Lancet* 2003;361:1149–1158.

Design: Prospective, randomized, double blind, multicenter trial. Primary end point was non-fatal MI and fatal CHD. Median follow-up: 33 years (trial stopped early).

Purpose: To assess the benefits of cholesterol lowering in primary prevention of CHD in hypertensive patients with normal cholesterol levels.

Population: 10,342 of 19,342 total ASCOT patients with TC ≤250 mg/dL; all were aged 40 to 79 years and with at least three other CRFs in addition to HTN.

Exclusion Criteria: Included prior MI, currently treated angina, CVA in past 3 months, and heart failure.

Treatment: Atorvastatin 10 mg or placebo.

Results: The atorvastatin group had 36% fewer primary events compared to placebo (1.9% vs. 3.0%, hazard ratio 0.64, $p = 0.0005$). This benefit emerged in the first year of follow-up. There were 13% fewer deaths in the atorvastatin group ($p = 0.16$).

Comments: The rest of the trial, which compares amlodipine ± perindopril with atenolol ± bendrofluazide for treating HTN, is reported elsewhere.

31. **Kastelein JJP,** et al. for the ENHANCE Investigators. Simvastatin with or without eze-timibe in familial hypercholesterolemia. *N Engl J Med* 2008;358:1431–1443.

Design: Prospective, randomized, double blind, multicenter trial. Primary end point was the change in the mean carotid-artery intima–media thickness at 24 months.

Purpose: To assess the effect on progression of atherosclerosis with the addition of ezetimibe to simvastatin in patients with familial hypercholesterolemia.

Population: A total of 720 men and women, ages 30 to 75 (average 46), with familial hyper-cholesterolemia, regardless of prior lipid-lowering therapy, with LDL cholesterol greater than 210 mg without lipid-lowering therapy.

Exclusion Criteria: Severe carotid artery disease or previous carotid revascularization, homozygous familial hypercholesterolemia, severe, symptomatic heart failure, arrhythmia, or recent cardiovascular event.

Treatment: Simvastatin 10 mg or placebo.

Results: There was no significant change in carotid-artery intima–media thickness (0.0058 mm in simvastatin-only, vs. 0.0111 mm in simvastatin-plus-ezetimibe, $p = 0.29$). The mean LDL cholesterol level was 192.7 mg/dL in the simvastatin-only group and 141.3 mg/dL in the simvastatin-plus-ezetimibe group at the end of the study ($p < 0.01$).

SECONDARY PREVENTION

32. **Coronary Drug Project.** Coronary Drug Project Research Group: clofibrate and niacin in coronary heart disease. *JAMA* 1975;231:360–381.

Design: Prospective, randomized, multicenter study. Primary end point was all-cause mortality. Mean follow-up was 74 months.

Purpose: To evaluate the effects of clofibrate and niacin on cholesterol levels and major cardiac events.

Population: 8,341 men age 30 to 64 years with ECG-documented prior MI.

Treatment: Clofibrate, 1.8 g/day, or niacin, 3 g/day.

Results: Clofibrate group had a nonsignificant 6% decrease in TC and 7% fewer MIs; niacin group had a 10% decrease in TC, 26% lower TGs, and significant decrease in nonfatal MIs (but not fatal MIs).

Comments: At 15-year follow-up, the niacin group had a significant 11% mortality reduction compared with placebo (52.0% vs. 58.2%; $p = 0.0004$).

33. **Buchwald H,** et al. Program on the Surgical Control of Hyperlipidemia (POSCH): changes in sequential coronary arteriograms and subsequent coronary events. *JAMA* 1992;268:1429–1433 (see also *Am J Cardiol* 1990;66:1293).

Design: Prospective, randomized, open-label, multicenter study. Mean follow-up period was 9.7 years.

Purpose: To evaluate whether cholesterol lowering induced by partial ileal bypass surgery would reduce mortality and morbidity due to CHD.

Population: 838 patients with an MI in the prior 6 to 60 months and TC ≥ 220 mg/dL or LDL = 140 mg/dL after 6 weeks of dietary therapy.

Exclusion Criteria: Obesity, HTN, and diabetes.

Treatment: Partial ileal bypass of distal 200 cm or one third of small intestine (whichever was greater); all patients were on the AHA phase II diet.

Results: Surgical group had lower TC and LDL cholesterol levels (4.71 vs. 6.14 mM; 2.68 vs. 4.30 mM); surgical group had 35% reduction in incidence of cardiovascular death and MI at 5 years (82 vs. 125 events; $p < 0.001$); surgical group had significantly less angiographic progression ($p < 0.001$ at 5 and 7 years). Fewer surgical patients underwent CABG surgery ($p < 0.0001$) and angioplasty ($p = 0.005$).

34. **Scandinavian Simvastatin Survival Study Group (4S).** Randomised trial of cholesterol lowering in 4444 patients with coronary heart disease: the 4S. *Lancet* 1994;344:1383–1389.

Design: Prospective, randomized, double-blind, placebo-controlled, multicenter study. Primary end point was all-cause mortality. Median follow-up period was 5.4 years.

Purpose: To evaluate whether simvastatin would improve survival of patients with CHD.

Population: 4,444 patients aged 35 to 70 years with angina pectoris or previous MI (≥6 months earlier) and serum cholesterol, 5.5 to 8.0 mM.

Exclusion Criteria: Unstable angina, secondary hypercholesterolemia, planned CABG surgery, or angioplasty.

Treatment: Simvastatin, 20 to 40 mg once daily, or placebo.

Results: Simvastatin group had 25% lower TC, 35% lower LDL, and 8% higher HDL levels; simvastatin patients had significant 30% RRR in overall mortality (8.2% vs. 11.5%; $p = 0.0003$), as well as 39% fewer nonfatal MIs (7.4% vs. 12.1%), 41% fewer IHD deaths (5.0% vs. 8.5%), and 34% fewer myocardial revascularization procedures (11.3% vs. 17.2%). A 35% risk reduction was noted among patients in the lowest quartile of baseline LDL. Cost analysis showed that simvastatin-treated patients had 34% fewer cardiovascular-related hospital days and that there was $3,872 savings/patient, reducing the effective drug cost by 88% to 28 cents/day. A subsequent analysis showed the annual cost of life gained (all costs, including lost wages) ranged from $3,800 (70-year-old man with a TC level of 309 mg/dL) to $27,400 (35-year-old woman with a TC level of 213 mg/dL).

35. **Sacks FM,** et al. Cholesterol and Recurrent Events (CARE): the effect of pravastatin on coronary events after MI in patients with average cholesterol levels. *N Engl J Med* 1996;335:1001–1009.

Design: Prospective, randomized, double-blind, placebo-controlled, multicenter study. Primary end point was CHD death and nonfatal MI. Median follow-up period was 5.0 years.

Purpose: To study the effectiveness in a typical population of lowering LDL-C levels to prevent coronary events after MI.

Population: 4,159 patients with MI within the prior 3 to 20 months, TC less than 240 mg/dL (mean, 209) and LDL, 115 to 174 mg/dL (mean, 139).

Exclusion Criteria: EF less than 25%; fasting glucose, 220 mg/dL; symptomatic HF.

Treatment: Pravastatin, 40 mg once daily, or placebo.

Results: Pravastatin group had 24% fewer cardiac deaths and nonfatal MIs (10.2% vs. 13.2%; $p = 0.003$), 26% lower rate of CABG surgery (7.5% vs. 10%; $p = 0.005$), 23% lower rate of balloon angioplasty (8.3% vs. 10.5%), 31% fewer strokes ($p = 0.03$), and nonsignificant 20% mortality reduction ($p = 0.10$). The reduction in primary events was restricted to those with a baseline LDL ≥125 mg/dL (>150 to 175 mg/dL, 35% reduction; 125 to 150 mg/dL,

26% reduction; less than 125 mg/dL, 3% *increase*). Subsequent analysis found pravastatin use associated with a 32% reduction in stroke (*p* = 0.03) and 27% reduction in stroke or TIA (*p* = 0.02). Another subsequent analysis found that among those with LDL less than 125 mg/dL, only diabetics had a significant reduction in primary events (see *Circulation* 2002;105:1424).

36. **The Long-term Intervention with Pravastatin in Ischaemic Disease (LIPID)** Study Group. Prevention of cardiovascular events and death with pravastatin in patients with coronary heart disease and a broad range of initial cholesterol levels. *N Engl J Med* 1998;339:1349–1357.

Design: Prospective, randomized, double-blind, placebo-controlled, multicenter study. Primary end point was cardiovascular mortality. Mean follow-up period was 6.1 years.
Purpose: To evaluate the effects of lipid-lowering therapy on overall mortality in patients with a history of CAD and average cholesterol levels.
Population: 9,014 patients aged 31 to 75 years with MI or unstable angina within 3 to 36 months before study entry and an initial TC of 155 to 271 mg/dL.
Exclusion Criteria: Renal or hepatic disease, use of cholesterol-lowering medications, and significant medical or surgical event in prior 3 months.
Treatment: Pravastatin, 40 mg daily, or placebo.
Results: Pravastatin group had significant reduction in death from CHD, 6.4% versus 8.3% (RRR, 24%; *p* < 0.001); pravastatin patients also had a lower overall mortality rate (11.0% vs. 14.1%; RRR, 22%; *p* < 0.001), fewer MIs (7.4% vs. 10.3%; RRR, 29%; *p* < 0.001), fewer strokes (3.7% vs. 4.5%; RRR, 19%; *p* = 0.048), and less revascularization (13% vs. 15.7%; RRR, 20%; *p* < 0.001); no significant adverse effects were associated with pravastatin.

37. **Rubins HB,** et al. Veterans Affairs HDL Cholesterol Intervention Trial **(VA-HIT)** Study Group. Gemfibrozil for the secondary prevention of coronary heart disease in men with low levels of high-density lipoprotein cholesterol. *N Engl J Med* 1999;341:410–418.

Design: Prospective, randomized, placebo-controlled, double-blind, multicenter study. Primary outcome was a combined incidence of CHD death or nonfatal MI. Mean follow-up was 5.1 years.
Purpose: To evaluate whether increasing HDL cholesterol levels and lowering TG levels would reduce major cardiac events in men with low HDL and LDL cholesterol.
Population: 2,531 men, aged 74 years, with CHD, HDL ≥40 mg/dL, LDL = 140 mg/dL, and TGs = 300 mg/dL.
Treatment: Gemfibrozil, 1,200 mg once daily, or placebo.
Results: Gemfibrozil therapy did not significantly reduce LDL levels, but did increase HDL by 6% and decrease TG levels by 31% at 1 year. The gemfibrozil group had a significant reduction in CHD-related death or MI (17.3% vs. 21.7%; RRR, 22%; *p* = 0.006). A nonsignificant 10% reduction was noted in all-cause mortality (15.7% vs. 17.4%; *p* = 0.23).

38. **Keech A,** for the FIELD study investigators. Effects of long-term fenofibrate therapy on cardiovascular events in 9795 people with type 2 diabetes mellitus (the FIELD study): randomised controlled trial. *Lancet* 2005;366:1849–1861.

Design: Prospective, randomized, placebo-controlled, double-blind, multicenter study. Primary outcome was a combined incidence of CHD death or nonfatal MI.
Purpose: To evaluate the effect of fenofibrate therapy on cardiovascular outcomes in patients with type 2 diabetes and dyslipidemia.
Population: A total of 9,795 patients ages 50 to 75, with type 2 diabetes mellitus and with a total-cholesterol concentration of 3.0 to 6.5 mmol/L and a total-cholesterol/HDL-cholesterol ratio of 4.0 or more or plasma TG of 1.0 to 5.0 mmol/L.
Treatment: Fenofibrate 200 mg daily, or placebo.
Results: In the fenofibrate group, 5.2% experienced a primary event versus 5.9% of patients taking placebo (relative reduction of 11%, *p* = 0.16). There was a significant reduction in the risk

of nonfatal MI in the fenofibrate group (24%, $p = 0.010$), and a nonsignificant trend toward increased CHD mortality (19%, $p = 0.22$).

Comments: In the placebo group, more patients began other lipid-lowering therapy (predominantly statins) during the trial than in the fenofibrate group (17% vs. 8%, $p < 0.0001$), making interpretation of the results difficult.

39. **The Accord Study Group**. Effects of combination lipid therapy in type 2 diabetes. *N Engl J Med* 2010;362:1563–1574.

Design: Multicenter, randomized, placebo-controlled trial. Primary endpoint was cardiovascular death, MI, or stroke at mean follow-up of 4.7 years.

Purpose: To assess the impact of fenofibrate for cardiovascular prevent, as supplemental therapy to a statin.

Population: 5,518 patients with type 2 diabetes mellitus.

Treatment: Simvastatin, plus either fenofibrate or placebo.

Results: Annual rates of the primary endpoint were 2.2% and 2.4% in the fenofibrate and placebo groups, respectively ($p = 0.32$). However, prespecified subgroup analyses did such heterogeneity of these effects, particularly according to sex, and possibly those with hypertriglyceridemia or low HDL cholesterol.

40. **MIRACL** (Myocardial Ischemia Reduction with Aggressive Cholesterol Lowering). Effects of atorvastatin on early recurrent ischemic events in acute coronary syndromes: the MIRACL study: a randomized controlled trial. *JAMA* 2001;285:1711–1718.

Design: Prospective, randomized, double-blind, placebo-controlled, multicenter trial. Primary end point was death, MI, cardiac arrest with resuscitation, or recurrent symptomatic ischemia with objective evidence requiring emergency hospitalization. Follow-up was 4 months.

Purpose: To evaluate the efficacy of early initiation of lipid-lowering therapy with atorvastatin in ACS patients.

Population: 3,086 conservatively managed patients with unstable angina/non-STEMI. Patients had the following: (a) chest pain for longer than 15 minutes at rest or with minimal exertion within 24 hours, and a change from a previous pattern of angina; (b) new or dynamic ST- or T-wave changes, or new wall-motion abnormality, or positive noninvasive test; (c) troponin or CK-MB greater than two times ULN for non-STEMI.

Exclusion Criteria: Serum cholesterol greater than 270 mg/dL, Q-wave MI within 4 weeks, CABG within 3 months, PCI within 6 months, left bundle branch block (LBBB) or paced rhythm, lipid-lowering drugs other than niacin at doses less than 500 mg daily, vitamin E (unless less than 400 IU daily), liver dysfunction [alanine aminotransferase (ALT) greater than twice ULN], insulin-dependent diabetes.

Treatment: Randomization within 24 to 96 hours to high-dose atorvastatin (80 mg/day), or matching placebo.

Results: The atorvastatin group had a significant 15% relative reduction in the composite primary end point compared with placebo (14.8% vs. 17.4%; $p = 0.048$), primarily because of fewer recurrent ischemic events with objective evidence (RR, 0.74; $p = 0.02$). No differences were found between the groups in death, MI, or cardiac arrest.

Stroke was significantly decreased in the atorvastatin group (RR, 0.41; $p = 0.02$). Lipid levels were decreased by approximately 40% with atorvastatin, but findings were not coupled to degree of lipid lowering. Only 3% had an increase in liver function tests to more than three times normal, and no cases of rhabdomyolysis were observed.

41. **LaRosa JC**, for the Treating to New Targets (TNT) Investigators. Intensive lipid lowering with atorvastatin in patients with stable coronary disease. *N Engl J Med* 2005;352:1425–1435.

Design: Prospective, randomized, active-controlled, double-blind, multicenter study. Primary outcome was a combined incidence of CHD death, nonfatal, non–procedure-related MI, resuscitation after cardiac arrest, or any stroke at a median of 4.9 years of follow-up.

Purpose: To examine the effects of lowering LDL cholesterol below 100 mg/dL in patients with stable CHD.

Population: A total of 10,001 patients, ages 35 to 75, with clinically evident CHD (a history of MI, a diagnosis of angina with objective evidence of CHD, or previous coronary revascularization), and LDL cholesterol levels below 130 mg/dL.

Treatment: Atorvastatin 10 mg daily or 80 mg daily.

Results: Patients receiving atorvastatin 80 mg daily had average LDL cholesterol levels of 77 mg/dL versus 101 mg/dL in the group receiving 10 mg daily. Primary events occurred in 8.7% of patients receiving 80 mg atorvastatin versus 10.9% in the 10 mg group (22% relative reduction, $p < 0.001$). Overall mortality was similar in the two groups, however there was a significantly higher incidence of liver enzyme elevation in the high-dose group (0.2% vs. 1.2%, $p < 0.001$).

42. **Pedersen TR,** et al. for the Incremental Decrease in End Points Through Aggressive Lipid Lowering (IDEAL) Study Group. High-dose atorvastatin vs. usual-dose simvastatin for secondary prevention after myocardial infarction: the IDEAL Study: a randomized controlled trial. *JAMA* 2005;294:2437–2445.

Design: Prospective, randomized, active-controlled, double-blind, multicenter study. Primary outcome was a combined incidence of CHD death, nonfatal MI, or resuscitation after cardiac arrest. Median follow-up was 4.8 years.

Purpose: To compare high-dose atorvastatin versus standard-dose simvastatin for secondary CVD prevention in patients with a previous MI.

Population: A total of 8,888 patients, 80 years or younger, with a history of acute MI.

Treatment: Atorvastatin 80 mg daily, simvastatin 20 mg daily.

Results: Patients receiving atorvastatin had average LDL cholesterol levels of 81 mg/dL versus 104 mg/dL in the group receiving simvastatin. Primary events occurred in 9.3% of patients receiving atorvastatin versus 10.4% in the simvastatin group (hazard reduction 11%, $p = 0.07$). There was a significant reduction in nonfatal MI in the atorvastatin group (7.2% vs. 6.0%, $p = 0.02$); however, there were no significant differences in the risk of overall or cause-specific mortality.

43. Study of the Effectiveness of Additional Reductions in Cholesterol and Homocysteine (SEARCH), presented at the American Heart Association, New Orleans, LA, November 2008.

This international trial randomized 12,064 men and women aged 18 to 80 years with a previous MI to either simvastatin 80 mg daily or 20 mg daily, and homocysteine-lowering therapy with folic acid and vitamin B_{12}, in a two-by-two factorial disease. Patients were followed for a mean of 6.7 years, with a composite primary endpoint of major coronary events (nonfatal MI, coronary revascularization, or CHD death), any stroke, or revascularization (including coronary and noncoronary surgery, angioplasty, or amputation). There was an average 14 mg/dL reduction in LDL cholesterol in the high-simvastatin group; however, there was no difference in the primary outcome between the statin groups (24.5% in the 80-mg simvastatin group vs. 25.7% in the lower-dose group, $p = 0.10$). Of note, there were five times as many cases of myopathy in the high-dose simvastatin group (53/6031 vs. 3/6033). In the folate/B12 group, homocysteine was reduced by an average of 3.8 μmol/L, yet there was no difference in incidence of primary-outcome events (25.5% in the treatment group vs. 24.8% in the placebo control).

COMBINED PRIMARY AND SECONDARY PREVENTION TRIALS

44. **Heart Protection Study** (HPS) Collaborative Group. MRC/BHF Heart Protection Study of cholesterol lowering with simvastatin in 20,536 high-risk individuals: a randomised placebo-controlled trial. *Lancet* 2002;360:7–22.

Design: Prospective, randomized, double-blind, placebo-controlled, multicenter trial. Primary end point was mortality and fatal or nonfatal vascular events (for subcategory analyses).

Purpose: To determine whether reducing LDL-C may reduce the development of vascular disease, irrespective of initial cholesterol concentrations.

Population: 20,536 U.K. men and women with coronary disease, other occlusive arterial disease, diabetes, or HTN in men older than 65 years.

Exclusion Criteria: Included chronic liver disease, impaired renal function, inflammatory muscle disease, severe HF.

Treatment: Simvastatin, 40 mg daily (average compliance, 85%), or matching placebo (average nonstudy statin use, 17%).

Results: The simvastatin group had a significant reduction in all-cause mortality compared with the placebo group (12.9% vs. 14.7%; $p = 0.0003$), because of a highly significant 18% relative reduction in coronary death rate (5.7% vs. 6.9%; $p = 0.0005$), a marginally significant reduction in other vascular deaths (1.9% vs. 2.2%; $p = 0.07$), and a nonsignificant reduction in nonvascular deaths (5.3% vs. 5.6%; $p = 0.4$). Simvastatin also was associated with lower rates of nonfatal MI or coronary death (8.7% vs. 11.8%; $p < 0.0001$), nonfatal or fatal stroke (4.3% vs. 5.7%; $p < 0.0001$), and coronary or noncoronary revascularization (9.1% vs. 11.7%; $p < 0.0001$). The reductions in major events were not significant in the first year, but were then highly significant for each subsequent year. The proportional reduction in the event rate was similar (and significant) in all subcategories, including those with cerebrovascular disease, PAD, diabetes, those either younger than or older than 70 years at entry, and even those who had an initial LDL-C less than 116 mg/dL (3.0 mM) or TC less than 193 mg/dL (5 mM). The annual excess risk of myopathy with this regimen was only about 0.01%. No significant adverse effects on cancer incidence were found.

Comments: This landmark study demonstrates that adding simvastatin to existing treatments safely provides substantial additional benefits for high-risk patients, irrespective of their initial cholesterol concentrations. After making allowance for noncompliance, actual use of this regimen would likely decrease major event rates by about one third.

45. **ALLHAT-LLT** (ALLHAT Lipid Lowering Trial): The ALLHAT officers and coordinators for the ALLHAT Collaborative Research Group. Major outcomes in moderately hypercholesterolemic, hypertensive patients randomized to pravastatin versus usual care. *JAMA* 2002;288:2998–3007.

Design: Prospective, randomized, active-controlled, multicenter trial. Primary end point was all-cause mortality. Secondary outcomes included nonfatal MI or fatal CHD (CHD events) combined, cause-specific mortality, and cancer. Mean follow-up was 4.8 years.

Purpose: To determine whether pravastatin compared with usual care reduces all-cause mortality in older, moderately hypercholesterolemic, hypertensive participants with at least one additional CHD risk factor.

Population: 10,355 individuals aged 55 years or older, with LDL-C of 120 to 189 mg/dL (100 to 129 mg/dL if known CHD) and TGs less than 350 mg/dL. During the trial, 32% of usual-care participants with and 29% without CHD started taking lipid-lowering drugs.

Treatment: Pravastatin, 40 mg/day versus usual care.

Results: At year 4, pravastatin group had 17% lower TC levels compared with an 8% reduction with usual care. Among those who had LDL-C levels assessed, levels were reduced by 28% with pravastatin versus 11% with usual care. All-cause mortality was similar for the two groups [14.9% (pravastatin); 15.3%; $p = 0.88$]. A nonsignificant 9% relative reduction was noted in CHD event rates in the pravastatin group [6-year incidence, 9.3% (pravastatin) vs. 10.4%; RR, 0.91; $p = 0.16$].

Comments: The lack of a significant difference between the usual-care group and those randomized to receive a statin may be explained by the inclusion of statins in the usual-care group for secondary prevention.

EARLY STATIN INITIATION TRIALS

46. **Cannon CP,** et al. for the Pravastatin or Atorvastatin Evaluation and Infection Therapy— Thrombolysis in Myocardial Infarction 22 Investigators. Intensive versus moderate lipid lowering with statins after acute coronary syndromes. *N Engl J Med* 2004;350:1495–1504.

Design: Prospective, randomized, active-controlled, multicenter trial. Primary end point was a composite of death from any cause, MI, documented unstable angina requiring rehospitalization, revascularization (at least 30 days after randomization), and stroke.

Purpose: The design was geared to establishing *noninferiority* of pravastatin, compared with atorvastatin, with respect to the primary endpoint over a mean follow-up time of 24 months.

Population: 4,162 men and women over the age of 18, hospitalized for an acute coronary syndrome within the previous 10 days. Enrollment was completed after any revascularization procedure and included patients naive to lipid-lowering therapy (if TC was less than 240 mg/dL), or those already on lipid-lowering agents (if TC was less than 200 mg/dL).

Treatment: Pravastatin, 40 mg daily (standard therapy) versus atorvastatin 80 mg daily (intensive therapy).

Results: Mean LDL values were 95 and 62 mg/dL in the standard and intensive-therapy groups, respectively ($p < 0.001$). There was a significantly lower rate of the primary event in the intensive therapy group (22.4%) versus the standard-therapy group (26.3%), with a 16% hazard reduction ($p = 0.005$).

Comments: This groundbreaking trial helped establish that lower is better for LDL cholesterol.

47. **De Lemos JA,** et al. for the A to Z Investigators. Early vs. a delayed conservative simvastatin strategy in patients with acute coronary syndromes. *JAMA* 2004;292:1307–1316.

Design: Prospective, randomized, double-blinded, active-controlled, multicenter trial. Primary end point was a composite of cardiovascular death, nonfatal MI, readmission for ACS, or stroke, over a median of 721 days of follow-up.

Purpose: To assess the advantage of early, intensive initiation of statin therapy in patients with ACS.

Population: 4,497 patients, ages 21 to 80 years, with acute MI (ST or non–ST elevation), with TC of 250 mg/dL or lower, who were not already on statin therapy.

Treatment: Simvastatin 40 mg daily for 1 month then 80 mg daily thereafter (intensive group) versus placebo for 4 months followed by simvastatin 20 mg daily.

Results: Median LDL cholesterol levels at 8 months were 63 and 77 mg/dL in the intensive and standard-therapy groups, respectively. 14.4% of patients in the intensive-therapy group and 16.7% of those in the standard-therapy group experienced an primary event (hazard ration 0.89, $p = 0.14$). There was a significant decline in cardiovascular death (4.1% vs. 5.4% favoring intensive therapy, $p = 0.05$), but no statistically significant differences in the remaining endpoints. Rates of myopathy were significantly higher in the intensive-therapy group (9 patients or 0.4% vs. 1 patient in the standard-therapy group, $p = 0.02$).

Comments: While this trial did not meet its primary endpoint, all the trends were consistent with previous and concomitant trials. Additionally, when assessed based on the degree of lipid-lowering, it appears to be consistent with similar trials (the differences in the LDL levels for the two groups in A to Z was less than for other trials).

48. **Patti G,** et al. Atorvastatin pretreatment improves outcomes in patients with acute coronary syndromes undergoing early percutaneous coronary intervention: results of the ARMYDA-ACS randomized trial. *J Am Coll Cardiol* 2007;49:1272–1278.

Design: Prospective, randomized, double-blinded, placebo-controlled, multicenter trial. Primary end point was a composite of death, MI, or unplanned revascularization at 30 days.

Purpose: To determine the advantage, if any, of early, aggressive statin therapy in the setting of PCI for NSTEMI.

Population: 171 patients with NSTEMI undergoing revascularization, who were statin-naive.
Treatment: Atorvastatin (80 mg 12 hour before PCI, and 40-mg preprocedure) versus placebo. All patients received long-term atorvastatin therapy (40 mg daily).
Results: A primary endpoint event occurred in 5% of patients in the atorvastatin group and 17% of those in the placebo group ($p = 0.01$), driven predominantly by a decreased incidence of recurrent MI. There was also a statistically significant reduction in incidence of postprocedure CK-MB elevation (7% vs. 27%, $p = 0.001$, respectively).

TRIALS OF RAISING HDL

49. **Kastelein JJP,** et al. for the RADIANCE Investigators. Effect of torcetrapib on carotid atherosclerosis in familial hypercholesterolemia. *N Engl J Med.* 2007;356(16): 1620–1630.

Design: Prospective, randomized, double-blinded, placebo-controlled, multicenter trial. Primary end point was a measure of increase in maximum carotid intima–media thickness, as assessed by B-mode ultrasonography, at baseline and at 2 years of follow-up.
Purpose: This was an early clinical trial of HDL-increasing therapy with torcetrapib, a novel cholesteryl ester transfer protein, using carotid intima–media thickness as a surrogate clinical endpoint.
Population: 850 patients with heterozygous familial hypercholesterolemia.
Treatment: Atorvastatin monotherapy versus atorvastatin with torcetrapib 60 mg daily.
Results: There was a significant difference in HDL levels between the two groups, 52.4 mg/dL in the atorvastatin monotherapy group versus 81.5 mg/dL in the combination therapy group. However, there was no significant difference in progression of carotid intima–media thickness in the two groups, 0.0053 mm per year in the atorvastatin monotherapy group versus 0.0047 mm per year in the torcetrapib–atorvastatin group ($p = 0.87$).
Comment: As confirmed in later studies, there was a significantly higher increase in SBP in the group receiving torcetrapib (1.3 mm Hg in the atorvastatin-only group and 4.1 mm Hg in the torcetrapib–atorvastatin group, $p < 0.001$).

50. **Nissen SE,** et al. for the ILLUSTRATE Investigators. Effect of torcetrapib on the progression of coronary atherosclerosis. *N Engl J Med* 2007;356:1304–1316.

Design: Prospective, randomized, double-blinded, placebo-controlled, multicenter trial. Primary end point was percent atheroma volume as measured by intravascular ultrasonography at baseline and after 2 years of follow-up.
Purpose: To assess the effect of torcetrapib on progression of coronary atherosclerosis, as measured by intravascular coronary ultrasound.
Population: 1,188 patients with known CAD.
Treatment: Torcetrapib 60 mg daily, or placebo; all patients were on atorvastatin therapy to target LDL-C of less than 100 mg/dL.
Results: Patients taking torcetrapib had significantly higher HDL levels, by nearly 60%, and lower LDL levels (by 20%). The percent atheroma volume increased in both groups, by 0.19% in the placebo group versus 0.12% in the torcetrapib group ($p = 0.72$).
Comment: Once again, torcetrapib was associated with a significant rise in BP.

51. **Barter PJ,** et al. for the ILLUMINATE Investigators. Effects of torcetrapib in patients at high risk for coronary events. *N Engl J Med* 2007;357:2109–2122.

Design: Prospective, randomized, double-blinded, placebo-controlled, multicenter trial. Primary end point was a composite of death from CHD, nonfatal MI, stroke, or hospitalization for unstable angina over median follow-up of 550 days.
Purpose: A study of torcetrapib for prevention of major adverse cardiovascular event in high-risk patients.
Population: 15,067 patients with stable CVD or with type 2 diabetes.

Treatment: Torcetrapib 60 mg daily, or placebo; all patients were on atorvastatin therapy to target LDL-C of less than 100 mg/dL.

Results: Patients taking torcetrapib had significantly higher HDL levels, by nearly 72.1%, and lower LDL levels (by 24.9%) at 12 months. However, there was a significantly higher rate of cardiovascular events (hazard ration 1.25, $p = 0.001$) and all-cause mortality (hazard ratio, 1.58, $p = 0.006$) in the *torcetrapib* group, compared with placebo (atorvastatin only). These were accompanied by significant decreases in serum potassium, and increases in serum sodium, bicarbonate, and aldosterone.

Comment: Development of torcetrapib was subsequently terminated; however, it is possible that its side effect of elevating BP is responsible for its poor clinical profile, and that this may not be a classwide effect. These questions remain unanswered. Other cholesteryl ester transfer protein inhibitors continue in development.

ANGIOGRAPHIC ANALYSES

52. **Blankenhorn DH,** et al. Cholesterol-Lowering Atherosclerosis Study (**CLAS-I**). Beneficial effects of combined colestipol–niacin therapy on coronary atherosclerosis and coronary venous bypass grafts. *JAMA* 1987;257:3233–3240.

This prospective, randomized, placebo-controlled, partially blinded, multicenter study enrolled 162 nonsmoking men aged 40 to 59 years who had undergone prior CABG surgery. Patients received colestipol (15 g twice daily) and niacin (3 to 12 g/day), or placebo. At follow-up (2 years), the drug group had 26% lower TC, 43% lower LDL, and 37% higher HDL; as well as higher atherosclerosis regression rate (16.2% vs. 2.4%; $p = 0.002$) and fewer new lesions or adverse changes in bypass grafts ($p < 0.04$ and $p < 0.03$, respectively).

53. **Brown G,** et al. Familial Atherosclerosis Treatment Study (**FATS**). Regression of coronary artery disease as a result of intensive lipid-lowering therapy in men with high levels of apolipoprotein B. *N Engl J Med* 1990;323:1289–1298.

This prospective, randomized, double-blind, placebo-controlled (or colestipol-controlled), multicenter study enrolled 146 men with documented CAD and family history of CAD. Patients were assigned to (a) lovastatin, 20 mg twice daily, and colestipol, 5 mg three times daily, for 10 days initially, then increased to 20 g three times daily; (b) niacin, 125 mg twice daily initially, gradually increased to 1 g four times daily at 2 months, and colestipol; or (c) placebo, lovastatin, and colestipol (although colestipol was given if LDL was elevated). At follow-up (2.5 years), group c (conventional therapy) had minimal changes in LDL and HDL (-7% and $+5\%$, respectively), whereas the changes were substantial in the treatment groups: colestipol and lovastatin, -46% and $+15\%$; niacin and colestipol, -32% and $+43\%$. Lesion progression in one of nine proximal coronary segments was seen in 46% in the conventional group, compared with 21% and 25% in the two treatment groups, respectively. Lesion regression was more frequently observed in the treatment groups (32% and 39% vs. 11%). Clinical events (death, MI, revascularization for worsening symptoms) occurred significantly less often in the treatment groups (6.5% and 4.2% vs. 19.2%).

54. **Post-CABG** Trial Investigators. The effect of aggressive lowering of LDL cholesterol levels and low-dose anticoagulation on obstructive changes in saphenous venous coronary artery bypass grafts. *N Engl J Med* 1997;336:153–162.

Design: Prospective, randomized, 2×2 factorial, multicenter study. Primary end point was substantial progression of graft atherosclerosis (defined as new lesions, progression of lesions present at baseline, new occlusions). Angiography was performed at an average of 4.3 years.

Purpose: To (a) determine whether aggressive lowering of LDL-C in patients with saphenous venous CABGs is more effective than moderate lowering in delayed progression of graft atherosclerosis; and (b) evaluate whether low-dose anticoagulation reduces bypass graft obstruction.

Population: 1,351 patients aged 21 to 74 years with LDL-C of 130 to 175 mg/dL who had undergone CABG surgery in prior 1 to 11 years and had one patent graft.

Exclusion Criteria: Likelihood of revascularization or death within 5 years, EF less than 30%, and unstable angina or MI within prior 6 months.

Treatment: Aggressive lipid-lowering therapy with lovastatin, 40 to 80 mg/day [goal LDL, less than 85 (actual, 93 to 97)] or moderate therapy with lovastatin, 2.5 to 5.0 mg/day [LDL goal, less than 140 (actual, 132 to 136)]. Cholestyramine was added if necessary. Second randomization to low-dose warfarin (mean international normalized ratio, 1.4), or placebo.

Results: Aggressive therapy group had less atherosclerotic progression (≥0.6 mm diameter decrease; 27% vs. 39%; $p < 0.001$) and 29% less revascularization (6.5% vs. 9.2%; p = 0.03). No difference was detected between warfarin and placebo groups, but at 7.5-year follow-up, low-dose anticoagulation patients had 31% lower incidence of death and MI.

55. **Brown BG,** et al. **HATS** (HDL-Atherosclerosis Treatment Study). Simvastatin and niacin, antioxidant vitamins, or the combination for the prevention of coronary disease. *N Engl J Med* 2001;345:1583–1592.

Design: Prospective, randomized, double-blind, placebo-controlled trial. Primary end point was mean change per patient in the most severe coronary stenosis from initial to final arteriogram. Primary clinical end point was the occurrence of a first cardiovascular event (death, MI, stroke, or revascularization). Follow-up was 3 years.

Purpose: To determine whether lipid-lowering and antioxidant therapy provide independent and additive benefits for patients with CAD and low HDL levels.

Population: 160 patients with clinical coronary disease (prior MI, coronary interventions, or confirmed angina), low HDL-C levels (men, less than 35 mg/dL; women, 40 mg/dL or less) and normal LDL-C levels (145 mg/dL or less).

Exclusion Criteria: Included previous CABG surgery, severe HTN, uncontrolled diabetes.

Treatment: Simvastatin plus niacin, vitamins, simvastatin–niacin plus antioxidants, or placebo [niacin placebo was active (only 50 mg), provoked flushing but did not affect lipids].

Results: In the simvastatin–niacin group, LDL decreased by 42% and HDL increased by 26%, whereas the levels were unchanged in antioxidant and placebo groups. The protective increase in HDL with simvastatin plus niacin was attenuated by concurrent therapy with antioxidants. The average stenosis progressed by 3.9% with placebos, 1.8% with antioxidants, and 0.7% with simvastatin–niacin plus antioxidants ($p = 0.004$), and regressed by 0.4% with simvastatin–niacin alone ($p < 0.001$). This study was not powered to evaluate clinical events, but they did observe that the incidence of the composite clinical end point was significantly lower in the simvastatin–niacin–alone group compared with the placebos (3% vs. 24%; $p = 0.003$); the incidence was an intermediate 14% in simvastatin–niacin plus antioxidants group.

TRIGLYCERIDES

Studies

56. **Criqui MH,** et al. Plasma triglyceride level and mortality from coronary heart disease. *N Engl J Med* 1993;328:1220–1225.

This study analyzed 7,505 patients in the Lipid Research Clinics Follow-up trial. The 12-year incidence of coronary death in both men and women increased with TG levels. However, after adjustment for potential covariates, this association was no longer statistically significant.

57. **Jeppensen J,** et al. Triglyceride concentration and ischemic heart disease. *Circulation* 1998;97:1029–1036.

This study of 2,906 Copenhagen Male Study participants initially free of CVD found that high fasting TG level is an independent risk factor for IHD. At 8-year follow-up, the risk factor–adjusted RRs of IHD were 1.5 (95% CI, 1.0 to 2.3; $p = 0.05$) and 2.2 (95% CI, 1.4 to 3.4; $p < 0.001$) for middle and higher thirds of TG levels. A clear gradient of risk was found with increasing TG levels within each level of HDL, including high HDL.

58. **Miller M,** et al. and PROVE IT-TIMI 22 Investigators. Impact of triglyceride levels beyond low-density lipoprotein cholesterol after acute coronary syndrome in the PROVE IT-TIMI 22 trial. *J Am Coll Cardiol* 2008;51:724–730.

This post hoc analysis of the PROVE IT-TIMI 22 study looked at the prognostic significance of TG levels, measured while on intensive statin therapy with LDL-C levels of less than 70 mg/dL. Through both univariate and multivariable analyses a TG level of less than 150 mg/dL on treatment with statins was associated with a significant reduction in death, MI, or recurrent ACS. This was a robust finding that persisted after adjustment of LDL-C levels, non-HDL levels, CRP, and other covariates.

LIPOPROTEIN(A)

Review Articles and Meta-analysis

59. **Danesh J,** et al. Lipoprotein(a) and coronary heart disease: meta-analysis of prospective studies. *Circulation* 2000;102:1082–1085.

This meta-analysis examined 27 prospective studies with at least 1 year of follow-up (mean, 10). Comparison of individuals in the top third of baseline plasma Lp(a) measurements with those in the bottom third resulted in a combined risk ratio of CHD death or nonfatal MI of 1.6 (95% CI, 1.4 to 1.8; $2 p < 0.00001$). The findings were similar when the analyses were restricted to the 18 studies of general populations (combined RR, 1.7; 95% CI, 1.4 to 1.9; $2 p < 0.00001$). Despite differences among studies in blood-storage techniques and assay methods, no significant heterogeneity was found among the 18 population-based studies or 9 studies of patients with previous disease.

Studies

60. **Schaefer EJ,** et al. Lipid Research Clinics Coronary Primary Prevention Trial (LRC-CPPT). Lipoprotein(a) levels and risk of coronary heart disease in men. *JAMA* 1994;271:999–1003.

This study enrolled 3,806 men aged 35 to 59 years with TC greater than 265 mg/dL and LDL greater than 190 mg/dL. Patients were randomized to cholestyramine or placebo. Lp(a) was measured in serum obtained (and frozen) before randomization from 233 patients who manifested CHD during the study (7 to 10 years), as well as from 390 CHD-free controls. Lp(a) levels were 21% higher in CHD cases (adjusted $p < 0.01$).

Antioxidants

STUDIES

61. **Cambridge Heart Antioxidant Study (CHAOS).** Randomised controlled trial of vitamin E in patients with coronary artery disease: CHAOS. *Lancet* 1996;347:781–786.

Design: Prospective, randomized, double-blind, placebo-controlled, single-center study. Primary end points were nonfatal MI and cardiovascular death plus nonfatal MI. The median follow-up period was 510 days.
Purpose: To evaluate whether high-dose α-tocopherol would reduce subsequent risk of MI and cardiovascular death in patients with known CAD.
Population: 2,002 patients with angiographically proven coronary atherosclerosis.
Exclusion Criteria: Prior use of vitamin supplements containing vitamin E.

Treatment: Vitamin E, 400 IU/day or 800 IU/day, or placebo.

Results: Treatment group had significant reduction in cardiovascular death and nonfatal MI (RR, 0.53; 95% CI, 0.34 to 0.083; $p = 0.005$). The beneficial effects on this composite end point were due to the 66% fewer nonfatal MIs (14 vs. 41 patients; $p = 0.005$); no difference in cardiovascular deaths was detected (27 vs. 23 patients; $p = 0.61$).

62. **Kushi LH,** et al. Dietary antioxidant vitamins and death from coronary heart disease in postmenopausal women. *N Engl J Med* 1996;334:1156–1162.

Prospective cohort study of 34,486 women without CVD who completed a diet questionnaire in 1986. At follow-up (7 years), increased vitamin E intake correlated with fewer CHD deaths; this association was strongest among nonusers of vitamin: RRs, 0.42 in two highest quintiles of vitamin E intake (vs. lowest quintile). Vitamin E from supplements was not shown to be beneficial, although high doses and duration of use were not definitively addressed. Vitamin A and C intake did not have significant associations with the risk of death from CHD.

63. **Rapola JM,** et al. Alpha-Tocopherol Beta-Carotene Cancer Prevention Study (**ATBC**). Randomised trial of alpha-tocopherol and beta-carotene supplements on incidence of major coronary events in men with previous MI. *Lancet* 1997;349:1715–1720 (editorial, 1710–1711).

Design: Prospective, randomized, double-blind, placebo-controlled study. Primary end point was cardiac death and MI. Follow-up period was 5.3 years.

Purpose: To evaluate the effects of α-tocopherol and β-carotene supplements on the frequency of major coronary events.

Population: 1,862 male smokers aged 50 to 69 years with a history of MI.

Exclusion Criteria: Malignant disease, severe angina, and significant use of vitamins A, E, or β-carotene supplements.

Treatment: α-Tocopherol, 50 mg/day; β-carotene, 20 mg/day; both; or placebo.

Results: No difference was detected between groups in incidence of cardiac death and MI, but the β-carotene and β-carotene plus α-tocopherol groups had more cardiac deaths (RRs, 1.75 and 1.58; $p = 0.007$; $p = 0.03$). α-Tocopherol group had fewer nonfatal MIs [adjusted RR, 0.62 (0.41 to 0.96)]. Authors speculated this to be owing to more fatal MIs.

Comments: β-Carotene serum levels were 19 times normal. Editorial points out that α-tocopherol dose used was one tenth that of CHAOS dose, and a synthetic form was used (CHAOS, natural form).

64. **GISSI-Prevenzione** Investigators. Dietary supplementation with n-3 polyunsaturated fatty acids and vitamin E after myocardial infarction: results of the GISSI-Prevenzione trial. *Lancet* 1999;354:447–455.

Design: Prospective, randomized, open-label, multicenter study. Primary end point was death, nonfatal MI, and stroke. Average follow-up was 3.5 years.

Purpose: To evaluate the independent and combined effects of n-3 polyunsaturated fatty acids (PUFAs) and vitamin E on morbidity and mortality after MI.

Population: 11,324 patients with a MI in the previous 3 months.

Treatment: n-3 PUFA (1 g daily), vitamin E (300 mg/day), both, or none.

Results: The n-3 PUFA group had a significant reduction in death, MI, and stroke [12.3% vs. 14.6% (control); $p = 0.023$]. All-cause mortality was 20% lower in the n-3 PUFA group (8.3% vs. 10.4%). The vitamin E group had a nonsignificant reduction in death, MI, and stroke (13.1% vs. 14.4%). Vitamin E use was associated with a significant 20% reduction in cardiovascular deaths.

65. **HOPE** (The Heart Outcome Prevention Evaluation Study Investigators). Vitamin E supplementation and cardiovascular events in high risk patients. *N Engl J Med* 2000;342:154–160 (see Ref. 228 for expanded summary/ramipril results).

This prospective, randomized, 2 × 2 factorial study of 9,541 high-risk patients aged 55 years or older with CAD, stroke, PVD, or diabetes plus one other CRF included a randomization to vitamin E (400 IU daily) or placebo. Vitamin E supplementation use was not beneficial [incidence of cardiovascular death, MI, and stroke was 16.0% vs. 15.4% (placebo)].

66. **Lee I-M,** et al. Vitamin E in the primary prevention of cardiovascular disease and cancer: the Women's Health Study: a randomized controlled trial. *JAMA* 2005;294:56–65.

Design: Prospective, randomized, double-blinded, multicenter study, with 2 × 2 factorial design evaluating vitamin E and aspirin, both compared with placebo. Primary end point was a composite of nonfatal MI, stroke, or cardiovascular death and total invasive cancer. Average follow-up was 10.1 years.

Purpose: To evaluate the efficacy of vitamin E supplementation for the prevention of CVD or cancer in women (the results of the aspirin arm were reported separately).

Population: 39,876 healthy women at least 45 years of age.

Treatment: Vitamin E 600 IU every other day versus placebo.

Results: There were no significant differences in outcomes between the two groups for incidence of MI (RR 1.01, $p = 0.96$), stroke (RR 0.98, $p = 0.82$), cancer (RR 1.01, $p = 0.87$), or all-cause mortality (RR 1.04, $p = 0.53$). There was significant lower cardiovascular mortality in the vitamin E group (RR 0.76, $p = 0.03$).

Comments: While cardiovascular mortality was lower in those taking vitamin E, this was not consistent with the other endpoints, and vitamin E was not recommended for cardiovascular or cancer prevention for women.

67. **Miller ER,** et al. Meta-analysis: high-dosage vitamin E supplementation may increase all-cause mortality. *Ann Intern Med* 2005;142:37–46.

This review of 135,967 patients in 19 clinical trials of vitamin E supplementation, both high-dose (^{3}400 IU daily) and standard-dose interventions. They found a pooled excess risk of all-cause mortality in the high-dose supplementation groups, at an overall rate of 39 per 10,000 persons ($p = 0.035$). There was a nonsignificant trend toward lower mortality in pooled analysis of low-dose trials, a reduction of 16 deals per 10,000 persons ($p > 0.2$). They identified a cutoff of 150 IU per day, over which an excess in mortality would be expected. Of note, these analyses did not include the WHS (above).

Special Diets

68. **de Lorgeril M,** et al. **Lyon Diet Heart Study**. A Mediterranean diet reduced mortality after MI. *Lancet* 1994;343:1454–1459.

This prospective, randomized, secondary prevention study enrolled 605 patients with a first MI (91% men). The diet group underwent a 1-hour educational session. At 8 weeks and annually, a diet survey and counseling were administered. At follow-up (average, 27 months), the Mediterranean diet group had a 73% lower incidence of death and nonfatal MI compared with the prudent Western-type diet group (2.7% vs. 11%; $p = 0.001$). A subsequent report with a mean follow-up of 46 months showed persistent benefits.

69. **Ascherio A,** et al. Dietary intake of marine n-3 fatty acids, fish intake and the risk of coronary disease among men. *N Engl J Med* 1995;332:977–982 (editorial, 1024–1025).

This analysis was performed on 44,895 Health Professionals Follow-up Study participants who completed detailed and validated dietary questionnaires. At 6-year follow-up, no significant associations were observed between dietary intake of n-3 fatty acids or fish intake and risk of coronary disease. The multivariate risk of CHD was 1.12 among men in the top quintile of n-3 fatty acid intake compared with men from the bottom quintile (95% CI, 0.96 to 1.31). The risk of CHD death was 0.74 among men who ate any amount of fish compared with those who ate no fish; this finding was significant (95% CI, 0.44 to 1.23), but the risk did not decrease as fish consumption increased. Editorial asserts that a little fish may still do some good, but a greater amount of fish is not necessarily better.

70. **Rimm EB,** et al. Vegetable, fruit and cereal fiber intake and risk of coronary heart disease among men. *JAMA* 1996;275:447–451 (editorial, 486–487).

   This observational study included 43,757 male physicians who filled out diet questionnaires. At 6-year follow-up, 41% fewer MIs were found in the highest-fiber quintile. The greatest risk reduction was associated with cereal fiber: RR, 0.71 for each 10-g increase. The editorial points out that the beneficial effect was confined to the highest quintile, probably the result of a healthy lifestyle (only 3.8% smokers, higher vitamin intake, etc.).

71. **Pietinen P,** et al. Intake of dietary fiber and risk of coronary heart disease in a cohort of Finnish men. *Circulation* 1996;94:2720–2727.

   This analysis focused on 21,930 ATBC patients (all male smokers aged 50 to 69 years). At follow-up (average, 6.1 years), MI and CHD deaths were found to be inversely associated with fiber intake. The highest quintile (34.8 g/day) versus lowest quintile (16.1 g/day) showed an RR of coronary death of 0.69 ($p < 0.001$ for trend). The same effect was evident after adjustment for CRFs and intake of β-carotene and vitamins C and E. The strongest association was seen with water-soluble and cereal (vs. vegetable or fruit) fibers.

72. **Wolk A,** et al. Long-term intake of dietary fiber and decreased risk of coronary heart disease among women. *JAMA* 1999;281:1998–2004.

   This analysis was performed on dietary data collected from NHS participants in 1984, 1986, and 1990 (semi-quantitative food-frequency questionnaire). The response rate among the 68,782 women was 80% to 90% during the 10-year follow-up period. Women in the highest quintile of total dietary fiber intake (median, 22.9 g/day) had nearly a 50% lower incidence of major CHD events (age-adjusted RR, 0.53; 95% CI, 0.40 to 0.69) compared with women in the lowest quintile (median, 11.5 g/day). This effect was attenuated after controlling for age, CRFs, dietary factors, and multivitamin supplement use (RR, 0.77; 95% CI, 0.57 to 1.04). The multivariate model found that a 10 g/day increase in total dietary intake resulted in a 19% RRR (95% CI, 1% to 34%).

73. **von Schacky C.** The effect of dietary omega-3 fatty acids on coronary atherosclerosis. *Ann Intern Med* 1999;130:554–562.

   This prospective, randomized, double-blind, placebo-controlled trial showed a modest reduction in angiographic progression of CAD with fish oil supplementation. A total of 223 patients with CAD by angiogram was randomized to fish oil concentrate (55% eicosapentaenoic and docosahexaenoic acids), 6 g/day for 3 months, and then 3 g/day, or placebo (fatty acid composition of average European diet), for 21 months. Pairs of angiograms (baseline and 2 years) were evaluated for 80 of 112 placebo recipients and 82 of 111 fish oil recipients. Angiographic analysis showed 48 coronary segments in the placebo group with changes (36 showed mild progression, 5 showed moderate progression, and 7 showed mild regression) and 55 coronary segments in the fish oil group with changes (35 showed mild progression, 4 showed moderate progression, 14 showed mild regression, and 2 showed moderate regression; $p = 0.041$). A trend toward fewer cardiovascular events was found in the fish oil group ($p = 0.10$), although LDL levels tended to be higher in the fish oil group.

74. **Liu S,** et al. A prospective study of dietary fiber intake and risk of cardiovascular disease among women. *J Am Coll Cardiol* 2002;39:49–56.

   This prospective cohort study used a semi-quantitative food-frequency questionnaire to assess dietary fiber intake among 39,876 female health professionals with no history of CVD or cancer. At 6-year follow-up, 570 incident cases of CVD had occurred, including 177 MIs. Comparing the highest quintile of fiber intake (median, 26.3 g/day) with the lowest quintile (median, 12.5 g/day), the RRs for CVD and MI, adjusted for age and randomized treatment status, were 0.65 (95% CI, 0.51 to 0.84) and 0.46 (95% CI, 0.30 to 0.72), respectively. After further adjustment for CVD risk factors, the RRs were a nonsignificant 0.79 and 0.68.

75. **Albert CM,** et al. Blood levels of long-chain n-3 fatty acids and the risk of sudden death. *N Engl J Med* 2002;346:1113–1118.

Prospective, nested case-control analysis of PHS participants (94 cases, 184 controls matched for age and smoking status). At follow-up (17 years), fatty acid composition in blood was analyzed by gas–liquid chromatography for 94 men in whom sudden death occurred as the first manifestation of CVD and for 184 controls matched for age and smoking status. Baseline blood levels of long-chain n-3 fatty acids were inversely related to the risk of sudden death both before and after adjustment for potential confounders (*p* values for trend, 0.004, 0.007). Compared with men whose long-chain n-3 fatty acid levels were in the lowest quartile, the RR of sudden death was significantly lower among men with levels in the third quartile (adjusted RR, 0.28; 95% CI, 0.09 to 0.87) and the fourth quartile (adjusted RR, 0.19; 95% CI, 0.05 to 0.71).

76. **Kris-Etherton PM,** et al. for the AHA Nutrition Committee. Fish consumption, fish oil, omega-3 fatty acids, and cardiovascular disease. *Circulation* 2002;106:2747–2757.

The AHA recommends that patients with documented CHD should consume about 1 g of omega-3 fatty acids per day. In those unable to eat sufficient amounts of fish to meet this requirement, it recommends daily supplementation with 1 g fish oil capsules that contain 180 mg of eicosapentaenoic acid and 120 mg of docosahexaenoic acid. In individuals with high TG levels, higher amounts (2 to 4 g/day) can be taken.

77. **Hooper L,** et al. Risks and benefits of omega 3 fats for mortality, cardiovascular disease, and cancer: systematic review. *BMJ* 2006;332:752–760.

The authors reviewed both randomized controlled trials (48 in total), as well as cohort studies (41 in total), that involved at least 6 months of omega 3 fat supplements. The pooled risk of total mortality was equivalent (relative risk 0.87, 95% CI 0.73 to 1.03), and the results of individual studies were inconsistent. The authors could not conclude that there was any benefit to omega 3 supplementation, either for all-cause mortality or cardiovascular outcomes. However, based on their analyses, they could not detect a signal of harm for patients taking omega 3 fat supplements.

78. **Appel LJ,** et al. for the OmniHeart Collaborative Research Group. Effects of protein, monounsaturated fat, and carbohydrate intake on blood pressure and serum lipids: results of the OmniHeart randomized trial. *JAMA* 2005;294:2455–2464.

Design: Prospective, randomized, crossover, multicenter study. Primary endpoints were measures of BP and LDL-C at baseline, following each diet, and at the end of the study period.
Purpose: To evaluate the effects on CRFs of various diets substituting saturated fats for alternative macronutrients.
Population: 164 adults with prehypertension or stage 1 HTN.
Treatment: A diet rich in carbohydrates, a diet rich in protein (about half from plant sources), and a diet rich in unsaturated fat (predominantly monounsaturated); each participant was exposed to each diet in a 6-week crossover feeding period.
Results: Overall, the protein and unsaturated fat diets both led to similar and lower 10-year CHD risk. There were significant reductions in BP, LDL-C, TGs, and increases in HDL-C for adults on the protein diet compared with the carbohydrate diet. For those on the unsaturated fat diet, there were significant reductions in BP and TGs, with increases in HDL-C (there was no effect on LDL-C, when comparing the carbohydrate and unsaturated fat diets).

Comment: The study represents strong evidence that dietary modification, over a period as short as 6 weeks, can modify long-term cardiovascular risk (if maintained).

79. **Dansinger ML,** et al. Comparison of the Atkins, Ornish, Weight Watchers, and Zone diets for weight loss and heart disease risk reduction: a randomized trial. *JAMA* 2005;293:43–53.

Design: Prospective, randomized, single-center study. Primary endpoints were changes in weight, measures of cardiac risk (cholesterol, BP, glucose), and self-selected dietary adherence at 1 year.

Purpose: To evaluate the comparative efficacy of four different fad diets in producing and maintaining meaningful changes in weight and/or cardiovascular risk.

Population: 160 adults ages 22 to 72 at an academic medical center in Boston, with mean BMI 35 kg/m^2, and known HTN, dyslipidemia, or fasting hyperglycemia.

Treatment: Randomization to four different popular diet groups, including the Atkins (carbohydrate restriction), Zone (macronutrient balance), Weight Watchers (calorie restriction), or Ornish (fat restriction) diets.

Results: Overall, each diet produced significant, yet modest, weight loss; adherence at 1 year was poor overall, yet reported better in patients with greater weight loss. There were significant improvements in LDL/HDL ratio from baseline for all diets (all $p < 0.05$), but not in BP or glucose as 1 year.

Diabetes and Metabolic Syndrome
EPIDEMIOLOGY

80. **Haffner SM,** et al. Mortality from coronary heart disease in subjects with type 2 diabetes and in nondiabetic subjects with and without prior MI. *N Engl J Med* 1998;339:229–234.

This Finnish-based population study found that diabetic subjects ($n = 1,059$) without a prior MI had a similar risk of subsequent MI compared with nondiabetic subjects ($n = 1,373$) with a prior MI. The 7-year incidence rates of MI among diabetics with and without a prior MI were 45.0% and 22%, compared with 18.8% and 3.5% in nondiabetics. The risk factor–adjusted HR for death from CHD for diabetics without prior MI as compared with nondiabetics with a prior MI was 1.2 (95% CI, 0.6 to 2.4).

81. **Gu K,** et al. Diabetes and decline in heart disease mortality in U.S. adults. *JAMA* 1999;281:1291–1297.

This analysis of data from the First National Health and Nutrition Examination Survey (NHANES I; 1971 to 1975) and NHANES I Epidemiologic Follow-up Survey (1982 to 1984) showed that the declines in heart disease mortality seen in the general population have not occurred in diabetics. The two cohorts were followed up for mortality at an average of 8 to 9 years. Comparing the 1982 to 1984 period with the 1971 to 1975 period, nondiabetic men had a 36.4% decline in age-adjusted heart disease mortality compared with only a 13% decline for men with diabetes. Among women, nondiabetics had a 27% decline, whereas a 23% increase occurred in diabetics. A similar pattern was found for all-cause mortality.

82. **Lotufo PA,** et al. Diabetes and all-cause and coronary heart disease mortality among U.S. male physicians. *Arch Intern Med* 2001;161:242–247.

This prospective cohort study found that the increased mortality risk conferred by diabetes is similar to that conferred by a history of CHD, whereas for CHD mortality, a history of CHD is a more potent predictor than is diabetes. The total cohort of 91,285 U.S. male physicians (aged 40 to 84 years) consisted of four groups: (a) reference group of 82,247 free of both diabetes and CHD (previous MI and/or angina) at baseline; (b) 2,317 with history of diabetes but not CHD; (c) 5,906 with history of CHD but not diabetes; and (d) 815 with a history of both diabetes and CHD. At follow-up (average 5.5 years), compared with men with no diabetes or CHD, the age-adjusted RR of mortality was 2.3 (95% CI, 2.0 to 2.6) among men with diabetes and without CHD, 2.2 (95% CI, 2.0 to 2.4) among men with CHD and without diabetes, and 4.7 (95% CI, 4.0 to 5.4) among men with both diabetes and CHD. The corresponding RRs of CHD death were 3.3, 5.6, and 12.0. Multivariate adjustment for BMI, smoking status, alcohol intake, and activity did not significantly alter these associations.

83. **Ford ES,** et al. Prevalence of the metabolic syndrome among U.S. adults: findings from the third National Health and Nutrition Examination Survey. *JAMA* 2002;287:356–359.

This analysis examined data on 8,814 participants in the Third National Health and Nutrition Examination Survey (1988 to 1994). The ATP III definition of the metabolic syndrome was used: three or more of the following: waist circumference, greater than 102 cm in men and greater than 88 cm in women; TGs, 150 mg/dL or greater; HDL, less than 40 mg/dL in men and less than 50 mg/dL in women; BP, greater than 130/85 mm Hg; glucose level, 110 mg/dL or more. Unadjusted and age-adjusted prevalences of metabolic syndrome were 21.8% and 23.7%, respectively. Prevalence increased from 6.7% in those aged 20 through 29 years to 43.5% and 42.0% for those aged 60 to 69 years and 70 years or older, respectively. Age-adjusted prevalences were similar in men (24.0%) and women (23.4%); however, among African Americans, women had a 57% higher prevalence than men, and among Mexican Americans, women had about a 26% higher prevalence than men.

84. **Lakka HM,** et al. The metabolic syndrome and total and cardiovascular disease mortality in middle-aged men. *JAMA* 2002;288:2709–2716.

This study analyzed data on 1,209 participants in a population-based, prospective cohort study of Finnish men who were initially free of CVD, cancer, or diabetes. At 11.4 years of follow-up, a total of 109 deaths was found, and the prevalence of the metabolic syndrome ranged from 8.8% to 14.3%, depending on the definition. After adjustment for conventional risk factors, the metabolic syndrome was associated with a significant 2.9- to 4.2-fold increased risk of CHD death (by both NCEP and WHO definitions). With the WHO definition, all-cause mortality was 1.9 times higher in those with the metabolic syndrome. The NCEP definition less consistently predicted CVD and all-cause mortality.

85. **Peterson JL,** et al. Metabolic syndrome is not associated with increased mortality or cardiovascular risk in nondiabetic patients with a new diagnosis of coronary artery disease. *Circ Cardiovasc Qual Outcomes* 2010;3:165–172.

In an observational analysis of patients with angiographically proven obstructive CAD, the researches assessed the prevalence of diabetes and the metabolic syndrome, and assessed rates of the primary outcome of death, MI, or stroke at 6 months, 1 year, and then annually to a median of 5 years. For these patients with newly diagnosed CAD, diabetes, but *not* the metabolic syndrome was significantly predictive of worse outcome, by all measures.

STUDIES

86. **Lewis EJ,** et al. The effect of angiotensin-converting-enzyme inhibition on diabetic nephropathy: the Collaborative Study Group. *N Engl J Med* 1993;329:1456–1462.

This prospective, randomized, placebo-controlled trial enrolled 409 patients with IDDM in whom urinary protein excretion was 500 mg/day or more and serum creatinine concentration was 2.5 mg/dL or less. Patients received captopril or placebo for a median of 3 years. Doubling of serum creatinine (primary end point) occurred less frequently in the captopril group (25 vs. 43 patients; $p = 0.007$). The reductions in creatinine doubling were 48% in the entire captopril group, 76% in the subgroup with baseline creatinine of 2.0 mg/dL, 55% in the subgroup with creatinine of 1.5 mg/dL, and 17% in the subgroup with creatinine of 1.0 mg/day.

Captopril also was associated with a 50% reduction in death, dialysis, or transplantation; this benefit was independent of the small difference in BP between the groups.

87. **UKPDS 38.** Tight blood pressure control and risk of macrovascular and microvascular complications in type 2 diabetes: UK Prospective Diabetes Study Group. *BMJ* 1998;317:703–713.

   This prospective, randomized, controlled, multicenter trial enrolled 1,148 type 2 diabetics with HTN (mean entry BP, 160/94 mm Hg). Patients were assigned to tight BP control (goal, 150/85 mm Hg or less) with use of captopril or atenolol as main treatment, or less tight control (goal, 180/105 mm Hg or less). At follow-up (median, 8.4 years), mean BP was significantly reduced in the group assigned tight BP control [144/82 vs. 154/87 mm Hg (looser control); $p <$ 0.0001]. Tight-control group had significant relative reductions of 24% in diabetes-related end points, 32% in deaths related to diabetes, 44% in strokes, and 37% in microvascular end points. A nonsignificant reduction was found in all-cause mortality. The tight-control group also had a 34% reduction in risk in the proportion of patients with deterioration of retinopathy by two steps and a 47% reduced risk of deterioration in visual acuity by three lines of the diabetic retinopathy study chart. In a predefined substudy of the tight-control patients (UKPDS 39, see *BMJ* 1998;317:713–720), captopril and atenolol were equally effective in reducing BP, risk of macrovascular end points, and deterioration in retinopathy.

88. **The Accord Study Group.** Effects of intensive blood-pressure control in type 2 diabetes mellitus. *N Engl J Med* 2010; 362:1575–1585.

   The trial tested the hypothesis (and guideline recommendations) that reducing SBP below 140 mm Hg in patients with diabetes is beneficial to cardiovascular health. They randomized 4,733 patients with type 2 diabetes mellitus to intensive BP therapy targeted to reduce SBP to less than 120 mm Hg, or conventional therapy with a goal of less than 140 mm Hg. At mean follow-up of 4.7 years, there was no statistically significant different in the rate of the primary endpoint of cardiovascular death, MI, or stroke (1.87% annually for intensive vs. 2.09% annually for standard, $p = 0.20$). There were, however, a surfeit of adverse events related to antihypertensive therapy in the intensive group (3.3% vs. 1.3%, $p < 0.001$).

89. **Parving HH,** et al. for the **IRMA II** (Irbesartan in patients with Type 2 Diabetes and Microalbuminuria) Study Group. The effect of irbesartan on the development of diabetic nephropathy in patients with type 2 diabetes *N Engl J Med* 2001;345:870–878.

   This prospective, randomized, double-blind, placebo-controlled, multicenter trial enrolled 590 hypertensive patients with type 2 diabetes and microalbuminuria. Primary end point was time to onset of diabetic nephropathy (urinary albumin excretion rate, more than 200 μg/min and 30% or more higher than baseline level). Patients received irbesartan, 150 mg daily or 300 mg daily, or placebo. At 2-year follow-up, irbesartan groups had a lower incidence of the primary end point compared with the placebo group [5.2% (300 mg) and 9.7% (150 mg) vs. 9.7% (placebo); HRs, 0.30 ($p < 0.001$) and 0.61 ($p = 0.081$)]. Average BPs were 141/83 mm Hg in the 300-mg group, 143/83 mm Hg in the 150-mg group, and 144/83 mm Hg in the placebo group [$p = 0.004$ (SBP placebo compared with SBP of combined irbesartan groups)]. Serious adverse events were less frequent among the patients treated with irbesartan ($p = 0.02$).

90. **Brenner BM,** et al. for the **RENAAL** (Reduction of End points in NIDDM with Angiotensin II Antagonist Losartan) Study Investigators. Effects of losartan on renal and cardiovascular outcomes in patients with type 2 diabetes and nephropathy. *N Engl J Med* 2001;345:861–869.

   This prospective, randomized, double-blind, placebo-controlled, multicenter trial enrolled 1,513 type 2 diabetics with nephropathy (urinary albumin-to-creatinine ratio of 300 or more and serum creatinine, 1.3 to 3.0 mg/dL). Patients received losartan, 50 to 100 mg once daily, or placebo. Both were taken in addition to conventional antihypertensive agents. At a mean follow-up of 3.4 years, the losartan group had a 16% RRR in primary events [doubling of baseline serum creatinine, end-stage renal disease (ESRD), or death] compared with the placebo group (43.5% vs. 47.1%; $p = 0.02$). Losartan reduced serum creatinine doubling by 25% ($p = 0.006$) and ESRD by 28% ($p = 0.002$) but had no significant effect on all-cause mortality. The benefits exceeded those attributable to changes in BP. Losartan also was associated with a lower rate of first hospitalization for HF (RRR, 32%; $p = 0.005$) and a 35% decline in proteinuria ($p < 0.001$ in comparison with placebo).

91. **The Action to Control Cardiovascular Risk in Diabetes Study (ACCORD) Group.** Effects of intensive glucose lowering in type 2 diabetes. *N Engl J Med* 2008;358:2545–2559.

Design: Prospective, randomized, multicenter study. The primary endpoint was a composite outcome of nonfatal MI, stroke, or death from cardiovascular causes.

Purpose: To test the hypothesis that more intensive glucose control would reduce cardiovascular events in patients with type 2 diabetes.

Population: 10,251 patients with type 2 diabetes and HbA1c 7.5% or greater, who were either aged 40 to 79 years with CVD or aged 55 to 79 and had anatomical evidence of significant end-organ damage or atherosclerosis risk factors.

Treatment: Intensive therapy targeting a HbA1c of less than 6.0% versus standard therapy targeting HbA1c of 7.0% to 7.9%. Counseling and lifestyle modification were employed in both groups, and there were no particular restrictions on the type of pharmacotherapy implemented.

Results: The difference in mean HbA1c achieved was significant at 1 year (6.4% in the intensive-therapy vs. 7.5% in the standard-therapy). After a mean follow-up period of 3.5 years, the study was discontinued due to the finding of higher mortality in the intensive-therapy group (257 deaths in the intensive arm vs. 203 in the standard group, $p = 0.04$). At the premature stopping point, a primary endpoint event occurred in 3.52 patients in the intensive-therapy group versus 371 in the standard-therapy group ($p = 0.16$). There were significantly more episodes of hypoglycemia requiring assistance in the intensive-therapy group ($p < 0.001$).

Comment: The results of this study came as a surprise, and the underlying mechanism(s) explaining such an outcome are not clear. The intensive-therapy arm may have had too aggressive of a goal, or perhaps the *type* of hypoglycemic therapy is important, as well.

92. **The Action in Diabetes and Vascular Disease: Preterax and Diamicron Modified Release Controlled Evaluation (ADVANCE) Collaborative Group**. Intensive blood glucose control and vascular outcomes in patients with type 2 diabetes. *N Engl J Med* 2008;358: 2560–2572.

Design: Prospective, randomized, multicenter-center study. The primary endpoint was a composite outcome of major macrovascular events (cardiovascular death, MI, stroke) and major microvascular events (nephropathy or retinopathy), both jointly and separately, after a median of 5 years of follow-up.

Purpose: To test the hypothesis that more intensive glucose control would reduce macro- and microvascular events in patients with type 2 diabetes.

Population: 11,140 patients with type 2 diabetes who were diagnosed at age 30 years or older, were 55 years or older at study entry, and had a history of major macro- or microvascular disease or at least one additional risk factor for vascular disease. Baseline HbA1c levels were not included in the inclusion or exclusion criteria.

Treatment: Intensive therapy targeting HbA1c of 6.5% or less using glipazide plus other drugs as needed versus standard glucose control.

Results: At the conclusion of the study, mean HbA1c level was lower in the intensive-therapy group (6.5%) than in the standard-therapy arm (7.3%). Combined major macro and microvascular events were lower in the intensive-therapy group (18.1% vs. 20.0%, $p = 0.01$), which was primarily driven by a reduction in major microvascular events (9.4% vs. 10.9%, $p = 0.01$), specifically nephropathy. There were no differences in outcomes with regard to retinopathy or major macrovascular events between the two groups.

Comment: The composite endpoint of this contemporary trial summarizes the combined outcomes of several previous trials—aggressive glucose control in type 2 diabetes can have significant effects on *micro*vascular disease (retinopathy, nephropathy), however, it is difficult to improve on *macro*vascular events (MI, stroke). Once again, it is unclear if more particular therapies (specifically, metformin), could have changed the outcome of this trial.

93. **Lewis EJ,** et al. **IDNT** (Irbesartan Diabetic Nephropathy Trial). Renoprotective effect of the angiotensin-receptor antagonist irbesartan in patients with nephropathy due to type 2 diabetes. *N Engl J Med* 2001;345:851–860.

This prospective, randomized, double-blind, placebo-controlled, multicenter, primary trial enrolled 1,715 hypertensive patients with nephropathy due to type 2 diabetes. Patients received irbesartan (300 mg daily), amlodipine (10 mg daily), or placebo. Target BP was 135/85 mm Hg or less. At mean follow-up of 2.6 years, irbesartan had 20% and 23% fewer primary events (doubling of baseline serum creatinine, ESRD, or death) than did the placebo and amlodipine groups [32.6% vs. 39% ($p = 0.02$) and 41.1%; $p = 0.006$]. Irbesartan was associated with 33% and 37% lower rates of serum creatinine doubling [16.9% vs. 23.7% ($p = 0.003$) and 25.4% ($p < 0.001$)] and 23% lower RR of ESRD than both other groups (14.2% vs. 17.8% and 18.3%; $p = 0.07$ for both comparisons). These differences were not explained by the achieved BP differences. No significant differences were noted between the groups in all-cause mortality or the cardiovascular composite end point.

94. **Gaede P,** et al. **STENO-2.** Multifactorial intervention and cardiovascular disease in patients with type 2 diabetes. *N Engl J Med* 2003;348:383–393.

This prospective, open, parallel trial randomized 160 type 2 diabetics with microalbuminuria to conventional treatment, in accordance with national guidelines, or intensive treatment, with a step-wise implementation of behavior modification and drug therapy that targeted hyperglycemia, HTN, dyslipidemia, and microalbuminuria, as well as secondary prevention of CVD with ASA. At follow-up (mean, 7.8 years), the intensive therapy group had a significantly lower risk of CVD (HR, 0.47; 95% CI, 0.24 to 0.73), nephropathy (HR, 0.39; 95% CI, 0.17 to 0.87), and retinopathy (HR, 0.42; 95% CI, 0.21 to 0.86).

Smoking

95. **Rosenberg L,** et al. The risk of MI after quitting smoking in men under 55 years of age. *N Engl J Med* 1985;313:1511–1514.

This prospective case-control study was composed of 1,873 patients with first MI and 2,775 controls. Among current smokers, defined as smoking within the prior 12 months versus never, the age-adjusted RR of MI was 2.9 (95% CI, 2.4 to 3.4). Among those who had quit smoking 12 to 23 months earlier versus never smokers, the RR of MI was 2.0 (95% CI, 1.1 to 3.8). Those who had quit 2 years earlier had a risk similar to that of never smokers (RR, 1.0).

96. **Willett WC,** et al. Relative and excess risks of coronary heart disease among women who smoke cigarettes. *N Engl J Med* 1987;317:1303–1309.

This analysis focused on 119,404 NHS participants with 6 years of follow-up; 30% were smokers. The number of cigarettes smoked per day was found to be associated with an increased risk of fatal CHD (in multivariate analysis, RR of 5.4 for 25 cigarettes/day), MI (RR, 6.3), and angina pectoris (RR, 2.3). If they smoked 1 to 14 cigarettes/day, RRs (in multivariate analysis) were 1.8 to 2.5; 15 to 24 cigarettes/day, RRs, 1.5 to 4.7; 45 cigarettes/day, RR of death and MI was 10.8. Overall, smoking was responsible for approximately 50% of events. The greatest absolute risks were seen with smoking in combination with other risk factors: smoking and HTN, RR, 22.2; smoking and hypercholesterolemia, RR, 18.9; smoking and diabetes, RR, 22.3.

97. **Kawachi I,** et al. Smoking cessation and time course of decreased risks of coronary heart disease in middle-aged women. *Arch Intern Med* 1994;154:169–175.

This prospective cohort study was composed of 117,006 nurses free of CHD in 1976. The average follow-up period was 11.7 years. In a multivariate analysis, among current smokers versus never smokers, the RR was 4.23 (95% CI, 3.60 to 4.96); among those who started smoking before age 15 years, RR, 9.25; among former smokers, RR, 1.48 (95% CI, 1.22 to 1.79). After quitting, one third of the excess risk was gone at 3 years, and normal risk was attained after 10 to 14 years.

98. **Steenland K,** et al. Environmental tobacco smoke and coronary heart disease in the ACS CPS-II cohort. *Circulation* 1996;94:622–628 (editorial, 596–599).

This prospective study was composed of 353,180 women and 126,500 male nonsmokers. A 22% higher CHD mortality rate (95% CI) was observed among men married to current smokers; the corresponding RR for women married to current smokers was 1.1 (95% CI, 0.96 to 1.22). The editorial provides an analysis of data from 14 studies that shows an approximate 20% increased risk of CHD death in nonsmokers married to smokers.

99. **Kawachi I,** et al. A prospective study of passive smoking and coronary heart disease. *Circulation* 1997;95:2374–2379.

This analysis focused on 32,046 NHS participants who did not smoke and were free of CHD in 1982. Exposure was assessed by self-report and only at baseline. At 10-year follow-up, the adjusted CHD risk (nonfatal MI and cardiac death) was significantly higher among those with frequent smoke exposure (RR, 1.91; 95% CI, 1.11 to 3.28), and a trend of increased risk with occasional exposure was noted (RR, 1.58; 95% CI, 0.93 to 2.68). No association was found between duration of living with a smoker and the incidence of CHD.

100. **He J,** et al. Passive smoking and the risk of coronary heart disease: a meta-analysis of epidemiologic studies. *N Engl J Med* 1999;340:920–926.

This analysis of 10 cohort and 8 case-control studies showed that nonsmokers exposed to environmental smoke had an RR of CHD of 1.25 (95% CI, 1.17 to 1.32) compared with that of nonsmokers with no such exposure. This association was significant in both men and women and present in those exposed at home or in the workplace. A significant dose–response relation was demonstrated: RR of CHD, 1.23 in those exposed to smoke of 1 to 19 cigarettes/day versus RR of 1.31 in those exposed to 20 cigarettes/day ($p = 0.006$ for linear trend).

101. **Alsever RN,** et al. Reduced hospitalizations for acute myocardial infarction after implementation of a smoke-free ordinance—City of Pueblo, Colorado, 2002–2006. *MMWR Morb Mortal Wkly Rep* 2009;57:1373–1377. Available athttp://www.cdc.gov/mmwr/PDF/wk/mm5751.pdf.

In this Colorado town, the authors identify significant declines in rates of acute MI after a city-wide smoking ban was implemented in July 1, 2003. They detected such a decline within only 18 months after the ban went into effect.

102. **Meyers DG,** et al. Cardiovascular effect of bans on smoking in public places. A systematic review and meta-analysis. *J Am Coll Cardiol* 2009;54:1249–1255.

The authors combine 11 studies from 10 smoking-ban locations to assess the impact of such ordinances on cardiovascular health. Risk of acute MI dropped by 17%, with progressive declines for each year the ban was in effect.

103. **The Varenicline Phase 3 Study Group.** See *JAMA* 2006;296(1):56–63, *JAMA* 2006;296(1):47–55, and *JAMA* 2006;296:64–71.

These three reports of the Varenicline Phase 3 Study Group compared varenicline, a partial nicotine receptor agonist, to placebo and sustained-release bupropion, for effectiveness at achieving smoking cessation. In several thousand adult smokers, these series of reports demonstrated that patients taking varenicline were significantly more like to abstain from cigarette smoking over follow-up periods up to 1 year. Abstinence was proven by use of carbon monoxide testing. Further reviews have demonstrated significant psychiatric side-effects leading to FDA warnings for patients at high-risk of such adverse events.

104. **Rigotti NA,** et al. Efficacy and safety of varenicline for smoking cessation in patients with cardiovascular disease: a randomized trial. *Circulation* 2010;121:221–229.

The investigators randomized 714 smokers with stable CVD to varenicline or placebo, with counseling for smoking cessation, over 12 weeks. Smoking abstinence higher for those on varenicline, and there was no difference in adverse cardiovascular events over 52 weeks of follow-up.

Hypertension

REVIEW ARTICLES/MISCELLANEOUS

105. **JNC 7,** Chobanian AV, et al. The seventh report of the Joint National Committee on prevention, detection, evaluation, and treatment of high blood pressure: the JNC 7 report. *JAMA* 2003;289:2560–2571.

JNC 7 defines HTN as SBP greater than 140 mm Hg and DBP as greater than 90 mm Hg, or taking hypertensive medication(s). JNC 7 introduced a new BP category called, "Prehypertensive," which includes those with SBP 120 to 139 mm Hg or DBP 80 to 89 mm Hg. When pharmacologic intervention is indicated, JNC 7 advocates the use of diuretics and β-blockers as first-line agents in most patients. As was the case with JNC VI, other therapies (e.g., ACE inhibitors) also are recommended for individuals with specific characteristics (see text for details, pages xx–xx). If BP is $>20 \neq 10$ mm Hg above targets ($<140 \neq 90$ or $<130 \neq 80$ if diabetic or chronic kidney disease present), initial therapy should be with two agents.

EPIDEMIOLOGY AND RISK FACTORS

106. **Kannel WB.** Blood pressure as a cardiovascular risk factor. **JAMA** 1996;275:1571–1576.

This analysis of 36-year follow-data from the Framingham Heart Study shows that from age 30 to 65 years, the average increases in SBP and DBP are 20 and 10 mm Hg, respectively. No evidence of a change was found in the prevalence of HTN over the past four decades. HTN occurs alone in only 20% (i.e., no diabetes, obesity, dyslipidemia). Hypertensive patients had increased RRs (M/F) of CAD (2.0/2.2), stroke (3.8/2.6), PAD (2.0/3.7), and CHF (4.0/3.0). See **Figure 1.2** of this chapter for estimated rates of CHD over a 10-year period according to different combinations of risk factors in men and women.

107. **O'Donnell CJ,** et al. Hypertension and borderline isolated systolic hypertension increase risks of cardiovascular disease and mortality in male physicians. *Circulation* 1997;95:1132–1137.

This prospective cohort analysis focused on 18,682 PHS participants, with a mean follow-up of 11.7 years. Isolated SBP (140 to 159 mm Hg) was associated with higher rates of

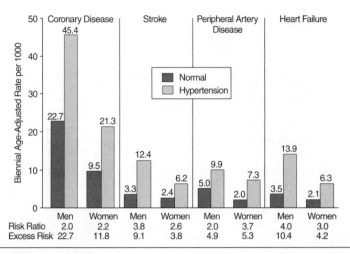

Figure 1.2 • Risk of cardiovascular events by hypertensive status in subjects aged 35 to 64 years, Framingham Study, 36-year follow-up. Coronary disease includes clinical manifestations such as myocardial infarction, angina pectoris, sudden death, other coronary deaths, and coronary insufficiency syndrome; peripheral artery disease is manifested as intermittent claudication. (Reprinted from Kannel WB. Lipids, diabetes, and coronary heart disease: insights from the Framingham Heart Study. *Am Heart J* 1985;110:1100–1107, with permission from Elsevier.)

stroke (RR, 1.42) and cardiovascular death (RR, 1.56), as well as a 22% higher all-cause mortality rate and nonsignificant increase in MI rate (RR, 1.26).

108. **Moster d'A,** et al. Trends in the prevalence of hypertension, antihypertensive therapy, and left ventricular hypertrophy from 1950 to 1989. *N Engl J Med* 1999;340: 1221–1227.

   This analysis focused on 10,333 Framingham Heart Study participants. From 1950 to 1989, the age-adjusted prevalence of SBP, 160 mm Hg, or DBP, 100 mm Hg, declined from 18.5% to 9.2% among men and from 28.0% to 7.7% among women. A decline was noted in ECG evidence of LV hypertrophy: 4.5% to 2.5% and 3.6% to 1.1%.

109. **Vasan RS,** et al. Residual lifetime risk for developing hypertension in middle-aged women and men: the Framingham Heart Study. *JAMA* 2002;287:1003–1010.

   Prospective cohort analysis of 1,298 Framingham Heart Study participants who were aged 55 to 65 years and free of HTN at baseline (1976 to 1998). The residual lifetime risks for developing HTN and stage 1 high BP or higher were 90% in both 55- and 65-year-old participants. The lifetime probability of receiving antihypertensive medication was 60%. The risk for HTN remained unchanged for women, but it was approximately 60% higher for men in the 1976 to 1998 period compared with the 1952 to 1975 period. In contrast, the residual lifetime risk for stage 2 high BP or higher (160/100 mm Hg or higher regardless of treatment) was lower in both sexes in the recent period (35% to 57% in 1952 to 1975 vs. 35% to 44% in 1976 to 1998), likely owing to a marked increase in pharmacologic treatment of individuals with substantially elevated BP.

META-ANALYSES

110. **Johnson AG,** et al. Do non-steroidal anti-inflammatory drugs affect blood pressure? A meta-analysis. *Ann Intern Med* 1994;121:289–300.

    This analysis was performed on data from 38 randomized, placebo-controlled trials and 12 randomized but not placebo-controlled trials (comparing two NSAIDs). NSAID use was associated with a 5.0 mm Hg higher elevated supine mean BP. NSAIDs also antagonized the antihypertensive effect of β-blockers (BP elevation, 6.2 mm Hg). Sulindac and ASA were found to have the least hypertensive effect.

111. **Schmieder RE,** et al. Reversal of left ventricular hypertrophy in essential hypertension: a meta-analysis of randomized double-blind studies. *JAMA* 1996;275:1507–1513.

    This meta-analysis of 39 trials showed that a decrease in LV mass correlated significantly with a decrease in SBP ($r = 0.46; p < 0.001$) and a longer duration of antihypertensive therapy ($r = 0.38; p < 0.01$). ACE inhibitors achieved a greater reduction in LV mass than did β-blockers and diuretics (-13% vs. $-6\%; p < 0.05; -13\%$ vs. $-7\%; p = 0.08$).

112. **Law MR,** et al. Use of blood pressure lowering drugs in the prevention of cardiovascular disease: meta-analysis of 147 randomised trials in the context of expectations from prospective epidemiological studies. *BMJ* 2009;338:b1665.

    The authors compile data from 147 randomized trials, including 464,000 patients to quantify the effect on BP of each class of antihypertensive medication. Overall, they found that the five different classes of medications (thiazide diuretics, β-blockers, ACE inhibitors, ARBs, and calcium-channel blockers) all had similar BP lowering effects. However, β-blockers had the additional benefit of lower risk of recurrent CAD events in those patients with a previous history of CAD. Similarly, calcium-channel blockers had a small advantage in lowering risk of stroke. However, in the general population, the authors could not identify meaningful clinical outcomes differences among the classes.

TREATMENT

β-Blocker and/or Diuretic Studies

113. Metoprolol Atherosclerosis Prevention in Hypertension (**MAPHY**). Primary prevention with metoprolol in patients with hypertension: mortality results from the MAPHY study. *JAMA* 1988;259:1976–1982.

    Design: Prospective, randomized, multicenter, open study. Median follow-up period was 4.2 years.
    Purpose: To investigate whether metoprolol lowers cardiovascular complications of high BP to a greater extent than do thiazide diuretics.
    Population: 3,234 white men aged 40 to 64 years.
    Treatment: Metoprolol (mean dosage, 174 mg/day) or thiazide [hydrochlorothiazide (mean dosage, 46 mg/day) or bendroflumethiazide (mean dosage, 4.4 mg/day)].
    Results: Metoprolol group had 48% lower all-cause mortality (4.8 vs. 9.3 deaths/1,000 patient years) and 58% lower CV mortality (2.6 vs. 6.2 deaths/1,000 patient years).

114. Systolic HTN in Elderly Program (**SHEP**). Prevention of stroke by antihypertensive drug therapy in older persons with isolated systolic hypertension. *JAMA* 1991;265: 3255–3264.

    Design: Prospective, randomized, multicenter, double-blind, placebo-controlled study. Primary outcome was nonfatal and fatal (total) stroke. Average follow-up period was 4.5 years.

Purpose: To assess the ability of antihypertensive drug therapy to decrease the risk of stroke in individuals with isolated systolic HTN.

Population: 4,736 patients aged $\geq$60 years (14% black, 57% women) with SBP, 160 to 219 mm Hg, and DBP, less than 90 mm Hg; 3,161 patients were taking antihypertensive drug(s).

Treatment: Step 1, chlorthalidone, 12.5 mg/day; dose, 2 25 mg/day; step 2, atenolol, 25 mg/day, and then 50 mg/day.

Results: At 5 years, 36% fewer strokes (5.2 vs. 8.2/1,000; $p = 0.0003$), lower SBP (143 vs. 155 mm Hg), and 27% decrease in nonfatal MI and coronary death were observed.

115. **Meade TW,** et al. Medical Research Council (**MRC**). MRC trial of treatment of hypertension in older adults: principal results. *BMJ* 1992;304:405–412.

Design: Prospective, randomized, single-blind, placebo-controlled study. Average follow-up period was 5.8 years.

Purpose: To determine whether antihypertensive therapy in men and women aged 65 to 74 years reduces mortality and morbidity due to stroke and CHD.

Population: 4,396 patients not taking any antihypertensive agents and with SBP, 160 to 209 mm Hg, and DBP, less than 115 mm Hg.

Exclusion Criteria: Stroke or MI in prior 3 months, diabetes, and asthma.

Treatment: HCTZ (25 to 50 mg/day), amiloride (2.5 to 5.0 mg/day), atenolol (50 mg/day), or placebo.

Results: Treated patients had 25% fewer strokes ($p = 0.04$) and 19% fewer coronary events ($p = 0.08$). β-Blockers induced nonsignificant reduction; diuretics induced 31% fewer strokes and 44% fewer coronary events.

116. **Neaton JD,** et al. Treatment of mild hypertension study (**TOMHS**): final results. *JAMA* 1993;270:713–724.

Design: Prospective, randomized, multicenter, double-blind, placebo-controlled study. Average follow-up period was 4.4 years.

Purpose: To compare five drug treatments with placebo for long-term management of mild hypertension.

Population: 902 patients aged 45 to 69 years and not taking any antihypertensive medications at initial screening, with DBP, 90 to 99 mm Hg (at two visits).

Treatment: Chlorthalidone, 15 mg/day (diuretic); acebutolol, 400 mg/day (β-blocker); doxazosin, 1 mg/day (α-1 agonist); amlodipine, 5 mg/day; enalapril, 5 mg/day; or placebo (all AM dosing). All patients received nutritional and hygienic advice (low weight, low sodium, low alcohol, increased exercise).

Results: Drug therapy reductions were sizable in all six groups (DBP decreased by 8.6 to 12.3 mm Hg). Drug groups had a nonsignificant reduction in death and MACE (5.1% vs. 7.3%; $p = 0.21$). Drug therapy also was associated with better quality of life and decreased resting ECG abnormalities; no differences were seen between the five drug groups in LV mass, lipid levels, and other outcome measures.

Calcium-channel Blocker and/or ACE Inhibitor–focused Studies

117. **Staessen JA,** et al. **Syst-Eur.** Randomised double-blind comparison of placebo and active treatment for older patients with isolated systolic hypertension. *Lancet* 1997;350:757–764.

Design: Prospective, randomized, double-blind, placebo-controlled, multicenter study. Primary end point was fatal and nonfatal stroke. Median follow-up period was 2 years.

Purpose: To investigate whether treatment of isolated systolic HTN could reduce stroke and cardiovascular complications.

Population: 4,695 patients aged ≥60 years with average sitting SBP of 160 to 219 mm Hg and DBP of less than 95 mm Hg.

Exclusion Criteria: CHF; creatinine, 180 μM; and MI in prior year.

Treatment: Nitrendipine, 10 to 40 mg/day, with the possible addition of enalapril, 5 to 20 mg/day; and HCTZ, 12.5 to 25 mg/day; or matching placebos.

Results: At 2 years, treated patients had 42% fewer total strokes (7.9 vs. 13.7 per 1,000 patient years; $p = 0.003$) and 31% fewer fatal and nonfatal cardiac end points ($p = 0.03$). Treated patients had significantly lower SBPs and DBPs than did placebo patients (-10.1 mm Hg and -4.5 mm Hg). A trend was seen toward lower CV mortality with active treatment (-27%; $p = 0.07$), but all-cause mortality was not influenced ($-14\%; p = 0.22$).

Comments: A subsequent study at mean follow-up of 3.9 years demonstrated a 55% reduction in the risk of dementia with nitrendipine treatment (see *Arch Intern Med* 2002;162:2046).

118. **Captopril Prevention Project (CAPPP)**. Effect of angiotensin-converting-enzyme inhibition compared with conventional therapy on cardiovascular morbidity and mortality in hypertension: the Captopril Prevention Project (CAPPP) randomised trial. *Lancet* 1999;353:611–616.

Design: Prospective, randomized, multicenter, open study. Primary composite end points were fatal and nonfatal MI, stroke, and other CV deaths. Mean follow-up period was 6.1 years.

Purpose: To compare the effectiveness of captopril with a conventional antihypertensive regimen of diuretics or β-blockers on cardiovascular morbidity and mortality.

Population: 10,985 patients aged 25 to 66 years with DBP ≥100 mm Hg on two occasions.

Exclusion Criteria: Secondary HTN and serum creatinine greater than 150 μM.

Treatment: Captopril, 50 mg once or twice daily; β-blockers (most common: metoprolol and atenolol); or diuretics (most common, HCTZ and bendrofluazide).

Results: Two groups had a similar incidence of composite end point (11.1 and 10.2 events per 1,000 patient years in captopril and conventional therapy groups); captopril group had a trend toward lower CV mortality (RR, 0.77; $p = 0.092$) but a higher incidence of fatal and nonfatal stroke (RR, 1.15; $p = 0.044$); MI rates were similar.

Comments: Lower stroke risk in conventional group probably was owing to lower initial BP (–2 mm Hg).

119. **Hansson L,** et al. Randomised trial of effects of calcium antagonists compared with diuretics and beta-blockers on cardiovascular morbidity and mortality in hypertension: the Nordic Diltiazem (**NORDIL**) study. *Lancet* 2000;356:359–365.

Design: Prospective, randomized, open, blinded end point, multicenter trial. Primary end point was fatal and nonfatal stroke, MI, and other CV death. Mean follow-up, 4.5 years.

Purpose: To compare the effects of calcium antagonists with those of diuretics and β-blockers on major outcomes in middle-aged hypertensive individuals.

Population: 10,881 patients aged 50 to 74 years with DBP of 100 mm Hg or more.

Treatment: Diltiazem (180 to 360 mg daily) versus diuretics, β-blockers, or both. Additional antihypertensives could be added to achieve DBP less than 90 mm Hg.

Results: SBP and DBP were lowered effectively in the diltiazem and diuretic and β-blocker groups (reduction, 20.3/18.7 vs. 23.3/18.7 mm Hg; difference in systolic reduction, $p <$ 0.001). No difference was found between the two groups in the incidence of the primary composite end point [16.6 (diltiazem) vs. 16.2 events per 1,000 patient years]. The diltiazem group had a lower incidence of fatal and nonfatal stroke compared with the diuretic and β-blocker group [6.4 vs. 7.9 events per 1,000 patient years; RR, 0.80 (95% CI, 0.65 to 0.99); $p = 0.04$], whereas the rates of fatal and nonfatal MI were not significantly different [7.4 vs. 6.3 events per 1,000 patient years; RR, 1.16 (0.94 to 1.44); $p = 0.17$].

120. **PROGRESS** (Perindopril pROtection aGainst REcurrent Stroke Study), PROGRESS Collaborative Group. Randomised trial of a perindopril-based blood-pressure-lowering

regimen among 6,105 individuals with previous stroke or transient ischaemic attack. *Lancet* 2001;358:1033–1041 (editorial, 1026–1027).

Design: Prospective, randomized, double-blind, placebo-controlled, multicenter trial. Primary end point was total stroke (fatal or nonfatal). Mean follow-up was 3.9 years.

Purpose: To determine the effects of a BP-lowering regimen in hypertensive and nonhypertensive patients with a history of stroke or TIA.

Population: 6,105 individuals with a stroke (hemorrhagic or ischemic) or TIA in the previous 5 years and no major disability.

Treatment: Active treatment [perindopril (4 mg daily) with addition of the diuretic indapamide (2.5 mg daily) at physicians' discretion], or placebo.

Results: At follow-up, active treatment reduced BP by 9/4 mm Hg. In active treatment group, 60% received both drugs, and 40% received perindopril alone. The active treatment group had a significantly lower incidence of stroke compared with the placebo group (10% vs. 14%; 28% RRR; $p < 0.0001$). Active treatment also reduced total major vascular events by 26%. Hypertensive and nonhypertensive subgroups had similar reductions in stroke (all values $p < 0.01$). Combination therapy with perindopril plus indapamide reduced BP by 12/5 mm Hg and stroke risk by 43%, whereas single-drug therapy reduced BP by 5/3 mm Hg and resulted in no significant reduction in stroke incidence.

Comments: Editorialists dispute study's conclusion that treatment with both agents be considered routinely for patients with a history of stroke or TIA, irrespective of BP, and advocate starting treatment with a diuretic, not with combination therapy. They also point out that the 5 mm Hg reduction in systolic BP seen in the perindopril group should translate into an approximate 20% reduction in stroke risk, as seen in many prior studies using diuretics and β-blockers.

121. **Dahlof B,** et al. for the **LIFE** (Losartan Intervention For Endpoint reduction in hypertension) Study Group. Cardiovascular morbidity and mortality in the losartan intervention for endpoint reduction in hypertension study (LIFE): a randomised trial against atenolol. *Lancet* 2002;359:995–1003.

Design: Prospective, randomized, placebo-controlled, blinded, parallel-group, multicenter trial. Primary end point: death, MI, or stroke. Mean follow-up, 4.8 years.

Purpose: Use of losartan compared with atenolol in patients with HTN and left ventricular hypertrophy (LVH).

Population: 9,193 patients aged 55 to 80 years with previously treated or untreated HTN (SBP, 160 to 200 mm Hg; DBP, 95 to 115 mm Hg; ECG signs of LVH).

Exclusion Criteria: Included secondary HTN; MI or stroke in previous 6 months; angina requiring β-blockers or calcium antagonists; HF or LVEF 40% or less; need for treatment with any angiotensin II–receptor antagonist, any β-blocker, HCTZ, or ACE inhibitor.

Treatment: Losartan-based or atenolol-based regimen after 1 to 2 weeks of placebo. Drugs were dosed to reach a target BP of less than 140/90 mm Hg per titration schedule.

Results: BP was reduced by 30.2/16.6 mm Hg in the losartan group and 29.1/16.8 mm Hg in the atenolol group (treatment difference, $p = 0.017$ for SBP and $p = 0.37$ for DBP). The losartan group had a significantly lower incidence of death, MI, or stroke compared with the atenolol group (11% vs. 13%; HR, 0.87; $p = 0.021$), primarily driven by fewer strokes (5% vs. 7%; HR, 0.75; $p = 0.001$). CV mortality rates were not significantly different (4% vs. 5%; HR, 0.89; $p = 0.21$). Losartan also was associated with a lower incidence of new-onset diabetes (6% vs. 8%; HR, 0.75; $p = 0.001$). A major LIFE substudy examined CV outcomes in 1,195 patients with diabetes, HTN, and ECG signs of LVH (*Lancet* 2002;359:1004). At a mean follow-up of 4.7 years, mean BP decreased to similar levels (losartan, 146/79 mm Hg; atenolol, 148/79 mm Hg). However, the losartan group had a significant 24% RRR in death, MI, or stroke. Losartan also had significant reductions in CV mortality (37% RRR; $p = 0.028$) and all-cause mortality (39% RRR; $p = 0.002$). These substudy results suggest that losartan has benefits beyond BP reduction. In the subgroup of patients with isolated systolic HTN (DBP, less than 90 mm Hg) and LVH (by ECG), the losartan group was associated with 25% fewer primary events compared with atenolol (see *JAMA* 2002;288:1491).

Comments: These results are in contrast to those of the CAPPP, NORDIL, and STOP-HTN2 trials, which compared ACE inhibitors or calcium-channel blockers with β-blockers and diuretics for treatment of HTN and found no difference in efficacy. Because this trial examined the efficacy of losartan in high-risk hypertensive patients with signs of LVH, one cannot extrapolate these results to lower-risk patients.

122. **Teo KK**, et al. for the ACE Inhibitors Collaborative Group. Effects of long-term treatment with angiotensin-converting-enzyme inhibitors in the presence or absence of aspirin: a systematic review. *Lancet* 2002;360:1037–1043.

This overview examined data on 22,060 patients from six long-term randomized trials evaluating ACE inhibitor (ACEI) therapy. Results from analyses of all trials, except SOLVD, found no significant differences between the risk reductions with ACEI therapy in the presence or absence of ASA in the composite of death, MI, stroke, CHF hospitalization, or revascularization, or in any of its individual components, except MI (interaction $p = 0.01$). Overall, ACEI therapy significantly reduced the risk of major clinical outcomes by 22% ($p < 0.0001$), with clear reductions in risk both among those receiving ASA at baseline (OR, 0.80; 99% CI, 0.73 to 0.88) and those who were not (OR, 0.71; 99% CI, 0.62 to 0.81; interaction $p = 0.07$).

123. Wing LM, et al. **ANBP-2 (Second Australian National Blood Pressure Study)**. A comparison of outcomes with angiotensin-converting enzyme inhibitors and diuretics for hypertension in the elderly. *N Engl J Med* 2003;348:583–592.

Design: Prospective, randomized, open, multicenter study. Primary end point was death or any cardiovascular event. Median follow-up was 4.1 years.
Purpose: To compare outcomes in older hypertensive subjects receiving ACE inhibitors with those treated with diuretics.
Population: 6,083 subjects aged 65 to 84 years with HTN.
Treatment: ACE inhibitor or diuretic (enalapril and hydrochlorothiazide recommended, but not mandated).
Results: ACE inhibitor group had a significant reduction in primary events compared to diuretic group (hazard ratio 0.89, 95% CI 0.71 to 1.00, $p = 0.05$). Among men, the HR was 0.83 (95% CI 0.71 to 0.97, $p = 0.02$), while in women HR was 1.00 for women.
Comments: Criticisms of this trial include the open label design, no restrictions on drugs used, and inclusion of "soft" endpoints. Also of note, the study enrolled few or no black patients (% not reported).

124. Pepine CJ, et al. A calcium antagonist vs. a non-calcium antagonist hypertension treatment strategy for patients with coronary artery disease. The International Verapamil-Trandolapril Study (INVEST): a randomized controlled trial. *JAMA* 2003;290:2805–2816.

Design: Prospective, randomized, open-label, multicenter study with blinded endpoints. Primary end point was the first occurrence of death, nonfatal MI, or nonfatal stroke at 24 months.
Purpose: To compare clinical outcomes with calcium antagonists versus noncalcium antagonists in patients with CAD and HTN.
Population: 22,576 patients ages 50 years or older, with CAD and HTN, 862 sites in 14 countries.
Treatment: Calcium antagonist (verapamil sustained release, with trandolapril if needed) or noncalcium antagonist (atenolol with hydrochlorothiazide if needed).
Results: At follow-up (mean 2.7 years), there was no difference between the arms (RR 0.98) in the incidence of death, nonfatal stroke, or nonfatal MI. Achievement of guideline-recommended

BP (systolic and/or diastolic) was roughly equivalent between the two strategies. The verapamil group did have a lower incidence of new onset diabetes (6.2% vs. 7.3%). This finding may be related to the use of hydrochlorothiazide as the second step in atenolol arm [vs. protective effect of trandolapril (second step in verapamil arm)].

125. **Dahlöf B**, et al. For the **ASCOT** Investigators. Prevention of cardiovascular events with an antihypertensive regimen of amlodipine adding perindopril as required versus atenolol adding bendroflumethiazide as required, in the Anglo-Scandinavian Cardiac Outcomes Trial-Blood Pressure Lowering Arm (ASCOT-BPLA): a multicentre randomized controlled trial. *Lancet* 2005;366:895–906.

Design: Multicenter, prospective, randomized trial. Primary endpoint was fatal CHD or MI at median follow-up of 5.5 years.
Purpose: To compare two regimens of BP control—a calcium-channel blocker with ACE-I addition versus β-blocker with diuretic addition.
Population: 19,257 patients , ages 40 to 79, with HTN and at least three other CVD risk factors.
Treatment: Amlodipine with perindopril as needed versus atenolol with bendroflumethiazide as needed.
Results: Based on significantly higher mortality in the atenolol group, the trial was halted early, at median 5.5 years of follow-up. At this time, there was a nonsignificant trend in the primary endpoint, favoring the amlodipine group (unadjusted HR 0.90, $p = 0.1052$). Additionally, stroke (0.77, $p = 0.003$) and all-cause mortality (0.89, $p = 0.025$) were both significantly lower in the amlodipine group.

126. **Jamerson K**, et al. for the **ACCOMPLISH** trial investigators. Benazepril plus amlodipine or hydrochlorothiazide for hypertension in high-risk patients. *N Engl J Med* 2008;359:2417–2428.

Design: Prospective, randomized, double-blind trial. Primary endpoint was the composite of cardiovascular death, nonfatal MI, nonfatal stroke, hospitalization for angina, resuscitation from sudden cardiac arrest, or coronary revascularization.
Purpose: To compare hydrochlorothiazide in addition to benazepril, with amlodipine, also in addition to an benazepril.
Population: 11,506 patients with HTN at high risk for cardiovascular events—they had previous events, revascularization, impaired renal function, PAD, LVH, or diabetes mellitus.
Treatment: Hydrochlorothiazide plus benazepril versus amlodipine plus benazepril.
Results: After a mean follow-up of 36 months, the trial was halted early when the primary outcome significantly favored the benazepril–amlodipine arm (9.6% vs. 11.8%, $p < 0.001$), with a relative risk reduction of 19.6%. The narrower secondary endpoint, a composite of death, nonfatal MI, or nonfatal stroke also significantly favored the amlodipine arm (hazard ration 0.79, $p = 0.002$).

127. **The ONTARGET Investigators**. Telmisartan, ramipril, or both in patients at high risk for vascular events. *N Engl J Med* 2008;358:1547–1559.

Design: Multicenter, randomized, double-blind, controlled trial. Primary endpoint was cardiovascular death, MI, stroke, or CHF hospitalization at median follow-up of 56 months.
Purpose: To compare ACE-I, ARB, or their combination, for BP control in prevention of cardiovascular events.
Population: 25,620 patients with CAD, PAD, cerebrovascular disease, or diabetes.
Exclusion Criteria: Those who could not tolerate ACE-I were randomized in a separate trial to ARB or placebo.
Treatment: Ramipril, telmisartan, or both.
Results: Primary endpoint events occurred in 16.5% of patients in the ramipril group versus 16.7% in the telmisartan group, and 16.3% in the combination therapy group (pair-wise

comparisons not significant). There was more BP lowering and higher incidence of adverse events (hypotensive symptoms, syncope, and renal dysfunction) in the combination group, compared with the ramipril group.

Multiple Agent Studies

128. **Materson BJ**, et al. **VA Cooperative Study**. Single-drug therapy for hypertension in men: a comparison of 6 antihypertensive agents with placebo. *N Engl J Med* 1993;328:914–921.

Design: Prospective, randomized, double-blind, placebo-controlled, multicenter study. Primary end point was DBP less than 95 mm Hg. Follow-up period was 1 year.

Purpose: To compare the effectiveness of several different classes of antihypertensive therapies as monotherapy based on age and race.

Population: 1,292 men aged ≥21 years with DBP from 95 to 109 mm Hg.

Treatment: HCTZ, 12.5 to 50 mg/day; atenolol, 25 to 100 mg/day; clonidine, 0.2 to 0.6 mg/day; captopril, 25 to 100 mg/day; prazosin, 4 to 20 mg/day; sustained-release diltiazem, 120 to 360 mg/day; or placebo.

Results: Overall success rates (DBP less than 95 mm Hg over a 1-year period) were as follows: diltiazem, 59%; atenolol, 51%; clonidine, 50%; HCTZ, 46%; captopril, 42%; prazosin, 42%; and placebo, 25%. Certain drugs appeared to be more effective in particular subgroups of patients: in blacks (young and old), diltiazem was best; in young whites, captopril was best; and in older whites, atenolol was best. Subsequent 1-year follow-up showed a significant reduction in LVH in those receiving HCTZ, captopril, and atenolol (−42.9, −38.7, and −28.1 g).

Comments: One possible explanation for these findings is that blacks and older patients may be less responsive to ACE inhibition and more responsive to diuretics and calcium-channel blockade because of a higher prevalence of low-renin HTN.

129. **Hansson L**, et al. for the Hypertension Optimal Treatment (**HOT**) study. Effects of intensive blood pressure lowering and low dose aspirin in patients with hypertension: principal results of the Hypertension Optimal Treatment (HOT) randomized trial. *Lancet* 1998;351:1755–1762.

Design: Prospective, randomized, partially open, partially blinded (ASA arm), multicenter study. Mean follow-up period was 3.8 years.

Purpose: To (a) assess the association between major CV events and three different target BPs as well as the actual DBP achieved during treatment; and (b) evaluate whether the addition of low-dose ASA to antihypertensive treatment reduces major CV events.

Population: 18,790 patients aged 50 to 80 years (mean, 61.5 years) with DBP, 100 to 115 mm Hg.

Treatment: Target DBP levels of ≥90 mm Hg, =85 mm Hg, or =80 mm Hg. A five-step approach was used: step 1, felodipine, 5 mg/day; step 2, addition of low-dose ACE inhibitor or β-blocker; step 3, felodipine increased to 10 mg/day; step 4, dose of ACE inhibitor or β-blocker increased; and step 5, addition of low-dose alternative agent or HCTZ. All patients were randomized in double-blinded fashion to ASA, 75 mg/day, or placebo.

Results: At 2 years, target DBP was achieved in 85%, 67%, and 75%. Mean DBPs were closely grouped: 85.2, 83.2, and 81.1 mm Hg. Incidence of primary composite end point did not significantly differ between the three groups, but significantly fewer CV events and deaths were noted among diabetic patients assigned to a target DBP of ≥80 mm Hg compared with =90 mm Hg ($p = 0.005$; $p = 0.016$). No differences were found in BP between ASA- and placebo-treated patients. ASA use was associated with 15% fewer major events ($p = 0.03$), 36% reduction in fatal or nonfatal MI ($p = 0.002$), and similar rates of hemorrhagic and ischemic stroke.

Comments: Study was underpowered for two reasons: (a) actual mean DBPs were approximately 2 mm Hg apart instead of 5 mm Hg apart; and (b) only 724 major CV events occurred over a 3.8-year period versus projected 1,100 over a 2.5-year period.

130. **Hansson L,** et al. **STOP-HTN2.** Randomised trial of old and new antihypertensive drugs in elderly patients: cardiovascular mortality and morbidity in the Swedish Trial in Old Patients with Hypertension-2 study. *Lancet* 1999;354:1751–1756.

Design: Prospective, randomized, open (blinded end point evaluation), multicenter study. Primary end point was fatal stroke, fatal MI, or other fatal CV disease.

Purpose: To compare the effects of conventional and newer antihypertensive drugs on CV mortality and morbidity in elderly patients.

Population: 6,614 patients aged 70 to 84 years with HTN (SBP, 180 mm Hg or greater; DBP, 105 mm Hg or greater; or both).

Treatment: Conventional antihypertensive drugs (atenolol, 50 mg; metoprolol, 100 mg; pindolol, 5 mg; or HCTZ, 25 mg plus amiloride, 2.5 mg daily) or newer drugs (enalapril, 10 mg; or lisinopril, 10 mg; or felodipine, 2.5 mg; or isradipine, 2 to 5 mg daily).

Results: BP was decreased similarly in all treatment groups. No difference was found between the treatment groups in the primary combined end point of fatal stroke, fatal myocardial MI, and other fatal CV disease [19.8 events per 1,000 patient years (conventional drugs) vs. 19.8 per 1,000 (newer drugs)]. A similar incidence also was noted in the two treatment groups of fatal and nonfatal stroke, fatal and nonfatal MI, or other CV mortality.

131. The **ALLHAT** (Antihypertensive and Lipid-Lowering Treatment to Prevent Heart Attack Trial) Officers and Coordinators for the ALLHAT Collaborative Research Group. Major outcomes in high-risk hypertensive patients randomized to angiotensin-converting enzyme inhibitor or calcium channel blocker versus diuretic. *JAMA* 2002;288:2981–2997 (editorials, 3039–3044).

Design: Prospective, randomized, active-controlled, multicenter trial. Primary end point was fatal CHD or nonfatal MI. Secondary outcomes were all-cause mortality, stroke, combined CHD (primary outcome, coronary revascularization, or angina with hospitalization), and combined CVD (combined CHD, stroke, treated angina without hospitalization, HF, and PAD). Mean follow-up was 4.9 years.

Purpose: To determine whether treatment with a calcium-channel blocker or an ACE inhibitor lowers the incidence of CHD or other CVD events versus treatment with a diuretic.

Population: 33,357 participants aged 55 years or older with HTN and at least one other CHD risk factor.

Exclusion Criteria: Included history of hospitalized or treated symptomatic HF and/or known LVEF less than 35%.

Treatment: Chlorthalidone, 12.5 to 25 mg/day ($n = 15,255$); amlodipine, 2.5 to 10 mg/day ($n = 9,048$); or lisinopril, 10 to 40 mg/day ($n = 9,054$).

Results: No significant differences were found between the treatment groups in the incidence of fatal CHD or nonfatal MI (overall rate, 8.9%). Compared with chlorthalidone, the RRs for amlodipine and lisinopril were 0.98 (95% CI, 0.90 to 1.07) and 0.99 (95% CI, 0.91 to 1.08), respectively. All-cause mortality rates also were similar. SBP at 5 years was significantly lower with chlorthalidone compared with that in the amlodipine and lisinopril groups (–0.8 mm Hg, –2 mm Hg; $p < 0.001$), whereas DBP was significantly higher with chlorthalidone compared with amlodipine (0.8 mm Hg; $p < 0.001$). For amlodipine versus chlorthalidone, secondary outcomes were similar except for a higher 6-year rate of HF with amlodipine (10.2% vs. 7.7%; RR, 1.38; 95% CI, 1.25 to 1.52). For lisinopril versus chlorthalidone, lisinopril had higher 6-year rates of combined CVD (33.3% vs. 30.9%; RR, 1.10; 95% CI, 1.05 to 1.16); stroke (6.3% vs. 5.6%; RR, 1.15; 95% CI, 1.02 to 1.30); and HF (8.7% vs. 7.7%; RR, 1.19; 95% CI, 1.07 to 1.31). The fourth arm of the trial testing the α-blocker doxazosin was discontinued in January 2000 because of increased CV events and CHF hospitalizations for this agent compared with chlorthalidone (see *JAMA* 2000;283:1967).

Comments: The results from this very large trial suggest that in patients in which CV events are the greater risk, a thiazide-type diuretic is clearly the preferred first agent; however, in patients with kidney disease or with major risk for renal events, ACE inhibitors should be considered. The study results contradict those observed in HOPE, especially the stroke protection that was touted to be independent of BP. Major criticisms of the ALLHAT study include (a) results have limited relevance because most patients require combination therapy for adequate BP control; (b) results appear driven by the experience in black patients → smaller BP reduction in lisinopril group (blacks respond poorly to ACE inhibitors); (c) add-on therapy to ACE inhibitor should have been a diuretic or calcium-channel blocker, not a β-blocker.

132. **Wright JT,** et al. for the **ALLHAT** Collaborative Research Group. ALLHAT Findings revisited in the context of subsequent analyses, other trials, and meta-analyses. *Arch Intern Med* 2009;169(9):832–842.

The ALLHAT investigators recently re-evaluated their results in the context of contemporary trials and meta-analyses. Overall, they conclude that the original trial's conclusions persist—that neither α-blockers, calcium-channel antagonists, or ACE inhibitors are superior to thiazide-type diuretics for the initial management of HTN. However, they add that the new-onset diabetes associated with the diuretics did not lead to worse outcomes in the timeframe studied.

133. The **ONTARGET** investigators. Telmisartan, ramipril, or both in patients at high risk for vascular events. *N Engl J Med* 2008;358:1547–1559.

Design: Prospective, randomized, active-controlled, three-arm, multicenter trial. Primary end point was death from cardiovascular causes, MI, stroke, or heart failure hospitalization at median follow-up of 56 months.
Purpose: To help determine the role of ARBs versus or in addition to ACE inhibitors, in patients with diabetes or vascular disease without heart failure.
Population: 25,620 patients with vascular disease or high-risk diabetes, without heart failure, who remained following a run-in period.
Treatment: Ramipril 10 mg daily (ACE group), telmisartan 80 mg daily (ARB group), or both (combination group).
Results: In the ACE group, 16.5% of patients experienced a primary endpoint versus 16.7% in the ARB group, and 16.3% in the combination group. However, adverse events, including hypotension, syncope, and renal dysfunction, were all higher in the combination group. This study did not support the combination use of ACE inhibitors and ARBs in this patient population, as it did not compare favorably for clinical outcomes, and had a higher rate of adverse events.

Other Pharmacologic Agent Studies
134. **Parving HH,** et al. for the AVOID Study Investigators. Aliskiren combined with losartan in type 2 diabetes and nephropathy. *N Engl J Med* 2008;358:2433–2446.

Aliskiren, a novel direct renin inhibitor, was added to the ARB losartan in half of the 599 patients enrolled in this prospective, international, double-blind, randomized trial. The population included patients with HTN and type 2 diabetes with nephropathy, and the primary endpoint was reduction in albumin to creatinine ratio at 6 months. Patients receiving aliskiren did have lower albumin-to-creatinine ratios and it may provide a renoprotective effect. There was a mild, nonsignificant trend to lower SBP in the aliskiren group, and the adverse events were similar.

Diet Studies
135. **Appel LJ,** et al. for the Dietary Approaches to Stop Hypertension (**DASH**) Research Group. A clinical trial of the effects of dietary patterns on blood pressure. *N Engl J Med* 1997;336:1117–1124.

This prospective, randomized study was composed of 459 adults with SBP less than 160 mm Hg and DBP, 80 to 95 mm Hg. For 3 weeks, all participants were fed a control diet that was low in fruits, vegetables, and dairy products. They were then randomized to the control diet or a diet rich in fruits and vegetables or a combination diet rich in fruits, vegetables, and low-fat dairy products and with reduced saturated fat and total fat. Body weight and sodium intake were not modified. The combination diet resulted in significant reduction in SBP and DBP compared with the control diet (11.4 and 5.5 mm Hg, respectively; both $p < 0.001$).

136. **Whelton PK,** et al. Trial of Nonpharmacologic Interventions in the Elderly (**TONE**). Sodium reduction and weight loss in the treatment of hypertension in older persons. *JAMA* 1998;279:839–846.

Prospective, randomized study of 875 individuals aged 60 to 80 years with SBP less than 145 mm Hg and DBP less than 85 mm Hg on a single antihypertensive medication. Obese patients ($n = 585$) were randomized to reduced sodium intake (≥ 1 g/day), weight loss, both, or usual care, whereas nonobese patients ($n = 390$) received reduced sodium or usual care. After 3 months of intervention, discontinuation of the antihypertensive medication was attempted. At a median follow-up of 29 months, reduced sodium intake compared with no reduction in sodium intake was associated with a significant reduction in the incidence of CV events (MI, HF, bypass surgery, angioplasty), recurrent HTN, or reinitiation of antihypertensive therapy (relative HR, 0.69; 95% CI, 0.59 to 0.81; $p < 0.001$), a difference driven by lower rates of the latter two end-point components. Obese patients assigned to weight loss also had a lower incidence of the combined outcome measures compared with those not assigned to weight loss (relative HR, 0.70; 95% CI, 0.57 to 0.87; $p < 0.001$). Overall, weight loss (average, 3.5 kg), and sodium restriction resulted in an approximate 30% decrease in the need for antihypertensive medication.

137. **Sacks FM,** et al. for the **DASH** Sodium Collaborative Research Group. Effects on blood pressure of reduced dietary sodium and the dietary approaches to stop hypertension (DASH) diet. *N Engl J Med* 2001;344:3–10.

This prospective trial randomized 412 participants to a control diet typical of intake in the U.S. or the DASH diet (rich in vegetables, fruits, and low-fat dairy products). Within the assigned diet, participants ate foods with high, intermediate, and low levels of sodium for 30 consecutive days each, in random order. Decreasing sodium intake from the high to intermediate level reduced SBP by 2.1 mm Hg ($p < 0.001$) during the control diet and by 1.3 mm Hg ($p = 0.03$) during the DASH diet. Decreasing intake from the intermediate to low level resulted in further reductions of 4.6 mm Hg during control diet ($p < 0.001$) and 1.7 mm Hg during DASH diet ($p < 0.01$). The effects of sodium were seen in those with and without HTN, blacks, and women and men. The benefits of the DASH diet and low sodium intake were additive, with the largest SBP difference seen between those on the control diet with high sodium intake and DASH diet with low sodium (latter, 7.1 mm Hg lower in those without HTN, 11.5 mm Hg lower in hypertensives). In summary, the reduction of sodium intake to levels below the current recommendation of 100 mmol/day and the DASH diet both reduce BP substantially, with greater effects in combination.

138. **Mente A,** et al. A systematic review of the evidence supporting a causal link between dietary factors and coronary heart disease. *Arch Intern Med* 2009;169(7):659–669.

The authors compiled prospective cohort or randomized studies of dietary interventions and CHD outcomes, using Bradford Hill Criteria to assess causation. Overall, 507 cohort studies and 94 randomized trials were included, yielding strong evidence to support the associations of protective dietary factors (vegetables, nuts, "Mediterranean" patterns) and harmful dietary factors (*trans*-fatty acids, high glycemic-index foods). There was moderate evidence to suggest fish (omega-3 fatty acids), folate, whole grains, dietary vitamins E and C, beta carotene, alcohol, fruit, and fiber may be protective. When restricted to randomized trials, the Mediterranean dietary pattern was found to be protective. However, overall the review provides strong evidence for the role of diet in the incidence of coronary disease.

139. **The Look AHEAD Research Group.** Reduction in weight and cardiovascular disease risk factors in individuals with type 2 diabetes. *Diabetes Care* 2007;30:1374–1383.

In 5,145 patients with type 2 diabetes, the researches randomized half to an intensive lifestyle intervention (vs. usual care) in an effort to assess cardiovascular effects of weight loss. Those in the intervention group lost significantly more weight than controls (8.6% lost vs. 0.7%, $p < 0.001$), and additionally had significant improvements in CRFs, such as LDL, HbA1c (7.6 to 6.6% vs. 7.3% to 7.2%), BP, TGs, HDL cholesterol. All of these effects were observed and significant at only 1 year of follow-up.

Invasive Therapy

140. **van Jaarsveld BC,** et al. for **DRASTIC** (Dutch Renal Artery Stenosis Intervention Cooperative) Study Group. The effect of balloon angioplasty on hypertension in atherosclerotic renal-artery stenosis. *N Engl J Med* 2000;342:1007–1014.

This prospective, randomized study enrolled 106 hypertensive patients (DBP more than 95 despite at least two drugs) with atherosclerotic renal artery stenosis (50% or more stenosis) and a serum creatinine 2.3 mg/dL or less. Patients underwent percutaneous transluminal renal angioplasty (PTRA) or received drug therapy. BP, doses of antihypertensive drugs, and renal function were assessed at 3 and 12 months, and patency of the renal artery was assessed at 12 months. At 3 months, BPs were similar (169/99 mm Hg [PTRA] and 176/101 mm Hg). PTRA patients were taking fewer daily doses of medication compared with the drug-therapy group (2.1 vs. 3.2; $p < 0.001$). In drug group, 22 patients underwent PTRA after 3 months because of persistent HTN despite treatment with three or more drugs or worsening renal function. At 1 year, no significant differences were found between the groups in SBP and DBP, daily drug doses, or renal function.

141. **Kalra P**. The Impact of Renal Artery Revascularisation in Atherosclerotic Renovascular Disease: The Angioplasty and Stenting for Renal Artery Lesions (ASTRAL) Trial. Presented at the SCAI-ACC i2 Summit/American College of Cardiology Annual Scientific Session, Chicago, IL, March/April 2008.

To evaluate the utility of percutaneous renal artery stenting versus medical therapy in patients with significant renal artery stenosis, the investigators randomized 806 patients to stenting versus medical therapy alone. There was no significant benefit to stenting based on the endpoints of overall mortality, SBP, serum creatinine measurement, or overall vascular events over the mean follow-up period of 27 months.

Obesity and Weight

142. **Willett WC,** et al. Weight, weight change and coronary heart disease in women: risk within the normal weight range. *JAMA* 1995;273:461–465.

This prospective cohort study was composed of 115,818 nurses aged 30 to 55 years with no history of CAD. Even modest weight gains after 18 years were associated with increased risk (end point was CHD death and nonfatal MI): RR, 1.25 for 5- to 7.9-kg gain; RR, 1.64 for 8- to 10.9-kg gain; 2.65 for 11- to 19-kg gain.

143. **Rextrode KM,** et al. Abdominal adiposity and coronary heart disease in women. *JAMA* 1998;280:1843–1848.

This analysis of 8-year follow-up data of 44,702 NHS participants showed that a higher waist-to-hip ratio and greater waist circumference were associated with an increased risk of

CHD. If the waist-to-hip ratio was 0.88, the adjusted RR of CHD death or MI was 3.25 (vs. waist-to-hip ratio less than 0.72). A waist circumference of 38 inches was associated with an adjusted RR of CHD death and MI of 3.06. The independent predictive value of waist-to-hip ratio and waist circumference also was present in a subgroup with a BMI of ≥ 25 kg/m^2.

144. **Bender R,** et al. Effect of age on excess mortality in obesity. *JAMA* 1999;281:1498–1504.

This prospective cohort study was composed of 6,193 obese patients with a mean BMI of 36.6 kg/m^2 and mean age of 40.4 years. At follow-up (median, 14.8 years), standardized mortality ratios showed that obesity was associated with significantly increased mortality (men, 1.67; women, 1.45). This increased risk associated with obesity decreased with advancing age among both men (18 to 29 years, 2.46; 30 to 39 years, 2.30; 40 to 49 years, 1.99; 50 to 74 years, 1.31) and women (18 to 29 years, 1.81; 30 to 39 years, 2.10; 40 to 49 years, 1.70; 50 to 74 years, 1.26) (trend test, $p < 0.001$).

145. **Wilson PW,** et al. Overweight and obesity as determinants of cardiovascular risk: the Framingham experience. *Arch Intern Med* 2002;162:1867–1872.

This study examined Framingham Heart Study participants aged 35 to 75 years, who were monitored for up to 44 years. The primary outcome was new CVD, which included angina pectoris, MI, CVD, or stroke. Analyses compared overweight (BMI, 25.0 to 29.9) and obese persons (BMI, 30 or more) with a reference group of normal-weight persons (BMI, 18.5 to 24.9). Overweight status was associated with significantly increased risks of HTN (age-adjusted RR: men, 1.46; women, 1.75). New hypercholesterolemia and diabetes mellitus were less highly associated with excess adiposity. The age-adjusted RR (CI) for CVD was increased among those who were overweight [men, 1.21 (1.05 to 1.40); women, 1.20 (1.03 to 1.41)] and obese [men, 1.46 (1.20 to 1.77); women, 1.64 (1.37 to 1.98)].

146. **Flegal KM,** et al. Prevalence and trends in obesity among U.S. adults, 1999–2000. *JAMA* 2002;288:1723–1727.

Information was obtained from 4,115 adult men and women who participated in the NHANES. The age-adjusted prevalence of obesity was 30.5% in 1999 to 2000 compared with 22.9% in NHANES III (1988 to 1994; $p < 0.001$). The prevalence of overweight also increased during this period from 55.9% to 64.5% ($p < 0.001$). Extreme obesity (BMI, 40 or more) also increased significantly in the population, from 2.9% to 4.7% ($p = 0.002$). Racial/ethnic groups did not differ significantly in the prevalence of overweight or obesity for men. Among women, overweight and obesity prevalences were highest among non-Hispanic black women (more than 50% over age were obese).

147. **Fontaine KR,** et al. Years of life lost due to obesity. *JAMA* 2003;289:187–193.

This study examined data from U.S. Life Tables (1999), the Third National Health and Nutrition Examination Survey (NHANES III; 1988 to 1994), First National Health and Nutrition Epidemiologic Follow-up Study (NHANES I and II; 1971 to 1992), and NHANES II Mortality Study (1976 to 1992). Among whites, a U-shaped association was found between overweight or obesity and years of life lost (YLL). The optimal BMI (associated with the least YLL or greatest longevity) is 23 to 25 for whites and 23 to 30 for blacks. For any degree of overweight, younger adults typically had greater YLL than did older adults. The maximum YLL for white men aged 20 to 30 years with a severe level of obesity (BMI more than 45) is 13 and is 8 for white women. Among blacks older than 60 years, overweight and moderate obesity were not associated with an increased YLL; only severe obesity resulted in YLL. However, younger blacks with severe levels of obesity had a maximum YLL of 20 for men and 5 for women.

148. **Bibbins-Domingo K,** et al. Adolescent overweight and future adult coronary heart disease. *N Engl J Med* 2007;357(23):2371–2379.

On the basis of obesity rates in adolescents in 2000, the investigators estimated the prevalence of obese 35-year-olds in 2020, and the subsequent incidence of CHD based on models.

Carrying the expected shortcomings of such a study, the authors conclude there could be as many as 100,000 excess cases of coronary disease in 2035, attributable to the current epidemic of adolescent obesity.

Activity and Exercise

149. **Leon AS,** Connett J. Physical activity and 10.5 year mortality in the Multiple Risk Factor Intervention Trial (**MRFIT**). *Int J Epidemiol* 1991;20:690–697.

This analysis focused on 12,138 male MRFIT subjects who had leisure time physical activity (LTPA) assessed by the Minnesota questionnaire. The level of LTPA was inversely related to all-cause mortality, CHD mortality, and CV mortality because those in the lowest LTPA tertile had excess mortality rates of 15%, 27%, and 22%, respectively, compared with men in the middle tertile. No significant further attenuation of risk was seen with additional LTPA (tertile 3).

150. **Mittleman MA,** et al. Triggering of acute MI by heavy physical exertion. *N Engl J Med* 1993;329:1677–1683.

This analysis focused on interviews with 1,228 patients an average of 4 days after MI. Heavy exertion (≥6 metabolic equivalents) within 1 hour had occurred in 4.4%. The RR of acute MI in the 1 hour after exertion was 5.9; however, risk correlated with the frequency of exercise (less than once per week: RR, 107; 1 to 2 times: RR, 19.4; 3 to 4 times: RR, 8.6; at least 5 times: RR, 2.4).

151. **Willich SN,** et al. Physical exertion as a trigger of AMI. *N Engl J Med* 1993;329:1684–1690.

This analysis focused on interviews with 1,194 patients at 13 ± 6 days after MI. An increased risk of MI was associated with strenuous activity (≥6 metabolic equivalents; 7.1% of patients) at onset of acute MI (RR, 2.1). The RR also was 2.1 for activity within 1 hour; infrequent exercise (less than four times per week) was associated with an RR of 6.9 (vs. 1.3).

152. **Kushi LH,** et al. Physical activity and mortality in postmenopausal women. *JAMA* 1997;277:1287–1292.

This prospective cohort study of 40,417 postmenopausal Iowa women, aged 55 to 69 years at baseline (1986), assessed physical activity with a mailed questionnaire. After adjustment for confounders and excluding women with heart disease and those who died in the first 3 years of follow-up, women with regular physical activity had a lower risk of death during follow-up (mean, 7 years), compared with women who did not (RR, 0.77; 95% CI, 0.66 to 0.90). Increasing frequency of moderate activity was associated with reduced risk of death, and a similar pattern was seen for vigorous physical activity. Women with moderate activity but no vigorous activity also benefited; even moderate activity only once per week was associated with lower mortality (RR, 0.78; 95% CI, 0.64 to 0.96).

153. **Manson JE,** et al. A prospective study of walking as compared with vigorous exercise in the prevention of coronary heart disease in women. *N Engl J Med* 1999;341:650–658.

This prospective cohort study of 72,488 NHS participants found brisk walking, as assessed by a self-administered questionnaire, was associated with fewer coronary events. In multivariate analyses, women in the highest quintile group [≥3 hours/week at a brisk pace (=3 mph)], had an RR of 0.65 (95% CI, 0.47 to 0.91) compared with those who walked infrequently. Regular vigorous exercise (≥6 METs) was associated with similar risk reductions (30% to 40%).

154. **Tanasescu M,** et al. Exercise type and intensity in relation to coronary heart disease in men. *JAMA* 2002;288:1994–2000.

This cohort analysis examined the 44,452 U.S. men enrolled in the Health Professionals' Follow-up Study. At follow-up (average, 10.7 years), 1,700 new cases of CHD were found. Total physical activity, running, weight training, and rowing were each inversely associated with risk of CHD. The adjusted RRs of nonfatal MI or fatal CHD corresponding to quintiles of METs for total physical activity were 1.0, 0.90 (95% CI, 0.78 to 1.04), 0.87 (0.75 to 1.00), 0.83 (0.71 to 0.96), and 0.70 (0.59 to 0.82; $p < 0.001$ for trend). Men who ran for an hour or more per week had a 42% RR (RR, 0.58; 95% CI, 0.44 to 0.77) compared with men who did not run ($p < 0.001$ for trend). Weight training for 30 minutes or more per week was associated with a 23% risk reduction (RR, 0.77; 95% CI, 0.61 to 0.98; $p = 0.03$ for trend), whereas rowing for 1 hour or more per week was associated with an 18% risk reduction (RR, 0.82; 05% CI, 0.68 to 0.99). Average exercise intensity was associated with reduced CHD risk, independent of the total volume of physical activity: moderate (4 to 6 METs) and high (6 to 12 METs) activity intensities were associated with 6% and 17% RRRs compared with low activity intensity (less than 4 METs; $p = 0.02$ for trend).

155. **Lichtenstein AH,** et al. Diet and lifestyle recommendations revision 2006: a scientific statement from the American Heart Association Nutrition Committee. *Circulation* 2006;114:82–96.

The committee reviewed the most recent data on diet and lifestyle as they relate to CVD. Highlights of their recommendations include a balanced diet limiting intake of saturated fat, trans fat, and cholesterol. They stop short of recommending alcohol intake, but stress its use in moderation.

156. **Carnethon MR,** et al. Cardiorespiratory fitness in young adulthood and the development of cardiovascular disease risk factors. *JAMA* 2003;290:3092–3100.

As part of the Coronary Artery Risk Development in Young Adults (**CARDIA**) study, participants aged 18 to 30 years who had completed the treadmill examination in 1985 to 1986 were followed up in 2000 to 2001. A subset had repeated the test in 1992 to 1993. Investigators measured the incidence of type 2 diabetes, HTN, metabolic syndrome, and hypercholesterolemia, stratified by cardiorespiratory fitness. After first adjusting for age, race, sex, smoking, and family history of risk factors (diabetes, HTN, premature MI), participants in the lowest quintile of fitness were significantly more likely to develop diabetes, HTN, and metabolic syndrome when compared with those in the top three quintiles ($p < 0.001$). Statistically, body mass index partially accounted for such an effect. Interval increase in fitness did improve a participant's risk of developing such CRFs; however, this effect was mitigate when controlling for change in weight over the same period.

157. **Sigal RJ,** et al. Effects of aerobic training, resistance training, or both on glycemic control in type 2 diabetes. *Ann Intern Med* 2007;147:357–369.

The investigators compared various exercise techniques (aerobic training, resistance training, and combined training) in 251 adults with type 2 diabetes; for control a sedentary group was included. The primary endpoint of this randomized, controlled trial was HbA1c values at 6 months. They found that the maximum change in HbA1c occurred in patients participating in combined aerobic plus resistance training exercise programs; however, changes in other CRFs, such as BP and lipids, did not differ among groups.

158. **Manini TM,** et al. Daily activity energy expenditure and mortality among older adults. *JAMA* 2006;296:171–179.

Using radiolabeled water and indirect calorimetry, investigators measured the "free-living activity" energy expenditure in 302 highly functional, older adults (aged 70 to 82 years). After adjusting for age, sex, race, study site, weight, height, body fat percentage, and sleep duration, they found a significant and inverse relationship between free-living activity energy expenditure and risk of death over mean follow-up of 6.15 years. Thus, in this most-scientific method of assessing physical activity in older adults, increased activity was strongly associated with lower mortality.

Nonmodifiable Risk Factors

159. **Wei JY.** Age and the cardiovascular system. *N Engl J Med* 1992;327:1735–1739.

This review discusses the impact of age on the myocardium, vasculature, cardiac output, diastolic function, BP regulation, and effects of exercise training.

160. **Marenberg ME,** et al. Genetic susceptibility to death from coronary heart disease in a study of twins. *N Engl J Med* 1994;330:1041–1046.

This analysis is composed of data taken from 21,004 Swedish twins in 1961 and 1963; average follow-up was 26 years. Among men, RRs (of death secondary to CHD) if the twin died of CHD at younger than 55 years were 8.1 (monozygous) and 3.8 (dizygous). Among women, RRs were 15.0 and 2.6, respectively; overall, RRs decreased with increased age.

161. **Andresdottir MB,** et al. Fifteen percent of myocardial infarctions and coronary revascularizations explained by family history unrelated to conventional risk factors: the Reykjavik Cohort Study. *Eur Heart J* 2002;23:1655–1663.

This prospective cohort study examined 9,328 men and 10,062 women aged 33 to 81 years in the Reykjavik area, from 1967 to 1996. During follow-up (18 to 19 years), in 2,700 men and 1,070 women, CHD developed. After adjustment for other CRFs, the HR of CHD was highly significant, 1.66 (95% CI, 1.51 to 1.82) and 1.64 (95% CI, 1.43 to 1.89) for men and women, respectively. Family history of MI was attributed to 15.1% of all cases of CHD in men and 16.6% in women, independent of other known risk factors.

162. **Nabel E.** Genomic medicine: cardiovascular disease. *N Engl J Med* 2003;349:60–72.

The then director of the NHLBI reviews the known contributions of genetic factors to the pathogenesis of CVD. These include familial hypercholesterolemia syndromes, and the known genetic determinants of HTN, renal disease, and hemostatic balance.

Alcohol

163. **Camargo CA Jr.** Moderate alcohol consumption and risk for angina pectoris or MI in U.S. male physicians. *Ann Intern Med* 1997;126:372–375.

This prospective cohort study of 22,071 patients confirms the substantial body of data correlating moderate ethanol consumption with decreased CHD risk. One drink/day versus less than one drink/week confers an RR of angina of 0.69 (95% CI, 0.59 to 0.81) and an RR of MI of 0.65 (95% CI, 0.52 to 0.81).

164. **de Lorgeril M,** et al. Wine drinking and risks of cardiovascular complications after recent acute myocardial infarction. *Circulation* 2002;106:1465–1469.

This analysis examined 437 survivors of a recent MI who had at least two reliable assessments of drinking (and dietary) habits. Average ethanol intake was 7.6% of the total energy intake, of which wine ethanol represented 92%. At 4-year follow-up, 104 CV complications (23.8%) had occurred. In comparison with abstainers, the adjusted risk of complications was significantly reduced by 59% in patients whose average ethanol intake was 7.7% of the total energy intake (about 2 drinks/day), and by 52% in those whose average ethanol intake was of 16% of energy (about 4 drinks/day).

165. **Mukamal KJ,** et al. Roles of drinking pattern and type of alcohol consumed in coronary heart disease in men. *N Engl J Med* 2003;348:109–118.

This study assessed alcohol intake by questionnaires in 38,077 male health professionals free of CVD and cancer at baseline. At 12 years of follow-up, men who consumed alcohol 3 to 4 or 5 to 7 days per week had decreased risks of MI compared with those who had less than one drink per week [multivariate RR, 0.68 (95% CI, 0.55 to 0.84) and 0.63 (95% CI, 0.54 to 0.74), respectively]. No single type of beverage conferred additional benefit. A 12.5-g increase in daily alcohol consumption over a 4-year follow-up period was associated with an RR of MI of 0.78.

166. **Maraldi C,** et al. Impact of inflammation on the relationship among alcohol consumption, mortality, and cardiac events: the health, aging, and body composition study. *Arch Intern Med* 2006;166:1490–1497.

This analysis of 2,487 septuagenarians without baseline coronary disease or heart failure, assessed alcohol consumption and serum inflammatory makers (IL-6 and CRP) at mean follow-up of 5.6 years. Light to moderate alcohol intake did not affect inflammatory markers, but was associated with significantly less cardiac morbidity and mortality.

167. **Bryson CL,** et al. The association of alcohol consumption and incident heart failure: the Cardiovascular Health Study. *J Am Coll Cardiol* 2006;48:305–311.

This prospective cohort study of 5,888 subjects older than 65 years assessed risk of heart failure and concomitant alcohol intake over 7 to 10 years of follow-up. Mild or moderate alcohol intake (1 to 6 or 7 to 13 drinks per week, respectively), was associated with a lower risk of incident heart failure, when compared with those who abstained from alcohol altogether. This conclusion persisted despite control for incident MI and other factors.

Hormone Status and Hormonal Replacement

168. **Stampfer MJ,** et al. Postmenopausal estrogen therapy and cardiovascular disease. *N Engl J Med* 1991;325:756–762.

This prospective cohort study was composed of 48,470 postmenopausal women without prior CVD or cancer. After adjustment for risk factors, at an average follow-up of 7 years, estrogen patients had a significant 11% lower total mortality, 28% lower CV mortality, and 44% RRR in the incidence of major coronary disease. No significant difference was found in stroke rates.

169. **Grodstein F,** et al. Postmenopausal estrogen and progestin use and the risk of cardiovascular disease. *N Engl J Med* 1996;335:453–461.

This prospective cohort analysis focused on 59,337 NHS participants who were aged 30 to 55 years and free of known CVD at baseline. At an average follow-up of 11.2 years, combined estrogen and progestin users had a lower incidence of major CHD (MI, death) compared with nonhormone and estrogen-only users (adjusted RRs, 0.39 and 0.60). Thus the addition of progestin does not appear to attenuate the cardioprotective effects of postmenopausal estrogen therapy. No significant differences in stroke rates were found.

170. **Hulley S,** et al. Heart and Estrogen/Progestin Replacement Study (**HERS**). Randomized trial of estrogen and progestin for secondary prevention of coronary heart disease in postmenopausal women. *JAMA* 1998;280:605–613.

Design: Prospective, randomized, blinded, placebo-controlled, multicenter study. Average follow-up period was 4.1 years.
Purpose: To determine whether estrogen plus progestin alters the risk for CHD events in postmenopausal women with known coronary disease.
Population: 2,763 women younger than 80 years (mean age, 66.7 years).
Exclusion Criteria: CHD event in previous 6 months, sexual hormone use in previous 3 months, history of pulmonary embolism (PE), deep venous thrombosis (DVT), breast cancer, and endometrial cancer.

Treatment: Conjugated equine estrogens (0.625 mg once daily) and medroxyprogesterone (one tablet once daily) or placebo.

Results: Compliance rates were 82% at 1 year and 75% at 3 years. No difference in primary outcome (MI plus CV death; RH, 0.99) was observed. Lack of effect was observed despite the hormone group having 11% lower LDL and 10% higher HDL (each $p < 0.001$). The hormone group had more events in year 1 and fewer in years 4 and 5. The hormone group had more venous thromboembolism (RH, 2.89; 95% CI, 1.50 to 5.58) and gallbladder disease (RH, 1.38; 95% CI, 1.00 to 1.92).

171. **Barrett-Connor E,** et al. for the **MORE** Investigators (Multiple Outcomes of Raloxifene Evaluation). Raloxifene and cardiovascular events in osteoporotic postmenopausal women: four-year results from the MORE (Multiple Outcomes of Raloxifene Evaluation) randomized trial. *JAMA* 2002;287:847–857.

Design: Prospective, randomized, double-blind, placebo-controlled, multicenter trial. Primary end point was MI, unstable angina, coronary ischemia, and stroke or TIA.

Purpose: To determine the effect of raloxifene on CV events in osteoporotic postmenopausal women.

Population: 7,705 osteoporotic postmenopausal women (mean age, 67 years); osteoporosis documented by prior vertebral fracture or bone mineral density score (T score of less than −2.5).

Exclusion Criteria: Stroke or venous thromboembolic disease in prior 10 years.

Treatment: Raloxifene, 60 mg/day; raloxifene, 120 mg/day; or placebo, for 4 years.

Results: No significant differences were noted between the three treatment groups in coronary and cerebrovascular events (raloxifene, 60 mg/day: 3.2%; raloxifene, 120 mg/day: 3.7%; placebo, 3.7%). Among the 1,035 women with increased CV risk at baseline, those assigned to raloxifene (either dose) had a significantly lower risk of CV events compared with placebo (RR, 0.60; 95% CI, 0.38 to 0.95). The number of CV events during the first year was not significantly different in the overall cohort, or among women at increased CV risk ($p = 0.86$) or with evidence of established CHD ($p = 0.60$).

172. **Grady D,** et al. for the HERS Research Group. Cardiovascular disease outcomes during 6.8 years of hormone therapy: Heart and Estrogen/Progestin Replacement Study Follow-up (**HERS II**). *JAMA* 2002;288:49–57.

Design: Prospective, randomized, blinded, placebo-controlled, multicenter trial of 4.1 years' duration (HERS) and subsequent unblinded follow-up for 2.7 years (HERS II). Primary end point was nonfatal MI and CHD death.

Purpose: To determine if the risk reduction observed in the later years of HERS persisted and resulted in an overall reduced risk of CHD events with additional years of follow-up.

Population: 2,763 postmenopausal women with CHD and an average age of 67 years at enrollment in HERS; 2,321 women (93% of those surviving) consented to follow-up in HERS II.

Exclusion Criteria: Included age 80 years or older and prior hysterectomy.

Treatment: Conjugated estrogens, 0.625 mg/day, and medroxyprogesterone acetate, 2.5 mg/day, or placebo ($n = 1,383$) during HERS; in HERS II, open-label hormone therapy was prescribed at physicians' discretion; at least 80% adherence to hormones declined from 81% (year 1) to 45% (year 6) in the hormone group, and increased from none (year 1) to 8% (year 6) in the placebo group.

Results: No significant differences were found between the groups in primary CHD events or secondary CV events in HERS, HERS II, or overall. The unadjusted RH for CHD events in HERS was 0.99 (95% CI, 0.81 to 1.22); HERS II, 1.00 (95% CI, 0.77 to 1.29); and overall, 0.99 (0.84 to 1.17). The overall RHs remained similar after adjustment for potential confounders and differential use of statins between treatment groups (RH, 0.97), and in analyses restricted to women who were adherent to randomized treatment assignment (RH, 0.96). In an accompanying report (*JAMA* 2002;288:58–66), data were presented on thromboembolic events, biliary tract surgery, cancer, fracture, and total mortality. Hormone therapy was associated with an increased risk of venous thromboembolism (unadjusted intention-to-treat RH, 1.40; 95% CI, 0.64 to 3.05; vs. RH of 2.66 in HERS I); the RH was 2.08 overall for the 6.8 years (95% CI, 1.28 to 3.40). The overall RH for biliary tract surgery was 1.48 (95% CI, 1.12 to 1.95); for any cancer, 1.19 (95% CI, 0.95 to 1.50); and for any fracture, 1.04 (95% CI, 0.87 to 1.25). There were 261 deaths among those assigned to hormone therapy and 239 among those assigned to placebo (RH, 1.10; 95% CI, 0.92 to 1.31).

173. Writing Group for the **Women's Health Initiative** Investigators. Risks and benefits of estrogen plus progestin in healthy postmenopausal women: principal results from the Women's Health Initiative randomized controlled trial. *JAMA* 2002;288:321–333 (editorial, 366–368).

Design: Prospective, randomized, controlled, multicenter, primary prevention trial. Primary end point was CHD death and nonfatal MI. Primary adverse outcome was invasive breast cancer. A global index included the two primary outcomes plus stroke, PE, endometrial cancer, colorectal cancer, hip fracture, and death due to other causes.

Purpose: To assess the major health benefits and risks of the most commonly used combined hormone preparation in the United States.

Population: 16,608 postmenopausal women aged 50 to 79 years with an intact uterus.

Exclusion Criteria: Included prior breast cancer, other prior cancer in previous 10 years, low hematocrit or platelet counts.

Treatment: Equine estrogens, 0.625 mg/day plus medroxyprogesterone acetate, 2.5 mg/day, in one tablet, or placebo.

Results: The estrogen/progestin arm of the trial was terminated early (at 5.2 years follow-up vs. planned 8.5 years) because of excessive risk of global index in hormone group compared with placebo (HR, 1.15; 95% CI, 1.03 to 1.28). The hormone group also had a significantly higher incidence of CHD [HR, 1.29 (1.02 to 1.63)], breast cancer [HR, 1.26 (1.00 to 1.59)], stroke [HR, 1.41 (1.07 to 1.85)], and PE [HR, 2.13 (1.39 to 3.25)], whereas lower rates of colorectal cancer [HR, 0.63 (0.43 to 0.92)] and hip factures [HR, 0.66 (0.45 to 0.98)] occurred, and a trend toward lower rates of endometrial cancer [HR, 0.83 (0.47 to 1.47)]. All-cause mortality rates were similar [HR, 0.98 (0.82 to 1.18)].

Comments: Although mortality rates were similar, the overall risk–benefit profile in this trial is not consistent with the requirements for a clearly safe and efficacious intervention for primary prevention of chronic diseases. The estrogen-only arm was not stopped.

174. **Barret-Connor E,** et al. For the Raloxifene Use for The Heart (RUTH) Trial Investigators. Effects of raloxifene on cardiovascular events and breast cancer in postmenopausal women. *N Engl J Med* 2006;355:125–137.

Design: International, multicenter, randomized, double-blind, placebo-controlled trial. The two primary endpoints were coronary events (coronary death, MI, hospitalization for ACS) and invasive breast cancer at median follow-up of 5.6 years.

Purpose: To evaluate the effects of raloxifene, an estrogen-receptor modulator, on CHD and breast cancer.

Population: 10,101 postmenopausal women (average age 67.5 years) with CHD or multiple risk factors.

Treatment: Raloxifene 60 mg daily or placebo.

Results: There was a similar number of coronary events in each arm (HR 0.95, 95% CI 0.84 to 1.07) over the follow-up period. Invasive breast cancer occurred in significantly fewer women in the raloxifene arm (40 vs. 70 events, respectively, HR 0.56, 95% CI 0.38 to 0.83). This finding was mainly driven by a reduction in estrogen receptor–positive invasive cancers. Overall mortality was similar between the two groups, however there were significantly increased rates of venous thromboembolism (HR 1.44) and stroke (HR 1.49) in the raloxifene arm.

Comment: While raloxifene did not contribute to coronary events and improved breast cancer outcomes, these benefits should be weighed against the risk for thromboembolic and cerebrovascular events.

175. **ESPRIT.** (EStrogen in the Prevention of ReInfarction Trial). The ESPRIT Team. Oestrogen therapy for prevention of reinfarction in postmenopausal women. *Lancet* 2002;360:2001–2008.

Design: Prospective, randomized, double-blind, placebo-controlled, multicenter, secondary prevention trial. Primary outcomes were reinfarction or cardiac death and all-cause mortality.
Purpose: To ascertain whether unopposed estrogen reduces the risk of further cardiac events in postmenopausal women who survive a first MI.
Population: 1,017 postmenopausal women aged 50 to 69 years who had survived a first MI.
Exclusion Criteria: Included use of HRT or vaginal bleeding in previous year; history of breast, ovarian, or endometrial cancer; history of DVT or PE; severe renal disease; active or chronic liver disease.
Treatment: Estradiol valerate, 2 mg once daily; or placebo, for 2 years. Compliance was poor in both groups [at 2 years, 43% (estradiol) and 63%].
Results: At 2 years, the incidence of cardiac death or reinfarction was similar between the two groups (both 12.1). Similarly, there was no significant difference in all-cause mortality between the estrogen and placebo groups (rate ratio, 0.79; 95% CI, 0.50 to 1.27; $p = 0.34$).

176. **Shetty KD,** et al. Hormone replacement therapy and cardiovascular health in the United States. *Med Care* 2009;47:600–606.

Following observational data associating hormone replacement therapy with increased rates of CVD (see WHI in *JAMA* 2002;288:321–333), the authors examine epidemiologic data on the use of HRT and rates of MI and stroke. They found a significant decline in use of HRT following publication of the WHI, and a concomitant decrease in rates of MI among women. However, there was no effect on stroke.

C-Reactive Protein

177. **Ridker PM,** et al. Inflammation, aspirin, and the risk of cardiovascular disease in apparently healthy men. *N Engl J Med* 1997;336:973–979.

Case-control study of 543 PHS participants who had an MI, stroke, or venous thrombosis, and 543 participants who did not have a vascular event at a long-term follow-up (more than 8 years). Baseline CRP concentrations were significantly higher in men who subsequently had an MI (1.51 vs. 1.13 mg/L; $p < 0.001$) or ischemic stroke (1.38 vs. 1.13 mg/L; $p = 0.02$), but not venous thrombosis (1.26 vs. 1.13 mg/L; $p = 0.34$) than among men without vascular events. Men in the highest quartile of CRP values had, as compared with those in the lowest quartile, an approximately threefold and twofold higher risk of MI and stroke, respectively (RR, 2.9; $p < 0.001$; RR, 1.9; $p = 0.02$). The use of ASA was associated with a substantial (55.7%) reduction ($p = 0.02$) in MI among men in the highest CRP quartile, but only a nonsignificant (13.9%) reduction among those in the lowest quartile.

178. **Ridker PM,** et al. C-reactive protein adds to the predictive value of total and HDL cholesterol in determining risk of first myocardial infarction. *Circulation* 1998;97:2007–2011.

This case-control study of PHS participants analyzed levels of CRP, TC, and HDL in 245 subjects who subsequently developed a first MI and among 372 controls. At follow-up (average period, 9 years), multivariate models incorporating CRP and lipid parameters provided a better method of predicting risk than did models using lipids alone. For example, among those with high levels of both CRP and TC, the risk of MI was increased fivefold ($p = 0.0001$) compared with more modest risk elevations with isolated elevations of CRP (RR, 1.5) or TC (RR, 2.3). CRP levels were predictive of risk for those with low as well as high levels of TC and TC/HDL.

179. **Ridker PM,** et al. Inflammation, pravastatin and the risk of coronary events after MI in patients with average cholesterol levels. *Circulation* 1998;98:839–844.

This nested case-control study was composed of 391 CARE patients with MI or cardiovascular death and 391 age- and sex-matched controls. Cases had higher CRP ($p = 0.05$) and serum amyloid A (0.006) levels; the highest quintiles had a significantly higher risk of recurrent events [RRs, 1.77 ($p = 0.02$), 1.74 ($p = 0.02$)]. The greatest risk was seen in placebo patients with elevated CRP and serum amyloid A (RR, 2.81; $p = 0.007$). Overall, the risk association between inflammation and risk was attenuated and nonsignificant in pravastatin patients [RR, 1.29 ($p = 0.5$) vs. RR, 2.11 ($p = 0.048$) in placebo patients].

180. **Koenig W,** et al. C-reactive protein, a sensitive marker of inflammation, predicts future risk of coronary heart disease in initially healthy middle-aged men. *Circulation* 1999;99:237–242.

This analysis focused on 936 men enrolled in MONICA (Monitoring Trends and Determinants in Cardiovascular Disease), a general population cohort study. At 8-year follow-up, the HR ratio of CHD events associated with a one standard deviation increase in the CRP level was 1.67 (95% CI, 1.29 to 2.17), and after adjustment for age and smoking, 1.50 (95% CI, 1.14 to 1.97).

181. **Albert MA,** et al. Effect of statin therapy on C-reactive protein levels: the Pravastatin Inflammation/CRP Evaluation (**PRINCE**): a randomized trial and cohort study. *JAMA* 2001;286:64–70.

Design: Prospective, randomized, placebo-controlled, partially double-blind, partially open, multicenter trial. Primary end point: change in high-sensitivity CRP (hsCRP) at 24 weeks.
Purpose: To determine the anti-inflammatory effects of pravastatin as measured by CRP reduction.
Population: 2,884 total patients: 1,702 individuals without CVD and an open-labeled study in 1,182 patients with known CVD off statins for at least 12 weeks.
Treatment: Primary prevention group received pravastatin, 40 mg once daily, or placebo. All patients in secondary prevention received pravastatin.
Results: In the primary prevention cohort, pravastatin reduced hsCRP by 16.9% (decrease of 0.02 mg) compared with no change with placebo. This effect was evident as early as 12 weeks and seen in all subgroups independent of other variables including gender, baseline, or on-treatment lipid levels, diabetes, and use of ASA and HRT. In the open-labeled CVD cohort, a similar 14.3% reduction in hsCRP was seen.

182. **Ridker PM,** et al. for Air Force/Texas Coronary Atherosclerosis Prevention Study Investigators. Measurement of C-reactive protein for the targeting of statin therapy in the primary prevention of acute coronary events. *N Engl J Med* 2001;344:1959–1965.

CRP was measured at baseline and 1 year in 5,742 AFCAPS/TexCAPS participants. At 5 years, higher baseline CRP levels were associated with higher coronary event rates. Lovastatin therapy reduced CRP levels by 14.8% ($p < 0.001$), an effect not explained by lovastatin-induced changes in the lipid profile. In particular, lovastatin was effective among those with a ratio of total-to-HDL cholesterol (TC/HDL) that was lower than the median and a CRP higher than the median ($p = 0.02$). In contrast, lovastatin was ineffective in those with TC/HDL cholesterol and a CRP level that were both lower than the median.

183. **Pradhan AD,** et al. Inflammatory biomarkers, hormone replacement therapy, and incident coronary heart disease: prospective analysis from the Women's Health Initiative observational study. *JAMA* 2002;288:980–987.

This prospective, nested case-control study of postmenopausal women examined the 304 cases in which CHD developed during the Women's Health Initiative; 304 controls were matched by age, smoking status, ethnicity, and follow-up time (median, 2.9 years). Cases had significantly higher median baseline levels of CRP and IL-6 compared with controls (0.33 vs.

0.25 mg/dL; $p < 0.001$; 1.81 vs. 1.47 pg/mL; $p < 0.001$). In matched analyses, the OR for incident CHD in the highest versus lowest quartile was 2.3 for CRP (95% CI, 1.4 to 3.7; p trend $= 0.002$) and 3.3 for IL-6 (95% CI, 2.0 to 5.5; p trend < 0.001). After additional adjustment for lipid and nonlipid risk factors, both inflammatory markers were significantly associated with a twofold increase in odds for CHD events. Current use of HRT was associated with elevated median CRP levels (no association with IL-6). In analyses comparing individuals with similar baseline levels of either CRP or IL-6, those taking or not taking HRT had similar CHD ORs. Thus use or nonuse of HRT had less importance as a predictor of cardiovascular risk than did baseline levels of either CRP or IL-6.

184. **Ridker PM,** et al. Comparison of C-reactive protein and low-density lipoprotein cholesterol levels in the prediction of first cardiovascular events. *N Engl J Med* 2002;347: 1557–1565.

This study measured baseline LDL-C and CRP in 27,939 WHS participants. At a mean follow-up of 8 years, both measures had a strong linear relation with the incidence of CV events, although the two were minimally correlated ($r = 0.08$). After adjustment for age, smoking status, diabetes, BP, use or nonuse of HRT, the RRs of first cardiovascular events (MI, ischemic stroke, coronary revascularization, or cardiovascular death) according to increasing quintiles of CRP, as compared with the women in the lowest quintile, were 1.4, 1.6, 2.0, and 2.3 ($p < 0.001$). Corresponding RRs in increasing quintiles of LDL-C, as compared with the lowest, were 0.9, 1.1, 1.3, and 1.5 ($p < 0.001$). Similar effects were observed in separate analyses of each component of the composite end point. Overall, 46% of major events occurred among those with LDL less than 130 mg/dL. Importantly, because CRP and LDL-C measurements tended to identify different high-risk groups, screening for both biologic markers provided better prognostic information than did screening for either alone.

185. **Mueller C,** et al. Inflammation and long-term mortality after non–ST elevation acute coronary syndrome treated with a very early invasive strategy in 1042 consecutive patients. *Circulation* 2002;105:1412–1415.

Prospective cohort study of 1,042 patients undergoing coronary angiography and subsequent culprit artery stenting within 24 hours. CRP levels were determined on admission. In-hospital mortality was significantly higher in patients with a CRP greater than 10 mg/L (3.7% vs. 1.2% with CRP less than 3 mg/L and vs. 0.8% with CRP of 3 to 10 mg/L; RR, 4.2 for more than 10 mg/L vs. CRP of 10 mg/L or less; $p = 0.004$). At follow-up (mean, 20 months), mortality was 3.4% with CRP less than 3 mg/L, 4.4% with CRP between 3 and 10 mg/L, and 12.7% with CRP more than 10 mg/L (RR, 3.8 for CRP more than 10 mg/L vs. CRP of 10 mg/L or less). In a multivariate analysis, CRP remained an independent predictor of long-term mortality.

186. **Ray KK,** et al. for the PROVE IT-TIMI 22 Investigators. Relationship between uncontrolled risk factors and C-reactive protein levels in patients receiving standard or intensive statin therapy for acute coronary syndromes in the PROVE IT-TIMI 22 trial. *J Am Coll Cardiol* 2005;46:1417–1424.

This additional analysis of the PROVE IT-TIMI 22 trial demonstrated that intensive statin therapy lead to lower CRP levels, independent of other risk factors. Furthermore, CRP level correlated significantly with a number of other, some modifiable, clinical risk factors such as age, gender, BMI, smoking, LDL-C, glucose, HDL-C, and TGs. This suggests that, in addition to pharmacotherapy, other means of reducing CRP, such as lifestyle intervention, may be appropriate in the secondary prevention of CHD.

187. **Tsimikas S,** et al. C-Reactive protein and other emerging blood biomarkers to optimize risk stratification of vulnerable patients. *J Am Coll Cardiol* 2006;47:C19–C31.

The authors review the role of CRP, and other up-and-coming biomarkers, in the global risk assessment and stratification of patients at risk for coronary disease. They provide insight in to the role of these biomarkers, and how they could come to help obviate unnecessary invasive testing, and identify patients who warrant the most aggressive interventions.

188. **Zacho J,** et al. Genetically elevated C-reactive protein and ischemic vascular disease. *N Engl J Med* 2008;359:1897–1908.

In subgroups of two observational cohorts, the authors compared the DNA polymorphisms of 2,238 patients with IHD with 4,474 controls and 612 patients with ischemic cerebrovascular disease with 1,224 controls. They identified four polymorphisms that were significantly linked with elevated CRP levels. However, while elevated CRP in the general population was predictive of ischemic events, patients with such polymorphisms were not at significantly increased risk of events. The authors conclude that these data demonstrate that CRP does not play a *causal* role in ischemic atherosclerotic disease.

189. **The Emerging Risk Factors Collaboration.** C-reactive protein concentration and risk of coronary heart disease, stroke, and mortality: an individual participant meta-analysis. *Lancet* 2010;375:132–140.

In a meta-analysis of 54 prospective studies with 160,309 participants without vascular disease, the investigators measured CRP and assessed risk for CVDs. After controlling for variation in risk factors among participants, CRP proved significantly predictive of CAD, ischemic, stroke, cardiovascular mortality, and death, as well as lung disease and several cancers. The predictive effect of CRP for CVD was significantly altered by conventional risk factors. These data support the idea of CRP as a marker of underlying inflammation of unclear pathophysiology, representing elevated risk for such disease processes.

Other

HOMOCYSTEINE

Meta-analysis

190. **Homocysteine Studies Collaboration.** Homocysteine and risk of ischemic heart disease and stroke: a meta-analysis. *JAMA* 2002;288:2015–2022.

This meta-analysis included data from 30 prospective or retrospective studies involving a total of 5,073 IHD events and 1,113 stroke events. Allowances were made for differences between studies, for confounding by known CRFs, and for regression dilution bias. Stronger associations were observed in retrospective studies of homocysteine measured in blood collected after the onset of disease than in prospective studies among individuals who had no history of CVD when blood was collected. After adjustment for CRFs in the prospective studies, a 25% lower than usual homocysteine level [about 3 mM (0.41 mg/L)] was associated with an 11% lower IHD risk (OR, 0.89; 95% CI, 0.83 to 0.96) and 19% lower stroke risk (OR, 0.81; 95% CI, 0.69 to 0.95).

Studies

191. **Nygard O,** et al. Total plasma homocysteine and cardiovascular risk profile. *JAMA* 1995;274:1526–1533.

This analysis focused on 16,176 patients aged 40 to 67 years without prior HTN, diabetes, CHD, or CVD. Homocysteine levels were higher in men and increased with age (age 40 to 42 years, 10.8 μM; age 65 to 67 years, 12.2 μM). A strong positive correlation was found, especially among women, with the number of cigarettes smoked per day (0 cigarettes, 1.5; $\geq$20 cigarettes, 11.7), TC (<155 mg/dL, 10.3; $\geq$310 mg/dL, 11.2), DBP (higher than 70 mm Hg, 10.3; higher than 100 mm Hg, 11.2), and heart rate (fewer than 60 beats/min, 10.4; more than 100 beats/min, 11.6). An inverse relation to physical activity was observed (none, 11.1; heavy, 10.4). The precise threshold for increased risk is still unclear.

192. **Morrison HI,** et al. Serum folate and the risk of fatal coronary heart disease. JAMA 1996;275:1893–1896.

This retrospective study of 5,056 patients showed that 15-year CHD mortality was correlated with serum folate levels (more than 6 ng/mL vs. less than 3 ng/mL meant a 69% increased risk). An accompanying editorial stresses the need for randomized trials to study whether folate (diet or supplements) would decrease CVD.

193. **Jacques PF,** et al. The effect of folic acid fortification on plasma folate and total homocysteine concentrations. *N Engl J Med* 1999;340:1449–1454.

This study analyzed blood samples of Framingham Offspring Study participants taken from January 1991 to December 1994 and compared them with subsequent samples obtained before fortification of enriched grain with folic acid (January 1995 to September 1996; control group) and after fortification was implemented (September 1997 to March 1998; study group). Among study-group subjects who did not use vitamin supplements, mean folate concentrations more than doubled from the baseline to follow-up visit (4.6 to 10.0 ng/mL; $p < 0.001$), and the prevalence of low folate levels (<3 ng/mL) markedly decreased from 22.0% to 1.7% ($p < 0.001$). The mean total homocysteine concentration decreased from 10.1 to 9.4 μM, and the prevalence of high homocysteine levels (more than 13 μM) decreased from 18.7% to 9.8% ($p < 0.001$). No significant changes were noted in folate or homocysteine concentrations in control group subjects.

194. **Bønaa KH.** For the **NORVIT** Trial Investigators. Homocysteine lowering and cardiovascular events after acute myocardial infarction. *N Engl J Med* 2006;354:1578–1588.

In 3,749 patients with recent acute MI, treatment with a randomized and variety of B vitamins (or placebo) lowered homocysteine levels, but had no effect on recurrent events (MI, stroke, or sudden CAD death).

195. **The Heart Outcomes Prevention Evaluation (HOPE) 2 Investigators**. Homocysteine lowering with folic acid and B vitamins in vascular disease. *N Engl J Med* 2006;354:1567–1577. [Epub 2006 Mar 12].

5,522 patients with CVD or diabetes were randomized to combination folate, vitamin B_6, vitamin B_{12}, or placebo. Over an average follow-up of 5 years, there was no significant effect of supplementation on the primary endpoint of cardiovascular death, MI, or stroke.

196. **Jamison RL.** Effect of Homocysteine lowering on mortality and vascular disease in advanced chronic kidney disease and end-stage renal disease a randomized controlled trial. *JAMA* 2007;298(10):1163–1170.

In 2,056 veterans with advanced chronic kidney disease and elevated homocysteine levels, researchers randomized each to either combination folate, vitamin B_6, vitamin B_{12}, or placebo. Despite homocysteine lowering, there was no difference in all-cause mortality at 3 months, or any of the additional secondary endpoints.

197. **Ebbing M,** et al. for the **WENBIT** Trial. Mortality and cardiovascular events in patients treated with homocysteine-lowering B vitamins after coronary angiography: a randomized controlled trial. *JAMA* 2008;300(7):795–804.

In patients undergoing coronary angiography (acutely or electively), 3,096 were randomized to combinations of folate, B_{12}, B_6, or placebo (in a factorial design), for the prevention of death, MI, UA, or stroke. No combination of the above vitamins or folate provided reduction in the primary endpoint.

198. **Bostom AG,** et al. Nonfasting plasma total homocysteine levels and all-cause and cardiovascular disease mortality in elderly Framingham men and women. *Arch Intern Med* 1999;159:1077–1080.

   Nonfasting plasma homocysteine levels were obtained in 1933 Framingham Study participants between 1979 and 1982; mean age was 70 years. At follow-up (median, 10.0 years), proportional hazards modeling showed that homocysteine levels in the upper quartile ($\geq$14.26 μM) compared with levels in the lower three quartiles were associated with RRs of all-cause and CV mortality of 2.18 and 2.17, respectively (95% CIs, 1.86 to 2.56 and 1.68 to 2.82). These RR estimates remained significant [1.54 (95% CI, 1.31 to 1.82), 1.52 (1.16 to 1.98)] after adjustment for age, sex, SBP, diabetes, smoking, TC, and HDL.

199. **Folsom AR,** et al. Atherosclerosis Risk in Communities (**ARIC**). Prospective study of coronary heart disease incidence in relation to fasting total homocysteine, related genetic polymorphisms, and B vitamins. *Circulation* 1998;98:204–210.

   This prospective analysis focused on 15,792 ARIC participants aged 45 to 64 years (at enrollment); average follow-up period was 3.3 years. Total plasma homocysteine (tHcy) was associated with increased age- and race-adjusted CHD incidence in women ($p < 0.05$) but not men. CHD was associated negatively with plasma pyridoxal 5-phosphate and, in women only, plasma folate and vitamin supplementation. After adjusting for other risk factors, only plasma pyridoxal 5-phosphate was associated with CHD incidence [RR of highest vs. lowest quintile, 0.28 (95% CI, 0.1 to 0.7)]. The C677T mutation of the methylenetetrahydrofolate reductase gene and three mutations of cystathionine B-synthase gene were not associated with CHD incidence.

200. **Nurk E,** et al. Plasma total homocysteine and hospitalizations for cardiovascular disease: the Hordaland Homocysteine Study. *Arch Intern Med* 2002;162:1374–1381.

   This prospective cohort study of 17,361 individuals aged 40 to 42 or 65 to 67 years was conducted from April 1992 to May 1998 (mean follow-up, 5.3 years) in western Norway. At baseline, those with preexisting CVD had higher mean tHcy values than did individuals without CVD. Risk of CVD hospitalizations increased significantly with increasing baseline tHcy only in the oldest age group. In this group, multiple risk factor–adjusted hospitalization rate ratios in 5-tHcy categories (less than 9, 9 to 11.9, 12 to 14.9, 15 to 19.9, and 20 mM or greater) were as follows: 1.00 (reference level), 1.00, 1.34, 1.67, and 1.94, respectively (p trend <0.001). The relation between tHcy level and CVD hospitalizations was significantly stronger among individuals with preexisting CVD than in those without (hospitalization rate ratio per 5-mM increment, 1.29 vs. 1.10; p for interaction, 0.02).

201. **Ridker PM,** et al. for Air Force/Texas Coronary Atherosclerosis Prevention Study (AFCAPS/TexCAPS) Investigators. Plasma homocysteine concentration, statin therapy, and the risk of first acute coronary events. *Circulation* 2002;105:1776–1779.

   A total of 5,569 AFCAPS/TexCAPS participants had homocysteine measured at baseline and 1 year. Median baseline homocysteine levels were significantly higher in those with subsequent acute coronary events [ACEs; 12.1 vs. 10.9 mM (no ACE); $p < 0.001$]. The RRs of future events from lowest to highest quartile of homocysteine were 1.0, 1.6, 1.6, and 2.2 ($p < 0.001$). This increased risk was only modestly attenuated after adjustment for other traditional risk factors. The subgroup of participants with elevated LDL-C and elevated homocysteine levels were at high risk and benefited significantly from lovastatin therapy (RR, 0.46; 95% CI, 0.29 to 0.75). However, in contrast to findings in this trial for CRP, homocysteine levels did not help to define low-LDL subgroups with different responses to lovastatin therapy.

202. **Ebbing M,** et al. Mortality and cardiovascular events in patients treated with homocysteine-lowering B vitamins after coronary angiography: a randomized controlled trial. *JAMA* 2008;300(7):795–804.

Design: Prospective, randomized, double-blind controlled trial, with a primary composite endpoint of all-cause mortality, nonfatal MI, hospitalization or unstable angina, or nonfatal thromboembolic stroke.

Purpose: To determine the effect of various homocysteine-lower therapies on clinical cardio-vascular outcomes following coronary angiography.

Population: 3,096 adults, mean age of 62 years, undergoing coronary angiography.

Treatment: A 2 × 2 factorial design to compare three interventions with placebo: folic acid plus vitamin B_{12} and vitamin B_6, folic acid plus vitamin B_{12}, or vitamin B_6 alone.

Results: The vast majority of patients in this trial had significant CAD (84% with stable angina, 60% with double- or triple-vessel disease, 15% with ACS). Mean serum homocysteine levels were reduced by 30% at 1 year in the groups receiving folic acid and vitamin B_{12}. However, the trial was terminated early out of concern for potential harm of one of the interventions, based on data form another trial. Over the median 38 months of follow-up, there were no significant differences in clinical outcomes (either all-cause mortality or cardiovascular outcomes), for patients in any of the intervention or placebo groups.

LIPOPROTEIN-ASSOCIATED PHOSPHOLIPASE A_2 (LP-PLA$_2$)

203. **O'Donoghue M,** et al. Lipoprotein-associated phospholipase A2 and its association with cardiovascular outcomes in patients with acute coronary syndromes in the PROVE IT-TIMI 22 (PRavastatin Or atorVastatin Evaluation and Infection Therapy—Thrombolysis In Myocardial Infarction) trial. *Circulation* 2006;113:1745–1752.

The investigators measured levels of Lp-PLA$_2$ in patients in the PROVE IT-TIMI 22 trial immediately following ACS, and again at 30 days. While levels in the setting of ACS were not useful in predicting clinical outcomes, elevation of Lp-PLA2 at 30 days following ACS was found to be associated with a higher risk of clinical cardiovascular events, independent of LDL-C or CRP.

204. **Mohler ER,** et al. for the **Darapladib** Investigators. The effect of darapladib on plasma lipoprotein-associated phospholipase A2 activity and cardiovascular biomarkers in patients with stable coronary heart disease or coronary heart disease risk equivalent: the results of a multicenter, randomized, double-blind, placebo-controlled study. *J Am Coll Cardiol* 2008;51:1632–1641.

Darapladib is a selective inhibitor of Lp-PLA$_2$; the investigators sought to measure its effect on other biomarkers of cardiovascular risk in 959 patients with CVD or its risk equivalents. All patients were already receiving atorvastatin. Darapladib at doses of 40, 80, and 160 mg daily inhibited Lp-PLA$_2$ activity in a dose–response fashion ($p < 0.001$); at the highest dose of 160 mg, darapladib significantly decreased interleukin-6 and hsCRP at 12 weeks. No clinical adverse effects or detrimental platelet function effects were detected during the brief study—this suggests therapy with darapladib as an inhibitor of Lp-PLA$_2$ may be beneficial in reducing the inflammation associated with CVD. Studies powered to detect differences in clinical events, as well as rare adverse effects, are needed.

205. **Herrmann J,** et al. Expression of lipoprotein-associated phospholipase A_2 in carotid artery plaques predicts long-term cardiac outcome. *Eur Heart J* 2009;30:2930–2938.

The authors sought to assess the significance of the local expression of Lp-PLA$_2$ in carotid artery plaques by quantify its expression in 162 patients undergoing elective carotid endarterectomy. Over a period of 48 months, they followed patients for cardiovascular death or MI and found, in addition to Lp-PLA$_2$ expression, the only other predictor of events was smoking; no other traditional risk factors yielded significant results in the Cox proportional hazard analysis. The authors offer the study as evidence of atherosclerosis as a systemic disease with local manifestations.

INFECTION

206. **Danesh J,** et al. *Chlamydia pneumoniae* IgG titres and coronary heart disease: prospective study and meta-analysis. *BMJ* 2000;321:208–213.

This nested case-control analysis (496 cases, 989 controls) found that the OR for CHD among those in the top third of *C. pneumoniae* IgG titers was 1.66 (95% CI, 1.25 to 2.21), but this decreased to 1.22 (0.82 to 1.82) after adjustment for smoking and indicators of socioeconomic status. A meta-analysis of these results with those of 14 other prospective studies of *C. pneumoniae* IgG titers, which included 3,169 cases, yielded a combined OR of 1.15 (95% CI, 0.97 to 1.36), with no significant heterogeneity among the separate studies.

207. **O'Connor CM,** et al. for the Investigators in the **WIZARD** (Weekly Intervention with Zithromax for Atherosclerosis and its Related Disorders) Study. *JAMA* 2003;290:1459–1466.

This prospective, randomized, placebo-controlled multicenter trial enrolled 7,747 post-MI patients with elevated *C. pneumoniae* titers. Patients received azithromycin (600 mg daily for the first 3 days, and then 600 mg/week for 11 weeks), or placebo. At 2-year follow-up, no significant difference was found between the two groups in the primary composite end point of all-cause mortality, recurrent MI, revascularization, and hospitalization for angina (7% reduction in azithromycin group; HR, 0.93; $p = 0.23$).

208. **Cannon CP,** et al. for the Pravastatin or Atorvastatin Evaluation and Infection Therapy—Thrombolysis in Myocardial Infarction 22 Investigators. Antibiotic treatment of *Chlamydia pneumoniae* after acute coronary syndrome. *N Engl J Med* 2005;352:1646–1654.

In the antibiotic arm of the PROVE IT-TIMI 22 trial, the 4,162 patients enrolled during hospitalization for ACS were randomized to treatment with gatifloxacin (a bactericidal antibiotic with known efficacy against *C. pneumoniae*), or placebo, in a randomized, double-blinded fashion. Subjects received therapy for an initial 2-week course beginning 2 weeks after randomization, then a 10-day course every month over the duration of the trial (a mean of 2 years). The primary endpoint was a composite of all-cause mortality, MI, hospitalization for unstable angina, revascularization, or stroke. There were no significant differences between the groups in this primary endpoint, or several secondary endpoints, over the follow-up period. This provided the most convincing data to date that, despite evidence suggesting a causal link, antibiotic therapy against *C. pneumoniae* is not an effective strategy to reduce CVDs.

209. **Grayston JT,** et al. ACES Investigators. Azithromycin for the secondary prevention of coronary events. *N Engl J Med* 2005;352(16):1637–1645.

In 4,012 patients with stable CAD, the investigators randomized them to 600 mg azithromycin weekly, or placebo, for 1 year. Over follow-up period of a mean of 3.9 years, there was no significant difference in the composite rate of CAD death, MI, coronary revascularization, or UA hospitalization between the azithromycin group (446 events) compared with placebo (449 events).

GENETICS AND MISCELLANEOUS

210. **Marenberg ME,** et al. Genetic susceptibility to death from coronary heart disease in a study of twins. *N Engl J Med* 1994;330:1041–1046.

This analysis focused on 21,004 Swedish twins, with 26-year follow-up data. The RRs of death due to CHD if one twin died of CHD at younger than 55 years were 8.1 (monozygous) and 3.8 (dizygous). For women, the RRs were 15.0 and 2.6. Overall, the RRs decreased with increasing age.

211. **Samani NJ,** et al. A meta-analysis of the association of the deletion allele of the ACE gene with MI. *Circulation* 1996;94:708–712.

This analysis focused on 15 studies with 3,394 MI cases and 5,479 controls. The incidence of genotypes was as follows: II, 22.7%; ID, 49%; and DD, 28.3%. The risk of MI was higher in the DD group versus the ID and II groups combined (OR, 1.26; $p < 0.001$). Pairwise ORs were 1.36 for DD and II, 124 for DD and ID, and 1.09 for ID and II ($p =$ NS).

212. **Ridker PM,** et al. PlA1/A2 polymorphism of platelet glycoprotein IIIa and risks of myocardial infarction, stroke, and venous thrombosis. *Lancet* 1997;349:385–388.

This nested case-control study of PHS participants showed no significant association between the PL allele and CVD. The 704 cases consisted of 374 men with a first MI, 209 with strokes, and 121 with venous thrombosis, as well as 704 matched controls. Mean follow-up was 8.6 years. The frequency of the PL allele was similar between cases (MI, 13.5%; stroke, 13.4%; venous thrombosis, 14.5%) and controls (14.8%).

213. **Laule M,** et al. A1/A2 polymorphism of glycoprotein IIIa and association with excess procedural risk for coronary catheter interventions. *Lancet* 1999;353:708–712 (commentary, 687–688).

This study was composed of 1,000 consecutive patients with CAD (by angiography) and 1,000 age- and sex-matched controls; 653 case patients underwent interventions (angioplasty, $n = 271$; stenting, $n = 280$; directional atherectomy, $n = 102$). No evidence was noted that the A2 allele was associated with an excess procedural risk, as assessed by a 30-day composite of death plus MI plus target vessel revascularization (RR, 1.36; $p = 0.37$). No association was found between the allele and the presence of CAD (OR, 0.99). Although these results contrast with the positive results seen in the smaller studies, they confirm those obtained from the larger PHS and the ECTIM group.

214. **Di Castelnuovo A,** et al. Platelet glycoprotein receptor IIIa polymorphism PLA1/PLA2 and coronary risk: a meta-analysis. *Thromb Haemost* 2001;85:626–633.

A total of 34 studies for CAD and six for restenosis after revascularization were identified, with a total of 9,095 cases and 12,508 controls. The overall OR of CAD for carriers of the PLA2 allele was 1.10 (95% CI, 1.03 to 1.18), suggesting a significant but weak association of this polymorphism with CAD.

215. **Humphries SE,** et al. Genetic testing for cardiovascular disease susceptibility: a useful clinical management tool or possible misinformation? *Arterioscler Thromb Vasc Biol* 2004;24:628–636.

Despite the availability of genetic tests to the general public for the advertised purpose of assessing their cardiovascular "risk," the authors of this review argue that the results are not yet helpful clinically. The results of such tests, thus far, do not add predictive value over and beyond that of routine clinical assessment, including demographics, physical exam, and serum lab testing.

216. **Palomaki GE,** et al. Association between 9p21 genomic markers and heart disease: a meta-analysis. *JAMA* 2010;303:648–656.

The authors compiled data from 22 articles, on 47 different data sets, including 35,872 cases and 95,837 controls. The 9p21 allele proved significantly related to cardiovascular risk, the magnitude of which varied by age of individual. Overall, the effect was small, particularly in the context of more traditional risk factors.

217. **Paynter NP,** et al. Association between a literature-based genetic risk score and cardiovascular events in women. *JAMA* 2010;303:631–637.

In 19,313 participants in the Women's Genome Health Study, the authors constructed genetic risk scores based on the National Human Genome Research Institute's catalog of genome-wide association results. In all, 101 single nucleotide polymorphisms had been found to be significantly associated with CVD. While the collective genetic score did significantly predict CVD risk after controlling for age (HR 1.02, $p = 0.006$), the effect was no longer significant after controlling for other traditional risk factors (HR 1.00).

Antiplatelet Drugs for Primary and Secondary Prevention

REVIEW ARTICLES AND META-ANALYSES

218. **Weisman SM, Graham DY.** Evaluation of the benefits and risks of low-dose aspirin in the secondary prevention of cardiovascular and cerebrovascular events. *Arch Intern Med* 2002;162:2197–2202.

This meta-analysis analyzed data from six trials (6,300 patients) that used low-dose ASA (<325 mg/day) in approved secondary prevention indications. ASA reduced the incidence of all-cause mortality by 18%, stroke by 20%, MI by 30%, and other "vascular events" by 30%. GI tract bleeding was 2.5 times more common in those taking ASA compared with placebo. Overall, the number needed to treat (NNT) for ASA to prevent one death from any cause was 67, whereas the NNT was 100 for detection of one nonfatal GI bleeding event. In summary, ASA use for the secondary prevention of thromboembolic events has a favorable benefit-to-risk profile and should be encouraged in those at high risk.

219. **Antithrombotic Trialists' Collaboration.** Collaborative meta-analysis of randomised trials of antiplatelet therapy for prevention of death, myocardial infarction, and stroke in high risk patients. *BMJ* 2002;324:71–86.

This analysis examined 287 randomized studies involving 135,000 patients in comparisons of antiplatelet therapy versus control and 77,000 in comparisons of different antiplatelet regimens. Among high-risk patients (e.g., acute MI, acute stroke, previous stroke or TIA, PAD, atrial fibrillation), antiplatelet therapy reduced the incidence of serious vascular events (nonfatal MI or stroke, vascular death) by approximately one fourth, nonfatal MI by approximately one third, nonfatal stroke by approximately one fourth, and vascular mortality by approximately one sixth (all p values <0.00001). No adverse effects were noted on other deaths. In each of the high-risk categories, the absolute benefits outweighed the absolute risks of major extracranial bleeding. Clopidogrel reduced serious vascular events by 10% compared with ASA. Among patients at high risk of immediate coronary occlusion, short-term addition of an intravenous GP IIb/IIIa antagonist to ASA prevented a further 20 vascular events per 1,000 ($p < 0.0001$) but caused 23 major (but rarely fatal) extracranial bleeds per 1,000.

220. **Antithrombotic Trialists' (ATT) Collaboration.** Aspirin in the primary and secondary prevention of vascular disease: collaborative meta-analysis of individual participant data from randomised trials. *Lancet* 2009;373:1849–1860.

Using individual patient-level data from the various trials included in the original meta-analysis (above), the ATT investigators reviewed the benefit in vascular events prevented versus the risks of bleeding events caused, when using aspirin for primary prevention. They found aspirin accountable for a 12% relative reduction in serious vascular events (MI, stroke, vascular death, $p = 0.0001$), largely due to a dramatic reduction in nonfatal MI (absolute reduction of 5%). The net effect on stroke incidence was not significant, given a nonsignificant increase in hemorrhagic strokes on aspirin. These effects appeared similar between men and women. However, aspirin increased all bleeding, GI and extracranial (0.10% vs. 0.07%, $p < 0.0001$). Thus, the authors conclude that aspirin for primary prevention, that is in patients without known vascular disease, the benefits of aspirin must be heavily weighed against a not-insignificant risk of adverse bleeding events.

221. **Berger JS,** et al. Aspirin for the primary prevention of cardiovascular events in women and men: a sex-specific meta-analysis of randomized controlled trials. *JAMA* 2006;295:306–313.

The authors analyzed six trials of aspirin for the primary prevention of CVD, to assess the sex-specific benefits. Overall, the trials included 95,456 participants, 51,342 women and 44,114 men. And while aspirin provided significant reductions in the risk of cardiovascular events (12% in women, 14% in men), they were driven by different events for each group. Aspirin provided no protection against cardiovascular mortality or MI for women, but yielded a significant reduction in ischemic stroke (OR, 0.76; p = 0.008). In contrast, aspirin did not protect men from stroke or cardiovascular death, there was a significant reduction in MI for the group (OR, 0.68; p = 0.001). Consistent with prior studies, aspirin significantly increased the risk of adverse bleeding events in both groups.

STUDIES

Primary Prevention

222. **Physicians' Health Study,** Steering Committee of the Physicians Health Study Research Group. Final report on aspirin component of the ongoing Physicians' Health Study. *N Engl J Med* 1989;321:129–135.

Design: Prospective, randomized, double-blind, placebo-controlled study. Average follow-up period was 5 years.
Purpose: To determine whether low-dose ASA decreases CV mortality.
Population: 22,071 male physicians aged 40 to 84 years.
Treatment: ASA, 325 mg every other day, or placebo.
Results: ASA group had a 44% reduction in the risk of MI (0.255%/year vs. 0.44%/year; p < 0.00001). This benefit was restricted to those older than 50 years. The ASA group also had a nonsignificant reduction in CV mortality (RR, 0.96), as well as a nonsignificant increase in stroke rate (RR, 2.1; p = 0.06). Among 333 patients with chronic stable angina, the risk of MI was reduced an astonishing 87%.
Comments: This study was stopped early because of the highly significant reduction in nonfatal MIs. However, as a result, the evidence regarding stroke and total CV deaths is inconclusive because of the very low event rates.

223. **Manson JE,** et al. A prospective study of aspirin use and primary prevention of cardiovascular disease in women. *JAMA* 1991;266:521–527.

This analysis of data on approximately 87,000 NHS participants showed that consumption of one to six tablets of ASA per week was associated with a 32% lower incidence of first MI (p = 0.005). This benefit was restricted to those older than 50 years and most substantial in smokers and those with HTN and hypercholesterolemia.

224. **Ridker PM,** et al. A randomized trial of low-dose aspirin in the primary prevention of cardiovascular disease in women. *N Engl J Med* 2005;352:1293–1304.

Design: Prospective, randomized, double-blind, placebo-controlled study. Average follow-up period was 10 years. Primary endpoint was a composite of nonfatal MI, nonfatal stroke, or cardiovascular death.
Purpose: To assess the efficacy of aspirin for primary prevention of CVD in apparently healthy women.
Population: 39,876 healthy women, aged 45 years or older.
Treatment: ASA, 100 mg every other day, or placebo.
Results: There was a nonsignificant reduction in the primary endpoint, favoring the aspirin group (relative risk, 0.91; p = 0.13). However, there was a significant 24% reduction in

ischemic stroke, favoring the aspirin group ($p = 0.009$), at the expense of a nonsignificant increase in hemorrhagic stroke (RR 1.24, $p = 0.31$). There were no significant differences in the risk of MI or cardiovascular death between the two groups. The risk of GI bleeding was significantly higher in the aspirin group (RR 1.40; $p = 0.02$).

225. Collaborative Group of the Primary Prevention Project. Low-dose aspirin and vitamin E in people at cardiovascular risk: a randomised trial. *Lancet* 2001;357:89–95.

Design: Prospective, randomized, open-label, 2×2 factorial, multicenter trial. Primary end point was CV death, nonfatal MI, and nonfatal stroke.

Purpose: To determine the benefit of ASA and vitamin E for primary prevention of cardiovascular events (CVDs) in a clinical practice setting.

Population: 4,495 patients aged 50 years or older with one or more CRFs including HTN, hypercholesterolemia, diabetes, obesity, family history of premature MI, or age 65 years or older; approximately 70% had two or more CRFs.

Treatment: Low-dose ASA (100 mg/day) and vitamin E (300 mg/day), either, or neither.

Results: Study was terminated prematurely at a mean follow-up of 3.6 years because the benefit of ASA was demonstrated in similar trials. ASA use was associated with a significantly lower incidence of CV death (0.8% vs. 1.4%; RR, 0.56) and CV death, MI, or stroke (6.3% vs. 8.2%; RR, 0.77). Bleeding occurred more frequently in the ASA group (1.1% vs. 0.3%). Vitamin E showed no effect on any end points.

Comments: The evidence in support of ASA for primary prevention of CV events has mounted and appears to be independent of dose (100 to 325 mg), age, gender, and CV risk status.

Secondary Prevention

226. **Gent M,** et al. Clopidogrel versus aspirin in patients at risk of ischaemic events (**CAPRIE**). A randomised, blinded trial of clopidogrel versus aspirin in patients at risk of ischaemic events (CAPRIE). *Lancet* 1996;348:1329–1339.

Design: Prospective, randomized, multicenter study. Primary end point was ischemic stroke, MI, and vascular death. Mean follow-up period was 1.9 years.

Purpose: To compare the effectiveness of clopidogrel with ASA in preventing major vascular events.

Population: 19,185 patients with a history of recent ischemic stroke (1 week to 6 months earlier), MI ($\geq$35 days earlier), or symptomatic PAD.

Treatment: Clopidogrel, 75 mg once daily, or ASA, 325 mg/day.

Exclusion Criteria: Carotid endarterectomy or severe deficit after stroke, uncontrolled HTN, and scheduled major surgery.

Results: Clopidogrel group had a 8.7% reduction in the primary composite end point (5.32 vs. 5.83%/year; $p = 0.043$). The PAD subgroup had a significant 23.8% reduction in the primary end point ($p = 0.003$), whereas the stroke patients had a nonsignificant 7.3% reduction ($p = 0.26$), and MI patients had a nonsignificant 3.7% increase (7.4% reduction if any prior MI). A subsequent analysis of all 8,446 patients with any history of MI showed that clopidogrel was associated with a statistically insignificant 7.4% decrease in the combined end point. No difference was found in incidence of side effects, including neutropenia (clopidogrel, 0.1%; ASA, 0.17).

227. **Bhatt DL,** et al. for the CHARISMA Investigators. Clopidogrel and aspirin versus aspirin alone for the prevention of atherothrombotic events. *N Engl J Med* 2006;354:1706–1717.

Design: Prospective, randomized, multicenter study. Primary end point was a composite of MI, stroke or cardiovascular death.

Purpose: To compare the effectiveness of dual antiplatelet therapy with clopidogrel with ASA versus ASA alone, in preventing major vascular events in a population of both primary and secondary prevention.

Population: 15,603 patients with either known CVD (secondary prevention group) or multiple risk factors (primary prevention group); they were not stratified.

Treatment: Clopidogrel, 75 mg daily, or placebo; both groups received low-dose aspirin (75 to 162 mg daily).

Results: A primary endpoint event occurred in 6.8% of patients in the clopidogrel plus aspirin group versus 7.3% in the aspirin only group ($p = 0.22$). Rates of severe bleeding were higher in the clopidogrel plus aspirin group (1.7% vs. 1.3%, $p = 0.09$). In the subgroup without known disease but multiple risk factors, those in the clopidogrel plus aspirin group had a similar number of primary endpoint events to the aspirin only group, but a significantly higher risk of cardiovascular death (3.9% vs. 2.2%, $p = 0.01$). In the subgroup with known disease, the addition of clopidogrel to aspirin yielded a 12% lower risk of cardiovascular events ($p = 0.046$).

Comment: While the overall primary endpoint of this trial was negative, it is important to note that results from the secondary prevention group (the "CAPRIE-like" cohort) were consistent with previous trials. However, it does not appear that dual antiplatelet therapy is appropriate for patients with multiple risk factors but no known CVD.

228. **Mangano DT,** et al. for the Multicenter Study of Perioperative Ischemia Research Group. Aspirin and mortality from coronary bypass surgery. *N Engl J Med* 2002;347:1309–1317.

This prospective, multicenter study of 5,065 patients undergoing CABG surgery found that early use of ASA is associated with a reduced risk of mortality and ischemic complications. During hospitalization, mortality was 3.2%, whereas the incidence of nonfatal cardiac, cerebral, renal, or GI ischemic complications was 16.0%. Among patients who received ASA (up to 650 mg) within 48 hours, mortality was nearly 70% lower [1.3% vs. 4.0% (no ASA); $p < 0.001$]. ASA therapy also was associated with a 48% lower incidence of MI (2.8% vs. 5.4%; $p < 0.001$), a 50% lower incidence of stroke (1.3% vs. 2.6%; $p = 0.01$), lower incidence of renal failure (0.9% vs. 3.4%; $p < 0.001$), and a 62% lower rate of bowel infarction (0.3% vs. 0.8%; $p = 0.01$). Multivariate analysis showed that no other factor or medication was independently associated with reduced rates of these outcomes. Furthermore, the risk of hemorrhage, gastritis, infection, or impaired wound healing was not increased with ASA use (OR, 0.63; 95% CI, 0.54 to 0.74).

Miscellaneous

229. **Gum PA,** et al. Aspirin use and all-cause mortality among patients being evaluated for known or suspected coronary artery disease: a propensity analysis. *JAMA* 2001;286:1187–1194.

This prospective, nonrandomized, observational, single-center cohort study consisted of 6,174 consecutive adults undergoing stress echocardiography for evaluation of known or suspected CAD. ASA was being taken by 2,310 (37%) patients. Patients with contraindications to ASA use (e.g., peptic ulcer disease, renal insufficiency, NSAID use) or significant valvular disease were excluded. At follow-up (median, 3.1 years), 276 (4.5%) patients had died. After adjustment for age, sex, standard CVRFs, use of other medications, CAD history, EF, exercise capacity, heart rate recovery, and echocardiographic ischemia, ASA use was associated with reduced mortality (HR, 0.67; 95% CI, 0.51 to 0.87; $p = 0.002$). After adjusting for the propensity for using ASA and other possible confounders and interactions, ASA remained associated with lower mortality (adjusted HR, 0.56; 95% CI, 0.40 to 0.78; $p < 0.001$). Patient characteristics associated with the largest ASA-related mortality reductions were older age, known CAD, and impaired exercise capacity.

Angiotensin-converting Enzyme Inhibition for Primary and Secondary Prevention

230. **HOPE.** The Heart Outcome Prevention Evaluation Study Investigators. Effects of an ACE inhibitor, ramipril, on cardiovascular events in high risk patients. *N Engl J Med* 2000;342:145–153 (see page xx for vitamin E results).

Design: Prospective, randomized, double-blind, 2 × 2 factorial, multicenter study. Primary end point was cardiovascular death, MI, or stroke. Mean follow-up, 4.5 years.

Purpose: To assess the role of an ACEI, ramipril, in patients who at high risk for CV events but without LV dysfunction or HF.

Population: 9,297 high-risk patients aged 55 years or older with CAD, stroke, PVD, or diabetes plus one other CVRF (HTN, elevated TC, low HDL, smoking, documented microalbuminuria).

Exclusion Criteria: Included HF, EF less than 40%, uncontrolled HTN, MI or stroke in previous 4 weeks, overt nephropathy.

Treatment: Ramipril (10 mg once per day orally), vitamin E (400 IU daily), both, or neither (placebo × 2).

Results: The ramipril group had a 22% relative reduction in CV death, MI, or stroke compared with the placebo group (14.0% vs. 17.8%; $p < 0.001$). Ramipril was associated with significantly lower rates of CV death (6.1% vs. 8.1%; RR, 0.74; $p < 0.001$), MI (9.9% vs. 12.3%; RR, 0.80; $p < 0.001$), stroke (3.4% vs. 4.9%; RR, 0.68; p < 0.001), all-cause mortality (10.4% vs. 12.2%; RR, 0.84; $p = 0.005$), revascularization procedures (16.3% vs. 18.8%; RR, 0.85; $p < 0.001$), cardiac arrest [0.8% vs. 1.3%; RR, 0.62; $p = 0.02$ (corrected)], HF (9.1% vs. 11.6%; RR, 0.77; $p < 0.001$), and diabetes-related complications (6.4% vs. 7.6%; RR, 0.84; $p = 0.03$). In the MICRO-HOPE substudy of 3,577 diabetics (see *Lancet* 2000;355:253), ramipril reduced primary events by 25%, MI by 22%, stroke by 33%, CV death by 37%, total mortality by 24%, and overt nephropathy by 24% ($p = 0.027$). After adjustment for the changes in SBP (2.4 mm Hg) and DBP (1.0 mm Hg), ramipril still reduced the risk of the combined primary outcome by 25%.

CHAPTER 2

Invasive Procedures and Revascularization

Christopher P. Cannon and Benjamin A. Steinberg

CORONARY ANGIOGRAPHY

Indications

1. Unstable angina and non–ST elevation myocardial infarction (NSTEMI; see Chapter 3) or STEMI (see Chapter 4).
2. Recurrent angina after percutaneous coronary intervention (PCI) or after coronary artery bypass graft (CABG) surgery.
3. Incapacitating angina pectoris despite medical therapy.
4. Complicated myocardial infarction [MI; e.g., recurrent ischemia, heart failure or hypotension, ventricular septal defect, mitral regurgitation, ventricular tachycardia (VT), failed thrombolysis].
5. Preoperative assessment (valve repair/replacement, other high-risk surgery).
6. Positive stress test result (e.g., exercise, echo, nuclear).
7. Miscellaneous: aortic dissection, unexplained ventricular failure, suspected congenital heart disease, postcardiac transplantation, pericardial tamponade or constriction, persistent precordial chest pain of unclear etiology.

Flow Grade

The Thrombolysis in Myocardial Infarction (TIMI) flow grade system is the most commonly used classification system to assess flow:

Grade 0, no anterograde flow beyond the point of occlusion.
Grade 1, contrast goes beyond occlusion but fails to opacify the entire distal bed.
Grade 2, entire vessel opacified, but the rate of entry to and clearance from the distal bed of the contrast is slower than normal.
Grade 3, normal flow.

The TIMI corrected frame count is a more precise method and allows quantitative assessment of flow as a continuous variable (1). The TIMI myocardial perfusion grade system (grades 0 through 3) provides additional prognostic information to epicardial flow assessment (TIMI grade flow) in acute MI patients receiving thrombolytic therapy (see *Circulation* 2000;101:125, Chapter 4).

Stenosis Morphology

The American College of Cardiology (ACC)/American Heart Association (AHA) Classification (2) is enumerated as follows:

Type A: discrete, concentric, readily accessible, nonangulated segment, smooth contour, little or no calcification, nonostial, no major side branch involved, no thrombus present, less than 10 mm in length.

Type B: tubular, eccentric, moderate tortuosity, moderately angulated segment (45 to 90 degrees), irregular contour, moderate to heavy calcification, total occlusion for ≤3 months, ostial location, bifurcation lesion, thrombus present, longer than 10 mm.

Type B1: one B characteristic.

Type B2: two B characteristics.

Type C: diffuse, excessive tortuosity, extremely angulated segment (>90 degrees), total occlusion for more than 3 months, inability to protect major side branch, degenerated vein graft lesion.

Procedural success rates are typically lower and restenosis rates higher for type B and especially type C lesions.

PERCUTANEOUS CORONARY INTERVENTION

Uses and Indications

1. Stable angina/coronary artery disease (CAD) with significant ischemia in medically optimized patients.
2. Unstable angina/non–ST elevation MI (see Chapter 3).
3. Acute ST-elevation MI (see Chapter 4).

Although stenting is almost always preferable to balloon angioplasty alone for these indications (see later section), stenting is especially effective (or required) for the following:

1. Dissection or abrupt closure.
2. High-risk lesions (e.g., left main disease in patients unable to have CABG).
3. Saphenous vein grafts. Lower restenosis rates have been reported in two retrospective analyses (17% vs. 50% with PTCA) (96,97), whereas the randomized Saphenous Vein de novo (SAVED) trial found a nonsignificant reduction in restenosis (37% vs. 46%).
4. Diabetic patients. One study found that stenting was associated with a 56% relative reduction in restenosis at 6 months compared with PTCA alone (27% vs. 62%, $p < 0.0001$); furthermore, the stent group had lower incidence of cardiac death and nonfatal MI at 4 years (14.8% vs. 26.0%, $p = 0.02$).

The superiority of stenting compared with balloon angioplasty alone is related mostly to a lower incidence of abrupt closure (<1% vs. 5%) and lower restenosis rates (15% to 20% for most lesions). Two disadvantages of stenting are difficulty in treating restenosis when it occurs and stent thrombosis [however, incidence is now less than 1% with antiplatelet regimens (see page 89)].

As compared with bare-metal stents (BMS), stents coated with antiproliferative agents or drug-eluting stents (DES) have markedly reduced the risk of restenosis in numerous trials (see Restenosis section later). However, the risk of stent thrombosis, especially after 1 year, is higher in DES versus BMS. Differences have now been seen with improved outcomes with the next-generation DES, especially the everolimus-eluting Xience stent (see below).

Operator and Hospital Volume

Substantial data accumulated in the early and mid-1990s showed better outcomes in patients undergoing PCI performed by high-volume operators and high-volume hospitals (7–10). The best outcomes were achieved by high-volume operators at high-volume facilities (more than 400 cases/year). The recent widespread use of stent technology and glycoprotein (GP) IIb/IIIa inhibitors has reduced overall major adverse event rates but has not attenuated the significant difference between high- and low-volume operators and hospitals (12). Current recommendations of the ACC/AHA Joint Committee and Society for Cardiac Angiography and Intervention (SCAI) suggest a minimum of 75 cases/year per operator, at a center performing more than 400 procedures yearly (200 minimum) to maintain proficiency (*J Am Coll Cardiol* 2008;51:172–209). In the treatment of acute MI with primary PCI, outcomes also are better in high-volume centers (recommended level is 36 or more cases/year); some of this benefit is likely related to the shorter door-to-balloon times obtained at such centers (see Chapter 4). Additionally, guidelines have continued to recommend PCI be performed only at centers with on-site cardiac surgery backup; exceptions have included research protocols investigating the safety of performing emergent primary PCI for STEMI (see Chapter 4). Observational data have demonstrated increased mortality in patients undergoing PCI at centers without on-side cardiac surgery backup (16).

Procedural Details

ACCESS

The right femoral artery is the most common arterial access site. If the patient has severe aortic or femoral vascular disease, radial or brachial artery access is often feasible. A 6-French (F) catheter is now most commonly used for diagnostic catheterization. In one study, the use of 6F catheters showed less bleeding and similar procedural success compared with 7F and 8F catheters (18). Additionally, more contemporary data hint that the use of radial access for angiography and PCI may reduce rates of bleeding complications (19,20).

Femoral closure devices are being used more frequently. Angioseal and Vasoseal are both collagen-mediated devices. Most studies have found they are associated with a shorter time to hemostasis and ambulation and earlier hospital discharge, but few studies have found significant reductions in major bleeding or vascular complications. One randomized trial directly compared the Angioseal and Vasoseal devices and found no significant differences in times to hemostasis and ambulation or the rates of device failure and vascular complications (see *Catheter Cardiovasc Interv* 2002;55:421–425). A third approved device is a Perclose, a suture-mediated device. One recent study found that it reduced time to hemostasis and ambulation and was associated with a lower incidence of major complications (*Am J Cardiol* 2000;85:864).

More recently, data on use of radial artery vascular access approaches have demonstrated impressive safety and efficacy with this approach. One recent meta-analysis included 12 different studies of 3,324 patients, comparing safety and efficacy of transradial versus transfemoral PCI for acute STEMI (see *Am Heart J* 2009;158:814–821). Transradial compared favorably, with less bleeding ($p = 0.0001$), as well as clinical outcomes of the composite of death, MI, or stroke ($p = 0.001$) and mortality alone (2.04% vs. 3.06%, $p = 0.01$). Importantly, these analyses included case–control and cohort studies, in addition to randomized trials; thus, confirmatory data are needed prior to making any conclusions regarding superiority of the transradial approach.

CONTRAST AGENT

Some observational and nonrandomized studies have found low-osmolar ionic contrast agents to result in fewer recurrent ischemic events than nonionic agents, whereas others found no significant reductions in major events with nonionic agents. Randomized trials also produced conflicting results (21–26); however, the data are consistent in regard to a significant reduction in hypersensitivity and allergic reactions with nonionic agents compared with ionic agents.

LESION EVALUATION

The severity of stenoses is typically first assessed by angiography. Subjective visual assessment and/or quantitative coronary angiography (QCA) are used to grade stenoses from 0 to 100%; the latter is used in clinical trials and usually performed by an independent core laboratory.

Intravascular ultrasound (IVUS) provides three-dimensional imaging, which can better estimate the severity of complex and eccentric lesions; it is more sensitive than fluoroscopy and angiography in detecting coronary calcification. IVUS can assess atheroma within the vessel walls, which often goes undetected by angiography because vascular "remodeling" due to outward displacement of the vessel wall allows early atheroma accumulation without impairing lumen diameter. IVUS also is used after stent deployment and can reveal suboptimal results due to edge dissections [if deep or long (longer than 5 mm), additional stenting is indicated] and malexpansion or malapposition (treated with balloon angioplasty with larger and/or higher pressure balloons).

In the REStenosis after IVUS-guided Stenting (RESIST) study, 155 patients who had successful stenting were randomized to no further balloon dilation or additional balloon dilation(s) until IVUS criterion was achieved for adequate stent expansion. At 6 months, the lumen cross-sectional area was 20% larger in the IVUS-guided group, but no significant differences were found between the groups in mean luminal diameter or restenosis (4.47 vs. 5.36 mm^2; $p = 0.03$). In the Can Routine Ultrasound Influence Stent Expansion (CRUISE) study (28), 522 patients from the Stent Anti-thrombotic Regimen Study (STARS) were enrolled in an IVUS substudy to determine whether IVUS-assisted stenting results in better outcomes when compared with angiography-assisted stenting. At 9 months, the IVUS-guided group had a larger minimal luminal diameter (MLD), a lower residual diameter stenosis, and a significantly lower target-vessel revascularization (TVR) rate (8.5% vs. 15.3%; $p < 0.05$), but no significant differences occurred in death or MI rates. In the OPTimization with ICUS to reduce stent restenosis (OPTICUS) study (33), a less selected group of 550 patients with a symptomatic coronary lesion or silent ischemia were assigned to either IVUS-guided or angiography-guided implantation of two or more stents. At 6-month angiography, no significant differences appeared between the two groups in minimal lumen diameter (MLD) or restenosis rate, and at 1 year, similar incidences were found of major adverse cardiac events (MACEs) and repeated PCI. Given these mixed results and the added expense and time, routine IVUS guidance for stenting is now not recommended.

Measurement of fractional flow reserve (FFR) is an effective method to evaluate stenoses of moderate severity. It can be performed immediately before a potential intervention and requires only the use of a pressure wire and administration of adenosine. FFR is defined as the maximal blood flow to the myocardium in a stenotic segment divided by the theoretic normal maximal flow in the same distribution. The normal value is 1.0, whereas an FFR of 0.75 or less is associated with inducible myocardial ischemia. In one study (27), all patients with an FFR less than 0.75 had reversible myocardial ischemia evident on at least one noninvasive test (bicycle exercise testing, thallium scintigraphy, dobutamine stress echocardiography). After revascularization was performed (PTCA or CABG surgery), all the positive test results reverted to normal. In contrast, 88% of patients with an FFR of 0.75 or more tested negative for reversible ischemia on all the noninvasive tests, and none underwent revascularization (more than 1 year follow-up). In a larger, randomized study of 325 patients (29), 144 patients with an FFR less than 0.75 underwent routine PTCA (reference group), whereas those with an FFR 0.75 or more were randomized to optimal intervention (performance group) or medical therapy (deferral group). At 2 years, the event-free survival was significantly higher in the performance and deferral groups (83% and 89%) compared with the reference group (78%). Additional, larger, contemporary randomized data have confirmed these findings—that is, percutaneous revascularization guided by angiography *and* FFR yielded better clinical outcomes when compared with angiography alone guiding revascularization (32). Subsequently, the most recent guidelines have made it a class IIa recommendation to measure FFR, and it is now a level of evidence "A" based on the most recent data (6).

Another alternative for noninvasive lesion evaluation is coronary flow velocity reserve (CFVR). A DEBATE II substudy (35) of 379 patients found that a low CFVR (<2.5) at the end of PCI was an independent predictor of MACEs at 30 days [odds ratio (OR), 4.71; $p = 0.034$)] and at 1 year (OR, 2.06; $p = 0.014$). In another study, a lower CFVR cutoff of less than 2.0 was a more accurate measure of major cardiac events than single-photon emission computed tomography (SPECT) imaging; also, a multivariate analysis found CFVR was the only significant predictor for cardiac events. Discordant results between CFVR and FFR have been observed in 25% to 30% of intermediate lesions. One recent study proposed that an index incorporating CFVR and FFR is a more accurate predictor than either method used alone (see *Circulation* 2002;106:441).

BALLOON ANGIOPLASTY

Balloon inflations are typically performed at 8 to 12 atm. Higher pressures are often used to perform poststenting dilatations and are often required during treatment of calcified lesions. Prolonged inflation (e.g., 5 minutes) has been shown in randomized studies to result in better procedural success but has no impact on major event rates or restenosis.

Success rates with balloon angioplasty of approximately 90% to 95% have been achieved in most institutions [vs. 64% success rate in the first major report (17)]. Failures occur when the lesion cannot be crossed, inadequate balloon dilatation is achieved, and abrupt closure occurs. Predictors of failure include chronic occlusion; stenoses that are long, angulated, eccentric, at an ostium or branch point, calcified, and/or associated with intraluminal thrombus; hospital with low volume; operator with low volume; saphenous vein grafts (especially if older than 3 years); female gender; and advanced age.

One specific type of balloon deserves mention. The cutting balloon, which consists of several microblades attached to a balloon, permits effective dilation at lower inflation pressures and thus, hypothetically, causes less vessel stretching and trauma. In the CUBA study, the cutting balloon was compared with conventional PTCA. Mean luminal diameter at 6 months was larger for the cutting balloon group, but there was no significant difference between groups in the incidence of death, MI, or any target-lesion revascularization. In the randomized CAPAS trial (55), lesions in smaller vessels were examined [less than 3.0 mm (mean, 2.2 mm), compared with 2.5 to 4.0 mm in CUBA]. The cutting-balloon group had a significantly lower 3-month restenosis rate than the PTCA group (25% vs. 42%) and a better 1-year event-free survival rate (72.8% vs. 61.0%). A third, larger randomized trial (1,238 patients) found the cutting balloon associated with a slightly lower TVR rate (11.5% vs. 15.4%; $p = 0.04$) but no difference in the rates of binary restenosis or MACEs (57). However, a more recent meta-analysis including several of the above-mentioned trials confirmed the lack of clinical benefit to routinely sectioning atheromas during PCI (60).

STENTING

First-generation stents [Palmaz–Schatz (PS) and Gianturco–Roubin] became available in the early 1990s and resulted in lower restenosis rates compared with PTCA in major randomized trials. As a result, subsequent second-generation stents were compared with the earlier stents (vs. PTCA) in trials designed to show "equivalence." A number of these trials were performed [examples: ASCENT (Multilink), BEST (BeStent), EXTRA (XT), GR-II (Gianturco–Roubin II), SCORES (Radius), SMART (Microstent II)] (48,52–54). The GR-II stent had inferior results compared with the PS stent (52), whereas the others were found to be equivalent but not superior to the PS. However, these trials excluded the most difficult lesion types (e.g., severe calcification and tortuosity) that compose the majority of stent targets. Because these difficult lesions were less amenable to PS stenting, the newer-generation stents were rapidly adopted. Randomized stent versus stent trials are similarly designed but have compared newer stents with second-generation stents [examples: TENISS (Tenax coated vs. Nir), MULTILINK-DUET (Multilink vs. Multilink Duet)]; numerous observational and registry studies also compared different stents.

The majority of currently available stents are balloon-expandable, slotted-tube stents, whereas there are a few self-expanding stents (Wallstent, Radius); the latter are very flexible and can be delivered through tortuous vessels, but accurate sizing and placement are challenging. In the past few years, lower profile and smaller stents have become available (2.5 mm, 2.25 mm, 2.0 mm). A post hoc analysis of 331 STRESS I-II patients found that stenting resulted in lower restenosis rates than did PTCA in vessels smaller than 3.0 mm (126). Data from several randomized trials, however, yielded conflicting results with small-vessel lesions, with three showing similar outcomes between stenting and PTCA (ISAR-SMART, SISA, and COAST studies) (127,129), whereas two found lower restenosis rates with stenting [BESMART (128)]. The more robust, significant benefits of stents compared with PTCA have been clearly demonstrated in larger vessels, total occlusions, and saphenous vein graft lesions (see later sections).

Medications

ASPIRIN

Aspirin, 325 mg daily for 1 month following BMS, 3 months after SES and 6 months after PES; then 75 to 162 mg daily thereafter and indefinitely (allergies and bleeding complications notwithstanding). Use of aspirin significantly reduces ischemic complications in PTCA (165); however, use in conjunction with a thienopyridine provides even better outcomes in stenting (see below). These recommendations are predominantly based on the dosing of aspirin used in clinical trials of stenting. Preliminary data from the CURRENT-OASIS 7 trial found no difference in CV death, MI, or stroke at 30 days between 75 and 325 mg of ASA in ACS patients managed invasively, including those who underwent PCI.

HEPARIN

Heparin: initial bolus, 50 to 60 U/kg when used in conjunction with a GP IIb/IIIa inhibitor; higher dosing typically is used when administered alone. The target activated clotting time (ACT) when used alone is 300 to 350 seconds; a low periprocedural ACT is associated with increased complications while higher ACTs (400 to 600 seconds) are associated with increased bleeding. One study found even less heparin (2,500 U; mean ACT, 185) appears safe in elective cases (73). Unless PCI is complicated (e.g., residual thrombus), a prolonged heparin infusion is not necessary because it is does not decrease ischemic complications and results in more frequent bleeding (71).

LOW-MOLECULAR-WEIGHT HEPARIN

Low-molecular-weight heparin (LWMH): Several studies have compared unfractionated heparin (UFH) with LWMH during coronary interventions. Conflicting data were found in studies in which LWMH were given for up to 1 month after the procedure. The ENTICES and REDUCE trials found a significant reduction in early ischemic events with enoxaparin or reviparin compared with UFH; these results were not confirmed in the ATLAST or ERA studies. Data regarding bleeding also are conflicting, with two of four studies showing reduced bleeding rates with LWMH. Observations from the NICE-1 and NICE-4 trials in which enoxaparin was used with and without GP IIb/IIIa inhibitors also show that the use of enoxaparin appeared safe and effective in the interventional setting.

The A to Z trial found no difference in bleeding with enoxaparin. The larger SYNERGY trial of over 10,000 patients with high-risk unstable angina or NSTEMI demonstrated noninferiority of enoxaparin in this setting, though the trial was open-label (74). A substudy of the ExTRACT-TIMI 25 trial (see Chapter 4) demonstrated superiority of enoxaparin in patients with STEMI undergoing subsequent PCI following fibrinolysis therapy (75). However, when necessary to monitor LMWH, this can be less convenient. Anti-Xa levels have been obtained in some studies but take longer to measure than does an ACT. Thus, despite significant clinic evidence of noninferiority and in certain situations superiority of enoxaparin over UFH, many operators continue to use UFH due to familiarity and easy, quick monitoring intra-procedure.

DIRECT THROMBIN INHIBITORS

In patients with known heparin-induced thrombocytopenia, direct thrombin inhibitors (e.g., argatroban or bivalirudin) are often administered. The 6,010-patient REPLACE 2 trial compared heparin plus eptifibatide or abciximab with bivalirudin alone (provisional GP IIb/IIIa inhibitor if needed) (106). Provisional IIb/IIIa-inhibitor treatment was given to only 7.2% of the bivalirudin group. The bivalirudin group had a nonsignificant reduction in death, MI, urgent revascularization at

30 days, and major in-hospital bleeding (primary end point) compared with heparin plus GP IIb/IIIa inhibitor (9.2% vs. 10.0%). Bivalirudin was associated with a significantly lower incidence of bleeding (2.4% vs. 4.1%), whereas there was a nonsignificant excess of MI with bivalirudin (7.0% vs. 6.2%). Contemporary data of bivalirudin, as compared with UFH, in stable or low-risk unstable coronary disease patients undergoing PCI with clopidogrel pretreatment were provided by the ISAR-REACT 3 trial (107). While there was no net clinical benefit (the combination of ischemic and bleeding events) of bivalirudin over UFH, patients receiving bivalirudin had lower bleeding events.

THIENOPYRIDINES/ADP RECEPTOR ANTAGONISTS

The first agent available was *ticlopidine* (250 mg twice daily for 2 to 4 weeks) which, when given in conjunction with aspirin and heparin, is more effective than an anticoagulant regimen (e.g., intravenous heparin followed by warfarin). In three randomized studies [Intracoronary Stenting and Antithrombotic Regimen (ISAR), Full Anticoagulation versus Aspirin and Ticlopidine (FANTASTIC), and Stent Anticoagulation Restenosis Study (STARS)] (76,77), 50% to 80% fewer cardiac end points were reached (**Fig. 2.1**).

Clopidogrel, now commonly is used as an alternative to ticlopidine (59,72,73). Results from one study showed 60% platelet inhibition [measured by using 5 μmol adenosine diphosphate (ADP)] is achieved within 2 to 4 hours of a loading dose of clopidogrel (300 mg) versus 4 to 5 days with regular dosing and 6 to 7 days with ticlopidine, 250 mg twice daily. Results of the Clopidogrel Aspirin Stent

Figure 2.1 • These data from major coronary stent studies show the superiority of a regimen consisting of aspirin and/or ticlopidine or clopidogrel. (Data from Refs. 73, 78, and 80.)

Figure 2.2 • The 2,658-patient Percutaneous Coronary Intervention-Clopidogrel in Unstable angina to prevent Recurrent ischemic Events **(PCI-CURE)** (81) study evaluated pretreatment and extended clopidogrel therapy and found it to be associated with a 31% relative reduction in cardiovascular death or nonfatal myocardial infarction. (Adapted from *The Lancet*, Vol. 358, Mehta SR, Yusuf S, Peters R, et al. Effects of pretreatment with clopidogrel and aspirin followed by long-term therapy in patients undergoing percutaneous coronary intervention: the PCI-CURe study, Pages 527–533, ©2001.)

International Cooperative Study (CLASSICS) showed clopidogrel (75 mg once daily for 4 weeks ± 300 mg loading dose) to be as effective as ticlopidine in preventing stent thrombosis and clinical events, but it is much better tolerated (81) **(Fig. 2.1)**. More important, as shown in the large Clopidogrel versus Aspirin in Patients at Risk of Ischaemic Events (CAPRIE) trial (see Chapter 1), the risk of neutropenia with clopidogrel is very low (0.1%) and similar to aspirin. Recent data suggest that up to 30% of patients do not respond to clopidogrel primarily due to low levels of enzyme CYP3A4; this drug resistance requires further study.

In the recent PCI-CURE study (82), pretreatment with clopidogrel before PCI was associated with a significantly lower incidence of cardiovascular death, MI, or urgent revascularization at 30 days compared with placebo [4.5% vs. 6.4%; relative risk (RR), 0.70; $p = 0.03$]. Long-term administration of clopidogrel also led to a 31% RR reduction in cardiovascular death or MI (8.8% vs. 12.6%; $p = 0.002$; see **Fig. 2.2**).

The Clopidogrel in Unstable Angina to Prevent Recurrent Events (CREDO) trial (87) found that a preprocedural loading dose followed by long-term treatment (1 year) with clopidogrel after elective PCI was associated with a 26.9% relative reduction in death, MI, or stroke compared with post-PCI clopidogrel therapy for 1 month [8.5% vs. 11.5% (placebo); $p = 0.02$]. An impressive further 37.4% relative reduction in major events occurred from day 29 to 1 year with clopidogrel ($p = 0.04$; **Fig. 2.3**). As for pretreatment, those given clopidogrel at least 6 hours before PCI had a 38.6% RR reduction in major events at 28 days ($p = 0.05$) compared with no reduction with treatment less than 6 hours before PCI. Among those

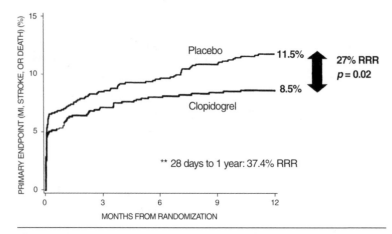

Figure 2.3 • The 2,116-patient Clopidogrel in Unstable angina to Prevent Recurrent Events **(CREDO)** (86) trial demonstrated a substantial 27% reduction in major events (death, myocardial infarction, stroke) at 1 year. Continued clopidogrel therapy from 28 days to 1 year was associated with a further 37% relative reduction in events compared with placebo. (Adapted from Steinhubl SR, Berger PB, Mann JT, et al. Early and sustained dual oral antiplatelet therapy following percutaneous coronary intervention: a randomized controlled trial. *JAMA* 2002;288:2411–2420.)

receiving a GP IIb/IIIa inhibitor (45%) and clopidogrel pretreatment, a 30% reduction in events was found [7.3% vs. 10.3% (no treatment, GP IIb/IIIa); $p = 0.12$]. Finally, a trend toward a higher incidence of major bleeding occurred with clopidogrel (at 1 year, 8.8% vs. 6.7%; $p = 0.07$).

Additionally, the PCI-CLARITY analysis looked at pretreatment with clopidogrel for an average of 3.5 days pre-PCI in patients initially presenting with STEMI. Clopidogrel reduced the risk of CV death, MI, or recurrent ischemia leading to urgent revascularization by 46% ($p < 0.001$) (88). A meta-analysis of the three trials (PCI-CURE, CREDO, and PCI-CLARITY) found a highly significant 29% reduction in death or MI post-PCI ($p = 0.004$) and a significant 31% reduction in MI pre-PCI ($p = 0.005$) (88), supporting the routine and *early* use of clopidogrel in patients subsequently undergoing PCI. In summary, the results of these three trials support preprocedural loading and long-term therapy with clopidogrel in those scheduled for or expected to undergo PCI. The significant benefits do not appear attenuated by use of GP IIb/IIIa inhibitors.

On the other hand, if high-dose clopidogrel is used, one study found it may eliminate the need for GP IIb/IIIa inhibition during PCI. A total of 2,159 low-risk patients (excluded if MI within 14 days, ACS or elevated troponin) undergoing elective PCI were all given 600 mg ≥2 hours before PCI and then randomized to abciximab or placebo (90). At 30 days, there was no difference in death, MI, or urgent TVR between the two groups (4% each in each group, $p = 0.82$).

Most recently, an additional and more potent thienopyridine has been approved, prasugrel. While approval was based largely on its use in acute coronary syndromes in the TRITON-TIMI 38 trial (see Chapter 4, page 215 for full details of the trial), prasugrel will likely find a role in routine use for patients undergoing PCI for ACS who have had poor outcomes despite therapy with both aspirin and clopidogrel. Furthermore, early data suggest some patients may have reduced response to clopidogrel based on their cytochrome P-450 genotypes; in these patients, prasugrel may provide a substantial benefit; however, this remains to be validated in large, prospective, randomized trials (89). A newer agent ticagrelor is a non-thienopyridine that has been seen to similarly reduce events in patients with ACS, many of whom underwent PCI (see Chapter 3).

GLYCOPROTEIN IIB/IIIA INHIBITORS

GP IIb/IIIa inhibitors have increasingly been used in patients with acute coronary syndromes and those undergoing PCI (**Fig. 2.4**). If used, lower heparin dosage is indicated, with a target ACT of approximately 250 seconds, as the use of a higher ACT target in early trials resulted in increased bleeding. The following agents are currently the most-widely used:

Abciximab

The monoclonal antibody fragment abciximab binds tightly to the GP IIb/IIIa receptor and has shown impressive results in patients undergoing PCI. In the Evaluation of 7E3 for the Prevention of Ischemic Complications (EPIC) trial (92),

Figure 2.4 • Glycoprotein IIb/IIIa inhibitors in percutaneous coronary intervention and acute coronary syndromes. (From Wiviott SD, Braunwald E, McCabe CH, et al. Prasugrel versus Clopidogrel in Patients with Acute Coronary Syndromes. *NEJM* 2007;357:2001–2015. © 2007 Massachusetts Medical Society. All rights reserved.)

composed of 2,099 high-risk patients [acute MI, postinfarct angina with electrocardiographic (ECG) changes, high-risk clinical or angiographic features], the group receiving abciximab, 0.25 mg/kg intravenous bolus, and then 10 mg/min infusion for 12 hours had 35% fewer end points compared with the placebo group. At 3-year follow-up, this benefit was still present. In the c7E3 Fab Antiplatelet Therapy in Unstable Refractory Angina (CAPTURE) trial (94), composed of 1,265 unstable angina patients, the abciximab group had a significant 29% reduction in primary composite end point at 30 days but not at 6 months. This loss of benefit is attributed to abciximab infusion being stopped 1 hour after PCI. In the Evaluation in PTCA to Improve Long-term Outcome with Abciximab Glycoprotein IIb/IIIa Blockade (EPILOG) trial (95), composed of 2,792 nonacute coronary syndrome patients, abciximab showed a greater than 50% reduction in primary composite end point at 30 days, and the reduction remained significant at 6 months and 1 year.

In the Evaluation of Platelet IIb/IIIa Inhibitor for Stenting (EPISTENT) trial (97), composed of 2,399 CAD patients randomized to stent plus placebo, stent plus abciximab, or balloon angioplasty plus abciximab, the two abciximab groups had a significantly lower incidence of death, MI, and urgent revascularization at 30 days (5.3% and 6.9% vs. 10.8%). One-year mortality was also lower. A recent meta-analysis of all abciximab trials showed a nearly 30% lower mortality during 6-month to 3-year follow-up ($p = 0.003$; see *J Am Coll Cardiol* 2002;37:2059). A study found intracoronary administration of abciximab in unstable angina or acute MI patients resulted in 50% fewer major cardiac events at 30 days compared with IV administration (see *Circulation* 2003;107:1840); similar findings have been seen with another GP IIb/IIIa inhibitor (103).

Although an antibody response develops in 6% to 7% of patients receiving abciximab after first administration, the Reopro Readministration Registry (R3) reported no significant differences in the incidence of adverse allergic or clinical events or thrombocytopenia in 500 patients receiving repeated abciximab compared with 23,000 patients treated for the first time.

Eptifibatide

In the Novel Dosing Regimen of Eptifibatide in Planned Coronary Stent Implantation (ESPRIT) study (99), which randomized 2,064 patients undergoing stenting to *double bolus* eptifibatide (two 180 μg/kg boluses 10 minutes apart, and then 2-μg/kg/min for 18 to 24 hours) or placebo, eptifibatide had a significantly lower incidence of death, MI, urgent TVR, and thrombotic bailout GP IIb/IIIa inhibitor therapy within 48 hours (6.4% vs. 10.5%; $p = 0.0015$). This benefit was consistent across different components of the primary end point, including death/MI/TVR [RR, 0.65; 95% confidence interval (CI), 0.47 to 0.87]; death/MI (RR, 0.60; CI, 0.44 to 0.82); and death (RR, 0.5; CI, 0.05 to 5.42). Kaplan–Meier survival curves appeared to separate over time, with most of the difference in mortality occurring between 30 days and 6 months (see *JAMA* 2001;285:2468–2473).

In the Platelet Glycoprotein IIb/IIIa in Unstable Angina Receptor Suppression Using Integrilin Therapy (PURSUIT) trial (see Chapter 3), a significant reduction in death or MI at 30 days of 31% was observed in patients undergoing PCI.

Tirofiban

The peptidomimetic tirofiban is currently approved by the U.S. FDA for use in acute coronary syndromes with or without PCI, but not in elective PCI. In the Randomized Efficacy Study of Tirofiban for Outcomes and Restenosis (RESTORE) (96), composed of 2,139 patients randomized to tirofiban, 10 μg/kg bolus, and then 0.15 μg/kg/min for 36 hours, or placebo, the tirofiban group had significantly fewer events at 2 days and 7 days but not at 30 days. In the Platelet Receptor Inhibition in Ischemic Syndrome Management in Patients Limited by Unstable Signs and Symptoms (PRISM-PLUS) trial (see Chapter 3), PCI patients showed a reduction in death or MI of approximately 35%. The TARGET trial (100) compared the safety and efficacy of tirofiban with abciximab, randomizing 5,308 patients scheduled for coronary stenting to tirofiban (10 μg/kg bolus, then 0.15 μg/kg/min for 18 to 24 hours) or abciximab. The tirofiban group had a significantly higher incidence of the primary composite end point of death, nonfatal MI, or urgent TVR at 30 days compared with the abciximab group (7.6% vs. 6.0%; p = 0.038). This significant difference did not persist at 6-month follow-up. Several investigators suggested that these results were due to under-dosing of tirofiban, and recent data documented only 70% platelet inhibition over the first hour, which could explain the poorer outcomes (*Am J Cardiol* 2002;89:647; *Circulation* 2002;106:1470). Accordingly, some newer trials used a higher loading dose of 25 μg/kg bolus, and found benefit (6,104).

A broad meta-analysis of 19 trials involving all available GP IIb/IIIa inhibitors (including those above) pooled 20,137 patients with death as the primary outcome. In these patients undergoing PCI (either urgently for acute MI or electively), use of a GP IIb/IIIA inhibitor significantly reduced overall mortality at 30 days (RR 0.69, 95% CI, 0.53 to 0.90), as well as at 6 months (RR 0.79, 95% CI, 0.64 to 0.97). Additional composite clinical outcome was also reduced, and there was little heterogeneity across the spectra of trials (102). See Chapters 3 and 4 for more detailed discussion of the use of GP IIb/IIIa inhibitors in UA/NSTEMI and STEMI, respectively.

Applications of PCI

STABLE ANGINA

Percutaneous Coronary Intervention versus Medical Therapy

The Angioplasty Compared to Medicine (ACME) study (36) compared PTCA with medical therapy in patients with stable, single-vessel CAD. The PTCA group had increased exercise time and less use of antianginal medications but had a higher frequency of MI (4%) and emergency coronary artery bypass surgery (2%).

The Veterans Administration Angioplasty Compared to Medicine (VA ACME) study (37) also showed that PTCA in patients with single-vessel CAD resulted in improved exercise time, less angina, and better quality-of-life score.

The Randomized Intervention Treatment of Angina (RITA-2) trial (38) showed that angioplasty was associated with less angina and longer treadmill time but with an increased incidence of death or MI due to procedure-related MI events. The most contemporary Clinical Outcomes Utilizing Revascularization and Aggressive Drug Evaluation (COURAGE) enrolled more than 2,000 patients with objective CAD by noninvasive testing and compared aggressive medical therapy alone with aggressive medical therapy with added PCI in all but the highest-risk patients with CAD (39). At the follow-up median time of 4.6 years, patients in the PCI group had no better rates of death, MI, or other cardiovascular events than those who were maximally medically managed (19% for PCI vs. 18.5% for medical management). The results of this trial underscored the pathophysiology of CAD—only medical management can reduce the burden of disease, whereas PCI is the therapy of choice for *acute* or *severe* coronary obstructions.

UNSTABLE ANGINA/NON–ST ELEVATION MYOCARDIAL INFARCTION

Recent major trials have shown that an early invasive strategy is superior to a conservative approach, especially in high-risk patients (e.g., ST-segment depression, positive cardiac troponin I; see Chapter 3).

ACUTE ST-ELEVATION MYOCARDIAL INFARCTION

In experienced centers with short door-to-balloon times, primary PCI has been associated with lower mortality than has thrombolytic therapy (see Chapter 4). However, the availability and institutional volume and experience are limiting factors.

AFTER THROMBOLYTIC THERAPY

Studies performed in the 1980s found that routine immediate PTCA PCI was harmful (TAMI I, TIMI IIA, and ECSG trials; see Chapter 4), whereas delayed PTCA (at 18 to 48 hours) was associated with similar outcomes (SWIFT and TIMI IIB; see Chapter 4). PTCA PCI is indicated in patients with high-risk features, such as cardiogenic shock, persistent pain or ischemia, and VT or ventricular fibrillation (VF). The data suggest that it can now be performed routinely and safely early after thrombolysis (PACT, TIMI 14, ExTRACT-TIMI 25; see also *Am J Cardiol* 2001;88:831–836; see Chapter 4). For high-risk patients, with extensive anterior MI, early transfer (<6 hours) post fibrinolysis is now recommended on the basis of the TRANSFER-AMI and CARESS-AMI studies (see Chapter 4).

STENTING VERSUS PERCUTANEOUS TRANSLUMINAL CORONARY ANGIOPLASTY: MAJOR TRIALS

All major trials have shown a substantial reduction in restenosis rates with stenting compared with balloon angioplasty alone. Important results include the following:

1. In the Stent Restenosis Study (STRESS) (40), composed of 410 patients, stenting was associated with higher procedural success, less restenosis at 6 months

(31% vs. 46%, $p = 0.046$), and a trend toward less revascularization ($p = 0.06$), but there was no significant reduction in clinical events.

2. In the EPISTENT study (94,95), composed of 2,399 patients, the rates of TVR at 6 months for stent and stent plus abciximab were significantly lower than those for PTCA and abciximab (10.6% and 8.7% vs. 15.4%; $p = 0.005$, $p < 0.001$).

Primary stenting versus percutaneous transluminal coronary angioplasty with stenting *has become the standard of care for coronary lesions, and balloon angioplasty* is typically only performed when stenting is not feasible.

DIRECT STENTING VERSUS BALLOON PREDILATATION

Direct stenting is now performed by many operators and potentially offers numerous advantages, including shorter procedure time, less radiation exposure and contrast use, and overall reduced costs. Possible disadvantages include increased risk of guide trauma and deployment failure. However, with the exclusion criteria used in several trials, such as excessive calcification, severe proximal tortuosity, and occlusion, crossover rates from direct stenting to predilatation have been low (3% to 6%). Most studies comparing direct stenting with predilatation followed by stenting have found no significant difference in major clinical outcomes (49,51; also *Heart* 2002;86:302); one study did find a lower TLR in a direct stenting group (18% vs. 28%; $p = 0.03$) (50). In summary, with careful lesion selection, direct stenting is typically successful, has at least similar clinical outcomes, and provides cost and procedural advantages compared with predilatation.

REPEATED INTERVENTION

Repeated PCI is performed only if recurrent symptoms emerge, because up to 50% with angiographic restenosis have no symptoms (see *Circulation* 2001;104:2289). PCI has a high initial success rate (95% to 100%) because restenosis is typically characterized by fibroproliferative tissue as opposed to atherosclerotic plaque. However, recurrent restenosis rates are high, exceeding 50% for diffuse ISR lesions. For treatment of restenosis after prior PTCA, stenting results in better outcomes compared with repeated PTCA; in the randomized REST study (157), the stent group had much lower restenosis and TVR rates compared with PTCA (18% vs. 32% and 10% vs. 27%, respectively).

For treatment of ISR, debulking techniques such as rotational atherectomy (RA) and directional atherectomy appear to be more effective than PTCA alone, but restenosis still occurs in about 30% of cases. Repeated stenting to treat ISR was examined in the RIBS (Restenosis Intrastent Balloon versus Stent) study (158). Results from this 450-patient study revealed that repeated stenting provided a larger MLD immediately after the procedure (2.77 mm vs. 2.25 mm; $p < 0.001$), and persisted to a lesser degree at 6-month follow-up (1.69 mm vs. 1.54 mm; $p = 0.046$). In a prespecified subgroup analysis, it was shown that patients whose target vessel was more than 3 mm in diameter had a lower restenosis rate and a better event-free survival with repeated stenting (27% vs. 49%, $p = 0.007$; 84% vs. 62%, $p = 0.002$). These findings were confirmed in long-term follow-up of the trial participants, up to 3 to 5 years, although many patients had events in each group and only large vessel diameter proved protective (see *J Am Coll Cardiol* 2005;46:756–760).

Contemporary data from the ISAR-DESIRE trial of 300 patients with in-stent restenosis demonstrated that DES were likely superior to balloon angioplasty in terms of recurrent restenosis at 6 months (160). The primary end point of angiographic restenosis based on "in-segment" analysis occurred in 44.6% in the balloon angioplasty group versus 14.3% in the sirolimus stent group, and 21.7% in the paclitaxel-stenting group ($p < 0.001$ for each stent compared with balloon angioplasty).

Complications

IN HOSPITAL

1. Death ($<0.2\%$) in elective PCI
2. MI ($<5\%$). Causes include distal embolization, side-branch occlusion, and obstructive lesion complications such as thrombus, abrupt closure, or severe dissection. Retrospective analyses suggest that even small non–Q-wave MIs [often occurring in the absence of symptoms or ECG changes and detected by routine creatine kinase (CK) and CK-MB measurement] result in increased incidence of ischemic complications and subsequent recurrent MI, revascularization, and death (134).

   Post-PCI elevations of the more sensitive troponin assays occur even more frequently. In the TOPSTAR study (137), more than half of patients had an elevated troponin-T level at 24 hours after PCI. In this study, use of a GP IIb/IIIa inhibitor significantly reduced the incidence of troponin elevation. Larger studies are needed to further investigate these findings, especially whether small troponin elevations with normal CK-MB levels are correlated with worse prognosis.
3. Severe dissection and abrupt closure ($<1\%$). Closure results from extensive dissection, thrombosis, or vasospasm. It may also result from stent embolization or mis-deployment (see *Am J Cardiol* 2001;88:634) and is more likely to occur if ACT is low (136). Aspirin has been proven to decrease its incidence, whereas GP IIb/IIIa inhibitor use has resulted in a lower incidence of urgent revascularization. Treatment options include (a) conservative medical therapy (reasonable if collateralization is adequate or the amount of jeopardized myocardium is small); (b) stent placement [restores flow in more than 90% of patients, but infarcts occur in up to 20% and reocclusion (over days to weeks) occurs in about 10%]; (c) repeated PTCA (50% success rate; perfusion catheter often is used, which allows balloon inflation for 10 to 30 minutes); or (d) emergency CABG (25% to 50% still have a Q-wave MI).
4. Perforation ($<0.5\%$). Small perforations can be sealed with prolonged balloon inflations and/or covered stent(s). Large perforations typically result in

pericardial tamponade. One major academic center reported a 0.12% incidence of tamponade in more than 25,000 PCIs (see *Am J Cardiol* 2002;90:1183). Delayed cardiac tamponade occurred in 45% of cases (mean time from PCI, 4.4 hours); thus tamponade should be considered a cause of late hypotension after PCI.

5. Emergency CABG surgery (<0.5%). Data from one large academic center found a decline in incidence from 1.5% in 1992 to 0.14% in 2000 (see *Circulation* 2002;106:2346), usually because of severe dissection, perforation, or recurrent acute closure.

6. Other acute complications: (a) allergic reactions: usually due to contrast agent; if severe, treat with epinephrine; if known, premedication is indicated with prednisone, diphenhydramine (Benadryl), and H_2 blocker; (b) hypotension: multiple causes include hypovolemia (inadequate hydration, blood loss), reduced cardiac output (ischemia, tamponade, arrhythmia), or severe arteriolar vasodilation [vasovagal reaction (especially with femoral sheath placement), excessive nitrates]; (c) arrhythmias: bradycardia (3%), most often due to vasovagal reaction; conduction disturbances (bundle branch block or complete AV block), prophylactic placement of temporary pacemaker is indicated for RA or rheolytic thrombectomy of right coronary; VT and VF (<0.5%), occurs most commonly from intracoronary contrast injection (especially right coronary artery).

IN HOSPITAL AND AFTER DISCHARGE

Stent Thrombosis

Subacute stent thrombosis occurs in 1% to 2% of procedures [used to be more than 5% before high-pressure balloon inflation and antiplatelet regimens were introduced] and typically results in MI or death. Some evidence suggests clopidogrel nonresponders are at significantly higher risk of stent thrombosis (see *Thromb Haemost* 2003;89:783); however, these data remain preliminary and whether such individuals respond to increased doses of clopidogrel and/or alternative agents requires further study. One study showed stent thrombosis had a 90% incidence of MI and a 17% mortality rate (142,143; see also *J Am Coll Cardiol* 2002;40:1567).

Subacute and *late* stent thrombosis is particularly a problem in the era of DES, as the same agents that inhibit neointimal hyperplasia also slow endothelialization over the stent (see later). For patients who receive DES, the number one predictor of stent thrombosis often is discontinuation of thienopyridine (clopidogrel) therapy (144,145). Additional data have shown that patients with STEMI secondary to stent thrombosis have worse outcomes than those with STEMI from de novo coronary lesions (146).

Restenosis

Restenosis is typically a subacute to chronic phenomenon that occurs anywhere from 2 months to years following PCI, and results from neointimal hyperplasia and vascular remodeling (less commonly progression of atherosclerosis). The incidence within the first year is approximately 30% to 40% for angioplasty alone (up to 50% to 60% for chronic occlusions), 15% to 20% bare-metal for stenting, and as low as 5% for DES (based on the need for repeat revascularization). Risk factors can be categorized as clinical (diabetes, unstable angina, smoking, male gender, hypertension, end-stage renal disease, high cholesterol), anatomic [angiographically visible thrombus (155), aorto-ostial or proximal location, saphenous vein graft, left anterior descending (LAD) artery, chronic occlusion, target-vessel diameter, target-lesion length], or procedural (residual stenosis more than 30%). Some studies have focused on the effect of stent strut thickness on restenosis rates. The ISAR-STEREO and ISAR-STEREO 2 trials (162,163) were randomized studies that found that thin-strut stents had lower rates of restenosis and TVR compared with thick-strut stents. Critics have asserted that potential confounders occur in these studies, such as stent-deployment pressure and other differences in design and mechanical properties of the tested stents. DES have been shown to reduce restenosis rates markedly (see later section).

Renal Dysfunction

Renal dysfunction: 5% have a transient increase in serum creatinine of 1 mg/dL. Risk is increased with excessive contrast dye load (more than 3 mL/kg); other risk factors include: diabetes, advanced age (over 75), peri-procedure dehydration, heart failure, comorbid cirrhosis, nephrosis, hypertension, proteinuria, use of NSAIDs, and intra-arterial injection (see *CMAJ* 2005;172(11):1461–1471; *N Engl J Med* 2006;354:379–386). If baseline creatinine is elevated, adequate pre- and posthydration is clearly beneficial (147). The use of *N*-acetylcysteine (Mucomyst) appears to provide protection in those with baseline renal dysfunction [150,151; also see *N Engl J Med* 2000;343:180; *J Am Coll Cardiol* 2002;40:1383; *Catheter Cardiovasc Interv* 2002;57:279 (no benefit in latter study)]. Fenoldopam, a selective agonist of the dopamine-1 receptor, showed protective benefit in some early studies (see *Am Heart J* 2002;143:894) but no benefit was observed in the randomized, 315 patient CONTRAST study (152). Early data suggested that hydration with sodium bicarbonate may be superior to normal saline (153); however, more recent clinical data have contradicted that finding (154). Finally, cholesterol embolization can cause a late increase in creatinine levels (weeks to months vs. 1 to 2 days with contrast nephropathy), and treatment is supportive, with frank renal failure developing in up to 50%.

Other Postprocedural Complications

Thrombocytopenia can be caused by either heparin (HIT) or GP IIb/IIIa inhibitors (incidence ~1%); if there is a known history of HIT, direct thrombin inhibitors (e.g., hirudin) should be used.

Infection: higher risk with brachial versus femoral approach; some centers administer prophylactic antibiotics when a delayed intervention after sheath exchange is performed.

Vascular complications include femoral or retroperitoneal hematoma, arteriovenous fistula, pseudoaneurysm (142).

Treatment and Prevention of Restenosis

DRUG STUDIES

Numerous therapies have shown no benefit in randomized trials, including aspirin (165), LWMH (167,174,185), subcutaneous (s.c.) UFH (171), abciximab (183), hirudin (170), 3-hydroxy 3-methyl-glutaryl coenzyme A (HMG-CoA) reductase inhibitors (168,175), angiotensin-converting enzyme (ACE) inhibitors, β-blockers (186), calcium-channel blockers (178,184), n-3 fatty acids (182), platelet-derived growth factor antagonists (169), thromboxane antagonists (166,172), nitric oxide donors, antibiotics (187), and antiallergic drugs [e.g., tranilast (188)].

Cilostazol, a platelet aggregation inhibitor (currently approved in the United States for treatment of claudication), also has shown promise in several small studies (179; also see *Int J Cardiol* 2001;78:285–291). In patients with diabetes undergoing PCI, cilostazol (when added to aspirin and clopidogrel) did reduce target-lesion revascularization at 9 months, when compared with only aspirin and clopidogrel (181). However, these findings remain to be validated in larger, broader studies.

RADIATION THERAPY

Intravascular radiation therapy (IVRT) yielded promising results in initial studies of ISR, with restenosis rates typically less than 20%. Gamma radiation sources were used in the Scripps Coronary Radiation to Inhibit Proliferation Post-Stenting (SCRIPPS) trials, Washington Radiation for In-Stent Restenosis Trial (WRIST), and GAMMA trials (189–191,193), whereas beta sources were used in the Beta Energy Restenosis Trial (BERT), BETA-WRIST, INHIBIT, START, and BRITE II trials (198,199,201,202). The LONG WRIST study examined lesions 36 to 80 mm in length and found gamma radiation reduced major cardiac events by one third at 1 year; additional benefit was seen with use of 18 Gy versus 15 Gy (22% vs. 42%, $p <$ 0.05) (196). Data from SVG WRIST demonstrated that the ability of gamma radiation to reduce restenosis also extends to saphenous vein grafts (195). The BRITE SVG trial evaluated beta radiation with a novel device in a small, nonrandomized cohort with good preliminary results (see *Am J Cardiol* 2003;92:312–314).

One issue noted early in the radiation experience was late (more than 1 month) stent thrombosis, which occurred in 6.6% of radiation-treated patients in one study (131). These late events likely occur because radiation delays the healing process. Subsequent studies, such as WRIST and WRIST 12 (192,194), used longer courses of thienopyridine therapy with lower stent thrombosis rates. Current recommendations are to avoid new stenting at the time of brachytherapy (if possible), and to continue dual antiplatelet therapy for at least 6 to 12 months following radiation.

Concern is expressed that radiation will have long-term sequelae including late development of restenosis and aneurysmal dilatation of treated segments. Two-year follow-up data from BERT showed a 15% incidence of restenosis from 6 months to 2 years [four of 30 patients (i.e., small sample size)], whereas no evidence was found of aneurysm or pseudoaneurysm formation (see *Circulation* 2002;106:539).

DRUG-ELUTING STENTS

The most promising development for the prevention of ISR has been the implantation of DES. These stents slowly release drugs that inhibit smooth-muscle cell proliferation, neointimal hyperplasia, and inflammation. Sirolimus (rapamycin) is a naturally occurring macrolide antibiotic that has immunosuppressive properties. It inhibits smooth-muscle cell proliferation and migration by blocking certain aspects of cellular metabolism and thereby preventing mitosis.

The Sirolimus-Eluting Stent in Coronary Lesions (SIRIUS) trial (205) examined the use of this stent in longer lesions (15 to 30 mm) and in a more typical patient population (28% with diabetes, 72% with hyperlipidemia, 70% with hypertension, 37% with previous PCI or CABG surgery). In 8-month angiographic data on the first 400 patients, the sirolimus stent group had only a 2% incidence of ISR versus 31.1% of controls; total in-segment restenosis rates were 9.2% and 32.3%, respectively. The proximal margin findings (similar 5.8% restenosis rates in both groups) suggest that balloon injury in this area is associated with pre/postdilation or stent delivery.

Long-term data were compiled in a 2009 meta-analysis of the four major SES trials (206). In this comparison of the SES to BMS in 1,748 patients who underwent nonemergent PCI, rates of TVR continued to favor SES (15.2% vs. 30.1%, $p <$ 0.0001), with no overall increase in death, MI, or stent thrombosis over 5 years. This stent is also being studied in an even broader array of lesions (SIRIUS excluded ostial lesions, total occlusions, thrombotic lesions), which are currently off-label uses based on the initial FDA approval (see below).

Paclitaxel-eluting stents were the next DES to hit the market. Paclitaxel is a taxane derivative that blocks mitosis by interfering with microtubule function; it is cytotoxic at higher doses. The TAXUS IV trial enrolled 1,314 patients with de novo lesions and compared the paclitaxel stent with an uncoated stent with the primary end point of angiographic follow-up at 9 months (209). Composite clinical end points of cardiac death, MI, or stent thrombosis were equal in the two groups, whereas rates of angiographic restenosis (26.6% for BMS vs. 7.9% for PES, $p <$ 0.001) and TLR (11.3% for BMS vs. 3.0% for PES, $p < 0.001$) were significantly reduced.

Thus, while initial trials may have hinted at improved MACE outcomes for DES, it has become increasingly clear that the major benefit of DES lies in prevention of repeat target-vessel revascularization (TVR); that is, in-stent restenosis is reduced. The second-generation DES has not necessarily led to reductions in deaths or MIs (210).

Importantly, DES were predominantly tested and approved for use in stable CAD in straightforward patient populations who have simple, de novo, short lesions in relatively large vessels. One exception was the TAXUS V trial, which randomized 1,156 patients with complex lesions (longer and narrower than previously studied) to either BMS or PES, often requiring multiple stents (211). At 9 months the primary end point of ischemia-driven TVR was significantly lower in the PES group (8.6% vs. 15.7%, $p < 0.001$). While additional data have yielded good results in alternative lesions and patient populations (e.g, those with diabetes, use in acute STEMI, use for in-stent restenosis), these remain 'off-label' uses of DES (212).

The latest DES on the market include a zotarolimus-eluting stent [ZES (Endeavor)] and an everolimus-eluting stent [EES (Xience, Promus)]. The Endeavor stent was the next to be approved, and demonstrated superiority to BMS in the Endeavor II trial (217); however, it was not superior to SES for angiographic outcomes at 8 months in the ENDEAVOR III trial (218). However, the latest DES to be approved, the Xience EES, has demonstrated superiority in reducing death or MI over first-generation DES in several studies (219). Advantages of the second-generation DES include refined pharmacokinetics of drug delivery from the polymer, and a stent delivery system that many intervention lists prefer.

Several trials of second-generation DES have demonstrated favorable results, particularly the Xience stent, when compared with its first-generation counterparts. In the SPIRIT III trial, use of the EES in 1,002 patients with stable CAD was compared with PES, for intervention in lesions less than 28 mm in length and with reference vessel diameter between 2.5 and 3.75 mm. Major cardiac events (including MI and TVR) were lower in the EES group at 9 months ($p = 0.03$) and 1 year ($p = 0.02$). At follow-up extended to 2 years, a signal of reduced stent thrombosis favoring EES was also detected. These data also seem to be supported by preliminary data from the SPIRIT IV trial.

These stents are now being compared with newer, biodegradable stents, which are resorbed by the body over time. Their advantages are that they provide the immediate scaffolding to maintain patency, can deliver drug to prevent in-stent restenosis, then dissolve over the long term to avoid late complications and imaging distraction. The latest is an everolimus-eluting stent build from a dissolvable polymer (219). Long-term results up to 2 years have demonstrated its safety and efficacy by multiple imaging techniques.

As previously mentioned, drugs released by the stents not only prevent restenosis, but also slow endothelialization of the stent, increasing the risk of stent thrombosis. These concerns led to multiple analyses of long-term data from DES trials. Pooled experience from the early nine trials of PES and SES demonstrated an increase risk of stent thrombosis at one year (216), when compared with their older, BMS counterparts (despite no difference in clinical outcomes at 4 years) (see **Fig. 2.5**). However, other long-term analyses have failed to detect this signal at a statistically significant level (206). It is based on these data and concerns over *late* stent thrombosis that current recommendations are for at least 1 year of dual antiplatelet therapy (aspirin plus thienopyridine) following DES implantation, bleeding risks notwithstanding.

Figure 2.5 • Rates of stent thrombosis, death, MI, and TLR in patients receiving SES (panel A, graphs 1–4) or PES (panel B, graphs 1–4) versus BMS. (From Stone GW, et al. Safety and efficacy of sirolimus-and paclitaxel-eluting coronary stents. *N Engl J Med* 2007;356:998–1008. © *2007 Massachusetts Medical Society. All rights reserved.*)

DIRECTIONAL ATHERECTOMY

Directional coronary atherectomy (DCA) is an effective debulking technique that uses a cutting device to excise atheromas. DCA requires an 8F or 9F sheath, results in frequent distal embolization, and is a difficult technique with a narrow therapeutic window. Eccentric, noncalcified, short lesions in nontortuous vessel segments are ideal lesions.

The Coronary Angioplasty versus Excisional Atherectomy Trial (CAVEAT) I and CAVEAT II (108) both showed that DCA achieved better initial success rates compared with balloon angioplasty within native vessel and saphenous vein graft lesions, respectively. However, the atherectomy groups did not have significantly lower restenosis rates, and the incidence of death and MI was higher. The Optimal Atherectomy Restenosis Study (OARS) and Balloon versus Optimal Atherectomy Trial (BOAT) (110,111) showed lower restenosis rates with atherectomy and similar major complication rates. In the BOAT, directional atherectomy was performed with adjunctive PTCA if indicated.

None of the trials mentioned earlier compared atherectomy with stenting. With the advent of DES, atherectomy as a strategy has waned. Data from the PrE Rapamycin-eluting stent FlExi-CuT (PREFECT) registry demonstrated that DCA prior to bifurcation-lesion stenting may be a reasonable strategy, but there remains a paucity of robust randomized data (112).

ROTATIONAL ATHERECTOMY

RA uses a diamond-coated burr that preferentially ablates atherosclerotic plaque while deflecting away from healthy elastic tissue ("differential cutting"). This technique can facilitate stent delivery and expansion by increasing arterial compliance and lumen diameter in complex, calcified, and diffusely atherosclerotic lesions.

RA was evaluated in the Excimer Laser, Rotational Atherectomy, and Balloon Angioplasty Comparison (ERBAC) trial in patients with type B or C lesions, and the atherectomy group was found to have a better procedural success rate than the balloon angioplasty (PTCA) or excimer laser groups, but the 6-month restenosis rate was higher compared with that observed with PTCA (57% vs. 47%; $p < 0.05$).

After this trial was completed, substantial technical improvements were made, so additional studies were performed. The Study to Determine Rotablator and Transluminal Angioplasty Strategy (STRATAS) randomized 497 patients to aggressive rotablator therapy (70% to 90% burr-to-artery ratio) or standard rotablator (50% to 70% burr-to-artery ratio). At 6 months, no significant differences were observed between the two groups in mean luminal diameter, restenosis, or clinical events. Similar results were seen in the COBRA study (113).

The Rotational Atherectomy Does Not Reduce Recurrent In-Stent Restenosis (ARTIST) study (114) examined the use of RA for the treatment of ISR. The RA and balloon angioplasty (PTCA) group had a higher restenosis at 6 months compared with PTCA alone (65% vs. 51%; $p = 0.039$).

NEWER TECHNIQUES

Thrombectomy

The Possis Angiojet catheter uses high-speed saline jets to generate intense local suction by the Venturi effect, which pulls thrombus into the jets, where it is macerated and then driven down the catheter lumen for external collection. The Vein Graft AngioJet Study randomized 352 patients with angina or MI more than 24 hours before the procedure and thrombus on angiography with intracoronary or graft urokinase (more than 6-hour infusion) or thrombectomy by using the AngioJet system (61). At 30 days, significantly fewer AngioJet patients had experienced MACEs (death, MI, revascularization; 16% vs. 33%; $p < 0.001$). Bradycardia occurred in 24% of those treated with AngioJet and was managed successfully with atropine and temporary pacing.

Additional data on the AngioJet rheolytic device, from the JETSTENT trial, were presented at ACC 2010. Five-hundred and one patients with STEMI and at least modest thrombus burden were randomized to either direct stenting or stenting following AngioJet rheolytic thrombectomy (62). Not only was the primary outcome (ST-segment resolution at 30 minutes) significantly improved in the AngioJet group, but so were clinical adverse cardiac events at 6 months.

Similar data from the TAPAS study support aspiration of thrombus during primary PCI (67). In 1,071 patients undergoing primary PCI, those randomly assigned to thrombus aspiration had more complete ST-segment resolution, improved myocardial blush, and better clinical outcomes in those with better myocardial perfusion grades. In summary, this technique allows rapid thrombus removal and stenting during the same catheterization session, and may be particularly beneficial in patients with acute MI who typically have a high thrombus burden.

Distal Protection

Distal embolization of friable debris is common during SVG interventions, is a main cause of no reflow, and frequently results in CK release. The Saphenous vein graft Angioplasty Free of Emboli Randomized (SAFER) trial (64) randomized 801 patients with a history of angina, evidence of myocardial ischemia, and more than 50% stenosis in the mid-portion of an SVG with a diameter of 3 to 6 mm, to the GuardWire (Medtronic/PercuSurge) balloon occlusion device or a conventional angioplasty guide wire. The embolic protection group had an impressive 42% relative reduction in MACEs at 30 days (9.6% vs. 16.5%; $p = 0.004$). This reduction was due primarily to fewer MIs (8.6% vs. 14.7%; $p = 0.008$) and "no-reflow" (3% vs. 9%; $p = 0.02$). The benefit of the distal protection device was evident both with and without the use of concomitant GP IIb/IIIa–receptor blockers.

Filter devices provide another method of distal protection that permits TIMI 3 flow during the intervention. In the FilterWireEX During Transluminal Intervention of Saphenous Vein Grafts (FIRE) trial, the FilterWireEX device was compared with the GuardWire; 30-day MACE rates were similar (9.9% vs. 11.6%) (65).

However, use of distal protection devices does not provide substantial benefit in urgent PCI, as demonstrated in the Enhanced Myocardial Efficacy and Recovery by Aspiration of Liberated Debris (EMERALD) trial (66). Two-hundred and fifty-two patients with STEMI undergoing primary PCI were randomized to routine PCI or balloon occlusion and aspiration distal microcirculatory protection system during PCI. Despite effectively retrieving embolic debris, the distal protection system did not affect microvascular flow, infarct dimensions, or clinical outcomes. Current recommendations are that distal embolic protection devices be used for SVG interventions, when technically possible.

CORONARY ARTERY BYPASS SURGERY

Risk factors for operative mortality include advanced age, female gender, smoking, left ventricular dysfunction, and the urgency of the operation, as well as anatomic variables.

Saphenous Vein Grafts

From 8% to 12% of SVGs occlude in the early postoperative period (most because of technical factors), and 12% to 20% more occlude in the first year (typically because of intimal proliferation and thrombosis), and then 2% to 4% per year (overall 50% at 10 years). Results of the Post-CABG trial (see Chapter 1) showed a 30% to 40% slowing of graft atherosclerosis with very aggressive low-density lipoprotein (LDL)-lowering therapy (average achieved, LDL 90 mg/dL).

Internal Mammary Artery

The patency rate for the internal mammary artery (IMA) is 85% to 95% at 10 years. Use is associated with improved long-term survival. A 27% lower mortality rate was observed in the Coronary Artery Surgery Study (CASS) registry analysis (248). In another analysis, IMA use was associated with a 40% lower 10-year mortality rate among triple-vessel disease patients (238).

Coronary Artery Bypass Surgery versus Medical Therapy

Three major clinical trials—the European Coronary Surgery Study (ECSS), CASS, and Veterans Administration (VA) study—helped to define the groups of patients that benefit from bypass surgery. These three studies were performed before the common use of the IMA for revascularization. The ECSS enrolled 768 men aged 65 years or younger and found that surgery resulted in improved survival compared with medical therapy. The majority of the benefit was seen in patients with proximal LAD artery stenoses (227). The CASS enrolled 780 patients aged 65 years or younger and found CABG to be associated with a trend toward lower mortality in patients with triple-vessel disease and an ejection fraction of 50% or less (228). Long-term follow-up showed better survival with CABG in patients with left main equivalent disease (severe proximal LAD and left circumflex disease) and left ventricular dysfunction. The VA study found no significant mortality difference between groups at 11-year follow-up, but CABG was beneficial in certain patients subgroups: (a) triple-vessel disease and left ventricular dysfunction, and (b) clinically high-risk patients (at least two of the following: resting ST depression, history of MI, or history of hypertension) (27).

An overview of 2,649 patients from these three trials and four smaller studies showed that CABG was associated with a significantly lower mortality rate at 5 years compared with initial medical management (OR, 0.61), 7 years (OR, 0.68), and 10 years (OR, 0.83) (223). The risk reduction was most marked in patients with left main disease and triple-vessel disease (Ors, 0.32 and 0.58). High-risk patients (defined as those with two of the following: severe angina, history of hypertension, prior MI, and ST-segment depression at rest) had a 29% mortality reduction with CABG at 10 years compared with a nonsignificant trend toward higher mortality in low-risk patients (no severe angina, hypertension, or prior MI). Overall these results demonstrate that patients with more severe coronary disease, poor LV dysfunction, and high-risk clinical characteristics derive a significant benefit from bypass surgery versus medical therapy.

Coronary Artery Bypass Surgery versus Percutaneous Coronary Intervention

The RITA-1, German Angioplasty Bypass Surgery Investigation (GABI), Emory Angioplasty versus Surgery Trial (EAST), Coronary Angioplasty versus Bypass Revascularization Investigation (CABRI), and Estudio Randomizado Argentino de Angioplastia versus Cirugia (ERACI) (230–233) all enrolled stable patients with single- to triple-vessel CAD. Overall they showed no mortality difference between CABG and PTCA groups. CABG patients did have longer hospitalizations, fewer repeated interventions, and better quality of life (e.g., less angina and better functional status) at follow-up. The Bypass Angioplasty Revascularization Investigation (BARI) study enrolled 1,829 patients (41% with triple-vessel CAD); the CABG group had an 85% lower revascularization rate at 5 years, but there was no significant mortality reduction (234). Importantly, a 44% lower rate of mortality ($p = 0.003$) was found among diabetic patients who underwent bypass surgery versus PTCA.

A meta-analysis of eight trials with 3,371 patients published through 1996 (225) showed no significant mortality differences between CABG and PTCA. CABG patients had 90% fewer interventions at 1 year. Only a small proportion of patients screened for these trials (5% to 10%) were actually randomized; thus these findings cannot be readily extrapolated to groups of patients with high-risk characteristics (e.g., left main disease, severe LV dysfunction, chronically occluded vessels). It also is important to note that these trials were completed before the frequent use of stenting.

The Arterial Revascularization Therapy Study (ARTS) (236), which compared stenting with bypass surgery in 1,200 patients with multivessel CAD, found similar rates of adverse outcomes at 30 days [6.8% (surgery) and 8.7% (stenting)] but a significantly lower incidence of repeated revascularization among bypass patients [0.8% vs. 3.7% (at 1 year: 3.5% vs. 16.8%)]. In the Stent or Surgery (SoS) trial, 988 patients with multivessel CAD were randomized to PCI (78% of lesions stented) or CABG. The CABG group had a lower 1-year revascularization rate (5.8% vs. 20.3%), whereas mortality rates were not significantly different (238). ERACI II was a similarly designed study, which enrolled 450 patients and also found a higher revascularization rate in the PCI group [at 18-month follow-up: 16.8% vs. 4.8% (CABG); $p < 0.002$]. However, the PCI group had a significantly lower 30-day and 18-month mortality (0.9% vs. 5.7%; $p < 0.013$; 3.1% vs. 7.5%; $p < 0.017$). A fourth study, the Angina with Extremely Serious Operative Mortality Evaluation (AWESOME), enrolled 554 high-risk VA patients (237). The PCI group had a slightly lower mortality at 30 days and 6 months, but the rates were similar at 3-year follow-up. Once again, the CABG group had a lower revascularization rate (4% vs. 11%). Subsequent meta-analyses of several of the above trials have confirmed the overall comparable safety between surgical and percutaneous approaches, with revascularization rates heavily favoring surgery (240–242) (see **Fig. 2.6**).

While it is reasonable to believe the use of DES will further narrow the gap between multivessel PCI and CABG surgery, this has not yet been observed in large randomized trials. Early data comparing CABG to DES are largely observational registries, and continue to demonstrate revascularization rates heavily favoring CABG. Perhaps the most notable yet comparison of CABG versus DES has been the Synergy between PCI with Taxus and Cardiac Surgery (SYNTAX) trial (246). Investigators prospectively randomized 1,800 patients with left main or triple-vessel CAD to either PCI with DES or CABG, the primary end point being a composite of death, stroke, MI, or repeat revascularization at 12 months. Notably, both an interventional cardiologist and cardiac surgeon were on hand to confirm that equivalent anatomic revascularization could be performed for each patient. Despite differences in medical management that favored the PCI group, outcomes of the primary end point favored CABG at 12 months (17.8 for PCI vs. 12.1 for CABG, $p = 0.0015$) and thus PCI failed the noninferiority test. Notably clinical end points of death or MI were not statistically different between the groups, and stroke rates favored PCI (0.6% for PCI vs. 2.2% for CABG, $p = 0.003$). As expected, the primary end point was driven by a highly significant excess of revascularizations in the PCI group (13.7% for PCI vs. 5.9% for CABG, $p < 0.0001$). The FREEDOM trial will further address this issue in approximately 1,500 patients (sirolimus-coated stenting vs. CABG).

Figure 2.6 • Outcomes of revascularization with either PCI or CABG, including mortality (**A**); death, stroke or MI (**B**); repeat revascularization (**C**); or the composite of death, stroke, MI, or repeat revascularization (**D**). (From Daemen J, Boersma E, Flather M, et al. Long-term safety and efficacy of percutaneous coronary intervention with stenting and coronary artery bypass surgery for multivessel coronary artery disease a meta-analysis with 5-year patient-level. Data from the ARTS, ERACI-II, MASS-II, and SoS Trials. *Circulation*. 2008;118:1146–1154.)

REFERENCES

Guidelines and Classification Articles

1. **Gibson CM,** et al. TIMI frame count. *Circulation* 1996;93:879–888.

This article describes a new method that quantifies coronary artery flow as a continuous variable [vs. assignment to one of four flow grades (i.e., TIMI grade 0, 1, 2, or 3)]. A total of 393 patients (315 TIMI-4 acute MI patients and 78 subjects without MI) were analyzed. The method was found to be reproducible (difference between two injections, 4.7 ± 3.9). Among normal patients, the LAD artery took 1.7 times longer to fill completely than did the right coronary artery and circumflex arteries (36.2 vs. 20.4, 22.2; both $p < 0.001$). After thrombolysis, mean corrected counts (LAD, divided by 1.7) were 39.2 at 90 minutes and 31.7 by 18 to 36 hours ($p < 0.001$); both were higher than those in patients without acute MI.

2. **Zaacks SM,** et al. Value of the ACC/AHA stenosis morphology classification for coronary interventions in the late 1990s. *Am J Cardiol* 1998;82:43–49.

   This prospective analysis was derived from 957 consecutive interventions in 1,404 lesions from June 1994 to October 1996. The overall procedural success rate was 91.9%. No significant differences in success rates were found between type A, B1, and B2 lesions (96.3%, 95.5%, 95.1%), but all were better than type C (88.2%; $p < 0.003$, $p < 0.004$, $p = 0.0001$, respectively). Multiple regression analysis showed that total occlusion and vessel tortuosity were predictive of procedural failure. Lesion type did not predict device use or complications. Actual predictors of complications were bifurcation lesions ($p = 0.0045$), presence of thrombus ($p = 0.0001$), inability to protect a major side branch ($p = 0.0468$), and degenerated vein graft lesions ($p = 0.0283$).

3. **Smith SC Jr,** et al. ACC/AHA/SCAI 2005 guideline update for percutaneous coronary intervention: a report of the American College of Cardiology/American Heart Association Task Force on Practice Guidelines (ACC/AHA/SCAI Writing Committee to Update the 2001 Guidelines for Percutaneous Coronary Intervention). American College of Cardiology Web Site. Available at: http://www.acc.org/clinical/guidelines/percutaneous/ update/index.pdf.

   These comprehensive guidelines discuss everything from the expected outcomes and standards for competency to the indications and medical management for patients undergoing angiography and PCI. They also address state-of-the-art percutaneous adjunctive technology.

4. **King SB III,** et al. 2007 focused update of the ACC/AHA/SCAI 2005 Guideline Update for Percutaneous Coronary Intervention: a report of the American College of Cardiology/American Heart Association Task Force on Practice Guidelines (2007 Writing Group to Review New Evidence and Update the 2005 ACC/AHA/SCAI Guideline Update for Percutaneous Coronary Intervention). *J Am Coll Cardiol* 2008;51:172–209. ACC-AHA-SCAI PCI guidelines.

   This focused update to the aforementioned 2004 guidelines predominantly focuses on invasive strategies for NSTEMI, complicated strategies for STEMI, as well as DES and recommendations for antiplatelet therapies.

5. **Eagle KA,** et al. ACC/AHA 2004 guideline update for coronary artery bypass graft surgery: a report of the American College of Cardiology/American Heart Association Task Force on Practice Guidelines (Committee to Update the 1999 Guidelines for Coronary Artery Bypass Graft Surgery). American College of Cardiology Web Site. Available at: http://www.acc.org/clinical/guidelines/cabg/cabg.pdf.

   In collaboration with the American Association for Thoracic Surgery and the Society of Thoracic Surgeons, the authors review outcomes and complications of surgery, comparisons with medical therapy and percutaneous revascularization, as well as perioperative and postoperative management of patients undergoing CABG. Special populations, such as the elderly, certain co-morbidities, poor LV function, or transplant patients are also discussed. This document is an update to the 1999 guidelines for CABG.

6. **Kushner FG,** et al. 2009 focused updates: ACC/AHA guidelines for the management of patients with STEMI (updating the 2004 guideline and 2007 focused update) and ACC/AHA/SCAI guidelines on percutaneous coronary intervention (updating the 2005 guideline and 2007 focused update): a report of the American College of Cardiology Foundation/American Heart Association Task Force on Practice Guidelines. *J Am Coll Cardiol* 2009;54:2205–2241.

   This most recent update to PCI guidelines predominantly focuses on selection and timing of adjunctive medication administration in patients undergoing PCI, particularly in the urgent/emergent settings of acute STEMI and in early-invasive approaches for UA/NSTEMI. Additionally, the authors amend their recommendations for measurement of FFR, PCI of unprotected left main CAD, as well as stent selection in acute STEMI.

Relation of Operator and Hospital Volume to Outcomes

7. **Jollis JG,** et al. The relation between the volume of coronary angioplasty procedures at hospitals treating Medicare beneficiaries and short-term mortality. *N Engl J Med* 1994;331:1625–1629.

   This analysis was conducted on 218,000 Medicare patients who underwent PTCA from 1987 to 1990. A significant mortality difference was found between the 10% treated at the highest- and lowest-volume (fewer than 50 procedures per year) centers (2.5% vs. 3.9%). A difference in the CABG surgery rate was found (2.8% vs. 5.3%).

8. **Kimmel SE,** et al. The relationship between coronary angioplasty procedure volume and major complications. *JAMA* 1995;274:1137–1142.

   This cohort study showed an association between low hospital volume and increased complications. The cohort consisted of 19,594 non-MI patients undergoing a first PTCA. Higher volume was associated with lower mortality ($p = 0.04$), emergency bypass surgery ($p < 0.001$), and major complications ($p < 0.001$). Multivariate analysis (adjusted for case mix) showed that the associations persisted, but the mortality difference was not significant. No difference was demonstrated in outcomes when comparing hospitals performing 200 versus more than 200 procedures. However, for hospitals performing 400 to 599 and 600 versus fewer than 200 procedures per year, the adjusted ORs for major complications were 0.66 and 0.54 ($p = 0.03; p = 0.001$).

9. **Jollis JG,** et al. Relationship between physician and hospital coronary angioplasty volume and outcome in elderly patients. *Circulation* 1997;95:2485–2491 (editorial, 2467–2470).

   This analysis focused on 97,478 Medicare patients treated by 6,115 physicians at 984 hospitals in 1992. Median procedure volume was only 13 per operator; hospital median was 98. After risk-factor adjustment, low-volume operators were associated with an increased rate of bypass surgery (fewer than 25, 3.8%; 25 to 50, 3.4%; more than 50, 2.6%; $p < 0.001$), and low-volume hospitals were associated with higher bypass surgery and mortality rates (fewer than 100, 3.9%/2.9%; 100 to 200, 3.5%/2.5%; more than 200, 3.0%/2.3%; $p < 0.001$). Improved outcomes were seen with up to 75 and 200 Medicare cases/year, respectively. The accompanying editorial points out that data were acquired in the early stent era and before the use of GP IIb/IIIa inhibition.

10. **Ritchie JL,** et al. Association between percutaneous transluminal coronary angioplasty volumes and outcomes in the Healthcare Cost and Utilization Project 1993–1994. *Am J Cardiol* 1999;83:493–497.

    This analysis of 163,527 procedures from 214 centers demonstrated superior outcomes in high-volume institutions (more than 400 cases/year) compared with low-volume centers (fewer than 200 cases/year).

11. **Ritchie JL,** et al. Coronary artery stent outcomes in a Medicare population: less emergency bypass surgery and lower mortality rates in patients with stents. *Am Heart J* 1999;138:437–440.

    Analysis of Medicare provider data for fiscal years 1994 and 1996. A total of 74,836 stents were placed during 300,000 coronary interventions. In both the conventional angioplasty and stent groups, a hospital volume of more than 200 cases/year was associated with better short-term outcomes.

12. **McGrath PD,** et al. Relation between operator and hospital volume and outcomes following percutaneous coronary interventions in the era of the coronary stent. *JAMA* 2000;284:3139–3144.

Analysis of Medicare patients aged 65 to 99 years who underwent PCI in 1997. Low-volume operators were defined as those who performed fewer than 30 Medicare interventions/year, whereas high-volume operators performed more than 60/year. Low-volume institutions were defined as those performing fewer than 80 Medicare interventions/year, whereas high volume was considered as more than 160/year. The lowest incidence of 30-day mortality and CABG (4.6%) occurred at high-volume hospitals with a high-volume interventionalist, whereas the highest incidence (6.1%) was seen at low-volume hospitals with low-volume interventionalists.

13. **Srinivas VS**, et al. Effect of physician volume on the relationship between hospital volume and mortality during primary angioplasty. *J Am Coll Cardiol* 2009;53:574–9.

Data from 7,321 patients in the New York State PCI Registry for acute MI demonstrated significant variation of outcomes based on physician experience and hospital volumes. Within high-volume hospitals, risk-adjusted mortality was higher for low-volume physicians than for high-volume physicians (OR 0.58, 95% CI, 0.39 to 0.86). While high-volume physicians in high-volume hospitals had a lower unadjusted mortality than low-volume physicians in low-volume hospitals (3.2% vs. 6.7%, $p = 0.03$), after risk adjustment this difference was no longer statistically significant (3.8% vs. 8.4%, $p = 0.09$).

14. **Vogt A**. Hospital mortality from PCI is unrelated to procedural volume. Presented at the European Society of Cardiology 2009 Congress.

Nationwide reporting of all in-patient PCIs in Germany included 236,849 cases in 474 hospitals. Overall in-hospital mortality was 2.2%, and after adjustment for age, gender, STEMI, shock, diabetes, renal failure, heart failure, and left main disease, there was no difference in mortality among hospital stratified by procedure volume. These preliminary data suggest that physician volume is likely more important than the volume of the center where he or she operates. However, caution should be used in applying German data to the US, where low-volume centers are *much* lower volume than those in Germany.

15. **Nallamothu BK,** et al. Relation between hospital specialization with primary percutaneous coronary intervention and clinical outcomes in ST-segment elevation: myocardial infarction national registry of myocardial infarction-4 analysis. *Circulation* 2006;113: 222–229.

The investigators stratified hospitals in NRMI by the proportion of STEMI patients who undergo primary PCI versus thrombolytics, and assessed outcomes based on this stratification. Centers with the highest proportion of patients undergoing primary PCI (>88.5%) had lower in-hospital mortality (adjusted RR 0.64, $p = 0.006$ for highest versus lowest quartiles). These differences did not extend to patients treated with fibrinolytic therapy. Additionally, door-to-balloon time was significantly shorter in the high-percentage-PCI group (99.6 versus 118.3 minutes, $p < 0.001$).

16. **Pride YB**, et al. Outcomes among patients with non–ST-segment elevation myocardial infarction presenting to interventional hospitals with and without on-site cardiac surgery. *JACC Cardiovasc Interv* 2009;2(10):944–952.

In the 100,071 patients with NSTEMI in NRMI from 2004 to 2006, the authors assessed in-hospital mortality in patients treated at hospitals with on-side cardiac surgery versus those without on-side cardiac surgery. In the overall population, irrespective of PCI, in-hospital mortality was significantly lower at centers with surgery (5.0% vs. 8.8%, $p < 0.001$), and patients at these centers were more likely to receive aspirin, beta-blockers, and statins ($p < 0.05$ for all). They were also more likely to undergo PCI at centers with on-side cardiac surgery (38.4% vs. 14.1%, $p < 0.001$); however, in propensity-adjusted analyses (including adjustment for medications and hospital characteristics), differences in mortality were nearly abolished (HR 0.98, $p = 0.050$) and mortality for patients undergoing PCI was nearly identical (1.3% vs. 1.0%, $p = 0.51$).

Technical Aspects

17. **Gruntzig AR,** et al. Nonoperative dilatation of coronary-artery stenosis: percutaneous transluminal coronary angioplasty. *N Engl J Med* 1979;301:61–68.

In this first major report of balloon angioplasty, 50 patients with angina (mean duration, 13 months) underwent angioplasty. All patients received aspirin, 1 g/day for 3 days (starting 1 day before), heparin and dextran during the procedure, and warfarin through follow-up (6 to 9 months). The procedural success rate was 64%. Five patients required CABG surgery, and three had an MI.

18. **Metz D,** et al. Comparison of 6F with 7F and 8F guiding catheters for elective coronary angioplasty: results of a prospective, multicenter randomized trial. *Am Heart J* 1997; 134:131–137.

This study showed that bleeding and procedural complications decreased with the use of 6F catheters. Four-hundred and sixty patients with an ejection fraction of 30% and target lesions that could accommodate a 6F catheter were enrolled. No differences were observed in procedural success rates (87%, 6F; 88%, 7F and 8F) or stenting rates (21%, 6F; 25%, 7F and 8F). The 6F group had approximately 40% fewer femoral access site complications (13.8% vs. 23.5%; $p < 0.01$), had shorter procedure and fluoroscopy times, used less contrast, and had shorter post–sheath removal femoral compression times (11.7 vs. 14.1 minutes; $p < 0.01$).

19. **Sciahbasi A,** et al. Arterial access-site-related outcomes of patients undergoing invasive coronary procedures for acute coronary syndromes (from the PRESTO-ACS vascular substudy). *Am J Cardiol* 2009;103:796–800.

The investigators examined access-related complications in a subset of patients in the PRESTO-ACS study undergoing PCI. All patients underwent PCI for NSTEMI ACS, and there was no difference in clinical events outcomes between those who had PCI via femoral site and those via radial approach (2.9% femoral vs. 2.6% radial, $p = 0.79$). Radial access was associated with less bleeding (2.4% vs. 0.7%, $p = 0.05$); at 1-year follow-up patients who underwent radial approach had significantly lower rates of death or MI (8.3% vs. 4.9%, $p = 0.05$) and bleeding (2.7% vs. 0.7%, $p = 0.03$). It is important to highlight that this is a post hoc analysis of a trial that did *not* randomly assign patients to each access site.

20. **Pristipino C,** et al. Major improvement of percutaneous cardiovascular procedure outcomes with radial artery catheterization: results from the PREVAIL study. *Heart* 2009;95:476–482.

This real-world observational study looked at 1,052 consecutive patients undergoing PCI at nine centers; 509 via radial access and 543 via femoral. The primary end point was a composite of major and minor bleeding, peri-procedural stroke, or access-site complication; a lower rate of such events occurred in the radial-access group (1.96% vs. 4.2%, $p = 0.03$). This result persisted in multivariable analysis (OR 0.37 for radial access, 95% CI, 0.16 to 0.84).

Contrast Agents

21. **Grines CL,** et al. A randomized trial of low osmolar ionic vs nonionic contrast media in patients with MI or unstable angina undergoing percutaneous transluminal coronary angioplasty. *J Am Coll Cardiol* 1996;27:1381–1386 (editorial, 1387–1389).

This randomized study of 211 patients with acute MI or unstable angina showed that the use of ionic low-osmolar contrast media reduced the risk of ischemic complications. Patients received nonionic or ionic low-osmolar contrast media during coronary angiography. The ionic media group had fewer recurrent ischemic events requiring repeated catheterization (3.0% vs. 11.4%; $p = 0.02$) and repeated angioplasty during initial hospitalization (1.0% vs.

5.8%; $p = 0.06$). At 1 month, the ionic contrast group had a reduced need for bypass surgery (none vs. 5.9%; $p = 0.04$) and reported fewer symptoms of any angina or angina at rest (8.5% vs. 20.0%; $p = 0.04$; none vs. 5.9%, $p = 0.04$).

22. **Schrader R,** et al. A randomized trial comparing the impact of nonionic (iomeprol) versus an ionic (ioxaglate) low osmolar contrast medium on abrupt vessel closure and ischemic complications after coronary angioplasty. *J Am Coll Cardiol* 1999;33:395–402.

This prospective, randomized trial was composed of 2,000 patients undergoing PTCA. The frequency of reocclusions requiring repeated intervention was similar in both groups [in laboratory, 2.9% (iomeprol) and 3.0% (ioxaglate); out of laboratory, 3.1% and 4.1%]. Major ischemic complication rates also were similar (emergency CABG, 0.8% and 0.7%; MI, 1.8% and 2.0%; in-hospital cardiac death, 0.2% and 0.2%). The iomeprol group had higher rates of dissection and stenting (31.6% vs. 25.7%, $p = 0.004$; 31.6% vs. 25.7%, $p = 0.004$), whereas allergic reactions requiring treatment occurred only in the ioxaglate group (0.9%; $p = 0.002$).

23. **Davidson CJ,** et al. Randomized trial of contrast media utilization in high-risk PTCA: the COURT trial. *Circulation* 2000:101;2172–2177.

A total of 856 patients undergoing high-risk interventions were randomized to a nonionic iso-osmolar contrast agent (iodixanol) or an ionic low-osmolar contrast agent (ioxaglate). Angiographic success was significantly better in the nonionic contrast patients (92.2% vs. 85.9%; $p = 0.004$). The nonionic contrast group had a significantly lower incidence of the primary composite end point of in-hospital MI, abrupt closure, recatheterization, or emergency revascularization (5.4% vs. 9.5%, $p = 0.027$). The difference persisted in multivariable analyses ($p = 0.01$).

24. **Bertrand ME,** et al. for the Visipaque in PTCA (**VIP**) Investigators. Influence of a non-ionic, iso-osmolar contrast medium (iodixanol) versus an ionic, low-osmolar contrast medium (ioxaglate) on major adverse cardiac events in patients undergoing percutaneous transluminal coronary angioplasty: a multicenter, randomized, double-blind study. *Circulation* 2000;101:131–136.

This prospective, randomized, parallel-group, double-blind study enrolled 1,411 patients. Patients received either iodixanol (a nonionic, iso-osmolar contrast medium) or ioxaglate (an ionic, low-osmolar contrast medium) during PTCA. No significant differences were found between the groups in the incidence of the primary composite end point, consisting of death, stroke, MI, CABG surgery, and repeated PTCA at 2 days (iodixanol, 4.7%; ioxaglate, 3.9%; $p = 0.45$) and at 1 month. However, the iodixanol group had a lower incidence of hypersensitivity reactions ($p = 0.007$) and adverse drug reactions ($p = 0.002$) compared with the ioxaglate group.

25. **Solomon RJ,** et al. Cardiac angiography in renally impaired patients (CARE) study a randomized double-blind trial of contrast-induced nephropathy in patients with chronic kidney disease. *Circulation* 2007;115(25):3189–3196. [Epub 2007 Jun 11].

The investigators performed a multicenter, randomized, double-blind comparison of iopamidol (796 mOsm/kg) and iodixanol (290 mOsm/kg) for patients with chronic kidney disease undergoing coronary angiography. In the 414 patients included, 4.4% in the iopamidol group and 6.7% in the iodixanol group had increases in serum creatinine of ≥5 mg/dL ($p = 0.39$ for the primary outcome); however, in the subgroup of patients with diabetes, such an increase occurred in 5.1% with iopamidol and 13.0% with iodixanol ($p = 0.11$). Though numerically trending in favor of iopamidol, the authors conclude the differences between the two agents are small and unlikely to be clinically significant.

26. **Mehran R,** et al. Ionic low-osmolar versus nonionic iso-osmolar contrast media to obviate worsening nephropathy after angioplasty in chronic renal failure patients: the ICON

(Ionic versus nonionic Contrast to Obviate worsening Nephropathy after angioplasty in chronic renal failure patients) study. *JACC Cardiovasc Interv* 2009;2(5):415–421.

In 146 patients with renal impairment (and at high-risk for contrast-induced nephropathy), the authors randomized each to iodixanol (nonionic iso-osmolar) or ioxaglate (ionic, low-osmolar), and compared median peak increase of serum creatinine from day 0 to day 3 after angiography. This primary end point did not differ between the two groups (0.09 mg/dL for iodixanol vs. 0.15 mg/dL for ioxaglate, $p = 0.07$). However, the authors cautioned that the use of medical-protective therapies (*n*-acetylcysteine) may have dampened any difference between agents, and larger studies are still needed.

Lesion Evaluation (Fractional Flow Reserve, Intravascular Ultrasound)

27. **Pijls NHJ,** et al. Measurement of fractional flow reserve to assess the functional severity of coronary-artery stenoses. *N Engl J Med* 1996;334:1703–1708.

A total of 45 consecutive patients with chest pain and a moderate coronary stenosis of approximately 50% underwent bicycle testing, thallium scintigraphy, dobutamine stress echocardiography, and coronary arteriography. In all patients (21) with an FFR less than 0.75, reversible ischemia was evident on at least one noninvasive test. After revascularization was performed (PTCA or CABG surgery), all positive test results reverted to normal. In contrast, 21 of 24 patients with an FFR of 0.75 or more tested negative for reversible ischemia on all the noninvasive tests. None of these patients underwent revascularization through 14 months of follow-up. The sensitivity of FFR in detecting reversible ischemia was 88%, specificity was 100%, positive predictive value was 100%, negative predictive value was 88%, and the accuracy was 93%.

28. **Fitzgerald PJ,** et al. Final results of the Can Routine Ultrasound Influence Stent Expansion (**CRUISE**) Study. *Circulation* 2000;102:523–530.

A total of 522 patients from 16 of 45 centers in the STARS were enrolled in this IVUS substudy to determine if IVUS-assisted stenting results in better outcomes when compared with angiography-assisted stenting. At 9 months, the IVUS-guided group had a larger MLD (2.9 mm vs. 2.7 mm; $p < 0.001$), a lower residual diameter stenosis (7.6% vs. 9.8%; $p < 0.001$), and higher final balloon size and inflation pressure (3.88 mm vs. 3.69 mm, and 18.0 atm vs. 16.6 atm; both $p < 0.001$). The IVUS group had a significantly lower TVR rate (8.5% vs. 15.3%; $p < 0.05$), whereas no differences were found in death or MI rates. Additional therapy based on IVUS information was used in 36% of patients (higher pressures in 59%, larger balloons in 33.7%, and an additional stent in 7%). In summary, IVUS-guided stent deployment results in improved stent expansion and a lower TVR compared with angiographic guidance alone.

29. **Bech GJW,** et al. Fractional flow reserve to determine the appropriateness of angioplasty in moderate coronary stenosis. *Circulation* 2001;103:2928–2934.

This study of 325 scheduled to undergo PTCA of a more than 50% native coronary artery stenosis in a larger than 2.5-mm vessel examined whether deferring PTCA, based on FFR of 0.75 or more, is safe and as least efficacious as performing PTCA. Patients were excluded if they had evidence of reversible ischemia in the previous 2 months. FFR was less than 0.75 for 144 patients, who underwent routine PTCA (reference group). Another 181 patients had an FFR of 0.75 or more and were randomized to optimal intervention (performance group) or medical therapy (deferral group) in a 1:1 fashion. Primary end point was absence of adverse cardiac events at 2 years, consisting of death, MI, PTCA, and any procedure-related complication requiring major intervention. At 2 years, event-free survival was significantly higher in the performance and deferral groups (83% and 89%) compared with the reference group (78%). The performance and deferral groups had similar rates of freedom from angina (50% vs. 49% at 1 year and 51% vs. 70% at 2 years), whereas the incidence was significantly higher in the reference group (67% at 1 year and 80% at 2 years).

30. **Bishop AH,** et al. Fractional flow reserve: critical review of an important physiologic adjunct to angiography. *Am Heart J* 2004;147(5):792–802.

The authors review the assessment of FFR, how its measurement is affected by factors other than epicardial disease (microvascular disease, LVH, diabetes, etc.), as well as its use for assessing outcomes after stenting. Additionally, the authors discuss how the FFR can be used to "triage" the most appropriate lesions for stenting.

31. **Christou MA,** et al. Meta-analysis of fractional flow reserve versus quantitative coronary angiography and noninvasive imaging for evaluation of myocardial ischemia. *Am J Cardiol* 2007;99(4):450–456. [Epub 2006 Dec 20].

A compilation of 31 studies comparing lesion assessment with FFR versus QCA and/or noninvasive imaging. The investigators assign sensitivity and specificity for each technique, as well as receiver–operator curves. The authors conclude that quantitative angiography does not predict functional stenosis, as predicted by FFR or dobutamine stress echocardiography.

32. **Tonino PAL,** et al. for the FAME Study Investigators. Fractional flow reserve versus angiography for guiding percutaneous coronary intervention. *N Engl J Med* 2009; 360(3):213–224.

Investigators from 20 centers randomized 1,005 patients with multivessel CAD to undergo PCI with routine angiography guiding DES placement, versus that guided by FFR along with angiography. Lesions initially identified for stenting on angiography were only stented in the FFR group if the FFR was 0.80 or less and the primary end point was a composite of death, MI, or repeat revascularization at 1 year. This occurred in 18.3% of patients in the angiography group, versus 13.2% in the FFR group ($p = 0.02$); additionally, the number of stents used was lower in the FFR group (2.7 vs. 1.3, $p < 0.001$), though the number of lesions stented was similar (2.7 vs. 2.8, $p = 0.34$). In this contemporary trial involving patients with multivessel diseases receiving DES, using FFR to guide stent placement not only reduced the number of stents used, but also improved clinical outcomes at 1 year.

33. **Mudra H,** et al. for the **OPTICUS** (OPTimization with ICUS to reduce stent restenosis) Study Investigators. Randomized comparison of coronary stent implantation under ultrasound or angiographic guidance to reduce stent restenosis (OPTICUS Study). *Circulation* 2001;104:1343–1349.

Prospective, randomized trial of 550 patients with a symptomatic coronary lesion or silent ischemia. Patients were assigned to either IVUS-guided or angiography-guided implantation of two or fewer stents. At 6-month angiography, no significant differences were seen between the two groups in MLD [1.95 mm (IVUS guided) vs. 1.91 mm] or restenosis rate (24.5% vs. 22.8%). At 1 year, the groups also had similar incidences of MACEs and repeated PCI.

34. **Chamuleau SA.** Prognostic value of coronary blood flow velocity and myocardial perfusion in intermediate coronary narrowings and multivessel disease. *J Am Coll Cardiol* 2002;39:852–858.

Prospective, multicenter study of 191 patients with stable angina and multivessel disease scheduled for PTCA. CFVR was measured distal to an intermediate lesion in another artery by using a Doppler guide wire. PTCA of the intermediate lesion was deferred when SPECT was negative or CFVR of 2.0 or more. Reversible perfusion defects were documented in the area of the intermediate lesion in 16%, whereas CFVR was positive in 24%. PTCA of the intermediate lesion was deferred in 182 patients. At 1-year follow-up, CFVR was a more accurate measure of major cardiac events than was SPECT; multivariate analysis showed CFVR as the only significant predictor for cardiac events.

35. **Albertal M,** et al. for the Doppler Endpoints Balloon Angioplasty Trial Europe (**DEBATE**) **II** Study Group. Coronary flow velocity reserve after percutaneous interventions is predictive of periprocedural outcome. *Circulation* 2002;105:1573–1578.

A total of 379 DEBATE II study patients underwent Doppler flow–guided angioplasty. CFVR measured before PTCA and CFVR in the reference artery were independent predictors of an optimal CFVR (2.5 or more) after balloon angioplasty. A low CFVR (<2.5) at the end of the procedure was an independent predictor of MACEs at 30 days (OR, 4.71; $p = 0.034$) and at 1 year (OR, 2.06; $p = 0.014$). After excluding MACE at 30 days, no difference in MACE at 1 year was observed between the patients with and without a CFVR less than 2.5 at the end of the procedure.

Comparison of Revascularization with Medical Therapy

36. **Parisi AF,** et al. Angioplasty compared to medicine (**ACME**): a comparison of angioplasty with medical therapy in the treatment of single-vessel coronary artery disease. *N Engl J Med* 1992;326:10–16.

Design: Prospective, randomized, multicenter study. Primary end point was changed in exercise tolerance, frequency of angina attacks, and nitroglycerin use.
Purpose: To compare medical therapy with balloon angioplasty in patients with one significant coronary artery stenosis.
Population: 212 patients with a single 70% to 99% stenosis.
Treatment: The drug therapy group included oral isosorbide dinitrate with sublingual glyceryl trinitrate and/or β-blockers and/or calcium antagonists. The balloon angioplasty group was given calcium antagonists before and for 1 month after the procedure, and heparin and glyceryl trinitrate during and until 12 hours after the procedure. All patients received aspirin, 325 mg orally daily.
Results: Balloon angioplasty (PTCA) was successful in 80% and reduced stenoses from 76% to 36%. The PTCA group had less angina (64% vs. 46%; $p < 0.01$), better exercise performance [+2.1 minutes (6 months vs. baseline exercise test) vs. +0.5 minutes; $p < 0.0001$], and more improvement in quality-of-life score (+8.6 units vs. +2.4 units; $p = 0.03$). However, the PTCA group did have more complications [emergency bypass surgery in two patients, MIs in five (vs. three), and repeated PTCA in 16].

37. **Folland ED,** et al. VA Angioplasty Compared to Medicine (**VA ACME**). Percutaneous transluminal coronary angioplasty vs medical therapy for stable angina pectoris. *J Am Coll Cardiol* 1997;29:1505–1511.

Design: Prospective, randomized, double-blind, multicenter study.
Purpose: To compare balloon angioplasty with medical therapy in patients with documented coronary disease and chronic stable angina.
Population: 328 patients with stable angina and positive exercise treadmill test; 101 patients had two-vessel disease ($\geq$70% stenosis in proximal two thirds), and 227 had single-vessel disease.
Exclusion Criteria: Medically refractory unstable angina, prior coronary revascularization, ejection fraction $\leq$30%.
Treatment: Medical therapy or balloon angioplasty.

Results: Among two-vessel patients, no significant changes were found between treatment groups in exercise treadmill test duration (performed at 2 to 3 years), or freedom from angina and quality of life. However, fewer angioplasty patients had improved perfusion imaging results (59% vs. 75%) and higher average stenosis of worst lesions (74% vs. 56%). Among single-vessel disease patients, the angioplasty group had more improvement in exercise time (+2.1 vs. +0.6 minutes; $p < 0.001$) and quality-of-life score (+7.1 vs. +1.5; $p = 0.01$), and were more angina free (63% vs. 48%; $p = 0.02$).

38. Randomized Intervention Treatment of Angina (**RITA**-2) Trial participants. Coronary angioplasty vs medical therapy for angina: the RITA-2 trial. *Lancet* 1997;350:461–468.

Design: Prospective, randomized, double-blind, multicenter study. Primary end point was death and nonfatal MI. Follow-up period was 2.7 years.

Purpose: To compare the effects of coronary angioplasty and conservative medical care in patients considered suitable for either treatment.

Population: 1,018 patients, 53% with grade 2 angina, 47% with prior MI, only 7% with three-vessel disease.

Exclusion Criteria: Unstable angina in prior 7 days, left main CAD, early revascularization necessary or planned.

Treatment: Medical therapy or balloon angioplasty (in the latter group, the procedure was performed in 93% at a median of 5 weeks).

Results: Angioplasty group had increased rates of death and MI (6.3% vs. 3.3%; $p = 0.02$). Benefit was attributable mostly to procedure-related events. However, the PTCA group had 7% less grade 2 angina at 2 years and longer exercise treadmill test time at 3 months (+35 seconds; $p < 0.001$).

39. **Boden WE,** et al. for the COURAGE Trial Research Group. Optimal medical therapy with or without PCI for stable coronary disease. *N Engl J Med* 2007;356:1503–1516.

Design: Prospective, randomized, multicenter trial. Primary outcome was a combined incidence of death or nonfatal MI at a median of 4.6 years of follow-up.

Purpose: To assess the advantage of stenting over optimal medical therapy to prevent clinical events in patients with stable CAD.

Population: A total of 2,287 patients with significant coronary disease (>70% stenosis of at least 1 epicardial vessel) and objective signs of ischemia (on ECG or by stress), without unstable angina.

Treatment: Patients were randomized to optimal medical therapy alone or in combination with revascularization by stenting. Optimal medical therapy included dual antiplatelet therapy in patients with stents, as well as long-acting metoprolol, amlodipine, isosorbide mononitrate, aggressive lipid lowering (to a goal LDL of 60 to 85 mg/dL), inhibitors of renin–angiotensin system, and additional HDL-raising therapy. In the group undergoing PCI, few received DES, as they were not approved until the final 6 months of the study.

Results: There was no statistical difference in the number of primary end points in the two groups (19.0% in the PCI group vs. 18.5% in the medical-therapy group, $p = 0.62$). This was true when stroke was added to the end point, as well as for comparisons of rates of hospitalizations for ACS or MI. There was a significantly higher rate of revascularization (PCI or CABG) procedures in the medical-therapy group (32.6% for the medical-therapy group vs. 21.1% for the PCI group, $p < 0.001$).

Comments: This pivotal study attempted to address the goals of stenting in patients with stable, fixed coronary disease. Significant caveats are that (a) few patients received DES and (b) patients were only randomized *after* their angiogram was done and viewed by the enrolling investigators (a potential source of significant enrollment bias). However, the trial does lend support to the idea that it is not the tight lesions identified at angiography that are rupturing to cause acute MIs.

Stent Studies

STENTING COMPARED WITH PTCA

40. **Fischman DL,** et al. Stent Restenosis Study (**STRESS**). A randomized comparison of coronary-stent placement and balloon angioplasty in the treatment of coronary artery disease. *N Engl J Med* 1994;331:496–501.

Design: Prospective, randomized, open-label, multicenter study. Primary end point was angiographic restenosis.

Purpose: To compare the results of elective balloon angioplasty with PS stent implantation on clinical outcomes and restenosis in patients with de novo coronary lesions.

Population: 410 patients with de novo 70% stenotic lesions ≤15 mm long and in vessels with a diameter of ≥3 mm.

Exclusion Criteria: MI in previous 7 days, EF less than 40%, diffuse coronary or left main artery disease, and angiographic evidence of thrombus.

Treatment: Balloon angioplasty or PS stent. All patients received aspirin, 325 mg daily. Stented patients received dextran (started 2 hours before the procedure); heparin, 10,000 to 15,000 U before the procedure and infusion for 4 to 6 hours after sheath removal; dipyridamole, 75 mg three times daily for 1 month; and warfarin for 1 month.

Results: Stent group had better procedural success (96.1% vs. 89.6%; $p = 0.011$), greater increase in lumen diameter (1.7 mm vs. 1.2 mm; $p < 0.001$; at 6 months, 1.56 mm vs. 1.24 mm; $p < 0.01$), and a lower rate of restenosis at 6 months (31% vs. 42%; $p = 0.046$). No significant difference in early clinical events (days 0 to 14) was observed between the two groups (19.5% vs. 23.8%). The stent group had a nonsignificant reduction in revascularization rate (10% vs. 15%; $p = 0.06$). At 1-year follow-up, 154 (75%) patients assigned to stent implantation and 141 (70%) to PTCA were free of all clinical events (death, MI, or any revascularization procedure).

Comments: The 1-year cost analysis showed the cost of stenting to be $800 more per patient despite lower costs during follow-up.

41. **Benestent I,** Serruys PW, et al. A comparison of balloon-expandable stent implantation with balloon angioplasty in patients with coronary artery disease. *N Engl J Med* 1994;331:489–495.

Design: Prospective, randomized, multicenter study. Primary end point was death, stroke, MI, CABG, or need for repeated percutaneous intervention during hospitalization.

Purpose: To compare elective balloon angioplasty with PS stenting in patients with stable angina and de novo coronary lesions.

Population: 520 patients aged 30 to 75 years with stable angina and one de novo coronary lesion shorter than 15 mm and in vessel larger than 3 mm in diameter.

Treatment: Balloon angioplasty or PS stenting. All patients received aspirin, 250 to 500 mg/day, and dipyridamole, 75 mg three times daily (started 1 day before procedure and continued for more than 6 months); heparin, 10,000 U was given before the procedure. Stented patients received dextran, 1,000 mL over 6 to 8 hours, and then warfarin for 3 months (target international normalized ratio, 2.5 to 3.5).

Results: No differences were observed between groups in incidence of death, stroke, MI, or subsequent revascularization during index hospitalization, and no differences were observed in composite end point of in-hospital clinical events (6.2% and 6.9%). At 7 months, the stent group had a significant reduction in primary composite end point (20.1% vs. 29.6%; $p = 0.02$), with the majority of this difference attributed to fewer second angioplasties (10% vs. 20.6%; $p = 0.001$). The stent group had more vascular complications (13.5% vs. 3.1%; $p < 0.001$) and longer hospital stays (8.5 vs. 3.1 days; $p = 0.001$). The 1-year follow-up data showed similar rates of death, stroke, MI, and CABG, but the stent group had 26% fewer primary end points (23% vs. 31%; $p = 0.04$), primarily because of approximately 50%

fewer repeated PTCAs (10% vs. 21%; $p = 0.001$). At 5-year follow-up, the stent group still had an approximate 10% absolute lower incidence of TVR (17.2% vs. 27.3%; $p = 0.008$; see *J Am Coll Cardiol* 2001;37:1598–1600).

Comments: Results suggest that stenting reduces repeated interventions but not major clinical events. Longer hospital stay with stenting was attributable to the aggressive antithrombotic regimen.

42. **Benestent II,** Serruys PW, et al. for the Benestent Study Group. Randomised comparison of heparin-coated stents with balloon angioplasty in selected patients with coronary artery disease (Benestent II). *Lancet* 1998;352:673–681.

Design: Prospective, randomized, double-blind, multicenter study. Primary end point was death, MI, and need for revascularization at 6 months.

Purpose: To compare elective balloon angioplasty with heparin-coated PS stents in patients with de novo coronary artery lesions.

Population: 827 patients with stable angina or stabilized unstable angina with one or more de novo lesions longer than 18 mm and in vessels ≥3 mm in diameter.

Exclusion Criteria: Left main disease, lesion at bifurcation with side-branch diameter greater than 2.0 mm, ejection fraction less than 30%, and MI in prior 7 days.

Treatment: Heparin-coated stents (10, 15, or 20 mm) or balloon angioplasty, and 1:1 subrandomization to clinical or angiographic follow-up. Stent patients received ticlopidine, 250 mg twice daily for 1 month.

Results: Stent group had an approximately one-third lower incidence of primary end point (12.8% vs. 19.3%; $p = 0.013$). The 30-day stent thrombosis rate was only 0.2%. In the subgroup undergoing angiographic follow-up, stented patients had a larger mean lumen diameter (1.89 mm vs. 1.66 mm; $p = 0.0002$) and less restenosis (16% vs. 31%; $p = 0.0008$). In the group assigned to clinical follow-up, the stent group had superior 1-year event-free survival [89% vs. 79%; $p = 0.004$ (RRs: cardiac events, 0.66; TVR, 0.60)]. The stent group patients with angiographic follow-up underwent 2.5 times more interventions (13.5% vs. 5.4%) than did clinical follow-up patients, whereas this ratio was only 1.5 among balloon angioplasty patients (18.7% vs. 12.4%).

43. **Betriu A,** et al. Randomized comparison of coronary stent implantation and balloon angioplasty in the treatment of de novo coronary artery lesions (**START**): a four-year follow-up. *J Am Coll Cardiol* 1999;34:1498–1506.

Design: Prospective, randomized, multicenter study. Primary end points were the rate of restenosis at 6 months and a composite of death, MI, and TVR at 4 years of clinical follow-up.

Purpose: To evaluate whether stent implantation in de novo coronary artery lesions would result in lower restenosis rates and better long-term clinical outcomes than balloon angioplasty.

Population: 452 patients with either stable or unstable angina.

Treatment: Stent implantation (229 patients) or standard balloon angioplasty (223 patients). Stent patients received aspirin, dipyridamole, dextran, calcium channel blocker, heparin, and warfarin; after the first 100 stents, oral ticlopidine replaced dextran, dipyridamole, and warfarin.

Results: Procedural success rate was achieved in 84% and 95% of angioplasty and stent patients, respectively. At 6 months, the stent group had a lower restenosis compared with the angioplasty group (22% vs. 37%; $p < 0.002$). At 4 years, no differences were found in mortality or nonfatal MI between the two groups. However, the stent group had a lower TVR rate (12% vs. 25% in the angioplasty group; $p = 0.0006$). Most of the repeated procedures (84%) were performed within 6 months.

44. **Witkowski A,** et al. on behalf of **AS** (Angioplasty or Stent) trial investigators. A randomized comparison of elective high-pressure stenting with balloon angioplasty: six-month angiographic and two-year clinical follow-up. *Am Heart J* 2000;140:264–271.

Design: Prospective, randomized, single-blind, multicenter study. Primary end points were restenosis at 6 months and event-free survival at 2 years.

Purpose: To determine whether routine high-pressure stenting with an antiplatelet regimen can show similar results.

Population: 400 patients with CCS class I to IV angina, single de novo lesion more than 50% and less than 15-mm length, and vessel diameter 2.5 mm or more.

Exclusion Criteria: Acute or recent MI, contraindication(s) to heparin, aspirin, or ticlopidine; left main lesions, bifurcation lesion, total occlusion.

Treatment: Balloon angioplasty or PS 153 stent using 14 atm or more after predilatation of target lesion. All received aspirin, 300 mg/day, and ticlopidine, 250 mg twice daily, started 2 or more days before the procedure and continued for 1 month.

Results: At 6 months, a trend toward a lower incidence of restenosis was found in the stent group (18.2% vs. 24.0%; $p = 0.055$). At 2 years, the stent group had a higher event-free survival rate compared with the angioplasty group (83.1% vs. 73.5%; $p = 0.017$). This difference was driven by a lower TVR rate in the stent group (17.2% vs. 25.5% in the angioplasty group; $p = 0.02$), whereas no significant differences were seen in the incidence of death or MI between the groups.

PROVISIONAL STENTING

45. **Weaver WD,** et al. Optimum percutaneous transluminal coronary angioplasty compared with routine stent strategy trial **(OPUS-1)**: a randomised trial. *Lancet* 2000;355:2199–2203.

Design: Prospective, randomized, open, multicenter study. Primary end point was death, MI, and TVR at 6 months.

Purpose: Whether routine implantation of coronary stents is the best strategy to treat flow-limiting coronary stenoses is unclear. An alternative approach is to do balloon angioplasty and provisionally use stents only to treat suboptimal results. The multicenter trial compared the outcomes of patients treated with these strategies.

Population: 479 patients aged 21 to 81 years with stable or unstable angina or MI more than 24 hours earlier and 70% coronary artery stenosis (≤ 2 mm length, vessel diameter ≥ 3 mm).

Treatment: Systematic stenting or provisional stenting (undertaken if greater than 20% residual stenosis, impending abrupt closure, ≥ 2 mm stenosis, or flow-limiting dissection). IVUS was used at the physician's discretion. Abciximab was used in fewer than 15% of patients. All patients received aspirin and ticlopidine.

Results: Stents were implanted in 98.7% of the routine stenting group, whereas 37% of patients assigned to initial PTCA had more than one stent placed because of suboptimal angioplasty results. At 6 months, the primary stenting group had a significantly lower incidence of death, MI, or TVR (6.1% vs. 14.9%; $p = 0.003$). The majority of this benefit was owing to a lower TVR rate (4% vs. 10%; $p = 0.007$). The provisional stent group had higher initial costs, but the overall costs at 6 months were similar in both groups.

46. **Lafont A,** et al. The French Randomized Optimal Stenting Trial **(FROST)**: a prospective evaluation of provisional stenting guided by coronary velocity reserve and quantitative coronary angiography. *J Am Coll Cardiol* 2000;36:404–409.

Design: Prospective, randomized, open, multicenter study. Primary end point was the 6-month angiographic MLD.

Purpose: To compare systematic stenting with provisional stenting guided by Doppler measurements of coronary velocity reserve and QCA.

Population: 251 patients undergoing elective PTCA.

Treatment: Provisional stenting (stenting performed if post-PTCA coronary velocity reserve was less than 2.2 and/or residual stenosis 35% or more or as bailout) or to systematic stenting.

Results: Stenting was performed in 48.4% of the provisional stenting group and all systematic stenting patients. At 6 months, no significant differences were found between the groups in

MLD [1.90 mm (provisional) vs. 1.99 mm; $p = 0.39$] or binary restenosis rate (27.1% vs. 21.4%; $p = 0.37$). The rates of TLR and MACEs (death, acute MI, and TLR) were similar in both groups (15.1% vs. 14.4%; 15.1% vs. 16.0%).

47. **Serruys PW,** on behalf of Doppler Endpoints Balloon Angioplasty Trial Europe (**DEBATE) II** Study Group. Randomized comparison of primary stenting and provisional balloon angioplasty guided by flow velocity measurement. *Circulation* 2000;102: 2930–2937.

Design: Prospective, randomized, double-blind, multicenter study. Primary end point was death, nonfatal MI, and TLR.

Purpose: To determine if provisional stenting is as effective as and less expensive than primary stenting.

Population: 620 patients scheduled to undergo angioplasty for stable or unstable angina pectoris and with documented myocardial ischemia due to a single de novo lesion shorter than 25 mm.

Exclusion Criteria: MI in prior week, total occlusion, ostial or bifurcation lesions, vessel with target lesion previously bypassed, vessel tortuous or containing thrombus.

Treatment: Primary stenting or balloon angioplasty guided by Doppler flow velocity and angiography. Patients in the latter group were further randomized after optimization to either additional stenting or termination of the procedure. Optimal result defined as flow reserve greater than 2.5 and diameter stenosis 35% or greater.

Results: Bailout stenting occurred in 25% of patients in the balloon angioplasty group. No differences were found between the two groups in event-free survival at 1 year (primary stenting, 86.6%; provisional angioplasty, 85.6%). Costs at 1 year were higher in the provisional angioplasty group (EUR 6573 vs. EUR 5885; $p = 0.014$), primarily because of longer hospitalizations and higher rate of surgical revascularization. After the second randomization, stenting was associated with better 1-year event-free survival after both optimal balloon angioplasty (93.5% vs. 84.1%; $p = 0.066$) and suboptimal balloon angioplasty (89.3% vs. 73.3%; $p = 0.005$).

Comments: An unexpected observation was a further reduction in MACEs in patients stented after optimal balloon angioplasty.

48. **Di Mario C,** et al. Randomized comparison of elective stent implantation and coronary balloon angioplasty and intracoronary Doppler. *Circulation* 2000;102:2938–2944.

Design: Prospective, randomized, double-blind, multicenter study. Primary end point was a composite of death, MI, and TLR at 1 year.

Purpose: To compare the outcomes of balloon angioplasty with provisional stenting with primary stenting.

Population: 738 patients with lesions suitable for stent implantation.

Exclusion Criteria: Recent MI (24 hours or less), prior MI with akinesis or dyskinesis in target-vessel territory, chronic total occlusion, graft and ostial stenoses, second restenosis after PTCA, stent restenosis, planned rotational or directional atherectomy.

Treatment: Elective stent implantations (370 patients, 386 lesions) or PTCA guided by QCA and Doppler CFR analysis (368 patients, 384 lesions). Balloon angioplasty result was considered "optimal" if the final lesion diameter by QCA was less than 35%; no type C through F dissections were found, and CFR distal to the stenosis was greater than 2.0.

Results: Optimal PTCA was achieved in 166 (43%) lesions. The main reasons for suboptimal PTCA were CFR 2.0 or less (62% cases) and significant residual stenosis (44% of cases). At 1 year, no significant difference was found in the primary composite end point of death, MI, and TLR (17.8% in elective stent group and 18.9% in guided PTCA group). When compared with provisional stenting, *optimal* PTCA was associated with a similar incidence of TLR (17.6% vs. 14.1% for provisional stenting; $p = $ NS) and death, MI, and TLR (20.1% and 18.0%, respectively; $p = $ NS).

Comments: Optimal PTCA achieved only in 43% of cases. Capacity to measure CFR is not available in every interventional laboratory, and it requires both operator and laboratory experience.

DIRECT STENTING

49. **Brito FS Jr,** et al. for The **DIRECT** Study Investigators. Comparison of direct stenting versus stenting with predilation for the treatment of selected coronary narrowings. *Am J Cardiol* 2002;89:115–120.

This prospective, multicenter trial randomized 411 patients to direct stenting or balloon predilatation followed by stent implantation. Lesions with severe calcification were excluded. Angiographic success rates were 100% with direct stenting (2.8% requiring balloon predilatation) and 98.6% with routine predilatation ($p = 0.12$). Direct stenting was associated with decreased use of balloons and a trend toward reduced procedure time (22.7 vs. 25.6 minutes; $p = 0.07$). Fluoroscopy time and contrast volume were not different between groups. At 6 months, mortality, MI, and TVR rates were similar in both groups. MACE-free survival rates were 87.5% for direct stenting and 85.5% for the predilatation group ($p = 0.0002$ for equivalence).

50. **Brueck M,** et al. Direct coronary stenting versus predilatation followed by stent placement. *Am J Cardiol* 2002;90:1187–1192.

This prospective, randomized study enrolled 335 symptomatic patients with single or multiple coronary lesions (severity, 60% to 95%; length, 30 mm or shorter; diameter, 2.5 to 4.0 mm). Lesion exclusion criteria: excessive calcification, severe proximal tortuosity, occlusion. Patients were assigned to direct stenting or stenting after predilatation. In the direct stent group, there was a 5% crossover rate to predilatation. Direct stenting was associated with shorter procedural time (42.1 vs. 51.5 minutes; $p = 0.004$), less radiation exposure time (10.3 vs. 12.5 minutes; $p = 0.002$), less contrast dye used (163 vs. 197 mL; $p < 0.0001$), and lower procedural costs. In-hospital complication rates were similar. At 6 months, direct stenting was associated with a lower rate of angiographic binary restenosis (20% vs. 31%; $p = 0.048$) and target-lesion revascularization (18% vs. 28%; $p = 0.03$).

51. **TRENDS** (Tetra Randomized European Direct Stenting). Preliminary results presented at the Transcatheter Cardiovascular Therapeutics meeting, Washington, DC September 2002.

This prospective, randomized, multicenter trial of 941 patients showed that direct stenting and stenting with predilatation yield comparable angiographic and clinical results. Both treatment groups had similar characteristics, with eccentric and type B lesions predominating. Exclusion criteria included chronic occlusions and unprotected left main stenoses. Only 5.7% of patients in the direct-stenting group crossed over to predilatation; this was because of failure to cross the target lesion in 25 of 31 cases. At 6-month angiography, no difference was found between the groups in MLD [2.91 mm (direct stenting) vs. 2.95 mm] or binary restenosis (11.6% vs. 11.4%). Resource use was less with the direct-stent approach, including shorter procedure time (34.3 minutes vs. 37.5 minutes; $p = 0.01$) and less contrast use (175 mL vs. 186 mL; $p = 0.05$). No significant difference was found between the groups in death, MI, and TLR (7.1% vs. 8.8%).

Bare-metal Stent versus Stent Studies

52. **Lansky AJ,** et al. Randomized comparison of GR-II stent and Palmaz–Schatz stent for elective treatment of coronary stenoses. *Circulation* 2000;102:1364–1368.

This prospective study randomized 755 patients to either Gianturco-Robin (GR)-II or PS stent implantation. At 30 days, the composite MACE rate was significantly higher in the

GR-II group compared with the PS group (4.2% vs. 1.3%; $p < 0.01$). This difference was mostly owing to more frequent subacute stent thrombosis in the GR-II group (3.9% vs. 0.3%; $p = 0.001$). At 1 year, the TLR rate (primary end point) also was significantly higher in the GR-II group (27.4% vs. 15.3%; $p < 0.001$).

53. **Baim DS,** et al. for the **NIRVANA** (NIR Vascular Advanced North American Trial) Investigators. Final results of a randomized trial comparing the NIR stent to the Palmaz–Schatz stent for narrowings in native coronary arteries. *Am J Cardiol* 2001;87:152–156.

This prospective study randomized 849 patients with single coronary lesions to the NIR stent or the PS. At 30 days, the two groups had a similar incidence of MACEs (death, MI, repeated TLR; 4.3% vs. 4.4%). The primary end point of target-vessel failure at 9 months occurred in 16.0% of NIR patients compared with 17.2% of PS patients, with the NIR proving to be equal or superior to the PS stent ($p < 0.001$ by test for equivalency). Angiographic restudy in 71% found no significant difference in restenosis rates [19.3% (NIR) vs. 22.4%].

54. **Baim DS,** et al. for the **ASCENT** Investigators (ACS MultLink Stent Clinical Equivalence in De Novo Lesions Trial). Final results of a randomized trial comparing the MULTI-LINK stent with the Palmaz–Schatz stent for narrowings in native coronary arteries. *Am J Cardiol* 2001;87:157–162.

This prospective, randomized, multicenter trial enrolled 1,040 patients with single, de novo native vessel lesions. Patients received ACS Multilink (ML) stent or PS stent. At 30 days, no significant differences were found between the groups in MACEs [5.0% (ML) vs. 6.5%]. The primary end point of target-vessel failure at 9 months occurred in 15.1% of ML-treated patients compared with 16.7% of PS-treated patients, with the ML proving to be equal or superior to the PS stent ($p < 0.001$ by test for equivalency). Angiographic restudy in a prespecified subgroup showed a nonsignificant trend toward reduced restenosis with the ML stent (16.0% vs. 22.1%).

Newer Devices/Techniques

CUTTING BALLOON

55. **Izumi M,** et al. Final results of the **CAPAS** trial. *Am Heart J* 2001;142:782–789.

A total of 248 type B/C lesions in small vessels (smaller than 3 mm diameter) were randomly assigned to cutting balloon angioplasty (CBA) or conventional balloon angioplasty (PTCA). At follow-up angiography (3 months), restenosis was significantly lower in the CBA group compared with the PTCA group (25.2% vs. 41.5%; $p = 0.009$). At 1 year, the event-free survival rate was 72.8% in the cutting balloon group and 61.0% in the PTCA group ($p = 0.047$).

56. **Adamian M,** et al. Cutting balloon angioplasty for the treatment of in-stent restenosis: a matched comparison with rotational atherectomy, additional stent implantation and balloon angioplasty. *J Am Coll Cardiol* 2001;38:672–679.

A total of 648 lesions with ISR were divided into four groups according to treatment strategy: CBA, RA, additional stenting, and PTCA. After the matching process, 258 lesions were entered into the analysis. Acute lumen gain was significantly higher in the stent group (2.12 mm) compared with the CBA, RA, and PTCA groups (1.70 mm, 1.79 mm, and 1.56 mm, respectively). However, the lumen loss at follow-up was lower for the CBA versus RA and stent groups (0.63 mm vs. 1.30 mm and 1.36 mm, respectively; $p < 0.0001$), resulting in a lower recurrent restenosis rate in CBA group (20% vs. 35.9% and 41.4%, respectively; $p < 0.05$). By multivariate analysis, predictors of TLR were CBA (OR, 0.17; $p = 0.001$) and diffuse restenosis at baseline (OR, 2.07; $p = 0.02$).

57. **Mauri L,** et al. Cutting balloon angioplasty for the prevention of restenosis: results of the Cutting Balloon Global Randomized Trial. *Am J Cardiol* 2002;90:1079–1083.

   This prospective, multicenter center randomized 1,238 patients to CB treatment or standard PTCA. At 6 months, binary angiographic restenosis rates (primary end point) were 31.4% for CB and 30.4% for PTCA. Freedom from TVR was slightly higher in the CB group (88.5% vs. 84.6%; log-rank $p = 0.04$). Coronary perforations occurred only in CB arm (0.8% vs. none; $p = 0.03$). At 270 days, the rates of MI, death, and total MACEs for CB and PTCA were 4.7% versus 2.4% ($p = 0.03$), 1.3% versus 0.3% ($p = 0.06$), and 13.6% versus 15.1% ($p = 0.34$), respectively.

58. **Albiero R,** et al. Cutting balloon versus conventional balloon angioplasty for the treatment of in-stent restenosis: results of the restenosis cutting balloon evaluation trial (RESCUT). *J Am Coll Cardiol* 2004;43(6):943–949.

   This prospective, randomized trial was conducted at 23 European centers and enrolled 428 patients with ISR of all types, the majority of which were short (<20 mm) lesions. Patients were assigned to CB or standard balloon angioplasty (PTCA). Total number of balloons used was less in the CB group, and a single balloon was used more often in the CB group (82.3% for CB vs. 75% for PTCA, $p = 0.03$). Balloon slippage also occurred much less often with the CB (6.5% vs. 25.%; $p < 0.01$), and there was a trend toward less stenting in the CB group (3.9% vs. 8.0%; $p = 0.07$). However, at 7 months, no significant differences were found between the CB and PTCA groups in the rates of binary restenosis by QCA (29.8% vs. 31.4%, $p = 0.82$) or a clinical-event composite of death, MI, or TLR (16.4% vs. 15.4%, $p = 0.79$).

59. **REDUCE II** (Restenosis Reduction by Cutting Balloon Evaluation). Preliminary results presented at Transcatheter Cardiovascular Therapeutics meeting, Washington, DC September 2002 [not subsequently published].

   This prospective, randomized, multicenter trial enrolled 466 patients with ISR. Patients were treated with the CB or a standard balloon. Procedural results were similar with both balloons, with no significant differences in QCA parameters. The CB group had a lower incidence of in-hospital death, MI, or TLR (4.0% vs. 8.2% for the standard balloon; $p = 0.049$). However, at 6-month angiographic follow-up, no significant differences were found between the groups in the rates of binary restenosis, percentage stenosis, and MLD.

60. **Bittl JA,** et al. Meta-analysis of randomized trials of percutaneous transluminal coronary angioplasty versus atherectomy, cutting balloon atherotomy, or laser angioplasty. *J Am Coll Cardiol* 2004;43:936–942.

   The authors review 16 trials of 9,222 patients to compare balloon angioplasty versus coronary atherectomy, laser angioplasty, or cutting balloon atherotomy. End points throughout the trials included both angiography improvement and clinical events. None of the adjunctive procedures improved 30-day mortality (OR 0.94, 95% CI, 0.46 to 1.92), angiographic restenosis rates (OR 1.06, 95% CI, 0.97 to 1.17), repeat revascularization (OR 1.04, 95% CI, 0.94 to 1.14), or cumulative adverse cardiac events at 1 year (OR 1.09, 95% CI, 0.99 to 1.20). There was an early (30-day), significant increase in periprocedural MI (OR 1.83, 95% CI, 1.43 to 2.34) and MACEs (OR 1.54, 95% CI, 1.25 to 1.89) in the adjunctive procedures group.

THROMBECTOMY

61. **Kuntz RE,** et al. Atrial comparing rheolytic thrombectomy with intracoronary urokinase for coronary and vein graft thrombus [the Vein Graft AngioJet Study (**VeGAS** 2)]. *Am J Cardiol* 2002;89:326–330.

   Design: Prospective, randomized, open, multicenter study. Primary end point was death, Q-wave MI, emergency coronary bypass surgery, TLR, stroke, or stent thrombosis at 30 days.

Purpose: To evaluate the safety and efficacy of rheolytic thrombectomy in CAD. Comparison of safety and efficacy of rheolytic thrombectomy (AngioJet) versus thrombolytic therapy (intracoronary urokinase).

Population: 352 patients with angina or MI more than 24 hours before the procedure and thrombus on angiography with discrete, mobile, intraluminal defect or a total occlusion with thrombus confirmed by multi-sidehole infusion catheter.

Exclusion Criteria: MI or thrombolytic therapy in previous 24 hours, more than two vessels requiring treatment, target vessel smaller than 2.0 mm diameter.

Treatment: Standard intracoronary or graft urokinase (more than 6-hour continuous infusion) or thrombectomy using the AngioJet system. Adjunctive thrombolytics and abciximab were discouraged, and crossover to AngioJet was prohibited. Short-term 30-day success was defined as more than 20% improvement in MLD, a final diameter stenosis of $\leq$50%, TIMI grade III flow, and freedom from major coronary events.

Results: Procedural success was significantly higher in the AngioJet group than in the urokinase group (86% vs. 72%; $p = 0.002$). Both treatments were equally effective with respect to the 30-day primary end point (AngioJet, 29%; urokinase, 30%). However, AngioJet patients had fewer MACEs (death, MI, revascularization; 16% vs. 33%; $p < 0.001$). Bradycardia occurred in 24% of those treated with AngioJet and was managed successfully with atropine and temporary pacing.

Comments: Trial was terminated early because of the growing safety difference between the two groups as well as reservations of investigators about using urokinase. Furthermore, mechanical thrombectomy allowed rapid thrombus removal and stenting during the same catheterization session.

62. Comparison of AngioJet Rheolytic Thrombectomy Before Direct Infarct Artery Stenting to Direct Stenting Alone in Patients with Acute Myocardial Infarction (**JETSTENT**). Presented by Dr. **David Antoniucci** at the ACC.10/i2 Summit, Atlanta, GA, March 2010.

The investigators randomized 501 patients with STEMI and at least modest thrombus burden to either direct stenting, or stenting following AngioJet rheolytic thrombectomy therapy. All patients received abciximab, and temporary pacing and balloon pre-dilatation were discouraged. Primary out of ST-segment resolution at 30 minutes significantly favored the AngioJet group (86% vs. 79%, $p = 0.043$). Additionally, the AngioJet group had significantly more favorable clinical outcomes of lower major cardiac events at 6 months (12.0% vs. 20.7%, $p = 0.012$). Though the AngioJet group had longer procedure times, peri-procedural complication rates, including bleeding, need for pacing, and perforation, were all similar in the two groups.

63. **Sardella G,** et al. Thrombus aspiration during primary percutaneous coronary intervention improves myocardial reperfusion and reduces infarct size: the EXPIRA (thrombectomy with export catheter in infarct-related artery during primary percutaneous coronary intervention) prospective, randomized trial. *J Am Coll Cardiol* 2009;53(4):309–315.

Design: Prospective, randomized, study. Primary end points were the occurrence of myocardial blush grade $\geq$2 and the rate of 90-min ST-segment resolution >70%.

Purpose: To evaluate the effect on infarct size and microvascular perfusion of mechanical thrombectomy during primary PCI for anterior STEMI.

Population: 175 patients with anterior STEMI were randomized to PCI or manual thrombectomy with PCI. Additionally, a subset underwent contrast-enhanced MRI at follow-up, to assess the resulting infarct.

Results: There was a lower rate of cardiac death in the thrombectomy group at 9 months (4.6% vs. 0%, $p = 0.02$). Additionally patients in the thrombectomy group more frequently had myocardial blush grade $\geq$2 (88% vs. 60%, $p = 0.001$) and ST-segment resolution (64% vs. 39%, $p = 0.001$). At 3 months, infarct size was reduced in the thrombectomy group.

Comment: Subsequent 2-year data suggested such mechanical aspiration may reduce mortality (presented at the American Heart Association, 2009).

DISTAL PROTECTION

64. **Baim DS,** et al. on behalf of Saphenous vein graft Angioplasty Free of Emboli Randomized (**SAFER**) Trial Investigators. Randomized trial of a distal embolic protection device during percutaneous intervention of saphenous vein aorto-coronary bypass grafts. *Circulation* 2002;105:1285–1290.

Design: Prospective, randomized, controlled, multicenter study. Primary end point was death, MI, emergency bypass surgery, or TVR (MACE) at 30 days.

Purpose: To compare clinical outcomes after SVG stenting plus GuardWire distal protection versus that performed over a conventional guide wire (control arm).

Population: 801 patients with a history of angina, evidence of myocardial ischemia, and greater than 50% stenosis in the mid-portion of an SVG with a diameter of 3 to 6 mm. In the first 142 patients, the lesion could not occupy more than one third of graft length.

Exclusion Criteria: Recent MI, ejection fraction less than 25%, creatinine greater than 2.5 mg/dL (unless receiving long-term hemodialysis), planned use of an atherectomy device.

Treatment: The 0.014-inch PercuSurge GuardWire balloon occlusion device or conventional 0.014-inch angioplasty guide wire. GP IIb/IIIa–receptor blocker could be used at the discretion of the operator.

Results: The embolic protection group had a 42% relative reduction in MACE at 30 days (9.6% vs. 16.5%; $p = 0.004$). This reduction was due primarily to fewer MIs (8.6% vs. 14.7%; $p = 0.008$) and "no-reflow" (3% vs. 9%; $p = 0.02$). The benefit of the distal protection device was evident both with and without the use of concomitant GP IIb/IIIa–receptor blockers.

Comments: The use of distal embolization protection devices in other territories, such as native coronary, carotid, and renal arteries, has yet to be fully examined.

65. **Stone GW,** et al. for the FilterWire EX Randomized Evaluation (FIRE) Investigators. Randomized comparison of distal protection with a filter-based catheter and a balloon occlusion and aspiration system during percutaneous intervention of diseased saphenous vein aorto-coronary bypass grafts. *Circulation* 2003;108:548–553.

This prospective, randomized, open, multicenter trial enrolled 651 patients with SVG lesion(s). Patients were treated using the GuardWire or FilterWireEx devices. Device success was 95.5% for FilterWire EX and 97.2% for GuardWire ($p = 0.25$), with postprocedure epicardial patency also similar. At 30 days, MACE rates were similar [9.9% (FilterWireEx) vs. 11.6%, p for superiority $= 0.53$, p for noninferiority $= 0.0008$].

66. **Stone GW,** et al. for the Enhanced Myocardial Efficacy and Recovery by Aspiration of Liberated Debris (EMERALD) Investigators. Distal microcirculatory protection during percutaneous coronary intervention in acute ST-segment elevation myocardial infarction: a randomized controlled trial. *JAMA* 2005;293:1063–1072.

Design: Prospective, multicenter, randomized, controlled trial. The primary end points were ST-segment resolution at 30 minutes after PCI and infarct size as measured by sestamibi imaging at 5 to 14 days post-PCI.

Purpose: To assess effects on infarct size and reperfusion of distal embolic protection during primary PCI.

Population: 501 patients with acute STEMI undergoing primary PCI or rescue intervention after failed thrombolysis.

Treatment: Routine PCI or PCI with a balloon occlusion and aspiration of distal microcirculatory protection system.

Results: Of the 252 patients who received distal protection, visible debris was aspirated in 73% of the cases. There was no difference in ST-segment resolution or infarct size between the two groups. MACEs at 6 months were also similar (10.0% for distal protection vs. 11.0% for routine PCI, $p = 0.66$).

67. **Svilaas T,** et al. Thrombus aspiration during primary percutaneous coronary intervention. *N Engl J Med* 2008;358(6):557–567.

Design: Prospective, single-center, randomized, controlled trial. The primary end point was myocardial blush grade of 0 or 1 (poor myocardial perfusion grades). Secondarily, outcomes of ST-segment resolution and clinical events were also recorded.

Purpose: To assess effects on microvascular perfection of thrombus aspiration during primary PCI for acute STEMI.

Population: 1,071 patients with acute STEMI undergoing primary PCI.

Treatment: Routine PCI or PCI with adjunctive thrombus aspiration (confirmed by histopathologic evidence of atherothrombotic material).

Results: Patients in the thrombus-aspiration group had a lower rate of myocardial blush grade of 0 or 1 (17.1% vs. 26.3%, $p < 0.001$) and improved resolution of ST-segments (56.6% vs. 442.%, $p < 0.001$). Independent of randomization category, rates of death and adverse events at 30 days were inversely related to myocardial blush grades—the lower the blush grade, the poorer the clinical outcomes ($p < 0.01$ for both death and adverse clinical events by blush grade).

68. **Haeck JDE,** et al. Randomized comparison of primary percutaneous coronary intervention with combined proximal embolic protection and thrombus aspiration versus primary percutaneous coronary intervention alone in ST-segment elevation myocardial infarction: the PREPARE (PRoximal Embolic Protection in Acute myocardial infarction and Resolution of ST-Elevation) study. *J Am Coll Cardiol Interv* 2009;2:934–943.

The investigators randomized 284 patients with STEMI undergoing primary PCI to the Proxis system of combined proximal embolic protection with thrombus aspiration or routine PCI. There was no significant difference in the primary end point of ST-segment resolution at 60 minutes (80% vs. 72%, $p = 0.14$). However, there were significant improvements in immediate complete ST-resolution (66% vs. 50%, $p = 0.009$) and lower ST-segment curve area; however, clinical cardiac and cerebral end points were similar at 30 days (albeit with a low number of events).

69. **Srinivasan M,** et al. Adjunctive thrombectomy and distal protection in primary percutaneous coronary intervention impact on microvascular perfusion and outcomes. *Circulation* 2009;119:1311–1319.

In light of the recent Thrombus Aspiration During Percutaneous Coronary Intervention in Acute Myocardial Infarction Study (see above), the authors review the prior evidence for and current role of mechanical thrombectomy and distal embolic protection in primary PCI.

Adjunctive Pharmacologic Therapy
ASPIRIN

70. **Schwartz L,** et al. Aspirin and dipyridamole in the prevention of restenosis after percutaneous transluminal coronary angioplasty. *N Engl J Med* 1988;318:1714–1719.

This prospective, randomized, double-blind, placebo-controlled study enrolled 376 patients undergoing planned PTCA. Patients received an aspirin–dipyridamole combination (330 to 75 mg t.i.d.), beginning 24 hours before PTCA and until follow-up angiography, or placebo. At follow-up angiography (249 patients), no differences were observed between the two groups in binary restenosis rates [37.7% vs. 38.6% (placebo)]. However, the aspirin–dipyridamole group had significantly fewer periprocedural Q-wave MIs compared with the placebo group (6.9% vs. 1.6%; $p = 0.0113$).

For additionally aspirin and antiplatelet studies, see below section on "Antithrombotic Regimens to Prevent Stent Thrombosis."

HEPARIN

71. **Garachemani AR,** et al. Prolonged heparin after uncomplicated coronary interventions: a prospective, randomized trial. *Am Heart J* 1998;136:352–356 (editorial, 183–185).

This prospective randomized trial was composed of 191 consecutive patients who underwent successful coronary angioplasty. Patients received prolonged intravenous heparin (12 to 20 hours) or no postprocedural heparin. Stents were used in 33% and 36% of patients. MIs occurred in 3% and 4%, whereas vascular complications were seen in 3% and 1%. Accompanying editorial contains results from a meta-analysis of six studies comprising 2,186 patients. Postprocedural heparin was associated with a nonsignificant OR of 0.91 (0.45 to 1.84) for ischemic complications and an OR of 2.54 (1.44 to 4.47) for bleeding complications (27 additional episodes/1,000 patients treated).

72. **Lincoff AM,** et al. Precursor to EPILOG (**PROLOG**) Investigators. Standard versus low-dose, weight-adjusted heparin in patients treated with the platelet glycoprotein IIb/IIIa receptor antibody fragment abciximab (c7E3 Fab) during percutaneous coronary revascularization. *Am J Cardiol* 1997;79:286–291.

This randomized 2×2 factorial pilot study was composed of a total of 103 patients undergoing PCI with concomitant abciximab (0.25 mg/kg intravenous bolus, and then 10 μg/min for 12 hours) who were randomized to standard or high-dose heparin (100 U/kg bolus before PCI and then hourly boluses to keep ACT 300 to 350 seconds, or continuous infusion at 10 U/kg/hr without further ACT measurements) or low-dose heparin (70 U/kg and then 30 U/kg boluses during the procedure, or continuous infusion at 7 U/kg/hr without further ACT measurements). There was a separate randomization to early or late sheath removal. The early sheath-removal group had heparin discontinued immediately after PCI and sheaths removed at 6 hours, whereas the late group had heparin continued for 12 hours and sheaths removed 4 to 6 hours later. No difference was found between the groups in the incidence of ischemic events at 7 days. The early sheath-removal group had a smaller decrease in mean hemoglobin from baseline ($p = 0.03$), and nonsignificant trends occurred toward less minor non-CABG bleeding with low-dose heparin and early sheath removal.

73. **Kaluski E,** et al. Minimal heparinization in coronary angioplasty: how much heparin is really warranted? *Am J Cardiol* 2000;85:953–956.

Prospective, randomized, open study of 341 consecutive patients undergoing nonemergency PTCA. Patients received 2,500 U of UFH before PTCA with the intention of no additional boluses. Mean ACT at 5 minutes was 185 seconds. Two in-hospital deaths and one Q-wave MI occurred. Six (2%) patients had abrupt coronary occlusion within 14 days after PTCA, requiring repeated TVR. Six-month clinical follow-up in 184 patients revealed three cardiac deaths (one arrhythmic, two after cardiac surgery), one Q-wave MI, and 9.7% repeated TVR. These results warrant larger, randomized, double-blind heparin dose-optimization studies.

LOW-MOLECULAR-WEIGHT HEPARIN

74. **The SYNERGY Trial Investigators.** Enoxaparin vs unfractionated heparin in high-risk patients with non–ST-segment elevation acute coronary syndromes managed with an intended early invasive strategy primary results of the SYNERGY randomized trial. *JAMA* 2004;292:45–54.

Design: Prospective, randomized, open, multicenter study. Primary end point was a composite of death or MI within 30 days. Safety outcomes of major bleeding or stroke were also assessed.
Purpose: To assess outcomes of patients with NSTEMI, undergoing an early invasive strategy with either UFH or enoxaparin.

Population: 10,027 patients with NSTEMI being treated with an intended early invasive strategy.
Treatment: Subcutaneous enoxaparin versus intravenous UFH, both started at the time of enrollment, and continued for a duration at the discretion of the treating physician.
Results: There was no difference in occurrence of the primary outcome for enoxaparin (14.0%) versus UFH (14.5%), or any other clinical ischemic outcomes. There were, however, increased rates of TIMI major bleeding in the enoxaparin group (9.1% vs. 7.6%, $p = 0.008$). The trial met the noninferiority margin for enoxaparin compared with UFH.

75. **Gibson CM,** et al. Percutaneous coronary intervention in patients receiving enoxaparin or unfractionated heparin after fibrinolytic therapy for ST-segment elevation myocardial infarction in the ExTRACT-TIMI 25 trial. *J Am Coll Cardiol* 2007;49:2238–2246.

The investigators performed a subgroup analysis of the 20,479 patients enrolled in the ExTRACT-TIMI 25 trial. The broader trial randomized patients with STEMI undergoing fibrinolytic therapy to either UFH or enoxaparin; however, a subgroup of 4,676 patients subsequently underwent PCI and were included in this analysis. It should first be noted that treatment remained blinded for the duration of hospitalization, and fewer patients initially randomized to enoxaparin actually underwent subsequent PCI. Of the group that did get PCI, those who received enoxaparin had a lower rate of death or MI at 30 days (10.7% vs. 13.8% for UFH, $p < 0.001$), the primary end point. Within this PCI subgroup, there were no differences in major bleeding rates (1.4% for enoxaparin vs. 1.6% for UFH, $p = $ NS). For additional details on the full ExTRACT-TIMI 25 study, see Chapter 4.
Additional data on LWMH can be found in Chapters 2 and 4.

THIENOPYRIDINES

76. **Schomig A,** et al. Intracoronary stenting and antithrombotic regimen (**ISAR**). A randomized comparison of antiplatelet and anticoagulant therapy after the placement of coronary artery stents. *N Engl J Med* 1996;334:1084–1089.

Design: Prospective, randomized, open, multicenter study. Primary cardiac end points were cardiovascular death, MI, bypass surgery, and repeated target-vessel intervention. Additional noncardiac end point was death from noncardiac causes, cerebrovascular accidents, severe hemorrhage, and peripheral vascular events.
Purpose: To compare the early outcome of patients given a combined antiplatelet regimen or conventional anticoagulation after coronary stent placement.
Population: 517 patients who underwent successful stenting.
Exclusion Criteria: Cardiogenic shock and stenting intended as a bridge to CABG surgery.
Treatment: Intravenous heparin for 12 hours; ticlopidine, 250 mg twice daily, and aspirin; or intravenous heparin for 5 to 10 days, phenprocoumon, and aspirin.
Results: At 30 days, the antiplatelet group had 75% fewer cardiac end points (1.6% vs. 6.2%), including a significant reduction in MI (0.8% vs. 4.2%; $p = 0.02$). The antiplatelet group had a 90% reduction in the primary noncardiac end point (1.2% vs. 12.3%; $p < 0.001$), including an 87% reduction in peripheral vascular events (0.8% vs. 6.2%; $p = 0.001$) and no bleeding complications (vs. 6.5%; $p < 0.001$). Antiplatelet therapy also was associated with 86% fewer stent reocclusions (0.8% vs. 5.4%; $p = 0.004$).

77. **Bertrand ME,** et al. Full Anticoagulation versus Aspirin and Ticlopidine (**FANTASTIC**). Randomized multicenter comparison of conventional anticoagulation versus antiplatelet therapy in unplanned and elective coronary stenting. *Circulation* 1998;98: 1597–1603.

Design: Prospective, randomized, multicenter study. Primary end point was bleeding and peripheral vascular complications. Secondary end points were death, MI, and stent occlusion.
Purpose: To compare the effects of aggressive antiplatelet treatment with anticoagulation after implantation of a Wiktor stent on bleeding rates and stent thrombosis rates.

Population: 485 patients undergoing elective (58%) or unplanned (42%) coronary stenting.

Exclusion Criteria: Platelet count less than 150,000, bleeding disorders, recent (<6 months) gastrointestinal bleeding, recent stroke, angiographic evidence of thrombus at target site, and allergy to aspirin or ticlopidine.

Treatment: Antiplatelet therapy with aspirin, 100 to 325 mg/day, and ticlopidine, 250 mg twice daily for 6 weeks [first dose (500 mg) given in catheterization laboratory], or anticoagulation with heparin (target activated partial thromboplastin time, 2.0 to 2.5 times control), and then warfarin for 6 weeks (target international normalized ratio, 2.5 to 3.0). The anticoagulation group also received aspirin. All patients received heparin, 10,000-U bolus before the procedure.

Results: Successful stent implantation was achieved in 99%. The antiplatelet group had fewer bleeding and peripheral vascular complications (13.5% vs. 21%; OR, 0.6; $p = 0.03$). Major cardiac events in electively stented patients were less common in the antiplatelet group (2.4% vs. 9.9%; OR, 0.23; $p = 0.01$). Antiplatelet patients had a shorter average hospital stay (4.3 vs. 6.4 days; $p = 0.0001$).

78. **Urban P,** et al. for the Multicenter Aspirin and Ticlopidine Trial after Intracoronary Stenting (**MATTIS**) investigators. Randomized evaluation of anticoagulation versus antiplatelet therapy after coronary stent implantation in high-risk patients. *Circulation* 1998;98:2126–2132.

Design: Prospective, randomized, multicenter study. Primary composite end point was cardiovascular death, MI, and repeated revascularization at 30 days.

Purpose: To compare antiplatelet therapy with anticoagulation in high-risk patients undergoing coronary stent implantation.

Population: 350 patients randomized within 6 hours of stent implantation who met the eligibility criteria: (a) stent(s) was placed to treat abrupt closure after balloon angioplasty; (b) suboptimal angiographic result was achieved; (c) the stented segment measured more than 45 mm (or was composed of three stents); (d) the vessel in question was small (i.e., largest balloon used was ≤2.5 mm). Eight different stent types were used by investigators.

Exclusion Criteria: Recent MI, persistent ischemia, administration of GP IIb/IIIa inhibitors before or during procedure, and intervention planned within 30-day follow-up period.

Treatment: Aspirin, 250 mg once daily, and ticlopidine, 250 mg twice daily for 30 days, or aspirin, 250 mg once daily, and oral anticoagulation (target international normalized ratio, 2.5 to 3.0).

Results: Antiplatelet group demonstrated a trend toward fewer cardiac end points (5.6% vs. 11%; $p = 0.07$) and significant reduction in major vascular and bleeding complications (1.7% vs. 6.9%; $p = 0.02$). The incidence of subacute stent thrombosis was not precisely known (no angiographic end point). In three patients (1.7%) treated with ticlopidine, asymptomatic agranulocytopenia developed.

79. **Leon MB,** et al. for the Stent Anticoagulation Restenosis Study (**STARS**) investigators. A clinical trial comparing three antithrombotic-drug regimens after coronary-artery stenting. *N Engl J Med* 1998;339:1665–1671.

Design: Prospective, randomized, open, multicenter study (54). The 30-day primary composite end point was death, MI, TLR, and angiographically evident thrombosis.

Purpose: To compare clinical outcomes for three antithrombotic regimens after elective coronary stenting.

Population: 1,653 patients who underwent successful stenting of a more than 60% stenosis in a native coronary artery with a diameter of 3 to 4 mm.

Exclusion Criteria: MI in prior 7 days, abciximab administration, and planned revascularization within 30 days.

Treatment: Aspirin, 325 mg daily; aspirin, 325 mg daily, and intravenous heparin followed by warfarin (target international normalized ratio, 2.0 to 2.5); or aspirin, 325 mg daily, and ticlopidine, 250 mg twice daily.

Results: Aspirin plus ticlopidine group had a significant reduction in the incidence of primary composite end points for aspirin and warfarin (0.5% vs. 2.7%) and for aspirin alone (3.6%; $p < 0.001$ for comparison of all three groups). Hemorrhagic and vascular surgical complications occurred less frequently with aspirin alone: 1.8% versus 5.5% (aspirin plus ticlopidine), and 6.2% (aspirin and warfarin) and 0.4% versus 2.0% and 2.0%. No significant differences were observed in the incidences of neutropenia or thrombocytopenia (overall incidence, 0.3%).

80. **Moussa I,** et al. Effectiveness of clopidogrel and aspirin versus ticlopidine and aspirin in preventing stent thrombosis after coronary stent implantation. *Circulation* 1999;99: 2364–2366.

This observational study was composed of 1,689 patients undergoing coronary stent implantation; 1,406 received ticlopidine (500 mg loading dose, and then 250 mg twice daily) and aspirin (325 mg once daily), and 283 received clopidogrel (300 mg loading dose and then 75 mg once daily) and aspirin. Exclusion criteria included requirement for oral anticoagulation, abciximab administration, and procedural failure. At 1-month follow-up, the two groups had a similar incidence of stent thrombosis [1.5% (ticlopidine plus aspirin) vs. 1.4%] and MACEs (3.1% vs. 2.4%). The clopidogrel plus aspirin group had a significantly lower incidence of side effects, consisting of neutropenia, diarrhea, or rash (5.3% vs. 10.6%; RR 0.53; $p = 0.006$).

81. **Bertrand ME,** et al. Double-blind study of the safety of clopidogrel with and without a loading dose in combination with aspirin, compared with ticlopidine in combination with aspirin after coronary stenting: the Clopidogrel Aspirin Stent International Cooperative Study (**CLASSICS**). *Circulation* 2000;102:624–629.

Design: Prospective, randomized, double-blind, placebo-controlled, multicenter study. The primary end point was a composite of major peripheral or bleeding complications, neutropenia, thrombocytopenia, or early discontinuation of the drug because of a noncardiac event. Secondary end point was cardiac events, consisting of cardiovascular death, MI, or TVR.

Purpose: To demonstrate that clopidogrel has an efficacy similar to and better tolerability than ticlopidine.

Population: 1,020 patients who had undergone successful planned or unplanned coronary stenting (one or two stents) in a single-vessel (reference vessel diameter, more than 2.8 mm) with the use of any non–heparin-coated stent(s).

Exclusion Criteria: Included acute ST-elevation MI; CK 2× normal or greater; stent(s) in left main coronary artery, vein grafts, or at a major bifurcation; oral anticoagulants, GP IIb/IIIa–receptor antagonists or other antiplatelet agents, except for aspirin, in previous month (or required after the procedure); percutaneous or surgical revascularization (PTCA, CABG) in the previous 2 months.

Treatment: Ticlopidine, 250 mg twice daily for 4 weeks; clopidogrel, 75 mg once daily for 4 weeks; or clopidogrel, 300 mg loading dose followed by 75 mg once daily (days 2 to 28). All patients received aspirin, 325 mg once daily.

Results: The clopidogrel groups had a significantly lower incidence of the primary composite end point, which consisted of major bleeding, neutropenia, thrombocytopenia, and early discontinuation of therapy: 2.9% (loading dose group) and 6.4% [clopidogrel, 75 mg/day (all clopidogrel patients, 4.6%) vs. 9.1% for ticlopidine ($p = 0.005$)]. No significant differences were seen among the three groups in the incidence of the secondary end point (0.9%, 1.5%, and 1.2% of patients, respectively).

Comments: Clopidogrel appears to have superior safety and tolerability compared with ticlopidine and acceptable efficacy in the prevention of MACEs after coronary stenting. Although this study was not developed to determine efficacy, the results support the use of clopidogrel as an alternative to ticlopidine after coronary stenting.

82. **PCI-CURE** (Clopidogrel in Unstable angina to prevent Recurrent ischemic Events), Mehta SR, et al. Effects of pretreatment with clopidogrel and aspirin followed by long-term therapy in patients undergoing percutaneous coronary intervention: the PCI-CURE study. *Lancet* 2001;358:527–533.

Design: Prospective, randomized, placebo-controlled, double-blinded, multicenter trial. Primary end point was 30-day composite of cardiovascular death, MI, or urgent TVR and cardiovascular death or MI to end of trial. Mean follow-up was 8 months.

Purpose: To determine if pretreatment with clopidogrel before PCI would be superior to placebo in preventing major ischemic events after PCI and if long-term treatment with clopidogrel for up to 1 year after PCI would result in additional benefit.

Population: 2,658 patients with mean age 61 years and acute coronary syndromes who were hospitalized within 24 hours of onset of symptoms. ECG evidence of new ischemia (but less than 1-mm ST elevation) or elevated concentrations of cardiac enzymes ($2\times$ normal or more) were required.

Exclusion Criteria: Contraindications to antithrombotic or antiplatelet therapy, high bleeding risk, NYHA class IV heart failure, need for oral anticoagulation, coronary revascularization in previous 3 months, GP IIb/IIIa–receptor inhibitors in previous 3 days.

Treatment: Clopidogrel, 300 mg loading dose, or matching placebo followed by 75 mg clopidogrel, or matching placebo once daily for 3 to 12 months (mean, 9 months). Patients underwent PCI at a mean 10 days after randomization. All received aspirin, 75 to 325 mg once daily. The use of GP IIb/IIIa–receptor antagonists was discouraged but allowed during PCI.

Results: Before PCI, the clopidogrel group had a lower incidence of MI or refractory ischemia compared with placebo (12.% vs. 15.3%; RR, 0.76; $p = 0.008$). At 30 days after PCI, the clopidogrel group had a lower incidence in the primary composite outcome of cardiovascular death, MI, or urgent revascularization (4.5% vs. 6.4%; RR, 0.70; $p = 0.03$). Long-term administration of clopidogrel after PCI was associated with a lower rate of the composite end point ($p = 0.03$) and cardiovascular death or MI ($p = 0.047$). Including events before and after PCI, the clopidogrel group was associated with a 31% lower incidence of cardiovascular death or MI (8.8% vs. 12.6%; $p = 0.002$; see **Fig. 2.3**). Clopidogrel use was associated with similar rate of major bleeding compared with placebo.

83. **Steinhubl SR,** et al. Ticlopidine pretreatment before coronary stenting is associated with sustained decrease in adverse cardiac events: data from the Evaluation of Platelet IIb/IIIa Inhibitor for Stenting (**EPISTENT**) Trial. *Circulation* 2001;103:1403–1409.

Design: Nonrandomized, multicenter study. Primary composite end points were all-cause mortality, nonfatal MI, or urgent revascularization at 30 days, and at 1 year, all-cause mortality, MI, and TVR.

Purpose: To determine whether pretreatment with ticlopidine before coronary stenting results in a sustained reduction in adverse cardiac events.

Population: Included 1,603 patients enrolled in the EPISTENT trial who were randomized to either placebo or abciximab. Of these, 932 patients received pretreatment with ticlopidine before stenting, at the discretion of the investigator.

Exclusion Criteria: see EPISTENT trial.

Treatment: Abciximab (bolus and 12-hour infusion) and stenting, placebo and stenting, or abciximab and balloon angioplasty. Investigators were encouraged to treat all patients with ticlopidine according to their usual practice before stenting. All were pretreated with aspirin.

Results: Among patients randomized to placebo, ticlopidine pretreatment was associated with a significant decrease in death, MI, or TVR at 1 year (adjusted HR, 0.73; 95% CI, 0.54 to 0.98; $p = 0.036$). At 30-day follow-up, the primary end point had occurred in 13.4% of patients in the no-abciximab or ticlopidine group, 8.9% of patients in the placebo + ticlopidine group, 5.5% of patients in the abciximab/no-ticlopidine group ($p = 0.028$ vs. placebo and plus ticlopidine) and 5.2% of patients in the abciximab + ticlopidine group. The benefit of pretreatment with ticlopidine in the placebo group was primarily attributable to a lower incidence of MI (8.4% vs. 12.5%; $p = 0.048$). At 1 year, fewer primary events occurred in the placebo group in patients pretreated with ticlopidine compared with patients not pretreated with ticlopidine (20.7% vs. 28.5%; $p = 0.008$), whereas no difference was related to pretreatment with ticlopidine in the abciximab group (19.5% for abciximab + ticlopidine vs. 20.9% for abciximab/no ticlopidine). Controlling for patient characteristics and for the propensity to use ticlopidine, Cox regression model identified ticlopidine pretreatment as an independent predictor of the need for TVR at 1 year (hazard ratio, 0.62; 95% CI, 0.43 to 0.89; $p = 0.01$) in both placebo-treated and abciximab-treated patients. By multivariate modeling, however, the beneficial effect of ticlopidine on TVR was diminished by treatment with abciximab.

Comments: Duration of pretreatment with ticlopidine was uncertain. Beneficial effect of ticlopidine in placebo-treated group may have been due to an antiplatelet effect in aspirin-resistant patients.

84. **Taniuchi M,** et al. Randomized comparison of ticlopidine and clopidogrel after intracoronary stent implantation in a broad patient population. *Circulation* 2001;104:539–543.

Design: Prospective, randomized, double-blind, placebo-controlled, parallel-group study. Primary end point was failure to complete the 2-week therapy.

Purpose: To determine the relative safety of a 2-week treatment with clopidogrel plus aspirin compared with ticlopidine plus aspirin in patients undergoing coronary stenting.

Population: 1,067 patients who had undergone successful stent implantation

Exclusion Criteria: Known intolerance to aspirin, ticlopidine, or clopidogrel.

Treatment: Loading dose of ticlopidine, 500 mg, followed by ticlopidine, 250 mg b.i.d., plus aspirin, 325 mg/day, for 14 days (522 patients), or a loading dose of clopidogrel, 300 mg, followed by clopidogrel, 75 mg/day, plus aspirin, 325 mg/day, for 14 days (494 patients).

Results: The primary end point occurred in 3.64% of patients in the ticlopidine group and in 1.62% of patients in the clopidogrel loading-dose group ($p = 0.04$). The most common adverse event requiring ticlopidine discontinuation was rash (0.96% in the ticlopidine group and 0.2% in the clopidogrel group). No significant differences were noted in rates of thrombocytopenia (0.57% in the ticlopidine group and 1.01% in the clopidogrel group) and neutropenia (0.38% and none, respectively). A trend toward a higher incidence of cardiac death was found in the ticlopidine group (1.53% vs. 0.61%), whereas the incidence of stent thrombosis was similar among the two groups (2.02% vs. 1.92%). The majority of stent thrombosis occurred during the first 8 days of treatment, whereas only one event per group occurred after the 2-week treatment period. At 30-day follow-up, the incidence of MACE was 4.6% in the ticlopidine group and 3.85% in the clopidogrel group.

85. **Bhatt DL,** et al. Meta-analysis of randomized and registry comparisons of ticlopidine with clopidogrel after stenting. *J Am Coll Cardiol* 2002;39:9–14.

Data were pooled and analyzed from published trials and registries comparing clopidogrel with ticlopidine in a total of 13,955 patients undergoing stenting. The pooled rate of MACEs was 2.10% in the clopidogrel group and 4.04% in the ticlopidine group. After adjustment for trial heterogeneity, the OR for ischemic events was lower with clopidogrel compared with ticlopidine (95% CI, 0.59 to 0.89; $p = 0.002$). The clopidogrel group also had a significantly lower mortality compared with the ticlopidine group (0.48% vs. 1.09%; OR, 0.55; 95% CI, 0.37 to 0.82; $p = 0.003$). The authors note that these findings may be due to the more rapid onset of an antiplatelet effect with the loading dose of clopidogrel, which was used in most of these studies, or to better patient compliance with clopidogrel therapy.

86. **Hongo RH,** et al. The effect of clopidogrel in combination with aspirin when given before coronary artery bypass grafting. *J Am Coll Cardiol* 2002;40:231–237.

This nonrandomized observational study of 224 consecutive patients undergoing non-emergency first-time CABG compared those with preoperative clopidogrel exposure within

7 days ($n = 59$) with those without exposure ($n = 165$). Groups had comparable baseline characteristics. The clopidogrel group had higher 24-hour mean chest tube output (1.2 L vs. 0.84 L; $p = 0.001$) and more transfusions of red blood cells (2.51 U vs. 1.74 U; $p = 0.036$), platelets (0.86 U vs. 0.24 U; $p = 0.001$), and fresh frozen plasma (0.68 U vs. 0.24 U; $p = 0.015$). Reoperation for bleeding was 10-fold higher in clopidogrel group (6.8% vs. 0.6%; $p = 0.018$). The clopidogrel group also had a trend toward less hospital discharge within 5 days (33.9% vs. 46.7%; $p = 0.094$).

87. **Steinhubl SR,** et al. for the Clopidogrel in Unstable angina to Prevent Recurrent Events **CREDO** Investigators. Early and sustained dual oral antiplatelet therapy following percutaneous coronary intervention. *JAMA* 2002;288:2411–2420.

Design: Prospective, randomized, double-blind, placebo-controlled, multicenter study. Primary end points were death, MI, or stroke at 1 year, and death, MI, or urgent TVR at 28 days in the per-protocol population.
Purpose: To evaluate long-term treatment (1 year) with clopidogrel after elective PCI and initiation of clopidogrel with a preprocedure loading dose, both in addition to aspirin therapy.
Population: 2,116 patients scheduled to undergo elective PCI or deemed at high likelihood of undergoing PCI.
Exclusion Criteria: Included contraindications to antithrombotic/antiplatelet therapy; failed PCI in previous 2 weeks; coronary anatomy not amenable to stenting or greater than 50% left main stenosis; planned staged procedure; administration of the following medications before randomization: GP IIb/IIIa inhibitors (within 7 days), clopidogrel (10 days), thrombolytics (24 hours).
Treatment: Clopidogrel loading dose (300 mg), or placebo, 3 to 24 hours before PCI. All patients then received clopidogrel, 75 mg/day, through day 28. From day 29 through 12 months, loading-dose patients received clopidogrel, 75 mg/day, and control patients received placebo. Both groups received aspirin throughout the study. GP IIb/IIIa inhibitors were administered in 45% of the per-protocol population. PCI was performed in 86%.
Results: At 1 year, long-term clopidogrel therapy was associated with a 26.9% relative reduction in death, MI, or stroke [8.5% vs. 11.5% (placebo); $p = 0.02$]. Although not a prespecified analysis, a further 37.4% relative reduction in major events occurred from day 29 to 1 year with clopidogrel ($p = 0.04$). At 28 days, clopidogrel pretreatment was associated with a nonsignificant 18.5% relative reduction in death, MI, or urgent TVR (6.8% vs. 8.3%; $p = 0.23$). However, in a prespecified subgroup analysis, those given clopidogrel at least 6 hours before PCI had a significant 38.6% RR reduction ($p = 0.05$) compared with no reduction with treatment less than 6 hours before PCI. Among those receiving a GP IIb/IIIa inhibitor and clopidogrel pretreatment, a 30% reduction in events was found [7.3% vs. 10.3% (no pretreatment, GP IIb/IIIa); $p = 0.12$]. A trend toward a higher incidence of major bleeding was found with clopidogrel (at 1 year, 8.8% vs. 6.7%; $p = 0.07$).
Comments: This trial, together with CURE and PCI-CURE, supports long-term use of clopidogrel plus aspirin post-PCI.

88. **Sabatine MS,** et al. Effect of clopidogrel pretreatment before percutaneous coronary intervention in patients with STEMI treated with fibrinolytics the PCI-CLARITY study. *JAMA* 2005;294:1224–1232.

This prospectively planned substudy of the CLARITY-TIMI 28 trial (see Chapter 4 for its complete details) evaluated the 1863 patients in the original trial who underwent PCI following mandated angiography. All patients were initially randomized to either clopidogrel or placebo (in addition to aspirin and other medical therapies) at enrollment; they subsequently underwent angiography (2 to 8 days later) and all patients requiring PCI subsequently received clopidogrel regardless of initial randomization assignment. However, in patients initially randomized to clopidogrel (thus, having been on it for 2 to 8 days prior to PCI), there was a significant reduction in MI or stroke prior to PCI (4.0% vs. 6.2%, $p = 0.03$), as well as a reduction in cardiovascular death, MI, or stroke after PCI (3.6% vs. 6.2%, $p = 0.008$). In this group undergoing PCI following fibrinolysis for STEMI, pretreatment with clopidogrel on presentation, prior to PCI, significantly reduced 30-day rates of cardiovascular death, MI, or stroke (7.5% vs. 12.0%, $p = 0.001$), without excess rates of major or minor bleeding (2.0% vs. 1.9%, $p > 0.99$).

89. **Mega JL,** et al. Cytochrome P-450 polymorphisms and response to clopidogrel. *N Engl J Med* 2009;360:354–362.

Based on previous data suggesting variable clinical response to clopidogrel based on cytochrome p-450 polymorphisms, the investigators of the TRITON-TIMI 38 trial (see Chapter 4) assessed clinical cardiovascular outcomes in patients with ACS, receiving clopidogrel, stratified by genotype. Among patients in the TRITON-TIMI 38 trial who were carriers of the CYP2C19 polymorphism, there was a relative increase over noncarriers of 53% in the primary end point, a composite of cardiovascular death, MI, or stroke (12.1% vs. 8.0%, $p = 0.01$). There was also, notably, a threefold increase in the risk of stent thrombosis in the carrier group (2.6% vs. 0.8%, $p = 0.02$). This represents one of the earliest studies to link pharmacogenomic status to clinical outcomes, and surely the beginning of more specific tailoring of pharmacotherapy to genetic profile.

90. **Kastrati A,** et al. for the Intracoronary Stenting and Antithrombotic Regimen–Rapid Early Action for Coronary Treatment (**ISAR-REACT**) Study Investigators. A clinical trial of abciximab in elective percutaneous coronary intervention after pretreatment with clopidogrel. *N Engl J Med* 2004;350:232–238.

Design: Randomized, double-blind, placebo-controlled trial. Primary end point was a composite of death, MI, or urgent TVR within 30 days.
Purpose: To compare abciximab versus placebo in stable patients undergoing elective PCI with clopidogrel pretreatment.
Population: 2,159 patients with stable CAD of low risk, undergoing elective PCI.
Exclusion Criteria: Recent MI (14 days), current ACS, positive troponin, or any of several other markers of higher risk.
Treatment: Abciximab infusion during PCI or placebo infusion; all patients were pretreated with 600 mg clopidogrel.
Results: There was no significant difference in rates of the primary end point between those who received abciximab and placebo (4% for abciximab vs. 4% placebo, $p = 0.82$). Bleeding end points were also roughly equivalent. The only significant difference between the groups was incidence of profound thrombocytopenia (1% for abciximab vs. 0% for placebo, $p = 0.002$).

91. **Kastrati A,** et al. for the Intracoronary Stenting and Antithrombotic Regimen: Rapid Early Action for Coronary Treatment 2 (**ISAR-REACT 2**) Trial Investigators. Abciximab in patients with acute coronary syndromes undergoing percutaneous coronary intervention after clopidogrel pretreatment: the ISAR-REACT 2 randomized trial. *JAMA* 2006;295:1531–1538.

Design: Randomized, controlled, double-blind, multicenter international trial. Primary end point was a composite of death, MI, or urgent TVR within 30 days. Bleeding complications were secondary end points.
Purpose: To assess the utility of adding abciximab to clopidogrel load in patients undergoing PCI for NSTEMI.
Population: 2,022 patients with NSTEMI undergoing PCI.
Treatment: PCI with abciximab bolus and infusion or PCI with placebo; both groups received pretreatment with 600 mg of clopidogrel.
Results: Rates of the primary end point significantly favored the abciximab group (8.9% vs. 11.9%, $p = 0.03$). However, this effect was confined to those patients with an elevated troponin. Bleeding rates were no different in the two groups.

GLYCOPROTEIN IIB/IIIA INHIBITORS

92. Evaluation of 7E3 for the Prevention of Ischemic Complications (**EPIC**). Use of a monoclonal antibody directed vs platelet glycoprotein IIb/IIIa receptor in high-risk percutaneous transluminal coronary angioplasty. *N Engl J Med* 1994;330:956–961.

Design: Prospective, randomized, double-blind, multicenter study. The 30-day primary composite end point was death, MI, CABG surgery, repeated PCI for acute ischemia, and stenting due to procedural failure, or placement of an intra-aortic balloon pump.

Purpose: To determine whether the monoclonal antibody c7E3 Fab provides clinical benefit in patients undergoing coronary angioplasty or atherectomy.

Population: 2,099 high-risk patients, defined as having experienced acute MI with onset of symptoms within previous 12 hours, two episodes of postinfarct angina within previous 24 hours with ECG changes, or high-risk clinical or angiographic features, who underwent percutaneous intervention (PTCA, 90%; directional atherectomy, 5%; both, 5%).

Exclusion Criteria: Included bleeding diathesis, major surgery in prior 6 weeks, and stroke in prior 2 years.

Treatment: Abciximab, 0.25 mg/kg intravenous bolus (started 10 minutes before procedure), and then 10 μg/min infusion for 12 hours, abciximab or placebo. All patients received heparin (10,000- to 12,000-U bolus; target ACT, 300 to 350 seconds).

Results: Abciximab bolus plus infusion group had 35% fewer end points (death, MI, unplanned surgical revascularization, repeated percutaneous procedure, need for intra-aortic balloon pump): 12.8% versus 11.4% (bolus only; $p = 0.43$) and 8.3% (placebo; $p = 0.008$). A significant reduction was observed in the MI rate only: 5.2% versus 8.6% for placebo ($p = 0.013$). Abciximab was associated with more bleeding episodes: 14% versus 7% ($p = 0.001$). Follow-up studies have shown abciximab to be associated with persistent significant reductions at 6 months (27% vs. 35.1%; $p = 0.001$) and 3 years [41.1% vs. 47.4% (bolus only) and 47.2% (placebo), $p = 0.009$]. Three-year follow-up also showed that the subgroup of patients with an evolving MI or refractory unstable angina (28% of patients) had a significant 60% reduction in mortality rate (5.1% vs. 12.7%; $p = 0.01$).

Comments: Significant bleeding likely was due to high heparin dosing.

93. Integrilin to Minimize Platelet Aggregation and Coronary Thrombosis II (**IMPACT II**). Randomised placebo-controlled trial of effect of eptifibatide on complications of percutaneous coronary intervention: IMPACT-II. *Lancet* 1997;349:1422–1428 (editorial, 1409–1410).

Design: Prospective, randomized, double-blind, multicenter study. The 30-day primary composite end point was death, MI, unplanned surgical or repeated percutaneous revascularization, or stenting for abrupt closure.

Purpose: To determine the effectiveness of eptifibatide in reducing ischemic complications in patients undergoing nonsurgical coronary revascularization.

Population: 4,010 patients who underwent elective, urgent, or emergency percutaneous intervention (PTCA, 91% to 93%).

Exclusion Criteria: Bleeding diathesis, major surgery in prior 6 weeks, and any history of stroke.

Treatment: Eptifibatide, 135 μg/kg intravenous bolus (10 to 60 minutes before procedure), and then 0.5 or 0.75 μg/kg/min for 20 to 24 hours; or placebo.

Results: At 30 days, a nonsignificant reduction in the primary composite end point was observed: 9.2% (135/0.5 group) and 9.9% (135/0.75 group) versus 11.4% (placebo) ($p = 0.063, 0.22$). On-treatment analysis showed that the 135/0.5 group had a significant 22% reduction in composite primary end point (9.1% vs. 11.6%; $p = 0.035$). No significant differences in bleeding or transfusion rates were observed.

94. c7E3 Fab Antiplatelet Therapy in Unstable Refractory Angina (**CAPTURE**). Randomized, placebo-controlled trial of abciximab before and during coronary intervention in refractory unstable angina: the CAPTURE study. *Lancet* 1997;349:1429–1435 (editorial, 1409–1410).

Design: Prospective, randomized, placebo-controlled, multicenter study. The 30-day primary end point was death, MI, or urgent intervention for recurrent ischemia.

Purpose: To assess whether abciximab given before and until briefly after PCI improves outcome in patients with refractory unstable angina.

Population: 1,265 patients with chest pain at rest with ST-segment depression or elevation or abnormal T waves, with one or more episodes (rest pain and/or ECG changes) occurring more than 2 hours after the start of intravenous heparin and nitrate therapy.

Exclusion Criteria: Recent MI, persisting ischemia that required immediate intervention, and left main stenosis as shown by angiography.

Treatment: After angiography, patients were randomized to abciximab (0.25 mg/kg bolus, and then 10 μg/min) or placebo for 18 to 24 hours before and 1 hour after PCI (balloon angioplasty with stenting only if necessary to maintain vessel patency). Goal ACT was 300 seconds.

Results: Trial was stopped early because of significant treatment effect (1,400 patients planned). The abciximab group had a 29% reduction in 30-day primary end points of death, MI, and ischemia requiring intervention (11.3% vs. 15.9%; $p = 0.012$). Most of this difference was due to fewer MIs (defined as CK or CK-MB 3 times the upper limit of normal in two samples): 4.1% versus 8.2% ($p = 0.002$). MIs occurred less frequently before and after PTCA in abciximab patients (0.6% vs. 2.1%; $p = 0.029$; 2.6% vs. 5.5%, $p = 0.043$). Importantly, no difference in event rates was seen at 6 months (31% vs. 30.8%). A twofold higher major bleeding rate was observed in the abciximab group (3.8% vs. 1.9%; $p = 0.043$). An ECG ischemia substudy (332 patients monitored from start of treatment to 6 hours after intervention) showed that the abciximab group had a lower incidence of two episodes of significant (≥ 1 mm) ST segment deviation (5% vs. 14%; $p < 0.01$).

Comments: In contrast to other studies, patients given abciximab for a substantial period before intervention and only briefly afterward had a reduction in events during the 18- to 24-hour interval before intervention. Lack of long-term benefits is likely owing to lack of 12-hour postintervention infusion.

95. Evaluation in PTCA to Improve Long-term Outcome with Abciximab Glycoprotein IIb/IIIa Blockade (**EPILOG**) investigators. Platelet glycoprotein IIb/IIIa receptor blockade and low-dose heparin during percutaneous coronary revascularization. *N Engl J Med* 1997;336:1689–1696 (editorial, 1748–1749).

Design: Prospective, randomized, double-blind, multicenter study. Thirty-day composite primary end point was death, MI, ischemia requiring urgent coronary bypass surgery, or repeated percutaneous coronary revascularization.

Purpose: To determine whether the clinical benefits of abciximab extend to all patients undergoing coronary intervention and to evaluate whether hemorrhagic complications are reduced by adjusting heparin dosing.

Population: 2,792 patients undergoing urgent or elective revascularization.

Exclusion Criteria: Acute MI or unstable angina with ECG changes in prior 24 hours, planned stenting or atherectomy, PCI in prior 3 months, anticoagulant therapy, major surgery or bleeding in prior 6 weeks.

Treatment: Abciximab [0.25 mg/kg intravenous bolus (10 to 60 minutes before procedure), and then 0.125 μg/kg/min for 12 hours] plus heparin (100 U/kg bolus), abciximab plus heparin, 70 U/kg, or placebo plus heparin, 100 U/kg.

Results: Abciximab groups had lower 30-day incidences of death, MI, and urgent revascularization: 5.4% and 5.2% versus 11.7% (OR, 0.45, 0.43; both $p < 0.001$). Fewer large non–Q-wave MIs also were observed (CK 5 times normal): 2.5% and 2% versus 5.6% ($p < 0.001$). Similar major bleeding rates were observed, but abciximab plus standard heparin was associated with more minor bleeds [7.4% vs. 4% (low heparin); $p < 0.001$]. At 6 months, similar rates of repeated revascularization and a smaller reduction in composite end points were observed (death, MI, and any revascularization): 22.3% and 22.8% versus 25.8% ($p = 0.04$). One-year follow-up showed persistent benefit in abciximab groups (incidences of primary end points were 9.6% and 9.5% in abciximab plus low-dose heparin and abciximab plus standard heparin groups, respectively, vs. 16.1% in placebo group).

Comments: In an effort to reduce bleeding rates, sheaths were removed as soon as possible, and no routine postprocedural heparin was administered.

96. Randomized Efficacy Study of Tirofiban for Outcomes and Restenosis (**RESTORE**) Investigators. Effects of platelet GP IIb/IIIa blockade with tirofiban on adverse cardiac events in patients with unstable angina or acute MI undergoing coronary angioplasty. *Circulation* 1997;96:1445–1453.

Design: Prospective, randomized, double-blind, placebo-controlled, multicenter study. Primary composite end point was death, MI, CABG due to failed PTCA or recurrent ischemia, repeated PTCA of target vessel due to ischemia or stenting for actual or threatened abrupt closure.

Purpose: To evaluate the effectiveness of tirofiban in patients undergoing high-risk coronary interventions.

Population: 2,139 patients seen within 72 hours of onset of symptoms with a 60% stenosis.

Exclusion Criteria: Included scheduled stenting or adjunctive rotablation.

Treatment: Tirofiban (10 μg/kg intravenous bolus over 3 minutes and then 0.15 μg/kg/min for 36 hours) or placebo. All patients were taking aspirin and heparin.

Results: For the initial procedure, PTCA was performed in 92% to 93%, and atherectomy in 7% to 8% of patients. At 30 days, a similar incidence of primary composite end points was observed (10.3% vs. 12.2%; $p = 0.16$). If only urgent/emergency CABG and PTCA are included, the rates are 8% versus 10.5% ($p = 0.052$). However, the tirofiban group had significantly fewer events at 2 days and 7 days (RR, 0.62; $p = 0.005$; RR, 0.73, $p = 0.022$), mostly because of less reinfarction and repeated PTCA [at 2 days, 2.7% vs. 4.4% ($p = 0.039$) and 1.1% vs. 3.2% ($p = 0.001$); at 7 days, 3.6% vs. 5.3% ($p = 0.055$) and 2.7% vs. 4.4% ($p = 0.034$)]. Similar rates of major bleeding and thrombocytopenia were observed [5.3% vs. 3.7% ($p = 0.096$) and 1.1% vs. 0.9%].

97. Evaluation of Platelet IIb/IIIa Inhibitor for Stenting (**EPISTENT**) Investigators. Randomized placebo-controlled and balloon-angioplasty-controlled trial to assess safety of coronary stenting with use of platelet glycoprotein IIb/IIIa blockade. *Lancet* 1998; 352:87–92.

Design: Prospective, randomized, double-blind, placebo-controlled multicenter study. Primary composite end point was death, MI, and urgent revascularization at 30 days.

Purpose: To evaluate the effects of platelet GP IIb/IIIa blockade with abciximab in conjunction with elective coronary stenting in patients with 60% coronary lesions.

Population: 2,399 patients with ischemic heart disease and suitable coronary artery lesions (e.g., stenosis $\geq$60%).

Exclusion Criteria: Unprotected left main stenosis, stroke within prior 2 years, PCI in past 3 months, systolic blood pressure (SBP) greater than 180 mm Hg, and diastolic blood pressure (DBP) greater than 100 mm Hg.

Treatment: Stent plus placebo, stent plus abciximab [0.25 mg/kg bolus up to 60 minutes before intervention, and then 0.125 μg/kg/min (maximum, 10 μg/min) for 12 hours], or balloon angioplasty plus abciximab. All patients were given aspirin and heparin (70 U/kg and 100 U/kg boluses in abciximab and placebo groups, respectively). Ticlopidine administration before enrollment was encouraged.

Results: Stent plus abciximab group had more than 50% reduction in 30-day composite end points compared with the stent plus placebo group (5.3% vs. 10.8%; $p < 0.01$), whereas the balloon angioplasty plus abciximab group had a 36% reduction (6.9%; $p = 0.007$). Death and large MIs (defined as CK greater than 5 times normal) occurred less frequently in the abciximab groups [3.0% and 4.7% vs. 7.8% (placebo)]. However, the rates of Q-wave MI were similar (0.9% to 1.5%). No significant differences were seen in major bleeding complications (1.4% to 2.2%).

98. **Lincoff AM,** et al. Complementary clinical benefits of coronary-artery stenting and blockade of platelet glycoprotein IIb/IIIa receptors. *N Engl J Med* 1999;341:319–327.

This report of the 6-month EPISTENT results demonstrates persistent benefits of stenting in combination with abciximab. The incidence of composite end points was 6.4% in the stent plus abciximab group, 9.2% in the angioplasty plus abciximab group, and 12.1% in the stent-alone group. The mortality rate with stent plus abciximab also was significantly lower than that with angioplasty plus abciximab [0.5% vs 1.8%; $p = 0.02$ (stent alone: 1.2%, $p = 0.12$)]. This mortality benefit persisted at 1 year.

99. The **ESPRIT** Investigators. Novel dosing regimen of eptifibatide in planned coronary stent implantation (ESPRIT): a randomised, placebo-controlled trial. *Lancet* 2000;356:2037–2044.

Design: Prospective, randomized, double-blind, placebo-controlled, multicenter study. Primary end point was death, MI, urgent TVR, and thrombotic bailout GP IIb/IIIa inhibitor therapy within 48 hours. Secondary end point was a composite of death, MI, and urgent TVR at 30 days.

Purpose: To determine whether double-bolus dosing of eptifibatide can improve outcomes of patients undergoing coronary stenting.

Population: 2,064 patients scheduled to undergo stent implantation.

Exclusion Criteria: These included ongoing chest pain necessitating urgent PCI, MI in prior 24 hours, PCI in prior 90 days, or planned staged PCI within 30 days, stroke or transient ischemic attack (TIA) in prior month, bleeding diathesis, major surgery in prior 6 weeks, SBP greater than 200 mm Hg or DBP greater than 110 mm Hg, platelet count less than 100,000, Cr greater than 350 μM.

Treatment: Placebo or eptifibatide (two 180 μg/kg boluses 10 minutes apart, and then 2 μg/kg/min for 18 to 24 hours). Bailout blinded GP IIb/IIIa receptor was available.

Results: The eptifibatide group had a significantly lower incidence of the primary composite end point (6.4% vs. 10.5%; $p = 0.0015$). This benefit was consistent across different components of the primary end point, including death/MI/TVR (RR, 0.65; 95% CI, 0.47 to 0.87), death/MI (RR, 0.60; CI, 0.44 to 0.82), and death (RR, 0.5; CI, 0.05 to 5.42). At 30 days, the eptifibatide group also had a reduction in the secondary end point of death, MI, and urgent TVR (6.8% vs. 10.5%; $p = 0.0034$). Eptifibatide group did have a higher incidence of major bleeding compared with placebo (1.3% vs. 0.4%; $p = 0.027$). No significant differences in major bleeding were found in the lowest tertile of ACT (ACT less than 244 seconds; 0.6% in both groups). At 6-month follow-up, the composite end point of death or MI had occurred in 7.5% of eptifibatide-treated patients and 11.5% of placebo-treated patients (RR, 0.63; 95% CI, 0.47 to 0.84; $p = 0.002$), whereas the composite of death, MI, or TVR had occurred in 14.2% and 18.2% of patients, respectively (RR, 0.75; 95% CI, 0.60 to 0.93). The 6-month mortality rate was 0.8% in the eptifibatide group and 1.4% in the placebo group (RR, 0.56; 95% CI, 0.24 to 1.34; $p = 0.19$). Kaplan–Meier survival curves appeared to separate over time, with most of the difference in mortality occurring between 30 days and 6 months (see *JAMA* 2001;285:2468–2473). At 1-year follow-up, the significant difference continued to persist (6.6% vs. 10.5%; $p = 0.015$), and a cost analysis found eptifibatide use associated with $1,407 per year of life saved (see *JAMA* 2002;287:618).

Comments: The persistent benefit observed at 6 and 12 months further supports the use of GP IIb/IIIa–receptor blockers as standard of care for patients undergoing stent implantation.

100. **Topol EJ,** et al. for the **TARGET** Investigators. Comparison of two platelet glycoprotein IIb/IIIa inhibitors, tirofiban and abciximab, for the prevention of ischemic events with percutaneous coronary revascularization. *N Engl J Med* 2001;344:1888–1894.

Design: Prospective, randomized, double-blind, double-dummy, multicenter study. Primary end points: death, nonfatal MI, or urgent TVR at 30 days.

Purpose: To compare the safety and efficacy of the two GP IIb/IIIa inhibitors, tirofiban and abciximab.

Population: 5,308 patients scheduled for coronary stenting with greater than 70% stenoses in either de novo or restenotic lesions in native coronary arteries or bypass grafts.

Exclusion Criteria: Cardiogenic shock, acute STEMI, serum creatinine 2.5 mg/dL or greater, high risk for bleeding or ongoing bleeding, platelet count less than 120,000.

Treatment: Tirofiban (10 μg/kg bolus, and then 0.15 μg/kg/min for 18 to 24 hours) or abciximab [0.25 mg/kg bolus and then 0.125 μg/kg/min (maximum, 10 μg/min) for 12 hours]. All received preprocedure aspirin (250 to 500 mg). Clopidogrel loading dose (300 mg) was given, when possible, 2 to 6 hours before PCI and then continued for 30 days (75 mg once daily). All were given initial heparin bolus of 70 U/kg, with a target ACT of 250 seconds.

Results: In both groups, 95% underwent stenting. The abciximab group had a significantly lower incidence of the primary composite end point of death, nonfatal MI, or urgent TVR compared with the tirofiban group (6.0% vs. 7.6%; $p = 0.038$). The abciximab group had fewer MIs (CK-MB, 3 times or more upper limit of normal or new Q waves; 5.4% vs. 6.9%; $p = 0.04$), whereas no significant differences were found between the two groups in 30-day mortality (0.4% vs. 0.5%; $p = 0.66$) or urgent TVR (0.7% vs. 0.8%; $p = 0.49$). Subgroup analysis showed superiority of abciximab in all subgroups, including age (younger than 65 or 65 years or older), gender, diabetes, and clopidogrel pretreatment. No significant differences were seen between the two groups in major bleeding complications or transfusions [0.7% (abciximab) vs. 0.9%; $p = $ NS], but tirofiban was associated with lower rates of minor bleeding episodes (2.8% vs. 4.3%; $p < 0.001$) and thrombocytopenia (<100,000/mm^3; 0.1% vs. 0.9%; $p < 0.001$). At 6 months, however, no significant difference was found between the groups in the incidence of the primary composite end point (14.8% vs. 14.3%; $p = 0.59$) (see *Lancet* 2002;360:355–360).

Comments: Two studies found the TARGET tirofiban dosing results in lower platelet inhibition levels compared those with abciximab, especially from 15 to 60 minutes after drug administration, which typically coincides with iatrogenic vessel injury (see *Am J Cardiol* 2002;89:647, 1293).

101. **PRICE** Investigators. Comparative 30-day economic and clinical outcomes of platelet glycoprotein IIb/IIIa inhibitor use during elective percutaneous coronary intervention: Prairie ReoPro versus Integrilin Cost Evaluation (PRICE) Trial. *Am Heart J* 2001; 141:402–409.

Prospective, randomized, double-blind study of 320 consecutive patients undergoing elective PTCA or stenting. Patients received adjunctive abciximab or eptifibatide therapy. The eptifibatide group had lower total in-hospital costs (primary end point) compared with the abciximab group (median, $7,207 vs. $8,268; $p = 0.009$). The eptifibatide group also had lower median costs at 30 days ($7,207 vs. $8,336; $p = 0.009$). No significant differences were found between the groups in incidence of death, nonfatal MI, and urgent revascularization [4.9% vs. 5.1% (hospital discharge), 5.6% vs. 6.3% (30 days)]. In a platelet-inhibition substudy (155 patients; Ultegra Rapid Platelet Function Assay), eptifibatide was associated with earlier and more durable platelet inhibition compared with abciximab ($p < 0.00001$).

102. **Karvouni E**, et al. Intravenous glycoprotein IIb/IIIa receptor antagonists reduce mortality after percutaneous coronary interventions. *J Am Coll Cardiol* 2003;41:26–32.

The authors compiled 19 randomized, placebo-controlled trials of 20,137 patients undergoing PCI with and without glycoprotein IIb/IIIa inhibition. The primary outcome was mortality, with secondary outcomes including MI, composite cardiac events, and major bleeding. The analysis included trials of both PTCA and stenting, in the elective as well as urgent/emergent setting (for acute MI). Postprocedure heparin was used in approximately half of the trials. At 30 days, there was a significant reduction in mortality favoring the glycoprotein IIb/IIIa group (RR 0.69, 95% CI, 0.53 to 0.90); this effect was persistent up to 6 months (RR 0.79, 95% CI, 0.64 to 0.97). This was a homogeneous effect across trials, for patients with and without acute MI, and regardless of continuous heparin infusion. Notably, excess bleeding was observed only in trials in which the heparin infusion was continued postprocedure (RR 1.70, 95% CI, 1.36 to 2.14).

103. **Deibele AJ,** et al. Intracoronary eptifibatide bolus administration during percutaneous coronary revascularization for acute coronary syndromes with evaluation of platelet glycoprotein IIb/IIIa receptor occupancy and platelet function: the Intracoronary Eptifibatide (**ICE**) Trial. *Circulation* 2010;121(6):784–791. [Epub 2010 Feb 1].

The investigators randomized 43 patients with ACS undergoing PCI to bolus, systemic eptifibatide versus intracoronary eptifibatide during catheterization. The primary end point was local coronary bed platelet GP IIb/IIIa saturation, as measured by coronary sinus sampling—this was significantly greater in the intracoronary group. Microvascular perfusion, as assessed by the TIMI frame count, also significantly favored the intracoronary eptifibatide group.

104. **Valgimigli M,** et al. for the Multicentre Evaluation of Single High-Dose Bolus Tirofiban vs Abciximab with Sirolimus-Eluting Stent or Bare Metal Stent in Acute Myocardial Infarction Study (**MULTISTRATEGY**) Investigators. Comparison of angioplasty with infusion of tirofiban or abciximab and with implantation of sirolimus-eluting or uncoated stents for acute myocardial infarction: the MULTISTRATEGY randomized trial. *JAMA* 2008;299:1788–1799.

Design: Randomized, controlled trial, with open-label therapies in a 2 × 2 factorial design. Primary end point differed for each comparison: in the drug comparison, it was ST-segment resolution at 90 minutes (with a noninferiority margin); in the stent comparison, it was a composite of death, reinfarction, or TVR at 8 months.
Purpose: To compare certain reperfusion strategies for STEMI, with respect to adjunctive IIb/IIIA therapy and stent selection.
Population: 745 patients with STEMI or new LBBB in Italy, Spain, and Argentina.
Treatment: Abciximab infusion versus tirofiban infusion during PCI, and BMS versus DES in PCI (2 × 2 factorial, open-label comparisons).
Results: There was no significant difference in the primary end point for the drug comparison, achieving the prespecified noninferiority margin (RR 1.020, $p < 0.001$ for noninferiority). Furthermore, bleeding complications were similar in the two groups. However, MACEs at 8 months, the primary end point, significantly favored the DES group in the stent comparison (7.8% vs. 14.5%, $p = 0.004$). This was driven by a decrease in revascularization rates in the coated stent group.

THROMBIN INHIBITORS

105. **Bittl A,** et al. Hirulog Angioplasty Study investigators (**HAS**). Treatment with bivalirudin (hirulog) as compared with heparin during coronary angioplasty for unstable or postinfarction angina. *N Engl J Med* 1995;333:764–769 (also see *Am Heart J* 2001;142:952–959).

Design: Prospective, randomized, double-blind, multicenter study. Primary composite end point was death in hospital, MI, abrupt vessel closure, or rapid clinical deterioration of cardiac origin. Follow-up period was 6 months.
Purpose: To evaluate whether bivalirudin is more effective than heparin in reducing mortality and ischemic events in unstable or postinfarction angina patients undergoing angioplasty.
Population: 4,098 patients undergoing coronary angioplasty (PTCA) for unstable angina or postinfarct angina.
Treatment: Bivalirudin, 1.0 mg/kg bolus, and then 2.5 mg/kg/hr for 4 hours and 1.0 mg/kg/hr for 14 to 20 hours, or heparin, 175 U/kg bolus, and then 15 U/kg/hr for 18 to 24 hours. Agents were started immediately before angioplasty, and doses were adjusted according to ACTs. All patients received aspirin (300 to 325 mg daily).

Results: Overall, no significant difference occurred between the groups in the incidence of the primary composite end point at 6 months (11.4% vs. 12.2%). At 7 days, however, fewer events were found in the bivalirudin group (6.2% vs. 7.9%; $p = 0.039$). Among postinfarction angina patients, bivalirudin was associated with a significant reduction in composite end points (9.1% vs. 14.2%; $p = 0.04$), although at 6 months, the cumulative rates of death, MI, and repeated revascularization were similar (20.5% vs. 25.1%; $p = 0.1$). Bivalirudin was associated with decreased bleeding (3.8% vs. 9.8%; $p < 0.001$).

106. **REPLACE-2.** Lincoff AM, et al. Bivalirudin and provisional glycoprotein IIb/IIIa blockade compared with heparin and planned glycoprotein IIb/IIIa blockade during percutaneous coronary intervention: the REPLACE-2 randomized trial. *JAMA* 2003;289:853–863.

This prospective, randomized, double-blind, triple-dummy, multicenter trial randomized 6,010 PCI patients to heparin plus a GP IIb/IIIa blocker (eptifibatide or abciximab) or to bivalirudin alone (0.75 mg/kg bolus plus 1.75 mg/kg/hr for duration of PCI) with the provisional addition of a GP IIb/IIIa blocker if needed in a double-blind, triple-dummy design. Provisional GP IIb/IIIa–blocker treatment was given to 7.2% of the bivalirudin group and 5.2% of the heparin and GP IIb/IIIa–blocker group. A nonsignificant reduction in death, MI, urgent revascularization at 30 days and major in-hospital bleeding (primary end point) with bivalirudin was found compared with heparin plus GP IIb/IIIa blockers (9.2% vs. 10.0%; $p = 0.32$). Among the four components, the only significant difference between the groups was a significantly lower incidence of bleeding with bivalirudin (2.4% vs. 4.1%). The secondary triple end point (death, MI, urgent revascularization) showed a trend toward fewer events in the heparin-plus-IIb/IIIa-blocker group [7.1% vs. 7.6% (bivalirudin)]; the difference was driven by a nonsignificant excess of MI with bivalirudin (7.0% vs. 6.2%). A cost analysis found that use of bivalirudin was associated with a cost savings of $448 per patient.

107. **Kastrati A,** et al. for the ISAR-REACT 3 Trial Investigators. Bivalirudin versus unfractionated heparin during percutaneous coronary intervention. *N Engl J Med* 2008;359:688–696.

Design: Prospective, randomized, double-blind, multicenter study. Primary composite end point of death, MI, urgent TVR for ischemia, or major bleeding at 30 days; this was designed as a net clinical benefit end point.

Purpose: To establish whether bivalirudin is superior to UFH in patients undergoing PCI after pretreatment with clopidogrel.

Population: 4,570 patients with stable or low-risk (normal cardiac markers) unstable angina undergoing PCI and pretreated with 600 mg clopidogrel at least 2 hours before PCI.

Treatment: Treatment during PCI with either bivalirudin or UFH.

Results: The primary end point occurred in 8.3% of patients in the bivalirudin group versus 8.7% in the UFH group ($p = 0.57$). The secondary end point of death, MI, or urgent TVR for ischemia occurred in 5.9% of the bivalirudin group compared with 5.0% in the UFH group ($p = 0.23$). Major bleeding occurred in 3.1% of patients receiving bivalirudin and 4.6% patients in the UFH group ($p = 0.008$). Thus, while there was no significant clinical benefit in terms of ischemic events, bivalirudin did reduce bleeding events in low-risk patients undergoing PCI.

See also the HORIZONS-AMI study in Chapter 4.

Directional Atherectomy Studies

108. **Topol EJ,** et al. Coronary Angioplasty versus Excisional Atherectomy Trial (**CAVEAT**). A comparison of directional atherectomy with coronary angioplasty in patients with coronary artery disease. *N Engl J Med* 1993;329:221–227.

Design: Prospective, randomized, controlled, multicenter study. Primary end point was angiographic restenosis at 6 months.

Purpose: To compare outcomes in patients undergoing balloon angioplasty (PTCA) with those having DCA.

Population: 1,012 patients with symptomatic CAD and no prior intracoronary interventions.

Treatment: PTCA or DCA.

Results: The atherectomy group had a higher initial success rate (≤50% stenosis; 89% vs. 80%) but was associated with a higher rate of early complications (11% vs. 5%) and higher hospital costs. At 6-month angiography, the atherectomy group showed a trend toward lower restenosis (50% vs. 57%; $p = 0.06$) and a higher probability of death or MI (8.6% vs. 4.6%; $p = 0$).

109. **Adelman AG,** et al. Canadian Coronary Atherectomy Trial (**CCAT**). A comparison of directional atherectomy with balloon angioplasty for lesions of the left anterior descending coronary artery. *N Engl J Med* 1993;329:228–233.

Design: Prospective, randomized, open-label, multicenter study. Primary end point was restenosis at follow-up angiography (median, 5.9 months).

Purpose: To compare restenosis rates for balloon angioplasty and directional atherectomy in lesions of the proximal LAD artery.

Population: 274 patients with de novo 60% stenosis of the LAD artery.

Treatment: Balloon angioplasty or directional atherectomy.

Results: Atherectomy group had a nonsignificantly higher success rate (94% vs. 88%; $p = 0.06$); no difference in complication rates was observed (5% vs. 6%). At follow-up angiography, restenosis rates and MLDs were similar [43% (angioplasty) vs. 46% (atherectomy); 1.61 vs. 1.55 mm].

110. **Simonton CA,** et al. Optimal directional atherectomy: final results of the Optimal Atherectomy Restenosis Study (**OARS**). *Circulation* 1998;97:332–339.

Design: Prospective, multicenter registry study. Primary end point was angiographic restenosis at 6 months.

Purpose: To determine if use of an optimal atherectomy technique would translate into a lower rate of late clinical and angiographic restenosis.

Population: 199 patients aged 18 to 80 years with angina or a positive functional study and after angiographic criteria: (a) target-vessel reference diameter, 3.0 to 4.5 mm; (b) culprit lesion(s) with 60% stenosis; and (c) mild to moderate tortuosity and mild or no target-lesion calcification. DCA and adjunctive angioplasty were performed if necessary to achieve less than 15% residual stenosis; 213 lesions met the criteria.

Treatment: DCA (7F device).

Results: Frequent (87%) postatherectomy angioplasty was performed. The short-term procedural success rate was 97.5%. The mean rate of residual stenosis was only 7%. The major complication rate was 2.5% (death, emergency bypass surgery, Q-wave MI). Non–Q-wave MI (CK-MB more than 3 times normal) occurred in 14%. At 1-year follow-up, the TLR rate was 17.8%. The 6-month restenosis rate was 28.9% (major predictor: smaller postprocedural lumen diameter).

Comments: A lower restenosis rate was observed than in prior directional atherectomy trials.

111. **Baim DS,** et al.. for the Balloon vs Optimal Atherectomy Trial (**BOAT**) Investigators. Final results of the Balloon vs. Optimal Atherectomy Trial (BOAT). *Circulation* 1998;97:322–331.

Design: Prospective, randomized, double-blind, multicenter study. Primary end point was restenosis rate at follow-up angiography (median, 6.9 months).

Purpose: To compare the optimal DCA technique with conventional balloon angioplasty on restenosis.

Population: 1,000 patients with single de novo, native vessel lesions in vessels larger than 3 mm in diameter.

Treatment: DCA (large device used) with aggressive tissue removal and use of adjunctive PTCA if indicated, or PTCA alone.

Results: DCA group had a higher procedural success rate (99% vs. 97%; $p = 0.02$) and a lower rate of residual stenosis (15% vs. 28%; $p < 0.0001$). Similar rates of major complication were observed (2.8% vs. 3.3%). However, DCA was associated with more frequent CK-MB elevations (more than 3 times normal; 16% vs. 6%; $p < 0.0001$). At follow-up angiography, the DCA group had a lower restenosis rate (primary end point): 31.4% versus 39.8% ($p = 0.016$). At 1-year follow-up, the DCA group had nonsignificant reductions in mortality (0.6% vs. 1.6%; $p = 0.14$), TVR (17.1% vs. 19.7%; $p = 0.33$), target-site revascularization (15.3% vs. 18.3%; $p = 0.23$), and target-vessel failure (death, Q-wave MI, or TVR; 21.1% vs. 24.8%; $p = 0.17$).

112. **Tsuchikane E,** et al. for the PERFECT Investigators. Pre-drug-eluting stent debulking of bifurcated coronary lesions. *J Am Coll Cardiol* 2007;50(20): 1941–1945. [Epub 2007 Oct 29].

The investigators recruited 99 patients undergoing PCI (with DES) of bifurcation lesions to this prospective, multicenter registry. Plaque debulking by DCA was performed in each case for the main and side branches (if feasible) prior to stent placement in the main branch only; each patient subsequently returned for repeat angiography 9 months later. The primary outcome of binary angiography restenosis was observed in 1.1% and 3.4% of main and side branches, respectively. No MACEs were observed in-hospital. This small, nonrandomized study suggests DCA prior to main-branch stenting with DES may be an acceptable alternative to complicated stenting for bifurcation lesions.

Rotational Atherectomy Studies

113. **Dill T,** et al. A randomized comparison of balloon angioplasty versus rotational atherectomy in complex coronary lesions (**COBRA** study). *Eur Heart J* 2000;21:1759–1766.

Design: Prospective, randomized, open-label, multicenter study. Primary end points were procedural success, 6-month restenosis rates in the treated segments, and major cardiac events during follow-up.

Purpose: To compare outcomes between RA and balloon angioplasty for the treatment of complex coronary artery lesions.

Population: 502 patients aged 20 to 80 years with angina and angiographic CAD with target-lesion stenosis of 70% to 99% and mean lumen diameter of 1 mm or less for a length of 5 mm or more. Lesions were required to be complex (calcified, ostial or bifurcational, eccentric, diffuse, or within angulated segment).

Exclusion Criteria: Unstable angina, MI in previous 4 weeks, prior PCI of target vessel within 2 months, left ventricular ejection fraction (LVEF) less than 30%.

Treatment: Rotablation (burr sizes, 1.25 to 2.5) or balloon angioplasty. All received ASA, nitroglycerin, nifedipine, and heparin (15 to 20 KU with target ACT, 350 seconds or more). Stenting allowed bailout for unsatisfactory outcomes.

Results: Procedural success was achieved more frequently with rotablation compared with angioplasty (85% vs. 78%; $p = 0.038$). No difference was found between PTCA and rotablation with respect to procedure-related complications such as Q-wave infarctions (both groups, 2.4%), emergency bypass surgery (1.2% vs. 2.4%), and death (1.6% vs. 0.4%). A higher incidence of stenting occurred after PTCA (14.9% vs. 6.4%; $p < 0.002$), mostly because of bailout or unsatisfactory results. If bailout stenting is included as an end point, procedural success rates were 84% for rotablation and were 73% for angioplasty ($p = 0.006$). At 6 months, the restenosis rates were similar in both groups (rotablation, 49%; PTCA, 51%).

114. **vom Dahl J,** et al. Rotational atherectomy does not reduce recurrent in-stent restenosis: results of the Angioplasty Versus Rotational Atherectomy for Treatment of Diffuse In-Stent Restenosis Trial (**ARTIST**). *Circulation* 2002;105:583–588.

Design: Prospective, randomized, multicenter (24 European sites). Primary end point was MLD assessed by QCA at 6 months.

Purpose: To determine the safety and efficacy of RA with balloon angioplasty (PTCA) compared with PTCA alone for the treatment of diffuse ISR.

Population: 298 patients with angina and/or objective evidence of target vessel–related ischemia and all of the following: documented ISR more than 70% within a stent ±5 mm of stent edges, stent diameter 2.5 mm or more, ISR as only lesion for treatment, length of ISR of 10 to 50 mm, lesion accessible for rotablation.

Treatment: RA with PTCA or PTCA alone. Rotablation was performed by using a stepped-burr approach followed by adjunctive PTCA with low (6 atm) inflation pressure. Use of GP IIb/IIIa inhibitors was discouraged.

Results: Initial procedural success rates (residual stenosis less than 30%) were similar in both groups (89% PTCA, 88% RA). However, at 6-month angiography, the PTCA group had superior results with a mean net gain in MLD of 0.67 mm versus 0.45 mm for RA ($p = 0.0019$). The mean gain in diameter of stenosis was 25% and 17% ($p = 0.002$), resulting in binary restenosis rates of 51% (PTCA) and 65% (RA; $p = 0.039$). Six-month event-free survival also was significantly higher after PTCA (91.3%) compared with RA (79.6%; $p = 0.0052$).

115. **Stankovic G,** et al. and AMIGO Investigators. Comparison of directional coronary atherectomy and stenting versus stenting alone for the treatment of de novo and restenotic coronary artery narrowing. *J Am Coll Cardiol* 2004;93:9

This prospective, multicenter (46 European sites) study randomized 753 patients to DCA plus stenting or stenting alone. The average lesion length was 14.6 mm in the DCA/stent group and 14.3 mm in the stent-only group. At 8 months, no significant overall difference was found in the subgroup (74%) with follow-up angiography available (26.7% in DCA/stent group vs. 22.1% in the stent-only group; $p = $ NS). Rates of mortality (1.3% vs. 0.8%, $p = 0.725$) and target-vessel failure, the composite of death, MI, or TVR (23.9% vs. 21.5%, $p = 0.487$) were similar between the two groups at 12 months.

Special Situations

CHRONIC TOTAL OCCLUSIONS

Angioplasty

116. **Violaris AG,** et al. Long-term luminal renarrowing after successful elective coronary angioplasty of total occlusion. *Circulation* 1995;91:2140–2150 (editorial, 2113–2114).

This analysis focused on 2,930 patients from four prospective restenosis trials, 7% with chronic occlusions. The occluded group had a higher restenosis rate (44.7% vs. 34.0%; RR, 1.58; $p < 0.001$), mostly due to more reocclusions (19.2% vs. 5.0%). The occluded group also had more absolute mean LD loss (0.43 vs. 0.31 mm; $p < 0.001$). The accompanying editorial points out that the occluded group had more prior MIs. Subsequent decreased distal bed flow could lead to slower flow, especially after angioplasty, causing increased reocclusion.

Stenting

117. **Rubatelli P,** et al. Gruppo Italiano di Studio sullo Stent nelle Occlusioni Coronariche (**GISSOC**). Stent implantation vs balloon angioplasty in chronic coronary occlusions: results from the GISSOC trial. *J Am Coll Cardiol* 1998;32:90–96.

This randomized study was composed of 110 patients who underwent successful PTCA of a chronically occluded vessel 3 mm in diameter. Patients were randomized to PS stenting and warfarin for 1 month, or to no other therapy. Repeated angiography (at mean 9 months) revealed that the stent group had a larger mean LD (1.74 mm vs. 0.85 mm; $p < 0.001$), lower restenosis rate (32% vs. 68%; $p < 0.001$), and less reocclusion (8% vs. 34%; $p = 0.003$). The stent group also had less recurrent ischemia (14% vs. 46%; $p = 0.002$) and TLR (5.3% vs. 22%; $p = 0.038$), although hospitalization was prolonged.

118. **Buller CE,** et al. Total Occlusion Study of Canada (**TOSCA**) Investigators. Primary stenting versus balloon angioplasty in occluded coronary arteries. *Circulation* 1999;100:236–242.

This prospective, multicenter, randomized trial of primary stenting (with heparin-coated PS stent) versus balloon angioplasty was composed of 410 patients with symptomatic nonacute total occlusion (TIMI grade 0/1 flow) of native coronary arteries. Randomization occurred after successful placement of a guide wire across the occlusion and was stratified by duration of occlusion (≤6 weeks vs. more than 6 weeks/unknown). The crossover rate to the stent arm was 10%. The overall incidence of the primary end point, failure of sustained TIMI grade 3 flow at 6 months (confirmed by angiography), was significantly lower in the stent group (10.9% vs. 19.5%; $p = 0.024$). The stent group also had a lower restenosis rate (<50% diameter stenosis; 55% vs. 70%; $p < 0.01$) and less TVR at 6 months (8.4% vs. 15.4%; $p = 0.03$).

119. **Hochman JS,** et al. for the Occluded Artery Trial (OAT) Investigators. Coronary intervention for persistent occlusion after myocardial Infarction. *N Engl J Med* 2006; 355:2395–2407.

Design: Prospective, randomized, multicenter trial with a primary–end point composite of death, MI, or NYHA class IV heart failure at 4 years.

Purpose: To determine the safety of the treatment of diffuse ISR.

Population: 2,166 patients with stable CAD who had total occlusion of an infarct-related artery 3 to 28 days after MI, and who had high-risk features (EF <50% or proximal occlusion). Patients in whom the infarct zone did not appear akinetic or dyskinetic were required to undergo stress testing prior to randomization—those with severe ischemia were excluded.

Treatment: PCI of infarct-related artery with stenting and optimal medical therapy, or optimal medical therapy alone.

Results: At 4 years of follow-up, a primary–end point event occurred in 17.2% of the PCI group and 15.6% of the medical therapy group (HR 1.16, $p = 0.20$). Rates of recurrent, non-fatal MI were 6.9% in the PCI group and 5.0% in the medical therapy arm ($p = 0.08$): notably, only 6 (0.6%) reinfarctions were attributed to the assigned PCI procedure. Based on these data, PCI does not appear to benefit patients who have had an evolved infarct without residual ischemia.

SAPHENOUS VEIN GRAFT LESIONS

Angioplasty

120. **Feyter PJ,** et al. Balloon angioplasty for the treatment of lesions in saphenous vein grafts. *J Am Coll Cardiol* 1993;21:1539–1549.

This review estimates an initial success rate of 90% and restenosis rate of 42%. The poorest outcomes were seen in patients with chronic total occlusions, diffuse SVG disease, and presence of chronic graft thrombus.

Stenting

121. **Savage MP,** et al. Saphenous Vein de novo (**SAVED**). Stent placement compared with balloon angioplasty for obstructed coronary bypass grafts. *N Engl J Med* 1997; 338:740–747.

Design: Prospective, randomized, multicenter study. Primary end point was restenosis.

Purpose: To compare stent implantation with balloon angioplasty for the treatment of obstructive disease of venous bypass grafts.

Population: 220 patients with obstructed coronary bypass grafts.

Exclusion Criteria: MI in prior 7 days, ejection fraction less than 25%, diffuse disease that would require more than stents, and presence of thrombus.

Treatment: PS stent or balloon angioplasty.

Results: Stent group had higher procedural efficacy, defined as residual stenosis less than 50% without cardiac complications (92% vs. 69%; $p < 0.001$). However, the stent group had more hemorrhagic complications (17% vs. 5%; $p < 0.01$). Restenosis rates were not significantly different [37% (stent group) vs. 46%; $p = 0.24$], but the stent group had a lower incidence in the composite end points of freedom from death, MI, repeated bypass surgery, and TLR (73% vs. 58%; $p = 0.03$).

122. **Vermeersch P,** et al. Randomized double-blind comparison of sirolimus-eluting stent versus bare-metal stent implantation in diseased saphenous vein grafts: six-month angiographic, intravascular ultrasound, and clinical follow-up of the RRISC trial. *J Am Coll Cardiol* 2006;48(12):2423–2431. [Epub 2006 Nov 28].

In 75 patients with 96 SVG lesions were randomized to PCI with either BMS or SES, and all underwent angiography 6 months later for the primary end point of in-stent late lumen loss. Lumen loss at 6 months was significantly lower in the SES group (0.38 mm vs. 0.79 mm, $p = 0.001$). Additionally, TLR (5.3% vs. 21.6%, $p = 0.047$) and TVR (5.3% vs. 27%, $p = 0.012$) rates were significantly lower for SES; however, MACE events were similar at 6 months. Notably, in the long-term follow-up study, mortality at mean follow-up of 32 months was lower in the BMS group (29% vs. 0%, $p < 0.001$), and the 6-month advantage of SES for repeat revascularization was lost (see DELAYED-RRISC, *J Am Coll Cardiol* 2007;50(3):261–267. Epub 2007 Jun 13).

123. **Brilakis ES,** et al. A randomized controlled trial of a paclitaxel-eluting stent versus a similar bare-metal stent in saphenous vein graft lesions the SOS (Stenting of Saphenous Vein Grafts) trial. *J Am Coll Cardiol* 2009;53(11):919–928.

Not to be confused with another SOS trial, these investigators randomized 80 patients with 112 SVG lesions, in a controlled, multicenter trial, to either BMS or PES for their SVG disease. Primary end point was binary in-segment restenosis at 12 months (by angiography). This was dramatically lower in the PES group (9% vs. 51%, $p < 0.0001$); over 18 months, TLR was significantly lower, as well (5% vs. 28%, $p = 0.03$). There were also nonsignificant trends toward reduced target-vessel failure and MI in the PES group, with similar mortality.

124. **Rodés-Cabau J,** et al. Comparison of plaque sealing with paclitaxel-eluting stents versus medical therapy for the treatment of moderate nonsignificant saphenous vein graft lesions: the moderate vein graft lesion stenting with the Taxus stent and intravascular ultrasound (VELETI) pilot trial. *Circulation* 2009;120(20):1978–1986. [Epub 2009 Nov 2].

The investigators randomized 57 patients with at least 1 SVG lesion of 30% to 60% to PCI with a PES or medical therapy alone, with IVUS and angiography at baseline and 12-month follow-up. Primary end points of the study were minimal SVG lumen by IVUS and changes in atheroma volume in disease-free SVG by ultrasound. At follow-up, patients in the medical therapy group had significant progression of disease within the index lesion compared with patients who received PES (22% vs. 0%, $p = 0.014$). Additionally, mean minimal lumen area also increased to a greater extent in the PES group ($p = 0.001$). At 12 months, incidence of MACE was 19% in the medical therapy group versus 3% in the PES group ($p = 0.091$).

SMALL VESSELS

125. **Akiyama T,** et al. Angiographic and clinical outcome following coronary stenting of small vessels. *J Am Coll Cardiol* 1998;32:1610–1618.

This analysis showed that stenting of small vessels is associated with poorer outcomes. A total of 1,298 consecutive patients with 1,673 lesions were identified; angiographic follow-up was done in 75%. Patients with smaller than 3-mm vessels versus 3 mm showed no difference in procedural success or subacute stent thrombosis rates (95.9% vs. 95.4%; 1.4% vs. 1.5%) but had a higher restenosis rate (32.6% vs. 19.9%; $p < 0.0001$) and a lower rate of event-free survival (63% vs. 71.3%; $p = 0.007$).

126. **Savage MP,** et al. Efficacy of coronary stenting versus balloon angioplasty in small coronary arteries: Stent Restenosis Study (STRESS) Investigators. *J Am Coll Cardiol* 1998;31:307–311.

Angiographic substudy of 331 STRESS I-II patients who had symptomatic CAD, de novo greater than 70% stenosis in native coronary vessel, lesion length less than 15 mm, and reference vessel diameter less than 3.0 mm by QCA. Patients underwent PS stenting (170) or balloon angioplasty. Compared with angioplasty, stenting was associated with a larger postprocedural lumen diameter (2.26 mm vs. 1.80 mm; $p < 0.001$), and this advantage persisted at 6 months (1.54 mm vs. 1.27 mm; $p < 0.001$). The binary restenosis rates at 6 months were 34% for stenting and 55% for angioplasty ($p < 0.001$). At 1 year, the event-free (death, MI, or revascularization) survival rate was better with stenting (78% vs. 67%; $p = 0.019$), primarily because of a lower TLR rate with stenting (16.1% vs. 26.6%; $p = 0.015$).

127. **Kastrati A,** et al. A randomized trial comparing stenting with balloon angioplasty in small vessels in patients with symptomatic coronary artery disease. **ISAR-SMART** Study Investigators. Intracoronary stenting or angioplasty for restenosis reduction in small arteries. *Circulation* 2000;102:2593–2598.

Design: Prospective, randomized, multicenter study. Primary end point was the incidence of angiographic restenosis at 6 months.
Purpose: To assess whether, compared with PTCA, stenting of small coronary vessels is associated with a reduction of restenosis.
Population: 404 patients with symptomatic CAD with lesions in vessels with 2.0- to 2.8-mm diameter.
Exclusion Criteria: Included acute MI in previous 3 days, left main stenoses, ISR.
Treatment: Stenting or PTCA. Adjunct therapy consisted of abciximab, ticlopidine, and ASA.
Results: In the PTCA group, 16.5% received at least one stent. Six-month angiographic restenosis rates were similar between the two groups [35.7% (stent) vs. 37.4% (PTCA); $p = 0.74$]. At 7 months, similar rates were found of death or MI (3.4% vs. 3.0%) and TVR (20.1% vs. 16.5%; $p = 0.35$).
Comments: In a prespecified subgroup analysis of the 98 (24%) patients with long lesions (15 mm), stenting was associated with a significant 41% relative reduction in restenosis compared with PTCA (35.6% vs. 60.6%; $p = 0.028$); however, 1-year TVR rates were not significantly different (see *Am J Cardiol* 2002;89:58).

128. **Koning R,** et al. for the **BESMART** (BeStent in Small Arteries) Trial Investigators. Stent placement compared with balloon angioplasty for small coronary arteries: in-hospital and 6-month clinical and angiographic results. *Circulation* 2001;104:1604–1608.

Design: Prospective, randomized, double-blind, multicenter study. Primary end point was angiographic restenosis rate at 6 months.
Purpose: To compare the results of balloon angioplasty with stenting in small arteries.
Population: 381 symptomatic patients with de novo focal lesions in small coronary vessels (<3.0 mm).

Exclusion Criteria: Ostial and/or bifurcation lesion, LVEF 30%, MI in previous 3 days, contraindication to ASA or ticlopidine.

Treatment: Stent implantation or standard balloon angioplasty.

Results: Angiographic success rates were similar [97.6% (stent), 93.9% (PTCA)]. At follow-up angiography (obtained in 91%), the stent group had a significant 55% relative reduction in restenosis (21% vs. 47%; $p = 0.0001$). Repeated TLR was less frequent in the stent group (13% vs. 25%; $p = 0.0006$).

129. **Doucet S,** et al. for the Stent In Small Arteries (**SISA**) Trial Investigators. Stent placement to prevent restenosis after angioplasty in small coronary arteries. *Circulation* 2001;104:2029–2033.

Design: Prospective, randomized, multicenter study. Primary end point was angiographic restenosis at 6 months (repeated angiography performed in 85.3%).

Purpose: To compare the effects of stenting and angioplasty in small vessels on restenosis rates and other major outcomes.

Population: 351 patients with stable angina, stabilized unstable angina, or documented silent ischemia with a de novo lesion and with reference vessel diameter between 2.3 mm and 2.9 mm.

Treatment: Balloon angioplasty (PTCA) alone or stent implantation.

Results: Angiographic success was achieved in 98.2% of stent patients versus 93.9% of PTCA patients ($p = 0.0065$). In the angioplasty group, 37 (20.3%) patients crossed over to stent implantation. Clinical success was higher in the stent group (95.3% vs. 87.9%; $p = 0.007$). No differences were found in major in-hospital cardiac complications including death (none), Q-wave MI (none), non–Q-wave MI (4.9% in the PTCA group vs. 1.8% in the stent group), CABG surgery (0.5% vs. 0.6%), and repeated angioplasty (2.7% vs. 0.6%). A trend toward fewer in-hospital events was seen in the stent group (3.0% vs. 7.1% in angioplasty group; $p = 0.076$), driven primarily by a lower incidence of non–Q-wave MI in the stent group. At 6 months, no significant differences were seen in the rates of angiographic restenosis [28% (stenting) vs. 32.9%] or TVR (17.8% vs. 20.3%).

DIABETES

130. **Kip KE,** et al. Coronary angioplasty in diabetic patients: the NHLBI PTCA Registry. *Circulation* 1996;94:1818–1825.

In this analysis of the 1985 to 1986 NHLBI Registry, 281 diabetic and 1,833 nondiabetic patients were studied. The diabetic group was older and had more triple-vessel coronary disease, atherosclerotic lesions, and comorbidities. At 9-year follow-up, diabetic patients had a twofold higher mortality rate (35.9% vs. 17.9%) and increased incidence of nonfatal MI (29% vs. 18.5%), CABG surgery (36.7% vs. 27.4%), and repeated PTCA (43.7% vs. 36.5%).

131. **Van Belle E,** et al. Effects of coronary stenting on vessel patency and long-term clinical outcome after percutaneous coronary revascularization in diabetic patients. *J Am Coll Cardiol* 2002;40:410–417.

A total of 314 diabetics undergoing stenting ($n = 157$) or balloon angioplasty ($n = 157$) were matched for gender, diabetes treatment regimen, stenosis location, reference diameter, and MLD. Other baseline characteristics were similar between groups. At 6 months, the stent group had a significantly lower restenosis rate (27% vs. 62%; $p < 0.0001$) and occlusion rate (4% vs. 13%; $p < 0.005$) than the angioplasty group. The ejection fraction in the stent group remained unchanged at 6 months, whereas the angioplasty group had a significant decrease ($p = 0.02$). At 4-year follow-up, the stent group had lower rates of cardiac death and nonfatal MI (14.8% vs. 26.0%; $p = 0.02$) and revascularization (35.4% vs. 52.1%).

132. **Sabaté M,** et al. for DIABETES Investigators. Randomized comparison of sirolimus-eluting stent versus standard stent for percutaneous coronary revascularization in diabetic patients:

the diabetes and sirolimus-eluting stent (DIABETES) trial. *Circulation* 2005;112: 2175–2183.

Design: Prospective, randomized, multicenter study. Primary end point was in-stent late lumen loss on angiography restenosis at 9 months.

Purpose: To compare the effects of stenting with BMS versus SES in patients with diabetes.

Population: 160 patients with diabetes, 33% of whom were on insulin, with de novo coronary stenoses.

Treatment: PCI with BMS or SES.

Results: At 9-month angiography, in-stent late lumen loss was significantly less in the SES group (0.06 mm) compared with the BMS group (0.47 mm, $p < 0.001$), as were TLR rates (7.3% vs. 31.3%, $p < 0.001$) and MACE rates (11.3% vs. 36.3%, $p < 0.001$). Outcomes were similar between patients on insulin and those off insulin.

Comment: Long-term follow-up demonstrated persistent differences in rates of TLR, and long-term safety of SES. However, they did observe stent thromboses in the SES group between 1 and 2 years, when patients had discontinued clopidogrel. (See *Eur Heart J* 2007 Aug;28(16):1946–1952. Epub 2007 Jun 11.)

133. **Lee S-W,** et al. A randomized comparison of sirolimus- versus paclitaxel-eluting stent implantation in patients with diabetes mellitus (The DES-DIABETES [Drug-Eluting Stent in patients with DIABETES mellitus] Trial). *J Am Coll Cardiol* 2008;52:727–733.

Design: Prospective, randomized, multicenter study. Primary end point was in-stent restenosis at 6 months.

Purpose: To compare the effects of stenting with PES versus SES in patients with diabetes.

Population: 400 patients with diabetes with native-vessel coronary stenoses.

Treatment: PCI with PES or SES.

Results: At 6-month angiographic follow-up, the SES had improved rates of in-stent restenosis (3.4% vs. 18.2%, $p < 0.001$), in-segment restenosis (4.0% vs. 20.8%, $p < 0.001$), as well as 9-month TLR rates (2.0% vs. 7.5%, $p = 0.017$). The groups had similar rates of death or MI at 9 months.

Comment: Long-term follow-up demonstrated similar findings at 24 months; that is, rates of death or MI were similar, but SES continued to carry an advantage for TVR (5.5% vs. 12.0%, $p = 0.014$) and TLR (3.5% vs. 11.0%, $p = 0.004$) (see *J Am Coll Cardiol* 2009; 53(9):812–813).

Complications

POSTINTERVENTION CK/CK-MB AND TROPONIN STUDIES

134. **Abdelmeguid AE,** et al. Significance of mild transient release of CK-MB fraction after percutaneous coronary interventions. *Circulation* 1996;94:1528–1536.

This retrospective analysis focused on 4,484 patients after PTCA or directional atherectomy. No elevations were detected in 3,776 patients; the CK level was 100 to 180 IU/L, and MB, greater than 4% in 450 patients, and CK, 181 to 360 IU/L, and MB, more than 4% in 258 patients. CK-MB elevation predictors included atherectomy (OR, 4.1) and catheterization laboratory complications (OR, 2.6). At 3 years, the group with elevated CK and CK-MB had more MIs (RR, 1.3), cardiac deaths (RR, 1.3), and ischemic complications (death, MI, revascularization; 48.9% vs. 43.3% vs. 37.3%).

135. **Kong TQ Jr,** et al. Prognostic implication of CK elevation following elective coronary artery interventions. *JAMA* 1997;277:461–466.

This retrospective cohort study was composed of 253 consecutive patients with CK and CK-MB elevations and 120 patients without CK elevations. The CK elevation group had increased cardiac mortality ($p = 0.02$), highest if more than 3 times normal (RR, 1.05 per 100 U/L CK increase). The effect was independent of procedure type and outcome. Top mortality predictors were peak CK and ejection fraction (both $p < 0.001$).

136. **Tardiff BE,** et al. Clinical outcomes after detection of elevated cardiac enzymes in patients undergoing percutaneous intervention. *J Am Coll Cardiol* 1999;33:88–96.

This analysis of the IMPACT-II database showed that even small elevations in cardiac enzymes are associated with an increased short-term risk of adverse outcomes. No CK-MB elevation was seen in 1,779 (76%) patients, whereas levels were elevated to 1 to 3 times the upper limit of normal (ULN) in 323 patients (13.8%), 3 to 5 times ULN in 3.6%, 5 to 10 times ULN in 3.7%, and more than 10 times ULN in 2.9%. For all devices, including stents, CK-MB elevations of any magnitude were associated with an increased incidence of the composite end point at 30 days and 6 months (at 6 months, normal CK-MB level was 20.2% to 27.3%; CK-MB, 1 to 3 times ULN was 29.6% to 40.0%). The degree of risk correlated with the increase in enzymes, even for patients who had undergone successful procedures without abrupt closure. As seen in other studies, atherectomy performed in conjunction with angioplasty was associated with a greater incidence of postprocedural CK-MB elevations than was angioplasty alone ($p < 0.0001$).

137. **Bonz AW,** et al. Effect of additional temporary glycoprotein IIb/IIIa receptor inhibition on troponin release in elective percutaneous coronary interventions after pretreatment with aspirin and clopidogrel (**TOPSTAR** Trial). *J Am Coll Cardiol* 2002;40:662–668.

This prospective, randomized, double-blind, placebo-controlled, single-center study enrolled 109 patients with stable angina undergoing PCI. All were pretreated with a loading dose of clopidogrel (375 mg) and ASA (500 mg) 1 day before PCI. Patients were randomized to received tirofiban (10 μg/kg bolus and then 0.15 μg/kg/min for 18 hours) or placebo. At 12, 24, and 48 hours after PCI, the tirofiban-treated patients had a lower incidence of troponin T release (12 hours, 40% vs. 63%; $p < 0.05$; 24 hours, 48% vs. 69%; $p < 0.05$; 48 hours, 58% vs. 74%; $p < 0.08$). At 9 months, the tirofiban group had a lower incidence of death, MI, and TVR (2.3% vs. 13.0%; $p < 0.05$). Future, larger studies are needed to confirm these findings, especially whether small troponin elevations with normal CK-MB levels are correlated with worse prognosis.

Also see *Ann Clin Biochem* 2002;39:392–397: troponin I 2.0 or more seen in 27% and correlated with an increased incidence of recurrent angina, repeated PCI, coronary bypass surgery, and cardiac death at 2 years.

138. **Ellis SG,** et al. Death following CK-MB elevation after coronary intervention: identification of an early risk period: importance of CK-MB level, completeness of revascularization, ventricular function, and probable benefit of statin therapy. *Circulation* 2002;106:1205–1210.

This analysis examined 8,409 consecutive nonacute MI patients with successful PCI and no emergency surgery or Q-wave MI; average follow-up was 3.2 years. Post-PCI CK-MB was above normal on routine ascertainment in 17.2%. Patients were prospectively stratified into those with CK-MB 1 to 5 times or CK-MB more than 5 times normal. No patient with CK-MB 1 to 5 times normal died during the first week after PCI, and excess risk of early death for patients with CK-MB elevation occurred mostly in the first 3 to 4 months. The actuarial 4-month risk of death was 8.9%, 1.9%, and 1.2% for patients with CK-MB greater than 5 times, CK-MB 1 to 5 times, and CK-MB more than 1 time normal ($p < 0.001$). Incomplete revascularization ($p < 0.001$), CHF class ($p = 0.005$), and no statin treatment at hospital discharge ($p = 0.009$) were associated with death at 4 months.

139. **De Labriolle A,** et al. Prognostic significance of small troponin I rise after a successful elective percutaneous coronary intervention of a native artery. *Am J Cardiol* 2009;103(5):639–645. [Epub 2009 Jan 17].

In a cohort of 3,200 consecutive elective PCI cases, the authors measured routine post-procedure troponin levels and assessed clinical outcomes to 1 year. Seven-hundred and fifty-one patients had troponin level to $>3\times$ the upper limit of normal, and elevation was associated with more complex anatomy and multivessel PCI. However, at 1 year, there were no differences in rates of death/MI (2.8% vs. 3.5%, $p = 0.3$) or MACE (9.6% or 10.4%, $p = 0.5$) among patients with and without significantly elevated ($>3\times$ the upper limit of normal) troponin levels. This study called into question the benefit of routinely measuring postprocedure troponin levels, a very sensitive assay.

140. **Prasad A,** et al. Prognostic significance of periprocedural versus spontaneously occurring myocardial infarction after percutaneous coronary intervention in patients with acute coronary syndromes: an analysis from the ACUITY (Acute Catheterization and Urgent Intervention Triage Strategy) trial. *J Am Coll Cardiol* 2009;54(5):477–486.

Investigators from the ACUITY trial (see Chapter 3, page 228) sought to assess the prognostic importance (if any) of periprocedure and/or spontaneous postprocedure MI in the 7,789 patients (56% of total) from the main trial who underwent an invasive strategy that included PCI for NSTEMI. They identified 466 (6.0%) periprocedural MIs and 200 (2.6%) spontaneous MIs unrelated to PCI. These patients had significantly higher rates of unadjusted 30-day mortality (5.0% vs. 3.2%, $p < 0.0001$) and 12-month mortality (16.0% vs. 6.0%, $p < 0.0001$). After risk adjustment, spontaneous MI (HR 7.49, $p < 0.0001$), and not periprocedure MI, remained a significant predictor of mortality. However, these results are difficult to draw and solid conclusions form, given that all patients presented in the acute setting of high-risk non–ST segment elevation ACS.

STENT THROMBOSIS

141. **Mak KH,** et al. Subacute stent thrombosis: evolving issues and current concepts. *J Am Coll Cardiol* 1996;27:494–503.

This excellent review discusses the advances in stenting technique and antithrombotic regimens that have led to a significant reduction in incidence of subacute stent thrombosis. The importance of antiplatelet therapy is emphasized.

142. **Hasdai D,** et al. Coronary angioplasty and intracoronary thrombolysis are of limited efficacy in resolving early intracoronary stent thrombosis. *J Am Coll Cardiol* 1996;28:361–367 (editorial, 368–370).

This retrospective analysis focused on 29 of 1,761 consecutive patients with early ($\leq$30 days) stent thrombosis occurring in 44 stents. Acute MI occurred in 90% of patients, and five (17%) patients died. Fourteen patients were treated with balloon angioplasty (PTCA), seven with PTCA and urokinase, and two with urokinase only. Among these treated patients, flow was restored in 48% (six of 14, four of seven, and one of two). Editorial points out that risk factors for stent thrombosis include emergency use and preexisting thrombus.

143. **Cutlip DE,** et al. Stent thrombosis in the modern era: a pooled analysis of multicenter coronary stent clinical trials. *Circulation* 2001;103:1967–1971.

These combined results from six stent trials and associated registries included 6,186 patients who received at least one coronary stent and adjunctive therapy with aspirin and ticlopidine. At 30 days, 0.9% developed stent thrombosis (0.7% documented on angiography). Significant, procedural predictors of thrombosis in this cohort receiving BMS included persistent dissection, total stent length, and final lumen diameter.

144. **Jeremias A,** et al. Stent thrombosis after successful sirolimus-eluting stent implantation. *Circulation* 2004;109:1930–1932.

In this singe-center observational study of 652 patients undergoing PCI with SES, the investigators followed patients prospectively for a median of 100 days. In all, seven stent thromboses occurred during the follow-up period; these patients had significantly smaller final nominal balloon diameters (2.75 vs. 3.00 mm, $p = 0.04$) and over half (4/7) had discontinued antiplatelet therapy after the procedure. Of these 7 patients with stent thrombosis, 1 died and 5 had resulting MIs.

145. **Iakovou I,** et al. Incidence, predictors, and outcome of thrombosis after successful implantation of drug-eluting stents. *JAMA* 2005;293:2126–2130.

In this multicenter, observational study in Europe, the investigators followed 2,229 patients who underwent PCI with either SES or PES. All patients received aspirin indefinitely, and clopidogrel or ticlopidine for at least 3 months after SES and at least 6 months after PES. Primary outcomes of subacute thrombosis (up to 30 days following PCI) and late thrombosis (after 30 days) occurred in 0.6% and 0.7%, respectively, at 9-month follow-up. Overall, 0.8% of patients with SES and 1.7% with PES had stent thrombosis ($p = 0.09$). Significant, independent predictors of stent thrombosis in this cohort included premature antiplatelet therapy discontinuation (HR **89.78,** $p < 0.001$), renal failure (HR 6.49, $p < 0.001$), bifurcation lesions (HR 6.42, $p < 0.001$), diabetes (HR 3.71, $p = 0.001$), and a lower EF (HR 1.09, $p < 0.001$ for each 10% decrease).

146. **Chechi T,** et al. ST-segment elevation myocardial infarction due to early and late stent thrombosis: a new group of high-risk patients. *J Am Coll Cardiol* 2008;51:2396–2402.

In this retrospective study of 190 patients with STEMI, the authors identified 115 definite cases of stent thrombosis. All patients underwent primary PCI for their acute index event. Compared with patients that had STEMI from de novo coronary lesions, patients with stent thrombosis were less likely to get successful reperfusion ($p < 0.0001$), had higher distal embolization ($p = 0.01$), and were more likely to have in-hospital major adverse cardiac or cerebrovascular events ($p = 0.003$). However, among patients who survived to hospital discharge, 6-month outcomes were no different ($p = 0.7$).

OTHER

147. **Solomon R,** et al. Effects of saline, mannitol, and furosemide on acute decreases in renal function induced by radiocontrast agents. *N Engl J Med* 1994;331:1416–1420.

Prospective, randomized study of 78 patients with chronic renal insufficiency (mean creatinine, 2.1 mg/dL) who underwent coronary angiography. Patients received 0.45% saline alone for 12 hours before and 12 hours after angiography, saline plus mannitol, or saline plus furosemide. Mannitol and furosemide were given just before angiography. An increase in the creatinine of 0.5 mg/dL or more after angiography was seen in 26%. The saline group had a lower incidence of elevated creatinine compared with the mannitol and furosemide groups (11% vs. 28% and 40%; $p = 0.05$). The mean increase in serum creatinine 48 hours after angiography was significantly greater in the furosemide group ($p = 0.01$) than in the saline group.

148. **Narins CR,** et al. Relation between activated clotting time during angioplasty and abrupt closure. *Circulation* 1996;93:667–671.

This study correlated low ACTs with adverse outcomes. The analysis focused on 62 of 1,290 consecutive nonemergency angioplasty patients with in- or out-of-catheterization laboratory closure and 124 matched controls. Abrupt closure patients had a lower initial and minimum ACT (350 vs. 380 seconds; 345 vs. 370 seconds). High ACTs were not associated with more major bleeding complications.

149. **Schaub F,** et al. Management of 219 consecutive cases of postcatheterization pseudoaneurysm. *J Am Coll Cardiol* 1997;30:670–675.

This analysis focused on 219 patients with postcatheterization pseudoaneurysm. A compression bandage was reapplied in 132 patients with 32% success [more likely if small pseudoaneurysm (10 mm; 71% vs. 95%) and patient not anticoagulated (72% vs. 93%)]. Ultrasound-guided compression repair was undertaken in 124 patients (primary treatment modality in 49). The success rate was 84%, higher if preceded by reapplied bandage (89% vs. 76%; $p = 0.04$). Overall, surgical repair was necessary in only 7% of patients.

150. **Kay J**, et al. Acetylcysteine for prevention of acute deterioration of renal function following elective coronary angiography and intervention: a randomized controlled trial. *JAMA* 2003;289:553–558.

Prospective, randomized, double-blind, placebo-controlled trial of 200 patients with stable moderate renal insufficiency (creatinine clearance, less than 60 mL/min) who underwent elective coronary angiography. Patients received oral acetylcysteine, 600 mg twice daily, or placebo, on the day before and the day of angiography. The acetylcysteine group had a significantly lower incidence of a greater than 25% increase in serum creatinine level within 48 hours compared with placebo (4% vs. 12%; relative $p = 0.03$). Average serum creatinine also was lower in the acetylcysteine group (1.22 mg/dL vs. 1.38 mg/dL; $p = 0.006$). The benefit of acetylcysteine was present in all patient subgroups and persisted for at least 7 days.

151. **Marenzi G**, et al. *N*-acetylcysteine and contrast-induced nephropathy in primary angioplasty. *N Engl J Med* 2006;354(26):2773–2782.

Investigators randomized 354 consecutive patients with STEMI undergoing primary angioplasty to either placebo, standard-dose, or high-dose *N*-acetylcysteine. In-hospital mortality was significantly higher among patients who developed contrast-induced nephropathy (26% vs. 1%, $p < 0.001$). Increase in creatinine of 25% or more occurred in 33% of patients receiving placebo, 15% in the standard-dose *N*-acetylcysteine, and 8% of the high-dose *N*-acetylcysteine group ($p < 0.001$).

152. **Stone GW**, et al. for the CONTRAST Investigators. Fenoldopam mesylate for the prevention of contrast-induced nephropathy: a randomized controlled trial. *JAMA* 2003;290(17):2284–2291.

This prospective, randomized, multicenter study enrolled 315 patients with baseline creatinine clearance (CrCl) of <60 cm³/min. Patients received fenoldopam (0.05 to 0.10 μg/kg/min) or placebo, starting 1 hour before angiography and continuing for 12 hours thereafter. There was no significant difference between the groups in primary end point of ≥2.5%. Serum creatinine increased in first 96 hours [33.6% (fenoldopam) vs. 30.1%, $p = 0.54$]. Additionally, there were no significant differences in death, new dialysis, or hospitalization at 30 days.

153. **Merten GJ**, Burgess WP, Gray LV, et al. Prevention of contrast-induced nephropathy with sodium bicarbonate: a randomized controlled trial. *JAMA* 2004;291(19):2328–2334.

The investigators randomized 119 patients undergoing radiologic or interventional procedure requiring intravenous contrast (e.g., CT scans, angiography, etc.) to receive pre-hydration with either normal saline or iso-osmolar sodium bicarbonate. Regardless of randomization assignment, patients received 3 mL/kg/hr for 1 hour prior to contrast, then 1 mL/kg/hr during and 6 hours after the procedure. The primary end point of ≥25% increase in creatinine within 2 days occurred in 13.6% of patients in the normal saline group versus 1.7% of those receiving sodium bicarbonate ($p = 0.02$). Notably, patients in the sodium chloride group had nonsignificantly higher creatinine levels at baseline (1.89 vs. 1.71, $p = 0.09$); however, contrast loads were similar between the two groups.

154. **Brar SS**, et al. Sodium bicarbonate vs sodium chloride for the prevention of contrast medium–induced nephropathy in patients undergoing coronary angiography: a randomized trial. *JAMA* 2008;300(9):1038–1046.

The investigators randomized patients with moderate to severe chronic kidney disease (estimated GFR $\leq$60 mL/min per 1.73 m^2) undergoing coronary angiography to either sodium bicarbonate or normal saline at similar volumes before, during, and after angiography. Additionally, patients had at least one of the following co-morbidities: diabetes, CHF, HTN, or age greater than 75 years. Rates of acute kidney injury ($\geq$25% increase in creatinine within 4 days) were similar in the two groups (13.3% for sodium bicarbonate vs. 14.6% for normal saline, p = 0.82). Rates of death, dialysis, MI, or cerebrovascular events were also similar at 30 days.

Restenosis

REVIEW ARTICLES AND MISCELLANEOUS

155. **Belle EV**, et al. Restenosis rates in diabetic patients. *Circulation* 1997;96:1454–1460 (editorial, 1374–1377).

This retrospective analysis showed an increased risk of restenosis among diabetic patients undergoing balloon angioplasty but not stenting. A total of 300 stented patients (one-native-vessel procedure, no high-pressure balloon inflation; 19% diabetics) and 300 balloon angioplasty (PTCA) patients were analyzed. The PTCA group had a nearly twofold higher restenosis rate (63% vs. 36%; p = 0.0002), whereas among stented patients, diabetics and nondiabetics had a similar rate of restenosis (25% vs. 27%). Editorial points out that these findings suggest that vascular remodeling (vs. neointimal proliferation) drives the excess in post-PTCA restenosis in diabetics. However, these findings contradict those of other studies that have shown no special benefit with stenting in diabetics. One possible explanation for the differences in results is that the lack of high-pressure balloon inflation in this stented population led to less vessel damage and subsequently less intimal proliferation (the latter may be especially important in the restenotic process in diabetics).

156. **Douglas JS**. Pharmacologic approaches to restenosis prevention. *Am J Cardiol* 2007;100(5A):10K–16K. [Epub 2007 Jun 26].

Despite the advances in reducing in-stent restenosis with DES, there remains a significant residual rate of restenosis even within DES. The author discusses systemic agents identified that may further reduce in-stent restenosis; these include probucol, AGI-1067, tranilast, trapidil, pioglitazone, as well as antiplatelet agents such as cilostazol.

REPEATED PERCUTANEOUS CORONARY INTERVENTION FOR RESTENOSIS AFTER PERCUTANEOUS TRANSLUMINAL CORONARY ANGIOGRAPHY

157. **Erbel R**, et al. **REST** (Restenosis Stent Study). Coronary-artery stenting compared with balloon angioplasty for restenosis after initial balloon angioplasty. *N Engl J Med* 1998;339:1672–1678.

Design: Prospective, randomized, multicenter study. Primary end point was angiographic evidence of restenosis at 6 months.

Purpose: To determine whether coronary stenting, as compared with balloon angioplasty, reduces restenosis after prior successful balloon angioplasty.

Population: 383 patients with clinical and angiographic evidence of restenosis after successful balloon angioplasty.

Treatment: Standard balloon angioplasty or PS stent implantation; crossover to stenting was allowed if symptomatic dissection occurred that could not be managed with repeated balloon inflations.

Results: Stent group had a significantly lower restenosis rate (18% vs. 32%; p = 0.03) and less TVR (10% vs. 27%; p = 0.001). The difference resulted from smaller MLD in angioplasty (1.85 vs. 2.04 mm; p = 0.01). The stent group had better event-free survival at 250 days

(84% vs. 72%; $p = 0.04$), but a nonsignificant increase was found in death and MI (at 6 months, 5.6% vs. 2.3%). Subacute thrombosis occurred more frequently in the stent group (3.9% vs. 0.6%).

Comments: These results are consistent with prior studies (35–38) that have shown a reduction in TVR but an excess of the hard end points of death and MI.

158. **Alfonsa F,** et al. for the Restenosis Intra-stent: Balloon Angioplasty Versus Elective Stenting (RIBS) Investigators. A randomized comparison of repeat stenting with balloon angioplasty in patients with in-stent restenosis. *J Am Coll Cardiol* 2003;42:796–805.

Design: Prospective, randomized, multicenter study. Primary end point was recurrent in-stent restenosis at 6 months.

Purpose: To compare the strategy of balloon angioplasty with re-stenting in patients with in-stent restenosis.

Population: 450 patients with in-stent restenosis more than 1 month out from prior stent placement.

Treatment: Balloon angioplasty or stent implantation.

Results: While immediate postprocedure mean luminal diameter was greater in the stenting group, at 6-month follow-up binary restenosis rates were similar in the two groups (38% for stenting vs. 39% for balloon). Additionally, 1-year survival was similar in the two groups (77% for stent vs. 71% for balloon, $p = 0.19$). However, in the prespecified group of patients with larger vessels (≥ 3 mm), restenosis rates (27% vs. 49%, $p = 0.007$) and survival (84% vs. 62%, $p = 0.002$) favored the stenting group.

Comment: Long-term results with follow-up up to a median of 4.3 years confirmed the similar clinical outcomes in the two groups, as well as persistence of vessel diameter as a significant predictor of outcome (see *J Am Coll Cardiol* 2005;46:756–760).

159. **Neumann FJ,** et al. Effectiveness and safety of sirolimus-eluting stents in the treatment of restenosis after coronary stent placement (TReatment Of Patients with an In-STENT REstenotic Coronary Artery Lesion [TROPICAL]). *Circulation* 2005;111: 2107–2111.

This prospective, multicenter registry followed 162 patients with in-stent restenosis who were treated with PCI with SES. A 6-month follow-up angiography, in-lesion late loss was 0.08 mm, with a binary restenosis rate of 9.7%. These data supported the use of DES for in-stent restenosis, leading to further clinical trials (see below).

160. **Kastrati A,** et al. for the ISAR-DESIRE Study Investigators. Sirolimus-eluting stent or paclitaxel-eluting stent vs balloon angioplasty for prevention of recurrences in patients with coronary in-stent restenosis a randomized controlled trial. *JAMA* 2005;293: 165–171.

Design: Prospective, randomized, multicenter study. Primary end point was recurrent in-stent restenosis at 6 months, as compared between stent groups and balloon angioplasty.

Purpose: To compare the strategy of balloon angioplasty with re-stenting using DES in patients with in-stent restenosis.

Population: 300 patients with in-stent restenosis of a BMS in a native coronary artery segment.

Treatment: Balloon angioplasty or PCI with either SES or PES. All patients received a clopidogrel loading dose prior to procedure.

Results: At follow-up angiography 6 months later, binary restenosis occurred in 44.6% of patients who underwent balloon angioplasty, compared with 14.3% in the SES group ($p < 0.001$ vs. balloon), and 21.7% in the PES group ($p = 0.001$ vs. balloon). In a prespecified comparison of SES and PES groups, restenosis ($p = 0.19$) and TVR rates (8% for SES vs. 19% for PES, $p = 0.02$) favored the SES group.

161. **ISAR-DESIRE 2.** Preliminary results presented at TCT 2009, San Francisco, CA.

In this subsequent study, 450 patients with in-stent restenosis of prior SES were randomized to re-stenting with either PES or repeat SES. Late lumen loss at 1 year was similar in the two groups (0.40 for SES and 0.38 for PES), as were rates of the composite end point of death, MI, or stent thrombosis (6.1% for SES vs. 6.3% for PES, p = NS).

EFFECT OF STENT DESIGN (STRUT THICKNESS)

162. **Kastrati A,** et al. Intracoronary stenting and angiographic results: Strut Thickness Effect on Restenosis Outcomes (**ISAR-STEREO**) Trial. *Circulation* 2001;103:2816–2821.

This prospective, randomized study of 651 patients examined whether stents with different strut thickness result in similar restenosis rates and clinical outcomes. Patients receive either a thin-strut stent (ACS MultiLink stent) or thick-strut stent (ACS MultiLink Duett stent). At 30 days, urgent TVR was the same in the two groups (both 1.5%); mortality and MI rates also were similar. At 6-month follow-up angiography [obtained in 79% (thin strut) and 82%], the primary end point of restenosis was significantly lower in the thin-strut group compared with the thick-strut group (15% vs. 25.8%; p = 0.003). At 1-year follow-up, 8.6% of the thin-strut stent patients and 13.8% of the thick-strut stent patients required TVR because of restenosis-related ischemia (p = 0.03). This study shows that even small changes in stent design can result in different angiographic and clinical outcomes.

163. **Pache J,** et al. Intracoronary stenting and angiographic results: Strut Thickness Effect on Restenosis Outcome (ISAR-STEREO-2) Trial. *J Am Coll Cardiol* 2003;41:1283–1288.

This prospective, randomized study also evaluated the effect of stent strut thickness on restenosis rates in 611 patients with stenoses in native coronary arteries 2.8 mm or more in diameter. Patients received a thin-strut stent (50 mm thickness) or thick-strut stent (140 mm thickness). Vessel size, lesion length, MLD, and GP IIb/IIIa platelet inhibitor use were similar in both groups. At 6 months, QCA showed that the thin-strut group had a greater MLD and less late lumen loss compared with the thick-strut group, as well as a significantly lower binary restenosis rate (17.9% vs. 31.4%; p < 0.001). Clinical restenosis (TVR) also was significantly lower in the thin-strut group (12.3% vs. 21.9%; p = 0.002). Combined death and MI rates were similar at 1 year.

164. **Briguori C,** et al. In-stent restenosis in small coronary arteries: impact of strut thickness. *J Am Coll Cardiol* 2002;40:403–409.

Retrospective analysis of 821 patients who had successful stenting in small native vessels (3.0-mm reference diameter) and had angiographic follow-up available. The thin-strut group (<0.10 mm) included 400 patients with 505 lesions, whereas the thick-strut group had 421 patients with 436 lesions. The thin-strut group had a significantly lower restenosis rate compared with the thick-strut group (28.5% vs. 36.6%; p = 0.009). When three subgroups were defined (2.50 mm or smaller, 2.51 to 2.75 mm, and 2.76 to 2.99 mm), strut thickness influenced restenosis only in the 2.76- to 2.99-mm subgroup [23.5% (thin) vs. 37%; p = 0.006]. By logistic regression analysis, predictors of restenosis were stent length, strut thickness, and diabetes.

DRUG STUDIES

165. **Schwartz L,** et al. Aspirin and dipyridamole in the prevention of restenosis after PTCA. *N Engl J Med* 1988;318:1714–1719.

Prospective, randomized, double-blind, placebo-controlled, multicenter study of 376 patients undergoing coronary angioplasty. Patients received aspirin, 330 mg/day, and dipyridamole, 75 mg three times daily (started 24 hours before angioplasty), or placebo. Dipyridamole was given by continuous intravenous infusion (10 mg/hr) from 16 hours before the procedure until 8 hours after. Among 249 patients who underwent follow-up angiography, similar restenosis rates [37.7% vs. 38.6% (placebo)] were observed. The drug therapy group had 77% fewer periprocedural Q-wave MIs (1.6% vs. 6.9%; $p = 0.01$).

166. **Serruys PW,** et al. Coronary Artery Restenosis Prevention on Repeated Thromboxane Antagonism (**CARPORT**). Prevention of restenosis after percutaneous transluminal coronary angioplasty with thromboxane A_2-receptor blockade. *Circulation* 1991;84:1568–1580.

Prospective, randomized, double-blind, placebo-controlled, parallel-group study of 697 patients who underwent successful balloon angioplasty of a de novo native coronary artery lesion. Patients received the thromboxane A_2–receptor antagonist, GR32191B, 80 mg before angioplasty and 40 mg/day for 6 months, or aspirin, 250 mg intravenously, before angioplasty and placebo for 6 months. At 6-month follow-up angiography (575 patients), no significant differences were found between the groups in lumen diameter or clinical events.

167. **Faxon DP,** et al. Enoxaparin Restenosis after Angioplasty (**ERA**). Low molecular weight heparin in prevention of restenosis after angioplasty: results of enoxaparin restenosis (ERA) trial. *Circulation* 1994;90:908–914.

Prospective, randomized, double-blind, placebo-controlled, multicenter study of 458 patients who underwent successful angioplasty. Patient received enoxaparin, 40 mg s.c. once daily for 1 month, or placebo. At 6 months, restenosis rates were similar in the two groups [51% (placebo) vs. 52%; $p = 0.63$]. Clinical event rates also were similar, except for minor bleeding, which was more frequent in the enoxaparin group.

168. **Weintraub WS,** et al. Lack of effect of lovastatin on restenosis after coronary angioplasty. *N Engl J Med* 1994;331:1331–1337.

Prospective, randomized, double-blind, placebo-controlled, multicenter study of 404 patients undergoing successful elective coronary angioplasty of native coronary vessels. Patients received lovastatin, 40 mg twice daily, started 7 to 10 days before angioplasty, or placebo. At 6-month angiography (321 patients), no significant reduction between the groups in luminal diameter was noted (preangioplasty, 64% vs. 63%; at 6 months, 44% vs. 46%; $p = 0.50$).

169. **Maresta A,** et al. Studio Trapidil versus Aspirin nella Restenosi Coronarica (**STARC**). Trapidil (triazolopyrimidine), a platelet-derived growth factor antagonist, reduces restenosis after PTCA. *Circulation* 1994;90:2710–2715.

Prospective, randomized, double-blind, comparative study of 254 patients younger than 75 years undergoing coronary angioplasty of de novo lesions. Patients received trapidil, 300 mg orally every 8 hours, or acetylsalicylic acid, 100 mg three times daily for 6 months. At 6-month angiography, the trapidil group had a significantly lower restenosis rate (24.2% vs. 39.7%; $p < 0.01$). Clinical events were similar in the two groups, except that recurrent angina occurred less frequently with trapidil (25.8% vs. 43.7%).

170. **Serruys PW,** et al. the **HELVETICA** Investigators. A comparison of hirudin with heparin in the prevention of restenosis after coronary angioplasty. *N Engl J Med* 1995;333:757–763.

Prospective, randomized, double-blind, multicenter study of 1,141 unstable angina patients in three groups. Group 1, heparin, 10,000-U bolus, continuous infusion for 24 hours, and then s.c. placebo twice daily for 3 days; group 2, hirudin, 40 mg, i.v. infusion for 24 hours, and then s.c. placebo twice daily for 3 days; group 3, same as group 2, except hirudin, 40 mg s.c. twice daily for 3 days. Hirudin-treated patients had decreased early (96-hour) cardiac events (7.9% and 5.6% vs. 11%), but no significant differences were seen in the primary end point of event-free survival at 7 months (67.3%, 63.5%, 68%). Mean MLDs at 6-month follow-up angiography were 1.54, 1.47, and 1.56 mm, respectively ($p = 0.08$).

171. Subcutaneous Heparin and Angioplasty Restenosis Prevention Trial (**SHARP**). The SHARP trial: results of a multicenter randomized trial investigating the effects of high dose unfractionated heparin on angiographic restenosis and clinical outcome. *J Am Coll Cardiol* 1995;26:947–954.

Prospective, randomized, parallel-group, open-label, multicenter study of 339 patients who had undergone successful coronary angioplasty of de novo lesions. Patients received heparin, 12,500 U s.c. twice daily for 4 months, or no treatment. At follow-up angiography (mean, 4.2 months), no significant differences were found between treatment groups in change in mean lumen diameter.

172. Savage MP, et al. for the Multi-Hospital Eastern Atlantic Restenosis Trial (**M-HEART II**) Study Group. Effect of thromboxane A$_2$ blockade on clinical outcome and restenosis after coronary angioplasty. *Circulation* 1995;92:3194–3200.

This prospective, randomized, double-blind, placebo-controlled, multicenter study enrolled 752 patients undergoing elective angioplasty. Patients received aspirin, 325 mg once daily; sulotroban, 800 mg four times daily; or placebo, started 1 to 6 hours before PTCA and continued for 6 months. The aspirin group had less angiographic restenosis (by lesion) than did the sulotroban group (39% vs. 53%; $p = 0.006$).

173. Cairns JA, et al. Enoxaparin MaxEPA Prevention of Angioplasty Restenosis (**EMPAR**). Fish oils and low-molecular-weight heparin for the reduction of restenosis after percutaneous transluminal coronary angioplasty. *Circulation* 1996;94:1553–1560.

Prospective, randomized, partially open, multicenter study of 814 patients undergoing elective angioplasty of de novo lesions. Patients received maxEPA, 18 capsules/day (5.4-g n-3 fatty acids) or placebo started a median 6 days before angioplasty and continued for 18 weeks. After sheath removal, 653 patients had one successfully dilated lesion and were randomized to enoxaparin, 30 mg s.c. twice daily or control (no treatment) for 6 weeks. At follow-up angiography (18 ± 2 weeks), no significant differences were observed in restenosis rates per patient and per lesion (fish oils, 46.5% vs. 39.7%; placebo, 44.7% vs. 38.7%; enoxaparin, 45.8% vs. 38.0%; control, 45.4% vs. 40.4%).

174. Karsch KR, et al. Reduction of Restenosis after PTCA: early Administration of Reviparin in a Double-Blind, Unfractionated Heparin and Placebo-Controlled Evaluation (**REDUCE**). Low-molecular weight heparin (reviparin) in percutaneous transluminal coronary angioplasty. *J Am Coll Cardiol* 1996;28:1437–1443.

Prospective, randomized, double-blind, multicenter study of 625 stable or unstable angina patients with single lesions suitable for elective PTCA. Patients received reviparin, 7,000 U, before PTCA, followed by 10,500 U over a 24-hour period, and then 3,500 U twice daily for 28 days, or heparin, 10,000 U over a 24-hour period, and then s.c. placebo. At 30 weeks, no significant differences were seen between groups in the primary composite end point of death, MI, reintervention, or CABG surgery [33.3% (reviparin) vs. 32%], loss of lumen diameter, and bleeding. The reviparin group had fewer acute events (3.9% vs. 8.2%; $p < 0.03$).

175. Bertrand ME, et al. Prevention of Restenosis by Elisor after Transluminal Coronary Angioplasty Trial (**PREDICT**). Effect of pravastatin on angiographic restenosis after coronary balloon angioplasty. *J Am Coll Cardiol* 1997;30:863–869.

Prospective, randomized, double-blind, placebo-controlled, multicenter study of 695 patients with total cholesterol, 200 to 310 mg/dL, undergoing elective angioplasty. Patients received pravastatin, 40 mg/day, or placebo for 6 months. No significant difference in mean lumen diameter was observed between the two groups [1.54 mm (pravastatin) vs. 1.54 mm; $p = 0.21$]. Late loss and net gain did not differ significantly between groups. Restenosis rates also were similar [39.2% (pravastatin) vs. 43.8%; $p = 0.26$].

176. **Kosuga K**, et al. Effectiveness of tranilast on restenosis after directional coronary atherectomy. *Am Heart J* 1997;134:712–718.

This nonrandomized study was composed of 192 patients who underwent successful DCA. After the procedure, 40 patients were given oral tranilast for 3 months, and 152 were not. Angiographic follow-up at 3 and 6 months showed that the tranilast patients had a significantly lower MLD (2.08 vs. 1.75 mm; $p = 0.004$; 2.04 vs. 1.70 mm; $p = 0.003$). The restenosis rate at 3 months was more than 50% lower in the tranilast group (11% vs. 26%; $p = 0.03$). At 1 year, the tranilast group also had experienced fewer clinical events ($p = 0.013$).

177. **Kastrati A**, et al. Restenosis after coronary stent placement and randomized to a 4-week combined antiplatelet or anticoagulant therapy. *Circulation* 1997;96:462–467 (editorial, 383–385).

This analysis of 432 ISAR patients who underwent 6-month angiography showed no favorable effects on restenosis in patients receiving an antiplatelet regimen. Antiplatelet versus anticoagulant therapy showed no significant differences in restenosis rate (26.8% vs. 28.9%), mean luminal diameter (1.95 vs. 1.90 mm), late lumen loss (1.10 vs. 1.15 mm), or TVR (14.6% vs. 15.6%). The accompanying editorial points out that this analysis was poorly powered to detect a restenosis difference.

178. **Dwens JA**, et al. Usefulness of nisoldipine for prevention of restenosis after percutaneous transluminal coronary angioplasty (results of the nisoldipine in Coronary Disease in Leuven (**NICOLE**) study). *Am J Cardiol* 2001;87:28–33.

This randomized, double-blind, placebo-controlled, single-center trial enrolled 826 patients who underwent successful intervention in native coronary arteries. Patients were randomized to nisoldipine (20 mg/day for 2 weeks and then 40 mg/day for 3 years) or placebo. At 6 months, no significant difference was found between groups in MLD, initial gain, late loss, diameter stenosis, or binary restenosis. The nisoldipine group had a lower incidence of unscheduled coronary angiography ($p = 0.006$), CABG surgery ($p = 0.012$), and repeated target-lesion PTCA ($p = 0.017$), which was likely driven by the lower incidence of recurrent angina in nisoldipine-treated patients (12% vs. 21%; $p = 0.004$).

179. **Tsuchikane E**, et al. Impact of cilostazol on restenosis after percutaneous coronary balloon angioplasty. *Circulation* 1999;100:21–26.

A total of 211 patients with 273 lesions who had successful PTCA were randomized to cilostazol (200 mg/day for 3 months) or aspirin (250 mg/day). At follow-up angiography (193 patients), the cilostazol group had significantly lower restenosis and TVRs compared with the aspirin group (17.9% vs. 39.5%; $p < 0.001$; 11.4% vs. 28.7%; $p < 0.001$).

180. **Douglas JS**, et al. Cilostazol for Restenosis Trial (CREST) Investigators. Coronary stent restenosis in patients treated with cilostazol. *Circulation* 2005;112:2826–2832.

Prospective, randomized, double-blind, placebo-controlled trial of cilostazol versus placebo to prevent in-stent restenosis in 705 patients with recent BMS placement. Primary outcome of restenosis at 6 months was lower in the cilostazol group (22.0% vs. 34.5%, $p = 0.002$), an effect that was consistent in patients with diabetes as well as those with small vessels, long lesions, and LAD lesion sites. Clinical outcomes of bleeding, rehospitalization, TVR, MI, or death were similar in the two groups.

181. **Lee S-W**, et al. Drug-eluting stenting followed by cilostazol treatment reduces late restenosis in patients with diabetes mellitus the DECLARE-DIABETES trial (A Randomized Comparison of Triple Antiplatelet Therapy With Dual Antiplatelet Therapy After Drug-Eluting Stent Implantation in Diabetic Patients). *J Am Coll Cardiol* 2008;51:1181–1187.

Prospective, randomized, multicenter trial of 400 patients with diabetes undergoing PCI with DES, randomized to cilostazol or placebo, in addition to standard dual antiplatelet therapy (aspirin and clopidogrel). After 6 months of therapy, in-stent and in-segment late loss were both significantly lower ($p = 0.025$ and $p = 0.031$, respectively). Binary restenosis rates were lower for cilostazol (8.0% vs. 15.6%, $p = 0.033$), as were 9-month TLR rates (2.5% vs. 7.0%, $p = 0.034$). There was a trend toward lower MACE rates as well (3.0% vs. 7.0%, $p = 0.066$).

182. Coronary Angioplasty Restenosis Trial (**CART**). n-3 Fatty acids do not prevent restenosis after coronary angioplasty: results from the CART study. *J Am Coll Cardiol* 1999;33: 1619–1626.

Prospective, randomized, double-blind, placebo-controlled study of 500 patients undergoing elective coronary angioplasty. Patients received n-3 fatty acids, 5.1 g/day, or corn oil (placebo) starting at least 2 weeks before and continued for 6 months after angioplasty. The restenosis rates were similar in the two groups (defined as MLD, less than 40%): 40.6% in the n-3 fatty acid group and 35.4% in the placebo group ($p = 0.21$).

183. Evaluation of Reopro and Stenting to Eliminate Restenosis (**ERASER**) Investigators. Acute platelet inhibition with abciximab does not reduce in-stent restenosis. *Circulation* 1999;100:799–806.

This prospective, multicenter, double-blind, placebo-controlled trial randomized 225 patients undergoing primary stent implantation to abciximab (12- or 24-hour infusion) or placebo. Target lesions were de novo 60% stenoses in native vessels with 3.0 mm to 3.5 mm diameter. At 6-month follow-up, no significant differences between groups were found in in-stent volume obstruction (primary end point).

184. **Jorgensen B,** et al. Restenosis and clinical outcome in patients treated with amlodipine after angioplasty: results from the Coronary AngioPlasty Amlodipine REStenosis Study (**CAPARES**). *J Am Coll Cardiol* 2000;35:592–599.

This prospective, randomized, double-blind, placebo-controlled, multicenter study enrolled 585 patients. Patients received amlodipine (5 to 10 mg/day) or placebo started 2 weeks before the procedure. Nonstudy calcium channel blockers were prohibited. Stenting was allowed only for bailout or unsatisfactory PTCA results (15.6%). At follow-up angiography, no significant differences were noted between groups in primary end point of mean loss in mean luminal diameter [0.30 mm (amlodipine) vs. 0.29 mm (placebo)]. At 4 months, the amlodipine group had a lower incidence of death, MI, CABG surgery, and repeated PTCA [9.4% vs. 14.5% (placebo group); $p = 0.049$]; this difference was primarily owing to fewer repeated PTCAs [3.1% vs. 7.3% (placebo group); $p = 0.02$].

185. **Meneveau N,** et al. Local delivery of nadroparin for the prevention of neointimal hyperplasia following stent implantation: results of the **IMPRESS** trial, a multicentre, randomized, clinical, angiographic and intravascular ultrasound study. *Eur Heart J* 2000;21:1767–1775.

Prospective, randomized, open-label, multicenter study of 250 patients who underwent PTCA followed by stenting. Patients were assigned to no local drug delivery (control group) or intramural delivery of nadroparin (2 mL of 2,500 anti-Xa-units/mL). Local nadroparin delivery was not associated with an increase in stent thrombosis, coronary artery dissection, side-branch occlusion, distal embolization, or abrupt arterial closure. At 6-month angiography, no significant differences were noted between groups in primary end point of late loss in lumen diameter [0.84 mm (control) vs. 0.88 mm (nadroparin)] and binary restenosis rate [20% (control) vs. 24% (nadroparin)]. An IVUS substudy found that the average area of neointimal tissue within the stent was similar between the groups (2.86 mm vs. 2.90 mm). MACE rates also were similar.

186. **Serruys PW,** et al. Carvedilol for prevention of restenosis after directional coronary atherectomy: final results of the European Carvedilol Atherectomy Restenosis (**EURO-CARE**) Trial. *Circulation* 2000;101:1512–1518.

    This prospective, double-blind, randomized, placebo-controlled trial enrolled 406 patients; 377 underwent attempted DCA with a 50% diameter stenosis achieved in 89% without stent use. Patients received carvedilol, 25 mg twice daily, starting 24 hours before scheduled DCA and for 5 months after a successful procedure, or placebo. At follow-up angiography (mean, 6 months), no significant differences were seen between the placebo and carvedilol groups in MLD (1.99 mm vs. 2.00 mm) or angiographic restenosis (23.4% vs. 23.9%). TLR and event-free survival also were similar at 7 months (16.2% vs. 14.5%; 79.2% vs. 79.7%).

187. **Neumann F,** et al. Treatment of *Chlamydia pneumoniae* infection with roxithromycin and effect on neointima proliferation after coronary stent placement (**ISAR-3**): a randomised, double-blind, placebo-controlled trial. *Lancet* 2001;357:2085–2089.

    Prospective, randomized, double-blind trial of 1,010 consecutive patients who underwent successful stenting. Patients received roxithromycin, 300 mg once daily for 28 days, or placebo. No difference was found between the groups in the primary end point of angiographic restenosis [31% (roxithromycin group) vs. 29%; $p = 0.43$] as well as TVR (19% vs. 17%; $p = 0.30$). Interestingly, in patients with high serum titers of *C. pneumoniae*, roxithromycin use was associated with a significantly lower restenosis rate [adjusted ORs at a titer of 1:512 were 0.44 (0.19 to 1.06) and 0.32 (0.13 to 0.81), respectively].

188. **Holmes DR Jr,** et al. Results of Prevention of REStenosis with Tranilast and its Outcomes (**PRESTO**) Trial. *Circulation* 2002;106:1243–1250.

    Design: Prospective, randomized, placebo-controlled, double-blind, multicenter study. Primary composite end point of death, MI, or ischemia-driven TVR at 9 months.
    Purpose: To determine whether tranilast reduces restenosis and major coronary events compared with placebo in patients undergoing successful PCI.
    Population: 11,484 patients who underwent successful PCI and had no evidence of MI.
    Treatment: Tranilast, 300 or 450 mg twice daily, for 1 or 3 months (four groups) or placebo.
    Results: At 9 months, the incidence of the composite primary–end point coronary was similar in the three groups (1-month tranilast group, 15.5%; placebo, 15.8%; 3-month tranilast group, 16.1%). In an angiographic substudy of 2,018 patients, the follow-up mean MLDs were similar (placebo, 1.76-mm group; tranilast, 1.72 to 1.78 mm); binary restenosis (>50%) rates also were similar (32% to 35%). In an IVUS substudy of 1,107 patients, plaque volume was not different between the placebo and tranilast groups (39.3 vs. 37.5 to 46.1 mm^3, respectively; $p = 0.16$ to 0.72).

RADIATION

Gamma Radiation

189. **Teirstein PS,** et al. Scripps Coronary Radiation to Inhibit Proliferation Post-Stenting (**SCRIPPS**). Catheter-based radiotherapy to inhibit restenosis after coronary stenting. *N Engl J Med* 1997;336:1697–1703 (editorial, 1748–1749).

    Fifty-five patients with restenosis (in-stent, 62%) were randomized to ^{192}Ir (20- to 45-minute exposure; dose of 800 to 3,000 cGy) or placebo. The iridium group had less diabetes mellitus. Angiographic follow-up in 53 patients at 6.7 ± 2.2 months showed that the iridium group had a larger mean luminal diameter (2.43 vs. 1.85 mm; $p = 0.02$) and an impressive 69% lower restenosis rate (17% vs. 54%; $p = 0.01$). No apparent complications were seen with iridium use, although long-term follow-up is necessary. At 2-year follow-up, the incidence of death, MI, or TLR was 55% lower in the radiation group (23.1% vs. 51.7%; $p = 0.03$). Most of this benefit was owing to a 75% lower TLR rate (15.4% vs. 44.8%; $p < 0.001$).

190. Washington Radiation for In-Stent Restenosis Trial (**WRIST**). *Circulation* 2000;101: 2165–2171.

Design: Prospective, randomized, blinded, placebo-controlled study. Primary clinical end point was cumulative composite of death, MI, repeated TLR.

Purpose: To evaluate the effectiveness of gamma radiation as adjunctive therapy for patients with ISR.

Population: 130 patients with ISR in native coronary arteries ($n = 100$) and saphenous vein grafts ($n = 30$) with reference diameter 3.0 to 5.0 mm and lesion length less than 47 mm.

Treatment: Catheter-delivered gamma radiation (^{192}Ir source; mean dwell time, 22 minutes) or placebo.

Results: At 6 months, the radiation therapy group had a significant reduction in the primary composite end point of death, MI, and TLR (29.2% vs. 67.6%; $p < 0.001$), primarily owing to a lower TLR rate (13.8% vs. 63.1%; $p < 0.001$). The death rates were 4.6% in the radiated group and 6.2% in the nonradiated groups; no patients had Q-wave infarcts. TLR also was lower in the radiation group (13.8%) versus the placebo group (63.1%), and the same pattern was seen at 12 months.

Comment: Most restenosis in the radiation group occurred at the edges of the stent.

191. **Leon MB,** et al. **GAMMA-1.** Localized intracoronary gamma-radiation therapy to inhibit the recurrence of restenosis after stenting. *N Engl J Med* 2001;344:250–256.

Design: Prospective, randomized, double-blind, multicenter study. Primary composite end point was death, MI, emergency CABG, or need for TLR at 9 months.

Purpose: To assess whether gamma radiation can prevent ISR.

Population: 252 patients with 60% restenosis of stented native vessels 2.75 to 4 mm in diameter and lesion length ≤45 mm.

Exclusion Criteria: Included MI in prior 72 hours, visible thrombus, ejection fraction less than 40%, and anticipated abciximab administration (actual use, less than 10%).

Treatment: Gamma radiation by using an ^{192}Ir ribbon or placebo. Lesions were irradiated with 800 to 3,000 cGy used (6, 10, or 14 seeds); delivery device dwell time was approximately 20 minutes. Most treated lesions (more than 70%) were complex (type B2 or C).

Results: Radiation group had a 58% lower stent restenosis rate ($p < 0.001$). At 9 months, the radiation group also had a significantly lower incidence of primary composite end point compared with the placebo group (28.2% vs. 43.8%; $p = 0.02$). Late thrombosis occurred in 5.3% (^{192}Ir) versus 0.8% (placebo; $p = 0.07$). A subsequent cost-effectiveness study found that initial costs were increased by nearly $4,100 per patient ($15,724 vs. $11,675; $p < 0.001$) and by $2,200 per patient at 1 year. However, if late thrombosis can be eliminated with extended antiplatelet therapy, long-term medical care costs will likely be lower with brachytherapy (see *Circulation* 2002;106:691–697).

192. **Waksman R,** et al. **WRIST PLUS**. Prolonged antiplatelet therapy to prevent late thrombosis after intracoronary gamma-radiation in patients with in-stent restenosis. *Circulation* 2001;103:2332–2335.

A total of 120 consecutive patients with diffuse ISR in native coronary arteries and vein grafts with lesions smaller than 80 mm underwent PCI, including stenting in 28.3%. After PCI, gamma radiation was administered (^{192}Ir seeds; 14 Gy to 2 mm). All received clopidogrel for 6 months. Late occlusion and thrombosis rates were compared with the 125 gamma radiation–treated patients and 126 placebo patients from WRIST and LONG WRIST (only 1 month of antiplatelet therapy). At 6 months, prolonged antiplatelet therapy resulted in total occlusion in 5.8%, and late thrombosis, in 2.5%; these rates were lower than those in the active gamma radiation group and similar to those in the placebo historical control group.

193. **SCRIPPS III** (Scripps Coronary Radiation to Inhibit Proliferation Post Stenting III). *N Engl J Med* 2001;344:297–299.

Design: Registry study of patients from SCRIPPS III and WRIST-Plus. Primary end points were stent thrombosis and mortality.

Purpose: To determine whether longer-term antiplatelet therapy is needed after stenting and beta-radiation brachytherapy to prevent late stent thrombosis.

Population: 500 patients with restenotic lesions within a stented area of a native coronary or bypass graft with vessel diameter of 2.75 to 4.0 mm and lesion length less than 80 mm. Of note, 25% in SCRIPPS-III and 29% in WRIST-Plus received new stents at the time of brachytherapy.

Treatment: Patients who received a 14-Gy fixed dose of beta radiation were given clopidogrel for 6 months. If a new stent was placed at the time of irradiation, clopidogrel was given for 12 months.

Results: At the time of the review of the Checkmate device for premarketing approval, 534 patients were registered in the two studies, of whom 206 (38.6%) had been followed up for 7 months. Late thrombosis had occurred in only three patients. In the combined population of these registries, the thrombosis-free survival rate was 99%.

194. **Waksman R,** et al. **WRIST 12.** Twelve versus six months of clopidogrel to reduce major cardiac events in patients undergoing gamma-radiation therapy for in-stent restenosis. *Circulation* 2002;106:776–778.

A total of 120 consecutive patients with diffuse ISR underwent PCI, including additional stent placement in 33%, followed by gamma radiation (^{192}Ir; 14 Gy at 2 mm). All patients received clopidogrel for 12 months. Clinical event rates at 15 months were compared with those of WRIST PLUS patients who received clopidogrel for 6 months. Late thrombosis rates were not significantly different [3.3% (12 months vs. 4.2%); $p = 0.72$]; no cases in the 12-month group were seen between 12 and 15 months. The 12-month group did have a significantly lower incidence of MACE (21% vs. 36%; $p = 0.01$) and TLR (20% vs. 35%; $p = 0.009$).

195. **Waksman R,** et al. **SVG WRIST.** Intravascular gamma radiation for in-stent restenosis in saphenous-vein bypass grafts. *N Engl J Med* 2002;346:1194–1199.

Design: Prospective, randomized, placebo-controlled, double-blind study. Primary end points were death from cardiac causes, Q-wave MI, TVR, and a composite of these events at 12 months.

Purpose: To examine the effects of i.v. gamma radiation in patients with ISR of saphenous vein bypass grafts.

Population: 120 patients with angina and evidence of ISR in saphenous vein grafts who underwent successful PTCA with provisional stenting, laser, or atherectomy.

Treatment: Gamma radiation (^{192}Ir source; 14 to 15 Gy in 2.5- to 4.0-mm vessels, and 18 Gy if diameter greater than 4.0 mm), or placebo.

Results: At 6 months, the gamma-radiation group had more than a 50% relative reduction in restenosis compared with placebo (21% vs. 44%; $p = 0.005$). Restenosis rates were significantly lower in all segments (i.e., stented, injured, irradiated). No significant differences were found between the groups in the incidence of death or Q-wave MI, but the radiation group had much lower revascularization rates (1 year TVR, 17% vs. 57%; $p < 0.001$). Late thrombosis rates were similar (both 1.7%).

196. **LONG WRIST.** Waksman R, et al. Intracoronary radiation therapy improves the clinical and angiographic outcomes of diffuse in-stent restenotic lesions. *Circulation* 2003;107:1744–1749.

Design: Prospective, randomized, placebo-controlled; registry group: open label. Primary 1 year clinical end point: deaths MI, target-lesion revascularization.

Purpose: To determine the safety and efficacy of vascular brachytherapy for the treatment of diffuse in-stent restenosis.

Population: 120 patients with lesions 36 to 88 mm in length; additional 120 patients were treated with 18 Gy (registry patients).
Treatment: [192]Ir with 15 Gy at 2 mm or placebo; registry group: 18 Gy.
Results: At 6 months, binary restenosis rates were 73%, 45%, and 38% in placebo, 15 Gy, and 18 Gy groups. One year primary event rates were 63% in placebo group compared with 42% in 15 Gy group ($p < 0.05$) and only 22% with 18 Gy.

197. **Limpijankit T,** et al. Long-term follow-up of patients after gamma intracoronary brachytherapy failure (from GAMMA-I, GAMMA-II, and SCRIPPS-III). *J Am Coll Cardiol* 2003;92:315–318.

The investigators combine outcomes from the GAMMA-1, GAMMA-II, and SCRIPPS-III studies report outcomes in a subset of 225 patients who failed brachytherapy for in-stent restenosis and subsequently survived to receive repeat PCI or CABG. They report worse total adverse events (including death, TVR, or MI) in the group that underwent PCI, as compared with CABG. It should be noted that these studies predate the use of DES for either de novo or in-stent lesions.

Beta Radiation

198. **King SB III,** et al. Beta Energy Restenosis Trial (**BERT**). Endovascular beta-radiation to reduce restenosis after coronary balloon angioplasty. *Circulation* 1998;97:2025–2030.

This small study (23 patients) demonstrated the safety and feasibility of beta radiation after angioplasty. A ^{90}Sr/Y source was used to deliver 12, 14, or 16 Gy at 2 mm. Source delivery was successful in 21 (91%) of 23 patients. No in-hospital morbidity or mortality occurred, and follow-up angiography in 20 patients showed a late lumen loss of only 0.5 mm and restenosis in 15%. A larger, randomized, double-blind study is ongoing. Subsequent 6-month follow-up data on 64 patients showed an overall restenosis rate of 14% (20% in the 12-Gy group and 11% in the 14- and 16-Gy groups).

199. **Waksman R,** et al. **BETA-WRIST.** Intracoronary β-radiation therapy inhibits recurrence of in-stent restenosis. *Circulation* 2000;101:1895–1898.

This small prospective study enrolled 50 patients with in-stent stenosis greater than 50%; lesion length, less than 47 mm; vessel diameter, 2.5 to 4.0 mm; and who had successful primary treatment (less than 30% residual stenosis without complications). Exclusion criteria were recent acute MI (<72 hours), ejection fraction less than 20%, angiographic thrombus, and multiple lesions in the same vessel. Patients received beta radiation with yttrium 90 at a dose of 20.6 Gy at 1.0 mm. At 6 months, the binary angiographic restenosis rate was 22%, the TLR rate was 26%, and the TVR rate was 34%.

200. **Serruys PW,** et al. Safety and performance of 90-strontium for treatment of de novo and restenotic lesions: the **BRIE** Trial (Beta Radiation in Europe). *Circulation* 2000;102:II-750.

This prospective, randomized, multicenter study enrolled 150 patients with de novo lesions. Patients were treated with the Novoste Betacath system (30-mm source) after angioplasty/stenting. At follow-up (**6 months**), angiographic restenosis had occurred in 33.6% and TVR in 15.4%. Geographic miss occurred in 41% of the patients and led to increased rates of restenosis (16.3% vs. 4.3%), especially at the edges of treated area (see *J Am Coll Cardiol* 2001;38:415–420). Geographic miss of stent-injured segments resulted in increased restenosis rates, whereas geographic miss of balloon-injured segments did not statistically increase restenosis.

201. **Waksman R,** et al. Use of localised intracoronary beta radiation in treatment of in-stent restenosis: the **INHIBIT** (Intimal Hyperplasia Inhibition with Beta In-stent Trial) randomised controlled trial. *Lancet* 2002;359:551–557.

Design: Prospective, randomized, blinded, multicenter study. Primary composite safety end point was death, Q-wave MI, and TLR at 9 months. Angiographic end point was binary restenosis.

Purpose: To evaluate whether beta-radiation brachytherapy with a P-32 source can reduce MACE and restenosis after treatment of ISR.

Population: 332 patients who underwent PTCA for single native vessel ISR. Reference vessel diameter was 2.4 to 3.7 mm, and lesion length, less than 45 mm.

Exclusion Criteria: Acute MI in previous 72 hours, previous radiation treatment to chest, thrombus by angiogram, multiple lesions in target vessel.

Treatment: P-32 beta emitter versus placebo delivered through a centering catheter via an automatic afterloader.

Results: The P-32 beta-irradiation group had a 56% reduction compared with the control group in the composite end point of death, Q-wave MI, and TLR (15% vs. 31%; $p = 0.0006$) and a 50% reduction in the angiographic binary restenosis rate (26% vs. 52% control; $p < 0.0001$).

202. **Popma JJ,** et al. for the Stents and Radiation Therapy (START) Investigators. Randomized trial of ^{90}Sr/^{90}Y ß-radiation versus placebo control for treatment of in-stent restenosis. *Circulation* 2002;106:1090.

This prospective, randomized, placebo-controlled, multicenter study enrolled 476 patients with native coronary ISR in lesions shorter than 20 mm. After angioplasty, patients were assigned to either 16 or 20 Gy of beta radiation (depending on diameter of vessel) or placebo. Primary end points at 8 months were restenosis, TLR, TVR, and MACE. Beta radiation was associated with significantly lower restenosis rates compared with placebo (in-stent 14% vs. 41%, analysis segment 28.8% vs. 45.2%). Radiation group also had improved clinical outcomes (TLR, 13.6% vs. 24.4%; TVR, 17% vs. 26.8%; and MACE, 18.6% vs. 27.7%).

DRUG-ELUTING STENTS

203. **Serruys PW,** et al. Coronary-artery stents. *N Engl J Med* 2006;354:483–495.

The authors provide a review of coronary stenting, specifically the genesis of implanting vascular stents, through to the pathophysiologic basis for DES, and the clinical data to support their use.

204. **Morice M-C,** et al. for the **RAVEL** (Randomized BX VELocity) Study Group. Randomized comparison of a sirolimus-eluting stent with a standard stent for coronary revascularization. *N Engl J Med* 2002;346:1773–1780.

Design: Prospective, randomized, double-blind, multicenter study. Primary end points were mean lumen diameter and late lumen loss at 6 months.

Purpose: To determine whether implantation of a sirolimus-eluting stent in de novo lesions will result in decreased restenosis compared with a bare stent.

Population: 238 patients with stable or unstable angina pectoris or silent ischemia who needed treatment of a single de novo lesion in a native vessel (2.5 to 3.5 mm or larger) that could be covered by a single 18-mm stent.

Exclusion Criteria: Included evolving MI, left main stenosis, ostial lesion location, calcified lesion that could not be completely dilated before stenting, angiographically visible thrombus within target lesion, ejection fraction less than 30%.

Treatment: Sirolimus-eluting stent or uncoated Bx Velocity balloon-expandable stent. All received ticlopidine or clopidogrel for 2 months.

Results: Rapamycin group had a mean late loss of 0.01 mm compared with 0.80 mm in the control group ($p < 0.0001$). Restenosis occurred in none of the rapamycin patients versus 26% of controls ($p < 0.0001$). Freedom from MACE (death, MI, repeated PCI, and CABG) was 96.7% in the rapamycin group compared with 72.9% in the control group ($p < 0.0001$). No cases of subacute stent thromboses were found.

205. **Moses JW**, et al. for the Sirolimus-Eluting Stent in Coronary Lesions (SIRIUS) Investigators. Sirolimus-eluting stents versus standard stents in patients with stenosis in a native coronary artery. *N Engl J Med* 2003;349:1315–1323.

Design: Prospective, randomized, double-blind, placebo-controlled, study. Primary end point was target-vessel failure defined as cardiac death, MI, or TVR at 9 months.

Purpose: To establish the safety and efficacy of the sirolimus-eluting BX Velocity stent in decreasing target-vessel failure in de novo native coronary artery lesions compared with the uncoated BX Velocity stent.

Population: 1,058 patients requiring single-vessel treatment of de novo higher-risk lesions (2.5 to 3.5 mm diameter and 15 to 30 mm long) in native vessels. Of note, 26% had diabetes, and 42% had multivessel disease. Most lesions were type B2 or C.

Exclusion Criteria: Included recent MI (<24 hours), unprotected left main disease, ostial location, total occlusion, angiographic evidence of thrombus, calcified lesion that could not be predilated; LVEF less than 25%, impaired renal function, pretreatment with devices other than balloon angioplasty, prior or planned intervention within 30 days.

Treatment: Sirolimus-eluting stent or uncoated stent. Antiplatelet therapy given for 3 months.

Results: Target-vessel failure (primary end point) was reduced by nearly 60% in the sirolimus group compared with the BMS group (from 21.0% to 8.6%; $p < 0.001$). The sirolimus stent group had a 91% reduction in ISR compared with BMS (3.2% vs. 35.4%; $p < 0.001$). ISR, which included the 5-mm segments proximal and distal to the stent, was reduced by 75% in the sirolimus group (8.9% vs. 36.3%; $p < 0.001$). Among diabetics, restenosis in the stent and in the segment was 8.3% and 17.6%, respectively, for sirolimus, compared with 48.5% and 50.5% for the bare stent. The distal margin had an equal treatment effect to that seen within the stent, whereas there was less intense effect but still significant effect in the proximal margin (late loss, 0.17 mm vs. 0.33 mm; $p < 0.001$). ISR increased by 13% for every additional 10 mm of implanted stent length in controls, compared with only 1.6% in the sirolimus group. Aneurysms occurred in two (0.6%) patients in the sirolimus group and in four (1.1%) patients in the control group. Stent thrombosis rates were also similar (0.6% and 1.1%). An IVUS study of 141 patients found an overall 90% reduction in neointimal volume in the coated-stent group; the lowest reduction was seen at the proximal margin in smaller vessels.

Comments: SIRIUS cohort had more patients with clinical characteristics associated with higher rates of restenosis as well as more complex lesions than the RAVEL cohort. However, several types of lesions were still excluded (see earlier), and ongoing studies are addressing these issues. The proximal margin findings suggest that balloon injury in this area is associated with pre/postdilation or stent delivery. However, the above findings in SIRIUS were confirmed Canadian cohorts in C-SIRIUS (see *J Am Coll Cardiol* 2004;43:1110–1115), as well as European cohorts in E-SIRIUS (see *Lancet* 2003;362:1093–1099). Results of cost-effectiveness analysis of the SIRIUS trial did not find DES implantation to be consistently cost-effective (see *Circulation* 2004;110:508–514).

206. **Caixeta A**, et al. 5-Year clinical outcomes after sirolimus-eluting stent implantation insights from a patient-level pooled analysis of 4 randomized trials comparing sirolimus-eluting stents with bare-metal stents. *J Am Coll Cardiol* 2009;54:894–902.

This combination of four trials of SES versus BMS (RAVEL, SIRIUS, E-SIRIUS, and C-SIRIUS) included 1,748 patients with follow-up to 5 years. While there was no difference in the rate of death or MI (15.15% for SES vs. 13.6% for BMS, $p = 0.36$), TVR was significantly reduced in the SES group (15.2% vs. 30.1%, $p < 0.0001$). Notably, rates of stent thrombosis, using a variety of definitions, were not different at 5 years (definite/probable stent thrombosis at 5 years: 2.1% vs. 2.0%, $p = 0.99$), using the Academic Research Consortium definition.

207. **ASPECT** (Asian Paclitaxel-Eluting Stent Clinical Trial). Park SJ, et al. A paclitaxel-eluting stent for the prevention of coronary restenosis. *N Engl J Med* 2003;348:1537–1545.

This prospective, randomized, triple-blind, multicenter study enrolled 177 patients with discrete coronary lesions (<15 mm in length, 2.25 to 3.25 mm in diameter). Patients received a low dose (1.3 mcg/mm^2) or high dose (3.1 mcg/mm^2) paclitaxel mounted on a nonpolymerized stent, or a BMS. At 4- to 6-month angiographic follow-up, the high-dose group had better results for the degree of stenosis (mean 14% vs. 39%, $p < 0.001$), late loss of luminal diameter (0.29 mm vs. 1.04 mm, $p < 0.001$), and binary restenosis (4% vs. 27%, $p < 0.001$).

208. **Colomboa A,** et al. for the TAXUS II Study Group. Randomized study to assess the effectiveness of slow- and moderate-release polymer-based paclitaxel-eluting stents for coronary artery lesions. *Circulation* 2003;108:788–794.

This prospective, randomized, multicenter trial enrolled a total of 536 patients and compared a bare stent with two formulations of a paclitaxel-eluting stent [slow-release (drug released over a 1-month period) or moderate-release (most released in the first 2 days)]. Lesions were standard-risk de novo lesions (average length, approximately 10 mm; average reference vessel diameter, approximately 2.75 mm). Patients received aspirin and clopidogrel for 6 months. Both paclitaxel-eluting stents demonstrated substantial reductions in the primary end point, percentage of in-stent net volume obstruction (by IVUS), compared with the bare stent group (60% reduction with slow-release and 62% with moderate-release version). At 12 months, MACE was significantly reduced with the DES [slow release, 10.9% vs. 22.0% (control); $p = 0.02$; moderate release, 9.9% vs. 21.4%; $p = 0.017$]. These reductions were driven by lower rates of TVR (slow release, 10.1% vs. 15.9%, $p = 0.20$; moderate release, 6.9% vs. 19.1%, $p = 0.005$) and TLR (slow release, 4.7% vs. 12.9%, $p = 0.03$; moderate release, 3.8% vs. 16.0%, $p = 0.002$). Importantly, no sign of edge effect was found, with nonsignificant *reductions* seen both in the proximal and in the distal segments of the segment with the DES versus controls.

209. **Stone G,** et al. for the TAXUS IV Investigators. A polymer-based, paclitaxel-eluting stent in patients with coronary artery disease. *N Engl J Med* 2004;350:221–231.

This prospective randomized, multicenter trial enrolled 1,314 patients undergoing stenting for de novo lesions and assigned them to either a BMS or slow-release PES, in a double-blind fashion. Angiographic follow-up at 9 months was prespecified in 732 patients. At 9 months, incidence of ischemia-driven TVR was 12% for the BMS group and 4.7% for the PES group ($p < 0.001$). Rates of TLR (11.3% vs. 3.0%, $p < 0.001$) and binary angiography restenosis (26.6% vs. 7.9%, $p < 0.001$) were also significantly reduced. However, rates of death or MI and stent thrombosis were similar.

210. **Malenka DJ,** et al. Outcomes following coronary stenting in the era of bare-metal vs the era of drug-eluting stents. *JAMA* 2008;299(24):2868–2876.

This observational study included 38,917 Medicare patients who received BMS prior to the release of DES, and 28,068 who underwent stenting after DES came about (61.5% received DES, 38.5% BMS). After risk adjustment, rates of repeat revascularizations at 2 years were significantly lower for patients treated in the DES era (HR 0.82, 95% CI, 0.79 to 0.85). Composite death or STEMI at 2 years was similar (HR 0.96, 95% CI, 0.92 to 1.01).

211. **Stone G,** et al. for the TAXUS V Investigators. Comparison of a polymer-based paclitaxel-eluting stent with a bare metal stent in patients with complex coronary artery disease: a randomized controlled trial. *JAMA* 2005;294:1215–1223.

Design: Prospective, randomized, double-blind, placebo-controlled, multicenter study. Primary end point was ischemia-driven TVR at 9 months.
Purpose: To establish the safety and efficacy of PES in more complex lesions, specifically those with narrower, longer stenoses, and those requiring multiple stents.

Population: 1,156 patients with de novo lesions of a single coronary artery, without evidence of recent MI.

Treatment: Paclitaxel-eluting stent or uncoated stent. Antiplatelet therapy given for 6 months.

Results: Rates of the primary end point, TVR, were significantly reduced in the PES group (17.3% vs. 12.1%, $p = 0.02$), as were rates of TLR (15.7% vs. 8.6%, $p < 0.001$). Overall, 78% of lesions were B2/C, and patients received a mean of 1.38 stents with an average reference vessel diameter of 2.69 mm and a lesion length of 17.2 mm. Binary angiography restenosis was reduced in the PES group (33.9% vs. 18.9%, $p < 0.001$), and this was a consistent effect for smaller vessels, larger vessels, as well as patients who received multiple stents. There were no differences in the rates of death or MI (5.5% vs. 5.7%) or stent thrombosis (0.7% for both).

212. **Marroquin OC,** et al. A comparison of bare-metal and drug-eluting stents for off-label indications. *N Engl J Med* 2008;358:342–352.

In this observational study of 6,551 patients in the National heart, Lung, and Blood Institute Dynamic Registry, the investigators looked at 1-year outcomes in patients who received either BMS or DES, and whether their use was off-label. This included stenting for restenosis, bypass groups, left main disease, ostial, bifurcated, or totally occluded lesions, or stenting in vessels with reference diameter of less than 2.5 mm, more than 3.75, or longer than 30 mm. This off-label use occurred in 54.7% of patients who received BMS and 48.7% of those who got DES. Those who received stents for an off-label indication had higher unadjusted 1-year mortality (5.3% vs. 2.7%, $p < 0.001$) and rates of MI (5.3% vs. 3.8%, $p = 0.0002$). However, these were lower for the DES off-label group, compared with the BMS off-label group. Overall, after risk-adjustment, rates of death or MI were no different for the DES group, compared with the BMS group. There were significantly lower rates of repeat PCI or revascularization in patients who received DES.

213. **James SK,** et al. Long-term safety and efficacy of drug-eluting versus bare-metal stents in Sweden. *N Engl J Med* 2009;360:1933–1945.

In a country-wide registry of patients undergoing PCI, the investigators examined 47,967 patients who received coronary stents, with mean follow-up of 2.7 years. In comparison between patients who received a single BMS (18,659) to those who received a single DES (10,294), there were no differences in the rates of death or MI, after risk adjustment. Rates of restenosis were significantly lower in the DES cohort (3.0 per 100 patient-years vs. 4.7, RR 0.43, 95% CI, 0.36 to 0.52).

214. **De Luca G,** et al. Efficacy and safety of drug-eluting stents in ST-segment elevation myocardial infarction: a meta-analysis of randomized trials. *Int J Cardiol* 2009;133: 213–22.

The authors combined 11 trials of DES versus BMS for primary PCI in STEMI, encompassing 3,605 patients. All trials had end points up to 12 months, and there were no differences in the combined rates of death (4.1% for DES vs. 4.4% for BMS, $p = 0.59$), recurrent MI (3.1% vs. 3.4%, $p = 0.38$), or stent thrombosis (1.6% vs. 2.2%, $p = 0.22$). Patients who got DES had significantly lower rates of TVR (5.0% vs. 12.6%, $p < 0.0001$). In a subset of four trials of 1,178, these outcomes were similar up to 18 to 24 months.

215. **De Luca G,** et al. Short and long-term benefits of sirolimus-eluting stent in ST-segment elevation myocardial infarction: a meta-analysis of randomized trials. *J Thromb Thrombolysis* 2009;28(2):200–210.

The authors assessed the efficacy and safety of SES for primary PCI in STEMI, by combing results of nine trials, including 2,769 patients randomized to either BMS or SES. Outcomes to 12 months were available, and patients who received SES had significantly lower rates of TVR (4.9% vs. 13.6%, $p < 0.0001$). Additionally, there was a trend to improved outcomes of mortality (2.9% vs. 4.2%, $p = 0.08$) and recurrent MI (3.0% vs. 4.3%, $p = 0.06$) for the SES group. No difference in stent thrombosis was identified at 12 months (1.9% vs. 2.5%, $p = 0.36$), and these findings were persistent up to follow-up of 2 to 3 years in a subset of four trials of 569 patients.

216. **Stone GW,** et al. Safety and efficacy of sirolimus- and paclitaxel-eluting coronary stents. *N Engl J Med* 2007;356:998–1008.

The investigators combined data from the early nine randomized trials of both SES (1,748 patients) and PES (3,513 patients) to assess clinical end points and, specifically, rates of late stent thrombosis in DES. At 4 years of follow-up, rates of death or MI were similar among the groups of SES, PES, and BMS; TLR rates were significantly lower in the DES groups, compared with the BMS groups. However, after 4 years, there were more stent thromboses in the SES group (1.2%) compared with the BMS group (0.9%, $p = 0.20$), as well as the PES group (1.3%, $p = 0.30$). Notably, of the five patients in the SES group who had stent thromboses within 1 year, only two were taking aspirin and clopidogrel, whereas two were taking only aspirin, and one was taking no antiplatelet agent at all. Similarly, in the PES group of nine patients with late stent thromboses, three were only taking aspirin and five were taking no antiplatelet agents at all (the medication status of one patient was unknown). Subsequently, guidelines have been updated to recommend a minimum of 1 year of dual antiplatelet therapy (aspirin plus a thienopyridine) following any DES implant.

217. **Fajadet J,** et al. for the ENDEAVOR II Investigators. Randomized, double-blind, multicenter study of the endeavor zotarolimus-eluting phosphorylcholine-encapsulated stent for treatment of native coronary artery lesions: clinical and angiographic results of the ENDEAVOR II trial. *Circulation* 2006;114:798–806.

This prospective, randomized, double-blind study assigned 1,197 patients with single, de novo coronary lesions to receive either a zotarolimus-eluting stent (ZES) or similar BMS. Mean reference vessel diameter was 2.75 mm and mean lesion length was 14.2 mm. At 9 months, the primary end point of target-vessel failure was lower in the ZES group (7.9% vs. 15.1%, $p = 0.0001$), as were rates of TLR (4.6% vs. 11.8%, $p = 0.0001$). In a subset of 531 patients with follow-up angiography, restenosis was lower for the ZES group (13.2% vs. 35%, $p < 0.0001$).

218. **Kandzari DE,** et al. for the ENDEAVOR III Investigators. Comparison of zotarolimus-eluting and sirolimus-eluting stents in patients with native coronary artery disease: a randomized controlled trial. *J Am Coll Cardiol* 2006;48:2440–2447.

The investigators randomized 436 patients undergoing PCI for stable de novo, native coronary lesions in a 3:1 fashion to receive either a new ZES or older SES. Primary end point was in-segment late lumen loss at 8-month angiography. This was significantly higher in the ZES group (0.34 mm vs. 0.13 mm, $p < 0.001$), as was binary in-segment restenosis (11.7% vs. 4.3%, $p = 0.04$). Rates of clinically driven TLR and target-vessel failure were similar between the ZES and SES groups. However, in-hospital MACE rates were lower in the ZES group (0.6% vs. 3.5%, $p = 0.04$).

219. **Stone G,** et al. for the SPIRIT III Investigators. Comparison of an everolimus-eluting stent and a paclitaxel-eluting stent in patients with coronary artery disease: a randomized trial. *JAMA* 2008;299:1903–1913.

Design: Prospective, randomized, single-blind study. Primary end point was in-segment late lumen loss on follow-up angiography at 8 months.

Purpose: To compare a contemporary everolimus-eluting stent (EES) to an older PES.

Population: 1,002 patients with stable CAD undergoing PCI for lesions less than 28 mm in length, and with reference vessel diameter between 2.5 and 3.75 mm.

Results: Late lumen loss was significantly lower for patients in the EES group versus PES (0.14 mm vs. 0.28 mm, $p \leq 0.004$). At 9 months, target-vessel failure was similar (7.2% vs. 9.0%, p for noninferiority <0.001). Based on fewer MIs and a lower rate of TVR, MACE rates were lower in the EES group at 9 months (4.6% vs. 8.1%, $p = 0.03$) and 1 year (6.0% vs. 10.3%, $p = 0.02$).

Comment: At 2-year follow-up, clinical outcomes continued to favor the EES group, including rates of stent thrombosis (see *Circulation* 2009;119:680–686). Results of the upcoming SPIRIT IV trial similarly favored EES over PES with a significantly lower rate of target lesion failure 4.2% vs. 6.8%, relative risk 0.62 $p = 0.001$. Stone et al. *NEJM* 2010;362:1663–1674.

220. **Ormiston JA,** et al. A bioabsorbable everolimus-eluting coronary stent system for patients with single de-novo coronary artery lesions (ABSORB): a prospective open-label trial. *Lancet* 2008;371:899–907.

In a prospective, open-label fashion the investigators implanted a novel absorbable, everolimus-eluting stent in 30 patients with stable, de novo coronary artery lesions. Previous studies had indicated 30% absorption (loss of stent mass) at 12 months, and 60% at 18 months. Stent sizes were limited to either 3.0×12 mm or 3.0×18 mm. One-year event rates were low, with only one patient (3.3%) experiencing MI and there were no TLRs or late stent thromboses. In-stent late loss was 0.44 mm on IVUS. Clinical events were confirmed in further analyses at 2 years, at which time the stent was bioabsorbed (see *Lancet* 2009;373:897–910).

221. **Vavry AA,** et al. Appropriate use of drug-eluting stents: balancing the reduction in restenosis with the concern of late thrombosis. *Lancet* 2008;371:2134–2143.

In light of significant data on late stent thromboses in patients who received DES without long-term dual-antiplatelet therapy, the authors review the indications for stenting as well as highlight patients who may be more appropriate for bare-metal stenting (e.g., those with poor access to medicines, at increased bleeding risk, or those likely to undergo invasive procedures in the near future). They emphasize the more-than-acceptable outcomes with BMS, specifically in patients at lower risk for in-stent restenosis.

CABG Surgery

REVIEW ARTICLES, META-ANALYSES

222. **Eagle KA,** et al. ACC/AHA 2004 guideline update for coronary artery bypass graft surgery: a report of the American College of Cardiology/American Heart Association Task Force on Practice Guidelines (Committee to Update the 1999 Guidelines for Coronary Artery Bypass Graft Surgery). *J. Am. Coll. Cardiol.* 2004;44;e213–e310 Available at: http://www.acc.org/clinical/guidelines/cabg/cabg.pdf.

223. **Yusuf S,** et al. Effect of coronary artery bypass graft surgery on survival: overview of 10-year results from randomised trials by the CABG Trialists Collaboration. *Lancet* 1994;344:563–570.

This review of data focuses on 1,324 patients assigned to CABG surgery and 1,325 patients who received medical management. The CABG group had a significantly lower mortality rate at 5 years (10.2% vs. 15.8%; OR, 0.61; $p = 0.0001$), 7 years (15.8% vs. 21.7%; OR, 0.68; $p < 0.001$), and 10 years (26.4% vs. 30.5%; OR, 0.83; $p = 0.03$). The risk reduction was most marked in patients with left main CAD and triple-vessel disease or single- or two-vessel disease [ORs, 0.32, 0.58 vs. 0.77 (two- and single-vessel disease)]. High-risk patients (defined as those with two of the following: severe angina, history of hypertension, prior MI, and ST-segment depression at rest) had a 29% mortality reduction at 10 years compared with a 10% reduction in patients at moderate risk and a nonsignificant trend toward higher mortality in low-risk patients [no risk factors (except ST depression) allowed].

224. **Nwasokwa ON.** Coronary artery bypass graft disease. *Ann Intern Med* 1995;123:528–545.

This thorough review of the literature showed only an approximate 50% patency of saphenous vein grafts at 10 years after bypass surgery versus more than 90% patency achieved with IMA grafts. The use of IMA grafts leads to less frequent symptoms, better LV function, decreased need for reoperation, and improved survival. The role of antiplatelet agents in decreasing graft occlusion rates also is reviewed.

225. **Pocock SJ,** et al. Meta-analysis of randomised trials comparing coronary angioplasty with bypass surgery. *Lancet* 1996;346:1184–1189.

This analysis of data was derived from 3,771 patients in eight trials (CABRI, RITA, EAST, GABI, MASS, ERACI, Toulouse, Lausanne). The average follow-up period was 2.7 years. No differences were demonstrated in overall cardiac mortality between PTCA and CABG. However, CABG patients had 90% fewer first-year reinterventions (3.3% vs. 33.7%) and less angina. A CABG was performed in 18% of PTCA patients within 1 year. The impact of longer follow-up is unknown (e.g., increased saphenous venous graft disease).

226. **Roach G,** et al. Adverse cerebral outcomes after coronary bypass surgery. *N Engl J Med* 1996;335:1857–1863.

This prospective study was composed of 2,108 patients, 6.1% with cerebral events: type I, 3.1% [focal injury, or stupor or coma at hospital discharge (D/C); 55 of 66 had nonfatal strokes] or type II, 3% (deterioration in intellectual function, memory deficit, or seizures). Events were associated with increased in-hospital mortality [21% (type I) and 10% vs. 2%], longer hospital stay (25 days, 21 days, 10 days), and more patients discharged to intermediate or long-term care (47%, 30%, 8%). Type I predictors included proximal aortic atherosclerosis, history of neurologic disease, and age; type II predictors included age, hypertension, pulmonary disease, and alcohol consumption.

STUDIES

CABG versus Medical Therapy

227. European Coronary Surgery Study (**ECSS**) Group. Long-term results of prospective randomised study of coronary artery bypass surgery in stable angina pectoris. *Lancet* 1982;320:1173–1180.

Design: Prospective, randomized, open study. Primary end point was all-cause mortality. Follow-up period was 5 to 8 years.
Purpose: To compare CABG surgery with initial medical management in patients with angina and multivessel CAD.
Population: 768 men aged ≤65 years with mild to moderate angina, ≥50% stenosis in two major vessels, and good LV function.
Treatment: CABG surgery or medical therapy.
Results: Surgery was beneficial in the total population (88.6% survival vs. 79.9% at 8 years), although most of the benefit was seen in patients with proximal LAD artery stenoses (10-year survival, 76% vs. 66%). No benefit was present if left main disease was present. Independent predictors of surgical benefit were abnormal rest ECG, ST depression 1.5 mm with exercise, peripheral vascular disease, and increased age.

228. Coronary Artery Surgery Study (**CASS**) Principal Investigators and their associates. Myocardial infarction and mortality in the CASS randomized trial. *N Engl J Med* 1984;310:750–758.

Design: Prospective, randomized, open, parallel-group study. Primary end point was all-cause mortality. Mean follow-up period was 6 years.

Purpose: To determine whether CABG surgery reduces mortality and MI rates in patients with mild angina and angiographically documented CAD.

Population: 780 patients aged ≤65 years with coronary artery stenosis ≥70%.

Exclusion Criteria: Prior CABG, unstable angina, heart failure (NYHA class III or IV).

Treatment: CABG surgery or medical therapy.

Results: Lower mortality trend was observed with CABG (1.1%/year vs. 1.6%/year), strongest in patients with EF ≤50% ($p = 0.085$) and triple-vessel disease and EF ≤50% ($p = 0.063$). Among patients with triple-vessel disease and EF of 35% to 49%, a significant mortality difference was found at subsequent follow-up [12% (CABG) vs. 35% mortality; $p = 0.009$]. At 10-year follow-up, CABG had been performed in 40% of medical patients, and no overall survival difference was noted (medical group, 79%; surgical group, 82%). However, the results of CABG were significantly better than medical therapy in patients with an EF less than 50% (79% vs. 61%; $p = 0.01$).

Comments: Long-term follow-up in 912 patients with left main equivalent disease (e.g., severe proximal LAD and left circumflex disease) showed that surgery prolongs life (13.1 vs. 6.2 years), but not if normal LV function is present (15-year survival, 63% vs. 54%; $p = $ NS), even with right coronary artery stenosis ≥70% (see *Circulation* 1995;91:2335).

229. **VA** Coronary Artery Bypass Surgery Cooperative Study Group. Eleven year survival in Veterans Affairs randomized trial of coronary bypass surgery for stable angina. *N Engl J Med* 1984;311:1333–1339.

Design: Prospective, randomized, multicenter, open study. Primary end point was all-cause mortality. Average follow-up was 11.2 years.

Purpose: To compare CABG with medical therapy in patients with stable angina.

Population: 686 patients with stable angina pectoris of longer than 6-month duration.

Exclusion Criteria: MI in prior 6 months, unstable angina, DBP greater than 100 mm Hg, uncompensated congestive heart failure.

Treatment: CABG surgery or medical therapy.

Results: Overall, a significant mortality difference was observed between groups at 7 years (77% survival in CABG group vs. 70%; $p = 0.043$) but not at 11 years (57% vs. 58%). Surgery was beneficial in the following subgroups: (a) triple-vessel disease plus LV dysfunction (per angiography), 50% versus 38% survival at 11 years ($p = 0.026$); (b) clinically high-risk patients (at least two of the following: resting ST depression, history of MI, history of hypertension), 49% versus 36% survival ($p = 0.015$); and (c) combined angiographic and clinically high risk, 54% versus 24% ($p = 0.005$). Patients with LV dysfunction (EF, less than 45%; end-diastolic pressure, more than 14 mm Hg; or any contraction abnormality) benefited from surgery at 7 years (survival, 74% vs. 63%; $p = 0.049$) but not at 11 years (53% vs. 49%).

Comments: Subsequent 18-year follow-up report showed no benefit of surgery, even in the high-risk subgroups. Overall, the benefits of surgery began to diminish after 5 years, a time course that parallels the development of graft disease.

Coronary Artery Bypass Graft Surgery versus Percutaneous Transluminal Coronary Angiography

230. Coronary angioplasty vs coronary artery bypass surgery: the Randomised Intervention Treatment of Angina (**RITA**) trial. *Lancet* 1993;341:573–580.

Design: Prospective, randomized, multicenter study. Primary end point was death and MI. Mean follow-up period was 2.5 years.

Purpose: To compare bypass surgery with coronary angioplasty in patients in whom equivalent myocardial revascularization could be achieved by either treatment method.

Population: 1,011 patients with multivessel coronary disease (55% with at least two diseases of the coronary arteries).

Exclusion Criteria: Left main disease, prior coronary angioplasty or bypass surgery, and significant valve disease.

Treatment: CABG surgery or PTCA.

Results: No difference was observed in the primary composite end point of death or MI at 5 years (8.6% vs. 9.8%; RR, 0.88; 95% CI, 0.59 to 1.29). CABG patients had a longer recovery but fewer additional measures. At 2 years, repeated angiography was performed in 7% versus 31% ($p < 0.001$), and revascularization or a primary event occurred in 11% versus 38% ($p < 0.001$). CABG patients also had less angina (22% vs. 31% at 2 years). A subsequent report showed that the PTCA group had a higher out-of-work rate at 2 years (26% vs. 22%) (see *Circulation* 1996;94:135).

231. **Hamm CW**, et al. German Angioplasty Bypass Surgery Investigation (**GABI**). A randomized study of coronary angioplasty compared with bypass surgery in patients with symptomatic multivessel coronary disease. *N Engl J Med* 1994;331:1037–1043.

Design: Prospective, randomized, multicenter study. Primary end point was freedom from angina at 1 year.

Purpose: To compare the clinical efficacy of bypass surgery with balloon angioplasty in patients with symptomatic multivessel CAD.

Population: 8,981 patients younger than 75 years were screened, and 359 were enrolled (total revascularization of at least two major vessels needed and feasible technically).

Exclusion Criteria: Totally occluded vessels, left main stenosis greater than 30%, MI in prior 4 weeks, and prior bypass or angioplasty.

Treatment: CABG surgery or PTCA.

Results: CABG group had longer hospitalization (19 vs. 5 days) and more MIs (8.1% vs. 2.3%; $p = 0.022$) owing to procedures. However, CABG patients had similar in-hospital mortality rates (2.5% vs. 1.1%), fewer interventions (6% vs. 44%; $p < 0.001$), and less angina at hospital discharge (7% vs. 18%; no difference at 1 year), and fewer patients were taking antianginal medications (12% vs. 22%; $p = 0.041$).

232. **King SB**, et al. Emory Angioplasty vs Surgery Trial (**EAST**). A randomized trial comparing coronary angioplasty with coronary bypass surgery. *N Engl J Med* 1994; 331:1044–1050 (editorial, 1086–1087).

Design: Prospective, randomized, multicenter study. Composite primary end point was death, Q-wave MI, and large defect on thallium scan at 3 years.

Purpose: To compare outcomes of bypass surgery with angioplasty in patients with multivessel disease.

Population: 392 patients with two- or triple-vessel CAD (5,118 patients screened; 842 eligible).

Exclusion Criteria: Prior bypass surgery or coronary angioplasty, recent myocardial infarction (<5 days), old chronic occlusions (more than 8 weeks), left main stenosis greater than 30%, and EF, less than 25%.

Treatment: CABG surgery or PTCA.

Results: No significant difference was observed between groups in 3-year mortality (7.1% vs. 6.3%) or primary composite end points (28.8% vs. 27.3%). However, CABG patients required fewer repeated CAGB surgeries (1% vs. 22%; $p < 0.001$) and fewer angioplasties (13% vs. 41%; $p < 0.001$), and reported less angina (12% vs. 20%).

233. CABRI Trial Participants. First year results of **CABRI** (Coronary Angioplasty vs Bypass Revascularization Investigation). *Lancet* 1995;346:1179–1184.

Design: Prospective, randomized, multicenter, open study. Primary outcomes were 1-year mortality and symptom status (based on angina class) at 1 year.

Purpose: To compare bypass surgery with angioplasty in patients with multivessel coronary disease requiring intervention.

Population: 1,054 patients aged ≤75 years with multivessel disease and typical angina or unstable angina, 62% with class III angina.

Treatment: CABG surgery or PTCA.

Exclusion Criteria: MI in prior 10 days; EF, less than 35%; and prior PTCA or CABG.

Results: At 1-year follow-up, mortality rates were similar between groups (2.7% for CABG, 3.9% for PTCA). The CABG group had 81% fewer reinterventions (6.5% vs. 33.6%; $p <$ 0.001) and 35% less angina, and patients were taking fewer medications. The 1-year mortality rate was highest in patients with grade IV angina or unstable angina (5% vs. 2.7%).

Comments: Complete revascularization was not required, and patients with total occlusions were not excluded.

234. **Frye RL,** et al. Bypass Angioplasty Revascularization Investigation (**BARI**). Comparison of coronary bypass surgery with angioplasty in patients with multivessel disease. *N Engl J Med* 1996;335:217–225 (editorial, 275–276).

Design: Prospective, randomized, multicenter study. Primary end point was all-cause mortality. Follow-up period was 5.4 years.

Purpose: To compare outcomes of bypass surgery with angioplasty in patients with multivessel disease and severe angina or ischemia.

Population: 1,829 patients; 41% had triple-vessel CAD.

Treatment: CABG surgery or PTCA.

Results: CABG and PTCA groups had similar in-hospital mortality rates [1.3% (CABG) vs. 1.1%] and 5-year survival rates (89% vs. 86%; $p = 0.19$). The CABG group had more in-hospital Q-wave MIs (4.6% vs. 2.1%; $p < 0.01$) but had an 85% lower 5-year revascularization rate (8% vs. 54%) and 44% better 5-year survival in patients with diabetes (19% of enrolled patients; 81% vs. 66%; $p = 0.003$). The PTCA group had a 31% 5-year CABG rate.

Comments: Accompanying editorial reports that combining data from the BARI, EAST, and CABRI trials, CABG is associated with nonsignificant 14% mortality reduction (95% CI, +16% to −37%). A subsequent cost and quality-of-life analysis of 934 patients showed that the initial costs were 35% lower in the PTCA group but only 5% lower at 5 years ($56,000 vs. $58,900; $p = 0.047$). The cost of surgery was −$26,000/year of life added, and surgical patients returned to work 5 weeks later but had better functional status at 3 years. Another analysis showed that more lesions were favorable for revascularization by CABG (92% vs. 78%; $p < 0.001$), especially 99% to 100% lesions (78% vs. 22%).

235. **Rodriguez A,** et al. ERACI II Investigators. Argentine randomized study: coronary angioplasty with stenting versus coronary bypass surgery in patients with multiple-vessel disease (**ERACI II**): 30-day and one-year follow-up results. *J Am Coll Cardiol* 2001;37:51–58.

Design: Prospective, randomized, multicenter study. Primary end point: death, MI, repeated revascularization procedures, and stroke at 30 days.

Purpose: To compare PTCR with stent implantation with conventional CABG surgery in symptomatic patients with multivessel CAD.

Population: 450 patients with multivessel CAD (2,759 screened) and an indication for revascularization.

Treatment: PTCR (225 patients) or CABG (225 patients).

Results: At 30 days, the PTCR group had fewer major adverse events compared with the CABG group (3.6% vs. 12.3%; $p = 0.002$), including a significantly lower mortality (0.9% vs. 5.7%; $p < 0.013$). At follow-up (mean, 18.5 months), the PTCR had a persistent mortality benefit (3.1% vs. 7.5%; $p < 0.017$). However, as seen in prior trials of similar design, the PTCR group had a much higher revascularization rate than did the CABG group (16.8% vs. 4.8%; $p < 0.002$).

236. **Serruys PW,** et al. for the Arterial Revascularization Therapies Study (**ARTS**) Group. Comparison of coronary-artery bypass surgery and stenting for the treatment of multivessel disease. *N Engl J Med* 2001;344:1117–1124.

Design: Prospective, randomized, parallel-group study. Primary end point: Freedom from death, MI, any cerebrovascular event, and any repeated coronary revascularization at 1 year.

Purpose: To compare coronary artery stenting with CABG surgery in patients with multivessel disease.

Population: 1,205 patients (average age, 61 years) who had not undergone bypass surgery or angioplasty with stable angina, unstable angina, or silent ischemia AND ≥two de novo lesions in different vessels and territories that were amenable to stenting. The average interval between randomization and treatment was 27 days for patients in surgery group and 11 days for the stenting group.

Exclusion Criteria: LVEF, 30% or less; overt congestive heart failure; history of cerebrovascular accident (CVA); transmural MI in previous week; severe hepatic or renal disease; diseased saphenous veins; neutropenia or thrombocytopenia; intolerance or contraindication to aspirin or ticlopidine; need for major surgery.

Treatment: Stenting or CABG surgery (randomized *after* a cardiac surgeon and an interventional cardiologist concurred that the same extent of revascularization could be achieved with either technique). The average interval between randomization and treatment was 27 days for patients in the surgery group and 11 days for the stenting group. Fewer than 4% were treated with GP IIb/IIIa inhibitors.

Results: At 1 year, no significant differences were seen between the two groups in death, stroke, or MI. Surgery was associated with a higher event-free survival compared with stenting (87.8% vs. 73.8%; $p < 0.001$). This difference was due to primarily the much higher rate of repeated revascularization in the stenting group; among those without a stroke or MI, the incidence was 16.8% versus 3.5% in the surgery group. No significant difference was noted between the two groups in the incidence of death (2.8% vs. 2.5%), stroke (2.0% vs. 1.5%), or MI (4.0% vs. 5.3%). The costs for the initial procedure were $4,212 less per patient for the stenting group, but this difference narrowed to $2,973 per patient by 1-year follow-up. Among CABG patients, an elevated CK-MB was observed in 61%, and an increase to more than 5 times normal in 12%, and was an independent predictor of adverse clinical events. A subsequent report (see *Circulation* 2001;104:533) found that diabetics who underwent stenting had the lowest event-free survival (63.4% vs. 84.4% diabetes and CABG, 76.2% no-diabetes and stenting, and 88.4% no-diabetes plus CABG); this was owing to an increased incidence of repeated revascularization. A nonsignificant trend toward a lower mortality rate was seen in the diabetic CABG group compared with the diabetic stenting group (3.1% vs. 6.3%).

Comments: GP IIb/IIIa inhibitors were used infrequently in this trial; higher use may have decreased the 2.8% stent thrombosis rate and the 30% CK-MB release in the stent group. Outcomes in the modern era of GP IIb/IIIa inhibition, clopidogrel, and coated stents and with longer follow-up to detect late graft failure are not known.

237. **Morrison DA,** et al. for the Investigators of the Department of Veterans Administration Affairs Cooperative Study 385, the Angina with Extremely Serious Operative Mortality Evaluation (**AWESOME**). Percutaneous coronary intervention vs. coronary artery bypass graft surgery for patients with medically refractory myocardial ischemia and risk factors for adverse outcomes with bypass: a multicenter, randomized trial. *J Am Coll Cardiol* 2001;38:143–149.

Design: Prospective, randomized, multicenter study. Primary end point was survival. Secondary end points were unstable angina, repeated hospitalization, repeated catheterization, and repeated revascularization with CABG or PCI.

Purpose: To compare PCI with CABG in high-risk patients with medically refractory MI.

Population: 554 patients (22,662 screened) with evidence of medically refractory MI and one or more of five high-risk clinical characteristics for CABG including prior open heart surgery, older than 70 years, LVEF less than 35, MI within 7 days, or intra-aortic balloon pump requirement.

Treatment: PCI or CABG surgery. The use of left IMA grafting increased from 57% in 1995 to 78% in 2000 (average, 70%), whereas stent use increased from 26% to 88% (average, 54%) and GP IIb/IIIa inhibitor use from 1% to 52% (average, 11%).

Results: The in-hospital and 30-day survival rates were 96% and 95%, respectively, for CABG, and 99% and 97% for PCI. At 6-month follow-up, the small difference in survival rates was still present (90% for CABG and 94% for PCI), whereas at 3-year follow-up, survival rates were similar (79% for CABG and 80% for PCI; $p = 0.46$). No significant differences were noted between the groups in freedom from unstable angina [65% (CABG) vs. 59%; $p <$ 0.16], whereas freedom from unstable angina and repeated revascularization was significantly better with CABG compared with PCI (61% vs. 48%; $p = 0.001$).

238. **SoS** (Stent or Surgery). SoS Investigators. Coronary artery bypass surgery versus percutaneous coronary intervention with stent implantation in patients with multivessel coronary artery disease (the Stent or Surgery Trial): a randomised controlled trial. *Lancet* 2002;360:965–970.

Design: Prospective, randomized, open, multicenter study. Primary outcome measure was rate of repeat revascularization. Median follow-up was 2 years.

Purpose: To assess the effect of stent-assisted PCI versus CABG in multivessel CAD patients.

Population: 988 patients with symptomatic multivessel CAD.

Exclusion Criteria: Previous CABG or PCI, acute MI in prior 48 hours, intervention of valves, myocardium, great vessels, carotids, or aorta scheduled for index revascularization procedure.

Treatment: Angioplasty with stenting (PCI) or CABG surgery; in PCI arm, mean number of vessels treated was 2.2, with 78% of lesions receiving stents.

Results: The PCI group had a higher revascularization rate compared with the CABG group (21% vs. 6%, $p < 0.0001$). The incidence of death or MI at 2 years was similar in both groups (PCI 9%, CABG 10%), though the mortality rate was significantly lower in the surgery group (2% vs. 5%, $p = 0.01$).

Comments: Although the revascularization rate was higher in the stent arm, the rates were about half those seen in the BARI and EAST trials.

239. **Diegeler A,** et al. Comparison of stenting with minimally invasive bypass surgery for stenosis of the left anterior descending coronary artery. *N Engl J Med* 2002;347:561–566.

A total of 220 symptomatic patients with high-grade proximal LAD lesions of the coronary artery were randomized to minimally invasive surgery (thoracotomy; no cardiopulmonary bypass) or stenting. At 6 months, the surgery group had a lower incidence of MACEs, consisting of cardiac death, MI, and TLR, compared with the stenting group (15% vs. 31%; $p = 0.02$). The difference was primarily owing to higher TLR for restenosis after stenting (29% vs. 8%; $p = 0.003$), as the combined rates of death and MI did not differ significantly between groups [6% (surgery) vs. 3%; $p = 0.50$]. The surgery group had more patients free from angina after 6 months compared with the stenting group (79% vs. 62%; $p = 0.03$). It should be noted that the stent group did not receive GP IIb/IIIa inhibitors.

240. **Bravata DM,** et al. Systematic review: the comparative effectiveness of percutaneous coronary interventions and coronary artery bypass graft surgery. *Ann Intern Med* 2007;147:703–716.

The investigators combine results from 23 randomized studies of 5,019 patients undergoing PCI (both balloon angioplasty and stenting with BMS, only one small trial with DES) and 4,944 undergoing CABG. Over 10 years of follow-up, mortality difference between the two groups was less than 1%. Consistent with previous findings, procedure-related stroke incidence was higher for the CABG group (1.2% vs. 0.6%, $p = 0.002$); however, repeat revascularization rates heavily favored CABG (33% reduction at 5 years, $p < 0.001$; absolute 5-year rates of 46.1% after balloon angioplasty, 40.1% after stenting, and 9.8% after CABG). Relief of angina also favored CABG. Importantly, specific patient co-morbidities possibly confounding data could not be assessed, and DES were used in a small minority of patients.

241. **Daemen J,** et al. Long-term safety and efficacy of percutaneous coronary intervention with stenting and coronary artery bypass surgery for multivessel coronary artery disease: a meta-analysis with 5-year patient-level data from the ARTS, ERACI-II, MASS-II, and SoS trials. *Circulation* 2008;118:1146–1154.

In a meta-analysis that included more stenting, the authors combined four randomized trials of 3,051 patients, following up at 5 years. Incidence of the primary end point, a composite of death, MI, stroke, was similar (16.7% for PCI vs. 16.9% for CABG, $p = 0.69$); however, repeat revascularization rates strongly favored CABG (29.0% vs. 7.9%, $p < 0.001$). Heterogeneity analysis did not reveal differing effects in patients with diabetes. However, importantly, the four trials included were of bare-metal stenting; DES were not part of this meta-analysis.

242. **Hlatky MA,** et al. Coronary artery bypass surgery compared with percutaneous coronary interventions for multivessel disease: a collaborative analysis of individual patient data from ten randomised trials. *Lancet* 2009;373:1190–1197.

The authors combined data from 10 randomized trials, six of balloon angioplasty versus CABG, and four with bare-metal stenting versus CABG; mean follow-up was 5.9 years. Mortality between any PCI and CABG was similar (16% vs. 15%, $p = 0.12$); however, in the subset of patients with diabetes, mortality rates favored CABG (HR 0.70, 95% CI, 0.56 to 0.87). Mortality also trended significantly to be lower as patient age increased ($p = 0.002$ for interaction). The authors conclude that patient-specific parameters should dictate which strategy they undergo, with the exception of older patients or those with diabetes in whom CABG may be more beneficial.

243. **Hannan EL,** et al. Long-term outcomes of coronary-artery bypass grafting versus stent implantation. *N Engl J Med* 2005;352:2174–2183.

In New York's cardiac registry, the authors identified patients with multivessel disease who underwent PCI with bare-metal stenting ($n = 22{,}102$) or CABG ($n = 37{,}212$) for revascularization. In this nonrandomized cohort, risk-adjusted survival rates significantly favored the CABG cohort, as stratified by disease: those with triple-vessel disease involving the proximal LAD had HR 0.64 (95% CI, 0.56 to 0.74); and 0.76 (0.60 to 0.96) for patients with two-vessel disease involving the LAD, but not proximally. Repeat revascularization rates were higher for stenting (7.8% underwent subsequent CABG and 27.3% subsequent PCI) compared with the original CABG group (0.3% repeat CABG, 4.6% repeat PCI).

244. **Hannan EL,** et al. Drug-eluting stents vs. coronary-artery bypass grafting in multivessel coronary disease. *N Engl J Med* 2008;358:331–341.

In a follow-up study (see above), the authors identified patients in the New York cardiac registry who underwent either PCI with DES or CABG for multivessel CAD. This included 9,963 patients in the PCI group and 7,437 in the CABG group, with overall follow-up at approximately 18 months. In risk-adjusted analysis of patients with triple-vessel disease, overall survival rates favored the CABG group (94% vs. 92.7%, $p = 0.03$), as did survival free of MI (92.1% vs. 89.7%, $p < 0.001$). Similar distinctions were found in patients with two-vessel disease; overall survival favored CABG (96% vs. 94.6%, $p = 0.003$), as did survival free of MI (94.5% vs. 92.5%, $p < 0.001$). In these observational data, mortality and MI rates favored CABG over PCI for patients with multivessel CAD.

245. **Seung KB,** et al. Stents versus coronary-artery bypass grafting for left main coronary artery disease (MAIN-COMPARE). *N Engl J Med* 2008;358:1781–1792.

The investigators compiled outcomes in patients with unprotected left main CAD who underwent either PCI ($n = 1{,}102$) or CABG ($n = 1{,}138$). In the PCI group, 318 (28.9%)

received BMS and 784 (71.1%) received DES; mean follow-up overall was 1,017 days. There was no overall difference in rates of death (HR for stenting 1.18, 95% CI, 0.77 to 1.80) or the composite of death, MI, or stroke (HR for stenting 1.10, 95% CI, 0.75 to 1.62). Rates of TVR were significantly higher in the stenting group (HR 4.76, 95% CI, 2.8 to 8.11). There was no difference in outcomes between patients who received BMS versus DES in the PCI group. These findings are persistent in long-term follow-up up to 3 years (see *J Am Coll Cardiol* 2009;54:853–859).

246. **Serruys PW,** et al. for the SYNergy between percutaneous coronary intervention with TAXus and cardiac surgery (SYNTAX) Investigators. Percutaneous coronary intervention versus coronary-artery bypass grafting for severe coronary artery disease. *N Engl J Med* 2009;360:961–972.

Design: Prospective, randomized, multicenter study. Primary end point was a composite of death, stroke, MI, or repeat revascularization at 12 months, for noninferiority.

Purpose: To assess the effect of PCI with DES versus CABG in patients with triple-vessel CAD and/or left main disease.

Population: 1,800 patients with previously untreated triple-vessel CAD or left main CAD, whom both a cardiac surgeon and an interventional cardiologist had agreed were anatomically appropriate for either surgical or percutaneous revascularization.

Treatment: Complete revascularization of all vessels at least 1.5 mm in diameter with stenoses of at least 50%, either by PCI with stenting or by CABG.

Results: Results of the primary composite end point heavily favored the CABG group (12.4% vs. 17.8%, $p = 0.002$), driven predominantly by a surfeit of repeat revascularization in the PCI group (5.9% vs. 13.5%, $p < 0.001$). The trial failed to meet its noninferiority margin. However, rates of guideline-recommended therapies were more frequently used in the PCI group (e.g., aspirin, thienopyridine, statin, and ACE inhibitor use at discharge). At 12 months, rates of death or MI were similar; rates of stroke favored the PCI group (2.2% for CABG vs. 0.6% for PCI, $p = 0.003$).

Comments: Each patient's anatomy was scored for complexity, using the SYNTAX score; stratification of patients by the SYNTAX score may help determine which patients are more likely to benefit from CABG and which could be more appropriate for PCI (see *Am J Cardiol* 2007;99:1072–1081).

247. **The BARI 2D Group.** A randomized trial of therapies for type 2 diabetes and coronary artery disease. *N Engl J Med* 2009;360:2503–2515.

Design: Prospective, randomized, multicenter trial of patients with diabetes and CAD. Primary outcomes were death, and a composite of death, MI, or stroke at 5 years.

Purpose: To assess identify the best management strategy for patients with type 2 diabetes and stable CAD.

Population: A total of 2,368 patients with type 2 diabetes and CAD who had not undergone revascularization in the previous 12 months were randomized following diagnostic angiography (ensuring they were suitable for either PCI or CABG but did not require urgent revascularization or have left main disease).

Treatment: Patients were randomized to either medical therapy or revascularization. Randomization was stratified by revascularization with PCI or CABG, and in a 2 × 2 factorial design, patients were also randomized to insulin-sensitization or provisional insulin (to target HbA1c <7%). Overall, 763 were found to be suitable for CABG (378 randomized to CABG and 378 to medical therapy), while 1,605 were selected for PCI (798 received PCI and 807 medical therapy). Overall, 977 were randomized to insulin sensitization and 967 to provisional insulin.

Results: There was no difference in mortality at 5 years between medical therapy and revascularization (88.3% for revascularization and 87.8% for medical therapy, $p = 0.97$), and between insulin sensitization or provisional therapy (88.2% for insulin sensitization and

87.9% for provisional insulin, $p = 0.89$). Freedom from major adverse cardiovascular events also was not different among the groups (77.2% for revascularization vs. 75.9% for medical therapy, $p = 0.70$; 77.7% for insulin sensitization and 75.4% for provisional insulin, $p = 0.13$). However, when stratified by revascularization patients who underwent CABG had lower rates of major adverse cardiovascular events than those who received medical therapy (22.4% for CABG vs. 30.5% for medical therapy, $p = 0.002$); this effect was not detected in the PCI group. Rates of severe hypoglycemia were higher in the insulin-sensitization group, compared with provisional insulin (9.2% vs. 5.9%, $p = 0.003$).

Comments: Adding evidence to the results of the COURAGE trial (see above), these findings provided additional data to support the more limited use of PCI for revascularization. It should be noted that only a minority of eligible patients in the BARI 2D study received DES (35%) and thienopyridine therapy (21%).

Graft and Patency Studies

248. **Loop FD,** et al. Influence of the internal mammary graft on 10 year survival and other cardiac events. *N Engl J Med* 1986;314:1–6.

This retrospective analysis focused on 5,931 patients who underwent CABG from 1971 to 1979; 3,625 patients had saphenous vein grafts only. IMA patients had better survival. Ten-year rates were 93.4% versus 88% ($p = 0.05$) for single-vessel disease; 90% versus 79.5% ($p < 0.0001$) for two-vessel disease; and 82.6% versus 71% ($p < 0.001$) for triple-vessel disease. A Cox multi-variate analysis was performed, and for the saphenous vein graft group, the RR of death was 1.61; late MI RR, 1.14; hospitalization for cardiac events RR, 1.25; and cardiac reoperation RR, 2.0.

249. **Cameron A,** et al. Coronary bypass surgery with internal thoracic artery grafts: effects on survival over a 15-year period. *N Engl J Med* 1996;334:216–219 (editorial, 263–265).

This analysis focused on 5,637 CASS registry patients, including 749 patients who received arterial grafts. In multivariate analysis, internal thoracic artery patients had a 27% lower mortality rate at 15-year follow-up. Benefit was seen in all major subgroups, with the mortality difference widening over time. The accompanying editorial refers to specific situations in which internal thoracic artery grafting is contraindicated: radiation damage, extensive brachiocephalic atherosclerosis, and subclavian steal.

250. **Fitzgibbon GM,** et al. Coronary bypass graft fate and patient outcome: angiographic follow-up of 5065 grafts related to survival and reoperation in 1388 patients during 25 years. *J Am Coll Cardiol* 1996;28:616–626.

This retrospective analysis focused on 1,388 patients (mostly male veterans) who underwent surgery between 1969 and 1994; 91% of grafts were venous. Saphenous vein graft patency was 88% at early angiography, 81% at 1 year, 75% at 5 years, and 50% at 15 years. At 15 years, 44% had more than 50% stenoses. Arterial patency rates were significantly better: early, 95%; late (5 years), 80%. Reoperative mortality (6.6% vs. 1.4% for isolated first CABG) and morbidity were mostly owing to vein graft atheroembolism.

251. **Goldman S,** et al. Predictors of graft patency 3 years after coronary artery bypass graft surgery. *J Am Coll Cardiol* 1997;29:1563–1568.

This retrospective analysis focused on 266 male VA patients with 656 grafts patent at 7 to 10 days. Multivariate analysis predictors of 3-year patency (related to operative technique vs. antiplatelet therapy) included total cholesterol ≤225 mg/dL ($p = 0.024$), no more than two proximal anastomoses ($p = 0.032$), vein preservation solution temperature ≤5°C ($p = 0.004$), and recipient artery diameter more than 1.5 mm ($p = 0.034$).

252. **Lopes RD,** et al. Endoscopic versus open vein-graft harvesting in coronary-artery bypass surgery. *N Engl J Med* 2009;361:235–244.

This was a retrospective pooled analysis of 3,000 patients in the PREVENT IV trial, a trial of vein graft treatment with E2F transcription factor decoy, edifoligide, in patients undergoing CABG. In the present study, the investigators assessed the primary outcome of vein-graft failure (stenosis of at least 75%) at 12 to 18 months postoperatively. Though the method of vein harvesting was at the surgeon's discretion (nonrandomized), baseline characteristics between the two groups were similar. However, vein-graft failure was higher in patients who underwent endoscopic vein harvesting, compared with those who underwent open harvesting (46.7% vs. 38.0%, $p < 0.001$). Clinical outcomes were also worse in the endoscopic group, with higher rates of death (7.4% vs. 5.8%, $p = 0.005$), death, or MI (9.3% vs. 7.6%, $p = 0.01$), and the composite of death, MI, or repeat revascularization (20.2% vs. 17.4%, $p = 0.04$). This study called into question the method of vein harvesting, and further, randomized data are needed.

253. **Jones RH,** et al. for the STITCH Hypothesis 2 Investigators. Coronary bypass surgery with or without surgical ventricular reconstruction. *N Engl J Med* 2009;360:1705–1717.

The investigators sought to test the hypothesis that surgical reduction of LV volume in patients with dilated, ischemic cardiomyopathy undergoing CABG would improve outcomes. They randomly assigned 1,000 patients with EF of ≤35% and CAD amenable to CABG and ventricular reconstruction to either routine CABG or CABG with LV reconstruction. At a median follow-up of 48 months, there was no difference in the primary outcome of death or cardiac hospitalization (59% for CABG alone vs. 58% for CABG plus reconstruction, $p = 0.90$). However, surgical reconstruction did significantly reduce end-systolic volume index by 19% (compared with 6%) for patients in that group; there was no difference in patients' symptoms.

254. **Shroyer AL,** et al. for the Veterans Affairs Randomized On/Off Bypass (ROOBY) Study Group. On-pump versus off-pump coronary-artery bypass surgery. *N Engl J Med* 2009;361:1827–1837.

Design: Prospective, randomized, multicenter study. Primary end point was a composite of death, stroke, MI, or repeat revascularization at 12 months, for noninferiority.
Purpose: To assess the effect on complication rate of CABG without cardiopulmonary bypass (off-pump), compared with the use of cardiopulmonary bypass (on-pump). Primary outcome was a composite of death, repeat revascularization, or MI at 1 year after surgery.
Population: 2,203 patients undergoing CABG (urgently or electively).
Treatment: CABG surgery either on-pump or off-pump
Results: One year after surgery, rates of the composite primary outcome favored the on-pump group (7.4% vs. 9.9%, $p = 0.04$), while rates at 30 days showed a similar, nonsignificant trend (5.6% for on-pump vs. 7.0% for off-pump, $p = 0.19$). One source of the difference in clinical outcomes may be that fewer planned grafts were able to be placed in the off-pump group (17.8% incomplete revascularization rate vs. 11.1%, $p < 0.001$). Graft patency on follow-up angiography was also lower in the off-pump group (82.6% vs. 87.8%, $p < 0.01$). On neuropsychological testing, there were no differences in short-term outcomes.

CHAPTER 3

Unstable Angina/Non–ST Elevation MI

Christopher P. Cannon and Benjamin A. Steinberg

EPIDEMIOLOGY

Each year in the United States, approximately 1,320,000 persons are admitted to hospitals for unstable angina and non–ST elevation myocardial infarction (UA/NSTEMI), and 2 to 2.5 million worldwide.

PATHOPHYSIOLOGY

UA/NSTEMIs are typically the result of nonocclusive coronary artery thrombus due to ruptured plaque(s). Other causes include vasoconstriction (e.g., Prinzmetal's angina, microcirculatory angina), progressive mechanical obstruction, and secondary causes (e.g., tachycardia, fever, thyrotoxicosis, anemia, and hypotension) (see **Fig. 3.1**).

Acute coronary syndrome (ACS) patients also have significant inflammation and plaque instability in nonculprit lesions and vessels, suggesting a widespread process. In an intravascular ultrasound of ACS patients, plaque ruptures were evident in other lesions and vessels in more than 70% of cases (4). One study examined neutrophil myeloperoxidase (MPO) levels in several types of patients and found that the UA subset had evidence of widespread inflammation [i.e., right and left coronary circulations with low MPO levels (indicative of enzyme depletion due to neutrophil activation)].

CLASSIFICATION

Unstable Angina

Canadian Cardiovascular Society (CCS) of angina and Braunwald classification of UA (see *Circulation* 2000;102:118–122) are the most commonly used classifications systems. In the CCS scale, class I is angina only with strenuous activity, class II is slight limitation with vigorous activity, class III patients have marked limitation

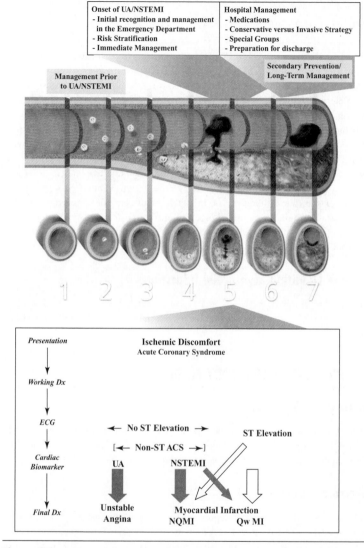

Figure 3.1 • Pathophysiology of acute coronary syndromes. **Top:** Schematic depiction of the progression of atherosclerotic CHD from natural endothelium with circulating lipids (frames 1-2), to deposition of lipids with formation of plaques (frames 3-4), leading to either unstable plaque rupture (frame 5) and/or stable, obstructive CHD (frame 6). **Bottom:** Clinical presentation of ACS, with correlation between ECG findings of "No ST Elevation" indicating only partial coronary occlusion, and "ST Elevation" indicating complete coronary occlusion yielding a Q-wave infarct. (Reprinted from Anderson JL, et al. ACC/AHA 2007 guidelines for the management of patients with unstable angina/non–ST-elevation myocardial infarction: a report of the American College of Cardiology/American Heart Association Task Force on Practice Guidelines (Writing Committee to Revise the 2002 Guidelines for the Management of Patients With Unstable Angina/Non–ST-Elevation Myocardial Infarction): developed in collaboration with the American College of Emergency Physicians, American College of Physicians, Society for Academic Emergency Medicine, Society for Cardiovascular Angiography and Interventions, and Society of Thoracic Surgeons. *J Am Coll Cardiol* 2007;50:e1–e157, with permission from Elsevier.).

with normal activity, and class IV patients are unable to perform activities of daily living and have episodes of rest angina. The Braunwald system is multitiered; severity of angina consists of three classes: class I, new-onset (<2 months), severe, or accelerated, with no rest pain in the preceding 2 months; class II, subacute (angina at rest more than 48 hours to 1 month previously); and class III, acute (at least one episode in the preceding 48 hours). Patients also are assigned a clinical class as follows: class A, secondary UA (e.g., triggered by anemia, infection, thyrotoxicosis); class B, primary UA; class C, postinfarction UA (<2 weeks after documented MI). Class IIIB patients are further subdivided into troponin-negative and troponin-positive patients. The third tier of the system is intensity of therapy: 1, absence of or minimal therapy; 2, occurring in the presence of standard therapy for chronic stable angina (e.g., oral β-blockers, nitrates, calcium antagonists); and 3, occurring despite maximal therapy [oral therapy and intravenous (i.v.) nitroglycerin (NTG)].

Non–ST Elevation Myocardial Infarction

One-third to one-half of patients in UA trials actually had an NSTEMI, defined as an elevation of cardiac markers of necrosis such as creatine kinase (CK)-MB or troponin.

CLINICAL AND LABORATORY FINDINGS

History and Symptoms

Chest discomfort typically occurs at rest or with increasing frequency and lasts 5 to 20 minutes but can last several hours. Temporary/incomplete relief is provided by sublingual NTG. Most chest pain episodes respond to sublingual NTG.

Electrocardiogram

In UA/NSTEMI, ST-segment depression is seen in approximately 20% to 30% of cases, and transient ST-segment elevation in 2% to 5%; these changes are predictive of adverse outcomes. T-wave inversions occur in approximately 20%; if present in five or more leads, they are associated with higher risk. Of NSTEMI patients, Q waves develop in 15% to 25%.

Cardiac Enzymes
CREATINE KINASE AND CREATINE KINASE-MB

These markers of myocardial necrosis are elevated in patients with NSTEMI. Both levels will typically increase approximately 6 hours after onset of ischemic symptoms and normalize within 48 to 72 hours.

TROPONINS T AND I

An elevated troponin is a qualifying criterion for MI. Because these markers are more sensitive than CK and CK-MB, the new MI definition will lead to higher MI rates, as one in three patients previously diagnosed with UA have had a small NSTEMI (some have called these "microinfarctions"). In a meta-analysis of 21 published studies, the two types of troponins were found to be equally sensitive and specific. In one study of patients with rest pain, troponin T was detected in 39%, whereas CK-MB was elevated in fewer than 10%. Troponin levels begin to increase within 4 to 6 hours after symptom onset, remain elevated for several days, and thus are a reliable marker for diagnosing MI within the preceding 2 to 7 days. For the same reason, however, CK-MB levels are usually necessary to diagnose reinfarction within the first several days of an index infarction.

MYOGLOBIN

Usefulness is limited by lack of cardiac specificity and period of brief elevation (<24 hours). However, in conjunction with other data, a negative myoglobin can be helpful in ruling out MI.

ESTIMATION OF EARLY RISK AT PRESENTATION

The Thrombolysis in Myocardial Infarction (TIMI) risk score (TRS) consists of seven predictor variables (each worth one point): age older than 65 years, three or more coronary artery disease (CAD) risk factors, prior coronary stenosis of more than 50%, ST-segment deviation on initial electrocardiography (ECG), two or more anginal events in prior 24 hours, use of aspirin in prior 7 days, and elevated serum cardiac markers. With TIMI 11B and Efficacy and Safety of Subcutaneous Enoxaparin in Non–Q-Wave Coronary Events (ESSENCE) data, the event rate (death, new or recurrent MI, ischemia requiring urgent revascularization) at 14 days increased from 4.7%, with a TRS of 0 or 1, to 40.9% for a score of 6 or 7 (**Fig. 3.2**) (73). This score has been validated in eight studies including the TIMI 3 Registry (see *Am J Cardiol* 2002;90:303), Platelet Receptor Inhibition in Ischemic Syndrome Management in Patients Limited by Unstable Signs and Symptoms (PRISM-PLUS) (see *Eur Heart J* 2002;23:223), and Clopidogrel in Unstable Angina to Prevent Recurrent Events (CURE) (see *Circulation* 2002;106:1622), where a higher risk also predicted greater benefit from glycoprotein (GP) IIb/IIIa inhibition. In a prespecified analysis in Treat Angina with Aggrastat and Determine Cost of Therapy with an Invasive or Conservative Strategy (TACTICS)-TIMI 18, those with higher TRSs were those found to have a significantly greater benefit from an early invasive strategy, whereas those with TRS of 0 to 2 had similar outcomes with an invasive or conservative strategy. In summary, this score with broad applicability is easily calculated and identifies patients with different responses to treatments for UA/NSTEMI (57).

Boersma et al. (see *Circulation* 2000;101:2557) also developed a risk-estimation score based on analysis of Platelet Glycoprotein IIb/IIIa in Unstable Angina

Figure 3.2 • This risk score is derived from data on TIMI 11B and ESSENCE patients, and shows a clear gradation of increasing risk with a higher risk score. (Adapted from Antman EM, et al. The TIMI risk score for unstable angina/non–ST elevation MI. A method for prognostication and therapeutic decision making. *JAMA* 2000;284:835–842.)

Receptor Suppression Using Integrilin Therapy (PURSUIT) trial data. The most important baseline features associated with death were age, higher heart rate (HR), lower systolic blood pressure (SBP), ST-segment depression, signs of heart failure, and elevated cardiac markers.

Lastly, a risk score to predict mortality was derived from the Global Registry of Acute Coronary Events (GRACE) registry of 15,007 patients in the derivation cohort (77). The model predicted 6-month mortality for patients with STEMI, NSTEMI, and UA based on nine clinical criteria: older age, history of MI, history of heart failure, tachycardia at presentation, hypotension at presentation, elevated initial creatinine, elevated initial biomarkers, ST-segment depression at presentation, and not having percutaneous coronary intervention (PCI) in-hospital. This score also could predict the risk of death or MI.

Treatment

ASPIRIN

Aspirin (160 to 325 mg initially, and then 81 to 325 mg daily) has been shown to reduce the risk of fatal or nonfatal MI by 50% to 70% during the acute phase in patients with UA or NSTEMI and by 50% to 60% at 3 months to 3 years (6,7). For chronic treatment, low-dose aspirin (e.g., 75 to 81 mg) has lower bleeding risk and similar efficacy compared with higher doses (11).

THIENOPYRIDINES/ADP RECEPTOR ANTAGONISTS

Three thienopyridines are commercially available, ticlopidine, clopidogrel, and prasugrel; clopidogrel and prasugrel are the preferred agents because of a lower incidence of hematologic side effects, especially neutropenia ($<0.1\%$ risk for clopidogrel vs. 1% risk with ticlopidine). A fourth agent, ticagrelor is a non-thienopyridine that binds reversibly to the ADP receptor.

In one early study of UA patients, ticlopidine (250 mg twice daily) reduced cardiovascular mortality and reinfarction rates by nearly 50% (10). Clopidogrel was evaluated in the recent CURE trial, which randomized 12,662 patients with unstable or NSTEMI to aspirin alone or clopidogrel, 300-mg loading dose and 75 mg once daily, and aspirin (11). At follow-up (mean, 9 months), the clopidogrel group had a significant 20% reduction in cardiovascular death, MI, or stroke compared with the aspirin-only group. An initial loading dose of clopidogrel (300 mg) was given, and the event curves separated within 2 hours. The clopidogrel group had a higher incidence of major bleeding at 1 year (3.7% vs. 2.7%).

Based on these results, the American College of Cardiology (ACC)/American Heart Association (AHA) guidelines have been modified and now advocate that clopidogrel should be given in addition to aspirin for ideally a year, for patients with UA/NSTEMI whether managed with revascularization or medically.

Prasugrel was evaluated in the 13,608-patient TRITON-TIMI 38 trial, in which patients with ACS, including STEMI patients, as well as those with UA/NSTEMI (74% of the total) were planned for PCI, and most often had undergone angiography without pretreatment with clopidogrel (12). The overall results found that prasugrel significantly reduced the risk of CV death MI or stroke by 19%, from 12.1% for clopidogrel to 9.9% for prasugrel ($p < 0.001$). In UA/NSTEMI patients undergoing PCI, prasugrel significantly lowered rates of the primary endpoint (a composite of CV death, MI, or stroke) at 15 months, when compared to clopidogrel (9.9% vs. 12.1%, hazard ratio 0.82, $p = 0.002$). Subsequently, prasugrel was approved for use in ACSs, but *only* at the time of PCI.

Ticagrelor was studied in the PLATO trial of patients with ACS (both UA/NSTEMI and STEMI). The PLATO (PLATelet Inhibition and Patient Outcomes) trial compared ticagrelor to clopidogrel in the prevention of cardiovascular events in 18,624 patients admitted to the hospital with ACS, with or without ST-segment elevation. The primary endpoint was the composite of death from vascular causes, myocardial infarction, or stroke at 1 year. The endpoint had occurred in 9.8% of patients receiving ticagrelor as compared with 11.7% of those receiving clopidogrel (hazard ratio 0.84; 95% CI, 0.77–0.92; $p < 0.001$). No significant differences in the overall rate of major bleeding rates were found between the two groups ($p = 0.43$), although ticagrelor was associated with a higher rate of major bleeding not associated with CABG than clopidogrel. Total mortality was reduced with ticagrelor, 4.5%, versus 5.9% with clopidogrel; $p < 0.001$.

HEPARIN

In a meta-analysis of six trials, unfractionated heparin [UFH; 60- to 70-U/kg bolus, and then 12 to 15 U/kg/hr; goal activated partial thromboplastin time (aPTT), 1.5 to 2.0 times control] showed a strong trend toward reducing rates of reinfarction and recurrent ischemia when used with aspirin [odds ratio (OR), 0.67; 95% confidence interval (CI) 0.44 to 1.02] (17). Increased rates of adverse events have been identified with heparin therapy for greater than 48 hours after admission for UA. After discontinuation of heparin infusion, a rebound phenomenon occurs, with patients at increased risk of reactivation of UA and MI (16).

LOW-MOLECULAR-WEIGHT HEPARINS

The ESSENCE and TIMI IIB trials showed enoxaparin (1 mg/kg subcutaneously twice daily) to be superior to UFH, resulting in 15% to 20% fewer major events (death, MI, and urgent revascularization) at 6 weeks (21,23). In the smaller EVET trial, enoxaparin was directly compared with another low-molecular-weight heparin (LMWH), tinzaparin; the enoxaparin group had a significantly lower incidence of recurrent UA or need for revascularization (see *J Am Coll Cardiol* 2001;37:365).

In the Fragmin during Instability in CAD (FRISC) trial (19), dalteparin (120 IU/kg subcutaneously twice daily for 6 days, and then 7,500 IU/day for 35 to 45 days) showed a significant reduction in death and MI at 6 days compared with placebo, whereas the Fragmin in Unstable Coronary Artery Disease (FRIC) trial showed equivalence between dalteparin and i.v. UFH (20). In FRISC II (22), extended use of dalteparin (120 IU/kg twice daily for 3 months) was associated with a significant reduction in death or MI at 30 days, but the reduction did not remain significant at 3 months. In the Fraxiparine in Ischemic Syndrome (FRAXIS) trial (24), fraxiparine showed no benefit compared with UFH; this study enrolled many low-risk patients.

It is not clear why enoxaparin is the only agent with a clear benefit, but it does have a higher ratio of antifactor Xa to antithrombin activity (3.8:1.0) than dalteparin or fraxiparine. The current ACC/AHA guidelines have a class Ia recommendation for either LMWH or UFH as treatment for UA/NSTEMI, and a class Ib recommendation for either fondaparinux or bivalirudin (for invasive strategy only) (**Figs 3.2 and 3.3**).

LMWH can be used in conjunction with GP IIb/IIIa inhibitors. In the Integrilin and Enoxaparin Randomized Assessment of Acute Coronary Syndrome Treatment (INTERACT) trial, 746 UA/NSTEMI patients receiving eptifibatide were randomized to heparin or enoxaparin, and the enoxaparin group had a significantly lower incidence of death and MI at 30 days (25). A to Z compared enoxaparin with UFH in a patient population that all received IIb/IIIa inhibitors and mainly involved a noninvasive approach. A total of 3,987 high-risk ACS patients, all of whom received aspirin and tirofiban, were randomized to enoxaparin or UFH; 60% of patients underwent angiography. The enoxaparin group had a 12% reduction in death, MI, or refractory ischemia compared to UHF (8.4% vs. 9.4%), which fulfilled the trial's noninferiority goal but did not demonstrate superiority ($p = 0.23$). Finally, the 10,000-patient SYNERGY trial compared the two agents in patients who are all going to the catheterization lab; enoxaparin was not superior, but was noninferior to heparin for death or MI at 30 days (see Chapter 2 for more details).

LMWHs stimulate platelets less than UFHs and have a lower incidence, compared with UFH, of heparin-induced thrombocytopenia (HIT). However, these agents also are associated with a higher incidence of minor bleeding compared with UFH.

An alternative to both UFH and LMWHs is the pentasaccharide factor Xa inhibitor fondaparinux, which was evaluated most extensively in the Organization to Assess Strategies for Ischemic Syndromes (OASIS) 5 trial (27). The investigators randomized 20,078 patients with UA/NSTEMI to either enoxaparin or fondaparinux for the primary endpoint of death, MI, or recurrent ischemia at 9 days. There were no statistically significant differences in the primary endpoint (5.8% for fondaparinux vs. 5.7% for enoxaparin). However, the incidence of catheter-related thrombus in patients undergoing PCI on fondaparinux let to hesitation about using this agent as sole anticoagulant during PCI, and most interventionalists will switch to UFH. Although included in the guidelines as an alternative, this agent is not yet approved for ACS management as of mid-2010.

A

(*Continued*)

Figure 3.3 • A, B: Management strategies for UA/NSTEMI. Guideline-recommended strategies of management for UA/NSTEMI by initial approach, invasive **(A)** or conservative **(B)**. (Data from Anderson JL, et al. ACC/AHA 2007 guidelines for the management of patients with unstable angina/non–ST-elevation myocardial infarction: a report of the American College of Cardiology/American Heart Association Task Force on Practice Guidelines (Writing Committee to Revise the 2002 Guidelines for the Management of Patients With Unstable Angina/Non–ST-Elevation Myocardial Infarction): developed in collaboration with the American College of Emergency Physicians, American College of Physicians, Society for Academic Emergency Medicine, Society for Cardiovascular Angiography and Interventions, and Society of Thoracic Surgeons. *J Am Coll Cardiol* 2007;50:e1–e157.)

DIRECT THROMBIN INHIBITORS

In the GUSTO IIb trial, hirudin use in patients with ACS (chest pain with ECG changes) resulted in a nonsignificant 11% reduction in death and MI at 30 days compared with heparin (35). In the OASIS-2 trial, medium-dose hirudin (0.4 mg/kg bolus and then 0.15 mg/kg/hr) resulted in a nonsignificant 16% reduction in cardiovascular death and MI at 7 days. A meta-analysis of the GUSTO IIb, TIMI 9B, OASIS 1, and OASIS 2 trials found that hirudin was associated with a significant 10% lower risk of death or MI at 35 days compared with heparin ($p = 0.015$) (38). Hirudin is currently indicated only for anticoagulation in patients with HIT, but these data show that additional trials of the direct antithrombins are warranted.

In addition to the data from the REPLACE-2 trial (see Chapter 2), bivalirudin was tested in the ACUITY trial, in which investigators randomized 13,819 patients with UA/NSTEMI undergoing invasive management to either a heparin (UFH or LMWH) plus GP IIb/IIIa, bivalirudin plus GP IIb/IIIa, or bivalirudin alone. The primary endpoints included a composite of ischemic events, bleeding, and net clinical benefit (ischemia and bleeding combined). For the comparison of either heparin or bivalirudin (both with GP IIb/IIIa agents), the bivalirudin group had similar rates of ischemic and bleeding. When used without a GP IIb/IIa inhibitor, bivalirudin was associated with significantly less bleeding when compared to a heparin with GP IIb/IIIa inhibition. This trial specifically enrolled patients undergoing aggressive, early invasive management. Thus, the use of bivalirudin as part of early management in patients with UA/NSTEMI is a class I (level of evidence B) recommendation only for those undergoing an invasive strategy.

GLYCOPROTEIN IIB/IIIA INHIBITORS

Intravenous Agents

The current ACC/AHA guidelines recommend (class IA) the use of either an i.v. GP IIb/IIIa antagonist or clopidogrel in UA/NSTEMI patients in whom catheterization and PCI are planned. Eptifibatide or tirofiban is preferred for "upstream" use (class IB); if it is only a short time to angiography, then abciximab can be used. Both clopidogrel and a GP IIb/IIIa may be used in some circumstances (class IIa). In patients being managed with a conservative strategy, a GP IIb/IIIa inhibitor could be considered (class IIb), but it would be also reasonable to add only if a patient developed recurrent ischemia (see **Fig. 3.3A and B**):

1. Tirofiban: In the PRISM-PLUS trial (39), tirofiban (0.4 μg/kg/min for 30 minutes, and then 0.10 μg/kg/min for 48 to 72 hours), heparin, and aspirin resulted in decreased death, MI, and refractory ischemia at 7 days compared with heparin alone (32), and death and MI were decreased by approximately 30% at 30 days.
2. Eptifibatide: In the large PURSUIT trial, eptifibatide (180 μg/kg bolus, and then 2.0 μg/kg/min) showed an approximately 10% reduction in death and MI at 30 days (41).

3. Abciximab (0.25 μg/kg bolus, and then 0.10 μg/min for 12 hours): The Evaluation of 7E3 for the Prevention of Ischemic Complications (EPIC), Evaluation in PTCA to Improve Long-term Outcome with Abciximab Glycoprotein IIb/IIIa Blockade (EPILOG), and c7E3 Fab Antiplatelet Therapy in Unstable Refractory Angina (CAPTURE) trials were interventional studies that enrolled some UA patients, and all showed substantial reductions (30% to 60%) at 30 days in the rates of death, MI, and ischemia-provoked intervention or revascularization (see Chapter 2). The 6-month results of the Evaluation of Platelet IIb/IIIa Inhibitor for Stenting (EPISTENT) trial, another interventional study comparing stenting alone versus stenting plus abciximab versus balloon angioplasty plus abciximab, showed a 10% absolute reduction in death and MI in the subgroup of patients with UA. However, the large Global Utilization of Streptokinase and Tissue Plasminogen Activator for Occluded Coronary Arteries (GUSTO) IV-ACS trial, which enrolled all ACS patients (7,800), abciximab was associated with no reduction in death or MI at 30 days compared with placebo, and the mortality rate was actually higher in the first 48 hours in the abciximab groups (45). Based on these results, abciximab is not recommended in ACS patients in whom PCI will be delayed. In the ISAR-REACT 2 trial abciximab retained its benefit after the addition of clopidogrel in patients with ACS undergoing PCI, though the advantage was confined to those patients with elevated troponin (46).

The question of timing of administration of GP IIb/IIIa inhibitors was addressed in the 9,492-patient EARLY ACS trial (49). The investigators randomized patients undergoing invasive management of UA/NSTEMI to either early eptifibatide (12 hours or more prior to PCI) or provisional eptifibatide after angiography (but before intervention). For the primary outcome composite of death, MI, recurrent ischemia requiring revascularization, or thrombotic complication during PCI (requiring "bailout" therapy), there was no statistical difference between the early or delayed groups (9.3% for early vs. 10.0% in delayed group, $p = 0.23$). Bleeding rates were higher in patients receiving early eptifibatide. As such, early initiation of GP IIb/IIIa inhibition could not be recommended on the basis of this trial.

Oral Agents

In contrast to the i.v. agents, several oral agents have shown an *increased* risk of death or bleeding events (see *Circulation* 2002;106:375; *Am J Med* 2002;112:647). The OPUS-TIMI 16 trial was terminated early because of an increased 30-day mortality in one of the orbofiban arms (42). In the SYMPHONY trial (43), sibrafiban was comparable to aspirin for major events but was associated with increased bleeding; these results prompted the early termination of the larger SYMPHONY II trial (44).

THROMBOLYTIC THERAPY

Thrombolytic therapy was not found to be beneficial in the TIMI 3 and the Unstable Angina Study Using Eminase (UNASEM) trials (50,51). Use was associated with increased bleeding and MI rates, and no benefit of adjunctive intracoronary thrombolytic therapy was observed during PTCA in the Thrombolysis and Angioplasty in Unstable Angina (TAUSA) trial (52).

ANTI-ISCHEMIC MEDICATIONS

β-Blockers

Limited randomized trial data are available on the use of β-blockers in specifically UA/NSTEMI. However, given the significant benefit demonstrated in STEMI, recent MI, heart failure, and stable angina with daily life ischemia, it is appropriate to extrapolate to UA/NSTEMI (see Chapter 4 for more details). They have been associated with lower mortality in patients undergoing PCI for ACS (see *J Interv Cardiol* 2003;16:299–305). Specific medication choices include metoprolol (5 mg i.v. every 5 minutes for three doses, and then 25 to 50 mg orally every 6 hours), propranolol (0.5 to 1.0 mg i.v., and then 40 to 80 mg orally every 6 to 8 hours), and atenolol (5 mg i.v., and then 50 to 100 mg orally daily). β-Blockers are contraindicated if marked first-degree atrioventricular (AV) block [PR interval, more than 0.25 second; any second- or third-degree block in the absence of a pacemaker; asthma; severe left ventricular dysfunction with congestive heart failure (CHF); HR <50; and SBP <90 mm Hg]. In 2007, the ACC/AHA guidelines added a class III recommendation that "It may be harmful to administer intravenous beta blockers to UA/NSTEMI patients who have contraindications to beta blockade (as noted above), signs of heart failure or low-output state, or other risk factors for cardiogenic shock, which include age greater than 70 years, systolic blood pressure less than 120 mm Hg, sinus tachycardia greater than 110 or heart rate less than 60, presentation more than 6 hour after symptom onset."

Nitrates

Nitrates are useful for treating episodes of recurrent ischemia (reducing both left ventricular end-diastolic pressure and SBP). If no relief is gained from three sublingual NTG tablets, i.v. NTG (5 to 200 μg/min) should be started. If nitrates do not provide adequate relief or if acute pulmonary congestion is found, consider morphine administration. Nitrates are contraindicated if a patient has hypotension (particularly in cases of right-ventricular infarction) or has taken sildenafil (Viagra) or related medications within 24 hours. Furthermore, there is a paucity of data demonstrating any improvement in clinical outcomes with nitrates, and, as such, current recommendations are for the use of nitrates to relieve ischemia, but should *not* preclude use with proven therapies (such as β-blockers or ACE inhibitors).

Calcium-channel Blockers

Calcium-channel blockers are as effective in relieving symptoms, but an overview of randomized trials showed no reduction in mortality or MI rates. Diltiazem confers a possible benefit in non–Q wave MI patients (majority with NSTEMI). In the Diltiazem Reinfarction Study, diltiazem use (90 mg, four times daily) was associated with a significant reduction in in-hospital mortality (29). However, no overall benefit was observed by the Multicenter Diltiazem Postinfarction Trial Research Group (60 mg, four times daily), although a post hoc analysis showed benefit in patients without evidence of left ventricular dysfunction. Similar to the effect of nitrates, calcium-channel blockers' benefit is largely confined to the reduction of ischemic discomfort and has not demonstrated a significant effect on clinical outcomes in UA/NSTEMI. Furthermore, clinicians should be aware of the potential for reflex tachycardia (and adverse events) in patients receiving dihydropyridine calcium-channel blockers (particularly immediate-release nifedipine) in the absence of β-blockade.

3-Hydroxy-3-methylglutaryl Coenzyme A Reductase Inhibitors (Statins)

In the Myocardial Ischemia Reduction with Aggressive Cholesterol Lowering (MIRACL) study, 3,086 conservatively managed UA/NSTEMI patients were randomized to high-dose atorvastatin (80 mg once daily) or placebo (64). In the atorvastatin group, mean low-density lipoprotein (LDL) cholesterol decreased from 124 to 72 mg/dL, and a significantly lower incidence of death, nonfatal MI, cardiac arrest with resuscitation, or ischemia requiring rehospitalization was found. Data from the CHAMP study found that if a statin was started in hospital, 91% were taking a statin at 1 year versus only 10% if not given in-hospital, and 58% had an LDL less than 100 mg/dL versus only 6% prior to institution of the quality improvement program (see *Am J Cardiol* 2001;87:819). Increasing data favors the more aggressive use of higher-dose statins earlier in patients with ACS, particularly those undergoing invasive management (see *J Am Coll Cardiol* 2009;54:2290–2295). For more data on statins, see Chapter 1.

INVASIVE STRATEGY

Coronary Angiography

With coronary angiography, multivessel disease is found in 40% to 50%, single-vessel disease in 30% to 35%, left main disease in 5% to 10%, and no critical obstruction in 10% to 20%.

The routine use of angiography has now been studied in nine randomized trials, with the five most recent studies all showing a significant benefit associated with an invasive strategy. The first trial, TIMI 3B, showed that early angiography followed by revascularization (if indicated) did not reduce major cardiac events but did result in fewer hospital readmissions (53), whereas the Veteran Affairs Non–Q-wave Infarction Strategies in Hospital (VANQWISH) study, which enrolled medium- to high-risk patients, showed no benefit of an invasive strategy and a trend toward higher mortality (54). The invasive group in the VANQWISH study had a high CABG operative mortality rate (12%). Both the TIMI 3B and VANQWISH trials were performed before GP IIb/IIIa inhibitors and coronary stenting was commonly used.

The FRagmin and Fast Revascularization during InStability in CAD study reported a significantly lower incidence of death or MI with an invasive strategy compared with a noninvasive strategy (at 6 months, 9.4% vs. 12.1%; $p = 0.031$) (56). A subgroup analysis showed that this benefit was restricted to men.

The TACTICS-TIMI 18 study enrolled 2,220 patients with at least one high-risk feature [ECG changes, elevated cardiac markers, or a history of CAD (prior catheterization, revascularization, or MI)] (57). Patients randomized to an early invasive strategy (routine catheterization within 4 to 48 hours and revascularization as appropriate) had a 22% lower incidence of death, nonfatal MI, and rehospitalization for an ACS at 6 months compared with a more conservative strategy (catheterization only if recurrent ischemia or abnormal stress test). Patients with an elevated troponin T had an even larger 39% reduction in the primary endpoint.

In the Randomised Intervention Trial of unstable Angina (RITA) 3 trial (58), 1,810 UA/NSTEMI patients were randomized to an early intervention or a conservative strategy. The intervention group had a 34% lower incidence of death, MI, or refractory angina at 4 months. Two other smaller randomized studies also found significant benefits with an early invasive strategy (TRUCS; see *Eur Heart J* 2000;21:1954; VINO, see *Eur Heart J* 2002;23:230).

The ICTUS trial tested the hypothesis of a "selectively invasive" strategy, randomizing 1,200 patients with NSTEMI at high risk (all patients had elevated troponin T and either ECG changes or a history of CAD) to either an early invasive strategy or a more conservative "selectively invasive" strategy whereby patients were taken to PCI only if they had refractory angina, hemodynamic or ECG instability, or significant ischemia on predischarge stress test (60). All patients received a contemporary in-hospital regimen, including aspirin, enoxaparin, and abciximab (at time of PCI); clopidogrel and aggressive lipid-lowering were recommended. While the trial did not demonstrate any reduction in the primary endpoint of death, MI, or rehospitalization for angina within 1 year, it should be noted that nearly half of the patients in the "selectively invasive" arm underwent revascularization.

In summary, after extensive investigation of management strategy in the current era, the latest ACC/AHA guidelines consider an early invasive strategy a class I indication if any of the following high-risk features are present: (a) recurrent angina/ischemia at rest or low-level activity despite intensive therapy; (b) elevated troponin T or troponin I; (c) new or presumably new ST-segment depression; (d) CHF signs or symptoms, new or worsening mitral regurgitation; (e) high-risk findings on noninvasive stress testing; (f) ejection fraction, less than 40%; (g) hemodynamic instability; (h) sustained ventricular tachycardia (VT); (i) PCI within previous 6 months or any prior CABG surgery; or (j) high risk score (e.g., the TRS or GRACE risk scores) (see **Figs. 3.2 and 3.3A**). With regard to timing of an early invasive strategy, the TIMACS trial compared early (median = 14 hours after randomization) with later (median = 50 hours) angiography. Overall, there was just a trend for reduction of the primary endpoint (death, MI, and stroke) in the group as a whole, but a significant reduction in patients with a high GRACE risk score. (See *N Engl J Med* 2009;360:2165–2175.) Thus, the highest risk, most unstable patients should be sent to cardiac catheterization within 12 to 24 hours, whereas others can go within 2 to 3 days.

Percutaneous Coronary Intervention

The success rate of PCI is 90% to 95%. Ischemic complications are reduced by concomitant administration of i.v. GP IIb/IIIa inhibitor (see earlier).

Coronary Artery Bypass Graft Surgery

The operative mortality rate with CABG surgery is typically 3% to 4% in patients with refractory UA (vs. approximately 2% for patients with chronic stable angina). Improved survival has been demonstrated in patients with left main disease and three-vessel disease with significant left ventricular dysfunction (see Chapter 2). An intra-aortic balloon pump may be needed for stabilization before surgery.

Noninvasive Evaluation

EXERCISE TREADMILL TEST

Treadmill testing should not be performed in the acute phase. In low-risk patients free of rest or low-level ischemia and CHF, the exercise treadmill test (ETT) can be performed after a minimum of 12 to 24 hours. In intermediate-risk patients, the wait should be at least 2 or 3 days. If the patient is high risk (e.g., $\geq$2-mm ST-segment depression), catheterization should be considered in place of ETT.

EXERCISE TREADMILL TESTING WITH NUCLEAR IMAGING

The ACC/AHA guidelines have a class I recommendation for the following patient subsets: baseline ST-segment abnormalities, bundle branch block, left ventricular hypertrophy, intraventricular conduction delay, paced rhythm, pre-excitation, and digoxin effect. Imaging also adds sensitivity to low-level/nondiagnostic ETT tests. The size of perfusion defect(s) is predictive of mortality and major cardiac events.

PHARMACOLOGIC STRESS TESTING WITH IMAGING

Pharmacologic stress testing with imaging is indicated in patients with severe physical limitations.

ECHOCARDIOGRAPHY

In patients with chest pain but no ECG changes or an obscured ECG picture [left bundle branch block (LBBB), paced rhythm], echocardiography can be used to evaluate whether a wall-motion abnormality is present.

CORONARY COMPUTERIZED TOMOGRAPHY ANGIOGRAPHY

In patients presenting with chest pain to the Emergency Department, but who are felt to have a low likelihood of actually having ACS, use of coronary computed tomography angiogram (CCTA) is now an option for "ruling out" coronary disease. Data from 368 patients in the ROMICAT trial demonstrated that in such low-risk patients (negative troponin and ECG), 64-slice coronary CTA (computed tomography angiogram) could effectively "rule out" patients for ACS during index hospitalization (68). That is, a finding of a normal CTA conferred extraordinary low risk for coronary disease. However, in patients with coronary plague or stenosis, further investigation is warranted.

Prognosis

UNSTABLE ANGINA

The hospital mortality rate is 1% to 2%; 1-year mortality rate, 7% to 10%; and 1-month reinfarction rate, approximately 5%. Twenty percent to 25% of patients are rehospitalized within 1 year. Recurrent ischemia is associated with a nearly threefold higher mortality.

NON–ST ELEVATION MYOCARDIAL INFARCTION

The in-hospital mortality rate is 3% to 4%; reinfarction rate, 8% to 10%; and 1-year mortality rate, 10% to 15%. (The latter is similar to that of ST-elevation patients.)

PRIOR ASPIRIN USE (ASPIRIN FAILURES)

Prior aspirin use is associated with an increased risk of death or MI at 30 days.

ELECTROCARDIOGRAPHY

A TIMI 3 Registry analysis showed an increased risk of death and MI at 1 year with LBBB on admission ECG [relative risk (RR), 2.8] and 0.5 mm of ST deviation (RR, 2.5). T-wave inversion alone was not associated with increased risk (99).

TROPONIN LEVELS

Troponin levels have been shown to provide substantial prognostic information. TIMI 3B and FRISC analyses showed a strong correlation between troponin T levels and adverse outcomes (83,84). In the FRISC trial, the benefit of LMWH over aspirin was limited to patients with elevated troponin T levels (83). In five trials (CAPTURE, PRISM, PRISM-PLUS, Paragon B, ISAR-REACT 2), the benefit of GP IIb/IIIa inhibition was magnified in patients with elevated troponin-T levels, with no benefit in troponin-negative patients (see also *J Thromb Thrombolysis* 2001;11:211; *Circulation* 2001;103:2891) (85,86). In the TACTICS-TIMI 18 trial, an elevated troponin level was associated with a 40% reduction in major cardiac events in the early invasive group versus conservative strategy group, whereas patients with normal levels (troponin I <0.1 ng/mL or troponin T <0.01 ng/mL) had no significant benefit from an early invasive strategy (87). The poor prognosis of elevated troponin even persisted in patients without significant angiographic CAD.

C-REACTIVE PROTEIN

Elevated levels of C-reactive protein (CRP) are found in patients who die. Multiple analyses have shown an additive, yet separate, effect of CRP and troponin in predicting mortality (90–93).

B-TYPE NATRIURETIC PEPTIDE

Brain (B-type) natriuretic peptide (BNP) is a neurohormone synthesized predominantly in ventricular myocardium.

A biomarker substudy of 2,525 ACS patients in the OPUS-TIMI 16 trial measured BNP in plasma samples at a mean of 40 ± 20 hours after the onset of symptoms (95). Baseline BNP level more than 80 pg/mL was significantly correlated with an increased risk of death, heart failure, and new or recurrent MI at 30 days and 10 months. Analysis of 1,676 TACTICS-TIMI 18 patients found similar findings; in addition, BNP was shown to add significant incremental prognostic information to troponin I measurement (96). Subsequent data from the A to Z trial demonstrated that serial, outpatient measurement of BNP following ACS predicted incidence of new heart failure or death (97).

REFERENCES

Review Articles and Pathophysiology

1. **Braunwald E.** Unstable angina: an etiologic approach to management. *Circulation* 1998;98:2219–2222.

   This editorial describes five different, though not mutually exclusive, causes of UA: (a) nonocclusive thrombus on preexisting plaques (most common); (b) dynamic obstruction (e.g., Prinzmetal's variant angina, microcirculatory angina); (c) progressive mechanical obstruction; (d) inflammation and/or infection; and (e) secondary causes (e.g., fever, thyrotoxicosis, hypotension).

2. **Libby P.** Current concepts of the pathogenesis of the acute coronary syndromes. *Circulation* 2001;104:365–372.

   This article provides a review of the underlying mechanisms of inflammation and acute thrombosis leading to ACSs. The article also addresses the myriad mechanisms by which agents such as statins and PPAR agonists mitigate such processes.

3. **Anderson JL,** et al. ACC/AHA 2007 guidelines for the management of patients with unstable angina/non-ST-elevation myocardial infarction: a report of the American College of Cardiology/American Heart Association Task Force on Practice Guidelines (Writing Committee to Revise the 2002 Guidelines for the Management of Patients With Unstable Angina/Non-ST-Elevation Myocardial Infarction): developed in collaboration with the American College of Emergency Physicians, American College of Physicians, Society for Academic Emergency Medicine, Society for Cardiovascular Angiography and Interventions, and Society of Thoracic Surgeons. *J Am Coll Cardiol* 2007;50:e1–e157.

   These guidelines provide a comprehensive approach to all aspects of risk assessment, and pharmacologic and interventional management for UA/NSTEMI.

4. **Rioufol G,** et al. Multiple atherosclerotic plaque rupture in acute coronary syndrome: a three-vessel intravascular ultrasound study. *Circulation* 2002;106:804–808.

   A total of 24 patients who underwent PCI after a first ACS with troponin-I elevation underwent intravascular ultrasound of the three major coronary arteries. Fifty plaque ruptures (mean, 2.08 per patient) were diagnosed by the association of a ruptured capsule with intraplaque cavity. Plaque rupture on the culprit lesion was seen in nine (37.5%) patients. At least one plaque rupture was found somewhere other than on the culprit lesion in 19 (79%) patients, and these lesions were in a different artery than the culprit artery in 70.8%. Thus, although one single lesion is clinically active at the time of ACS, the syndrome appears associated with overall coronary instability.

5. **Thygesen K,** et al. Joint ESC/ACCF/AHA/WHF Task Force for the Redefinition of Myocardial Infarction. Universal definition of myocardial infarction. *Eur Heart J* 2007;28:2525–2538.

With newer biochemical techniques and novel markers, the task force addresses the increasing specificity with which infarction can be detected. They update the definition to include the pathophysiologic basis, clinical scenario, as well as biochemical analysis for a complete assessment of myocardial necrosis.

Drugs and Studies

ASPIRIN

6. **Lewis HD Jr,** et al. **VA Cooperative Study.** Protective effects of aspirin against acute MI and death in men with unstable angina. *N Engl J Med* 1983;309:396–403.

Design: Prospective, randomized, double-blind, placebo-controlled, multicenter study. Primary endpoint was death or MI at 12 weeks.

Purpose: To determine whether aspirin can decrease death and acute MI in patients with UA.

Population: 1,266 men with pain at rest, beginning within the previous month, and present within the last week and evidence of CAD, defined as one or more of the following: history of MI, ST depression $\geq$1 mm, angiogram showing 75% stenosis of at least one vessel, exercise test with $\geq$1-mm ST depression, and exertional angina relieved by NTG within 5 minutes.

Exclusion Criteria: Included new Q-waves or ST elevation, elevated enzymes (more than twice normal level), severe heart failure (NYHA class IV), ventricular arrhythmia, oral anticoagulation, bleeding diathesis, allergy or intolerance to aspirin, recent aspirin ingestion (on more than 3 days of the previous 7), MI within the previous 6 weeks, bypass surgery in the previous 12 weeks, and cardiac catheterization in the prior week.

Treatment: Buffered aspirin, 324 mg once daily, or placebo for 12 weeks.

Results: At 12 weeks, the aspirin group had a 51% lower incidence of death and MI (5% vs. 10%; $p < 0.0005$), with both death and nonfatal MI being reduced by 51% (3.4% vs. 6.9%, $p = 0.005$; 1.6% vs. 3.3%, $p = 0.054$). No difference was observed in gastrointestinal symptoms or evidence of blood loss between the two treatment and placebo groups.

7. **Cairns JA,** et al. Aspirin, sulfinpyrazone, or both in unstable angina: results of a Canadian multicenter trial. *N Engl J Med* 1985;313:1369–1375.

Design: Prospective, randomized, double-blind, placebo-controlled, multicenter study. Primary endpoint was cardiac death and nonfatal MI. Mean follow-up period was 18 months.

Purpose: To evaluate the efficacy of aspirin, sulfinpyrazone, or both in the acute management of UA.

Population: 555 patients aged 70 years with evidence of myocardial ischemia (exertional angina, transient ST- or T-wave changes with pain, or relief with sublingual NTG in less than 10 minutes on at least three occasions in hospital) and unstable pain pattern (crescendo pain or pain 15 minutes in duration).

Exclusion Criteria: Included MI in preceding 12 weeks, contraindications to study medications, new Q waves on ECG, severe chest pain lasting $\geq$30 minutes, and elevated [more than twice the upper limit of normal (ULN)] enzymes (at least two of following: serum aspartate aminotransferase, lactic dehydrogenase, CK), with positive CK-MB fraction or MB more than 5%.

Treatment: Aspirin, 325 mg four times daily; sulfinpyrazone, 200 mg four times daily; both; or neither.

Results: Aspirin groups had 51% less cardiac death and MI than did nonaspirin groups (8.6% vs. 17%; $p = 0.008$). The aspirin groups also had 71% lower all-cause mortality rates (3.0% vs. 11.7%; $p = 0.004$). Intention-to-treat analysis showed aspirin groups to have 30% lower rates of cardiac death and nonfatal MI ($p = 0.072$), 56% fewer cardiac deaths ($p = 0.009$), and 43% lower all-cause mortality rate ($p = 0.035$). Sulfinpyrazone showed no benefit for any outcome event.

8. **Peters RJG,** et al. Effects of aspirin dose when used alone or in combination with clopidogrel in patients with acute coronary syndromes: observations from the Clopidogrel in Unstable angina to prevent Recurrent Events (CURE) study. *Circulation* 2003;108:1682–1687.

Patients in the CURE trial of clopidogrel in UA/NSTEMI (see below) were randomized to clopidogrel or placebo, in addition to therapy with varying doses of aspirin (75 to 325 mg daily). While clopidogrel benefited patients in all groups of aspirin dosing, bleeding risk increased significantly with increasing aspirin dose, without observed benefit in reduced ischemic events. The authors conclude that optimal dosing of aspirin is 75 to 100 mg daily, regardless of clopidogrel use.

9. **Lopes RD,** Alexander KP. Antiplatelet therapy in older adults with non-ST-segment elevation acute coronary syndrome: considering risks and benefits. *Am J Cardiol* 2009;104(5 suppl):16C–21C.

The authors review the risks and benefits of multiple antiplatelet agents [aspirin, P2Y(12) blockers, GP IIb/IIIa inhibitors] in elderly patients with NSTEMI. Relevant trials and their specific benefits to elderly patients, as well as the increased risks of bleeding, are reviewed.

THIENOPYRIDINES

10. **Balsano F,** et al. Antiplatelet therapy with ticlopidine in unstable angina: controlled, multicenter clinical trial. *Circulation* 1990;82:17–26 (editorial, 296–298).

In this randomized trial, 652 patients received conventional therapy (without aspirin) or ticlopidine, 250 mg twice daily. At 6 months, the ticlopidine group had 46% fewer primary endpoints, consisting of vascular death or nonfatal MI (7.3% vs. 13.6%; $p = 0.009$). A 53% reduction in risk of fatal or nonfatal MI was found (5.1% vs. 10.9%; $p = 0.006$).

11. The Clopidogrel in Unstable Angina to Prevent Recurrent Events (**CURE**) Trial Investigators. Effects of clopidogrel in addition to aspirin in patients with acute coronary syndromes without ST segment elevation. *N Engl J Med* 2001;345:494–502.

Design: Prospective, randomized, double-blind, placebo-controlled, multicenter trial. Primary endpoint composite was cardiovascular death, MI, or stroke. Mean follow-up was 9 months (range, 3 to 12 months).

Purpose: To evaluate the efficacy and safety of the antiplatelet agent clopidogrel when given with aspirin in ACS without ST-segment elevation.

Population: 12,562 patients with UA or NSTEMI with ECG changes, positive serum cardiac markers, or history of CAD, and seen within 24 hours of symptom onset.

Exclusion Criteria: Age younger than 60 years, contraindication to antithrombotic therapy, ST elevation, high bleeding or CHF risk, oral anticoagulation, coronary revascularization in previous 3 months, and GP IIb/IIIa inhibitor in previous 3 days.

Treatment: Aspirin (75 to 325 mg once daily) and clopidogrel (300-mg loading dose, and then 75 mg once daily) or aspirin and placebo.

Results: The clopidogrel group had a 20% relative reduction in cardiovascular death, nonfatal MI, or stroke at 1 year compared with the placebo group (9.3% vs. 11.4%; $p < 0.001$).

Clopidogrel group also had a significantly lower incidence of the primary composite end-point or refractory ischemia (16.5% vs. 18.8%; RR, 0.86; $p < 0.001$; at 24 hours: 1.4% for clopidogrel vs. 2.1%; 34% RR reduction; $p = 0.002$). The incidence of in-hospital refractory or severe ischemia, heart failure, and revascularization procedures was also significantly lower with clopidogrel. The clopidogrel group experienced more major bleeding at 1 year than the placebo group (3.7% vs. 2.7%; RR, 1.38; $p = 0.001$), but no significant excess of life-threatening bleeding occurred (2.1% vs. 1.8%; $p = 0.13$) or hemorrhagic strokes. Bleeding was lower in patients treated with aspirin, 75 to 100 mg once daily, compared with aspirin, 200 to 325 mg once daily (2.0% vs. 4.0%, respectively, in aspirin-only group; 2.6% vs. 4.9% in clopidogrel and aspirin group), indicating that bleeding appeared lower with clopidogrel and low-dose aspirin versus 325 mg of aspirin alone.

Comments: Benefits associated with clopidogrel occurred within 2 hours. The benefits were consistent in low-, intermediate-, and high-risk patients, as stratified by TRS (see *Circulation* 2002;106:1622).

12. **Wiviott SD,** et al. for the TRITON-TIMI 38 Investigators. Prasugrel versus clopidogrel in patients with acute coronary syndromes. *N Engl J Med* 2007;357:2001–2015.

Design: Prospective, randomized, double-blind, active-controlled, multicenter, international study. The primary endpoint was a composite of cardiovascular death, reinfarction, or stroke at 15 months. The safety endpoint was bleeding.
Purpose: To compare a new thienopyridine, prasugrel, with clopidogrel in patients undergoing PCI for ACSs.
Population: 13,608 patients with moderate-to-high-risk ACSs and scheduled to undergo PCI; 10,074 patients had moderate-to-high-risk UA or NSTEMI and 3,534 had STEMI.
Treatment: Clopidogrel (300-mg loading dose, followed by 75 mg daily) versus prasugrel (60-mg loading dose, followed by 10 mg daily).
Results: Prasugrel reduced the primary composite endpoint by an absolute 2.2% (9.9% vs. 12.1%, $p < 0.001$). However, major bleeding occurred in 2.4% of patients on prasugrel, versus 1.8% in the clopidogrel group ($p = 0.03$), and there was a similar increase in life-threatening bleeding (1.4% vs. 0.9%, $p = 0.01$).
Comment: Based heavily on this study, the FDA approved prasugrel for use in patients with high-risk ACSs *at the time of PCI.* However, they attached a black-box warning, advising physicians to consider a dose-reduction (to 5 mg daily) in patients at a high risk of bleeding.

13. **Wallentin L,** et al. for the **PLATO** Investigators. Ticagrelor versus clopidogrel in patients with acute coronary syndromes. *N Engl J Med* 2009;361:1045–1057.

Design: Prospective, randomized, double-blind, active-controlled, multicenter, international study. The primary endpoint was a composite of cardiovascular death (CV), myocardial infarction (MI), or stroke through 12 months. The safety endpoint was total major bleeding.
Purpose: To compare the new reversible and direct-acting, oral P2Y12 receptor antagonist, ticagrelor with clopidogrel in patients with ACS.
Population: 18,624 patients hospitalized for ACS (with or without ST elevation) in the PLATelet inhibition and patient Outcomes (PLATO) trial, treated with aspirin.
Treatment: Ticagrelor (180-mg loading dose, 90 mg twice daily thereafter) and clopidogrel (300- to 600-mg loading dose, 75 mg daily thereafter).
Results: Ticagrelor reduced the rate of CV death, MI, or stroke by 16%, from 11.7% for clopidogrel to 9.8% for ticagrelor, $p < 0.001$. Total mortality was also reduced from 5.9% for clopidogrel to 4.5% for ticagrelor, $p < 0.001$. No significant difference in the rates of major bleeding was found between the ticagrelor and clopidogrel groups (11.6% and 11.2%, respectively; $p = 0.43$) but had a higher rate of non-CABG-related bleeding (3.8% for clopidogrel vs. 4.5% for ticagrelor).

UNFRACTIONATED HEPARIN AND WARFARIN

14. **Theroux P,** et al. **Montreal Heart Study.** Aspirin, heparin, or both to treat acute unstable angina. *N Engl J Med* 1988;319:1105–1111.

Design: Prospective, randomized, double-blind, placebo-controlled, dual-center study. Major endpoints were death, MI, and refractory angina.

Purpose: To evaluate the usefulness of aspirin, i.v. heparin, and their combination in the early management of UA.

Population: 479 patients aged ≤75 years with accelerating pattern of chest pain occurring at rest or with minimal exercise, or pain lasting 20 minutes with the last episode in the previous 24 hours. Their ECG changes had to be consistent with ischemia; if absent, diagnosis had to be confirmed by two cardiologists. CK levels had to be less than twice the ULN.

Exclusion Criteria: Included regular use of aspirin, contraindications to heparin or aspirin, coronary angioplasty within the previous 6 months, and bypass surgery within the previous 12 months (or scheduled).

Treatment: Aspirin, 325 mg twice daily, or i.v. heparin, 1,000 U/hr (given for average 6 days).

Results: Incidence of MI was significantly reduced in groups receiving aspirin [3% vs. 12% (placebo); $p = 0.01$], heparin ($0.8\%; p < 0.001$), and aspirin plus heparin ($1.6\%; p = 0.003$). No deaths occurred in these three treatment groups. Heparin was associated with a trend toward refractory angina compared with aspirin (RR, 0.47; 95% CI, 0.21 to 1.05; $p = 0.06$). Combination therapy was associated with more serious bleeding [3.3% vs. 1.7% (heparin alone)].

Comments: An additional 245 patients were randomized to either aspirin or heparin to allow an adequately powered comparison. A total of 484 patients was randomized to these two treatments, and the heparin group demonstrated a 78% lower MI rate at 5.7 ± 3.3 days (0.8% vs. 3.7%; $p = 0.035$). Only one death occurred (aspirin patient).

15. **Wallentin LW,** et al. Research on Instability in CAD (**RISC**). Risk of MI and death during treatment with low dose aspirin and intravenous heparin in men with unstable coronary artery disease. *Lancet* 1990;336:827–830.

Design: Prospective, randomized, double-blind, placebo-controlled, 2 × 2 factorial, multicenter study. Primary endpoint was death and MI.

Purpose: To evaluate the efficacy of aspirin and/or heparin in acute treatment of unstable and non–Q wave MI and to assess the long-term effects of aspirin compared with placebo in these patients.

Population: 796 men younger than 70 years with non–Q wave MI or increasing angina within the previous 4 weeks, with the last episode of pain within 72 hours and ischemia on resting ECG or predischarge exercise test.

Exclusion Criteria: Included Q-wave MI, myocardial dysfunction due to prior MI, previous CABG surgery, LBBB or pacemaker, concurrent anticoagulant or aspirin therapy, and increased bleeding risk.

Treatment: Aspirin, 75 mg daily for 1 year, or placebo, and i.v. heparin boluses (10,000 U every 6 hours for four doses, and then 7,500 U every 6 hours for 4 days), or placebo alone.

Results: Trial was stopped early due to publication of ISIS-2 results (minimum follow-up reduced to 3 months vs. 12 months). Aspirin patients had a markedly reduced risk of MI and death at 5 days (OR, 0.43; $p = 0.033$), 1 month (OR, 0.31; $p < 0.0001$), and 3 months (OR, 0.36; $p < 0.0001$). No benefits were seen with heparin alone. The aspirin and heparin group had fewer events in the first 5 days [1.4% vs. 3.7% (aspirin alone), $p =$ NS; 5.5% (heparin alone), $p = 0.045$; 6.0% (both placebos), $p = 0.027$]. Gastrointestinal symptoms with aspirin became more frequent after 3 months.

16. **Theroux P,** et al. Reactivation of unstable angina after the discontinuation of heparin. *N Engl J Med* 1992;327:141–145.

This study demonstrated a clear rebound effect with discontinuation of heparin in patients not taking aspirin. Four hundred and three patients were randomized to i.v. heparin, aspirin, both, or neither, and completed 6 days of treatment without refractory angina or MI. After discontinuation of therapy, heparin-only patients had more frequent reactivation of UA or MI in the subsequent 96 hours: 14 of 107 patients versus only 5 patients in each of the other three groups ($p < 0.01$). Eleven of 14 of these reactivations required urgent interventions (thrombolysis, angioplasty, or bypass surgery) versus only 2 in the other groups combined ($p < 0.01$).

17. **Oler A,** et al. Adding heparin to aspirin reduces the incidence of MI and death in patients with unstable angina: a meta-analysis. *JAMA* 1996;276:811–815.

This meta-analysis was derived from six randomized trials enrolling 1,353 patients. Aspirin and heparin tended to be preferable to aspirin alone (RR of death and MI, 0.67; 95% CI, 0.44 to 1.02). Combination therapy also was associated with nonsignificant reduction in recurrent ischemia (RR, 0.82; 95% CI, 0.40 to 1.17). No difference in revascularization rates was observed (RR, 1.03; 95% CI, 0.74 to 1.43), whereas aspirin and heparin were associated with a nonsignificant increase in major bleeding (RR, 1.99; 95% CI, 0.52 to 7.65).

18. Organization to Assess Strategies for Ischemic Syndromes (**OASIS**) Investigators. Comparison of the effects of two doses of recombinant hirudin compared with heparin in patients with acute myocardial ischemia without ST elevation. *Circulation* 1997;96:769–777.

Design: Prospective, randomized, open, multicenter study. Primary endpoint was cardiovascular death, MI, or refractory angina at 7 days.
Purpose: To compare the effects of a 3-day treatment with hirudin versus heparin on clinical outcomes in UA and NSTEMI patients.
Population: 909 patients with UA or suspected NSTEMI within 12 hours of the most recent episode of chest pain and with either ECG evidence of ischemia or previous objective documentation of CAD.
Treatment: UFH (5,000 IU bolus + 1,000 to 1,200 U/hr), low-dose hirudin (0.2 mg/kg bolus and then 0.10 mg/kg/hr infusion), or medium-dose hirudin (0.4 mg/kg bolus and then 0.15 mg/kg/hr infusion) for 72 hours.
Results: At 7 days, cardiovascular death, new MI, or refractory angina (primary outcome) occurred in 6.5% in heparin group, 4.4% in low-dose hirudin group, and 3.0% in medium-dose hirudin group ($p = 0.27$, heparin vs. low-dose hirudin; $p = 0.047$, heparin vs. medium-dose hirudin). The incidence of new MI was lower in the hirudin groups: 2.6% and 1.9% versus 4.6% ($p = 0.14$. heparin vs. low-dose hirudin; $p = 0.046$, heparin vs. medium-dose hirudin). An increase in ischemic events was seen in the low-dose hirudin group at around 24 hours after treatment cessation and at approximately 5 days in the medium-dose group, but the differences between hirudin and heparin persisted at 180 days.

LOW-MOLECULAR-WEIGHT HEPARINS

19. **Wallentin L,** et al. Fragmin during Instability in CAD (**FRISC**). Low molecular weight heparin during instability in coronary artery disease. *Lancet* 1996;347:561–568.

Design: Prospective, randomized, double-blind, placebo-controlled, multicenter study. Primary endpoint was death or MI at 6 days.
Purpose: To evaluate whether subcutaneous dalteparin provides an additive benefit to that provided by aspirin and antianginal drugs in patients with UA or non–Q wave MI.
Population: 1,506 patients (men aged 40 years, women more than 1 year after menopause) with chest pain in the previous 72 hours. All had newly developed or increasing angina or angina at rest during the previous 2 months or persisting chest pain with a suspicion of MI and ST depression ≥ 1 mm or T-wave inversion ≥ 1 mm in two adjacent leads without Q waves in ischemic leads.
Exclusion Criteria: Included increased bleeding risks.

Treatment: Dalteparin, 120 IU/kg subcutaneously twice daily for 6 days, and then 7,500 IU daily for 35 to 45 days; or placebo.

Results: At 6 days, the dalteparin group had a 63% lower rate of death and new MI (1.8% vs. 4.8%; $p = 0.001$); a nonsignificant reduction was observed at 40 days (8% vs. 10.7%; $p = 0.07$).

Comments: Subsequent analysis showed the additive value of troponin T to predischarge ETT in providing risk stratification.

20. **Klein W,** et al. Fragmin in Unstable Coronary Artery Disease **(FRIC).** Comparison of low molecular weight heparin with unfractionated heparin acutely and with placebo for 6 weeks in the management of unstable coronary artery disease. *Circulation* 1997;96:61–68.

Design: Prospective, randomized, partially open-label, parallel, multicenter study. Primary endpoint was death, MI, or recurrent angina.

Purpose: To compare the efficacy and safety of weight-adjusted subcutaneous dalteparin with UFH in the acute treatment of UA or non–Q wave MI and the value of prolonged dalteparin compared with placebo in those initially given anticoagulants.

Population: 1,482 patients with chest pain in the preceding 72 hours and admission ECG with temporary or persistent ST depression ≥ 1 mV in at least two adjacent leads and/or temporary or persistent T-wave inversion ≥ 1 mm in two adjacent leads.

Exclusion Criteria: Included new Q waves, LBBB, indication for thrombolytic therapy, oral anticoagulation, diastolic blood pressure (DBP) greater than 120 mm Hg or SBP less than 90 mm Hg, bleeding diathesis or recent surgery, and history of cerebrovascular event.

Treatment: Phase 1 (open label, days 1 to 6)—dalteparin, 120 IU/kg subcutaneously twice daily, or i.v. UFH. Phase 2 (double-blind, days 6 to 45)—dalteparin, 7,500 IU subcutaneously once daily, or placebo.

Results: In the first 6 days, no significant differences were observed between groups in death, MI, or recurrent angina [7.6% (heparin) vs. 9.3% (dalteparin); 95% CI, 0.84 to 1.66]; death and MI (3.6% vs. 3.9%), or revascularization (5.3% vs. 4.8%). For days 6 to 45, similar incidences of composite endpoints (both 12.3%) and revascularization [14.2% (placebo) vs. 14.3%] were observed. The dalteparin group had a higher phase 1 mortality rate (11 vs. 3 deaths; RR, 3.37; 95% CI, 1.01 to 11.24).

Comments: Lack of benefit with dalteparin may be due to the low ratio of anti-factor Xa to antithrombin activity (only 2.0).

21. **Cohen M,** et al. Efficacy and Safety of Subcutaneous Enoxaparin in Non-Q wave Coronary Events **(ESSENCE).** A comparison of low molecular weight heparin with unfractionated heparin for unstable coronary artery disease. *N Engl J Med* 1997;337: 447–452 (editorial, 492–494).

Design: Prospective, randomized, double-blind, placebo-controlled, parallel-group, multicenter study. Primary endpoint was death, MI, or recurrent angina at 14 days.

Purpose: To compare the efficacy and safety of enoxaparin with UFH in patients with UA or non–Q wave MI.

Population: 3,171 patients with rest pain 10 minutes in the preceding 24 hours accompanied by one of the following: (a) new ST depression ≥ 1 mm, transient ST elevation, or T-wave changes in at least two contiguous leads; (b) documented prior MI or revascularization procedure; or (c) noninvasive or invasive tests suggesting ischemic heart disease. Only about one-third had ST-segment changes on admission.

Exclusion Criteria: Included LBBB or pacemaker, persistent ST elevation, angina with an established precipitating cause (e.g., heart failure), contraindications to anticoagulation, and creatinine clearance less than 30 mL/min.

Treatment: Enoxaparin, 1 mg/kg subcutaneously twice daily, or UFH for 2 to 8 days (mean duration, 2.8 days).

Results: Enoxaparin group had a 16% lower rate of death, MI, and recurrent angina at 14 days (16.6% vs. 19.8%; $p = 0.019$); at 30 days, the benefit persisted (19.8% vs. 23.3%; $p = 0.016$).

Enoxaparin also was associated with a lower 30-day revascularization rate (27% vs. 32.2%; $p = 0.001$). Similar rates of major bleeding were observed at 30 days (6.5% vs. 7.0%), but overall bleeding was higher in the enoxaparin group (18.4% vs. 14.2%; $p = 0.001$) because of injection-site ecchymoses.

22. FRagmin and Fast Revascularization during InStability in Coronary artery disease **(FRISC II)** Investigators. Long-term, low-molecular-mass heparin in unstable coronary artery disease: FRISC II prospective randomized multicenter study. *Lancet* 1999;354:701–707.

Design: Prospective, randomized, partially blinded parallel-group, multicenter study. Primary endpoint was death or MI at 3 months.

Purpose: To assess the effects of long-term treatment with dalteparin compared with a placebo in patients undergoing a noninvasive treatment strategy.

Population: 2,267 patients (median age, 67 years) with ischemic symptoms in the previous 48 hours accompanied by ECG changes (ST depression or T-wave inversion ≥ 0.1 mV) or elevated markers (e.g., CK-MB, more than 6 mg/L; troponin T, more than 0.10 mg/L).

Exclusion Criteria: Included angioplasty in previous 6 months, indication for or treatment with thrombolysis in past 24 hours, scheduled revascularization procedure.

Treatment: After 5 or more days of open-label dalteparin, patients randomized to subcutaneous dalteparin, 120 IU/kg twice daily, or placebo for 3 months.

Results: At 30 days, the dalteparin group had a significant reduction in death or MI (3.1% vs. 5.9%; $p = 0.002$), but at 3 months, the reduction was nonsignificant (6.7% vs. 8.0%; $p = 0.17$). A significant reduction was found in the 3-month incidence of death, MI, or revascularization (29.1% vs. 33.4%; $p = 0.031$), but this benefit did not persist at 6 months (38.4% vs. 39.9%; $p = 0.50$). Mortality was significantly reduced at 1 year (*Lancet* 2000;356:9).

23. **Antman E,** for the **TIMI 11B** Investigators. Enoxaparin prevents death and cardiac ischemic events in unstable angina/non–Q-wave MI: results of the TIMI 11B trial. *Circulation* 1999;100:1593–1601.

Design: Prospective, randomized, double-blind, placebo-controlled, multicenter study. Primary endpoint was death, MI, or urgent revascularization at 8 and 43 days.

Purpose: To evaluate the benefits of an extended course of enoxaparin compared with standard UFH for preventing death and cardiac events in patients with UA or non–Q wave MI.

Population: 3,910 patients with ischemic discomfort at rest within the past 24 hours and ST-segment deviation or positive CK-MB or troponin.

Exclusion Criteria: Included planned revascularization within 24 hours, treatable cause of angina, evolving Q-wave MI, CABG surgery within 2 months, or PTCA within 6 months, UFH infusion for more than 24 hours before enrollment, history of heparin-induced thrombocytopenia (HIT), contraindications to anticoagulation.

Treatment: Enoxaparin [1 mg/kg subcutaneously twice daily (acute phase), and then 60 mg (≥ 65 kg) or 40 mg (<65 kg) twice daily] during both acute (2 to 8 days) and chronic phases (through day 43) or i.v. UFH (acute phase only).

Results: Enoxaparin-treated patients had a significant 12% reduction in the primary composite endpoint of death, MI, or urgent revascularization at day 43 (17.3% vs. 19.7%; $p = 0.048$). This benefit was apparent by day 8 (12.4% vs. 14.5%; $p = 0.048$). During the first 72 hours and entire initial hospitalization, no difference was noted in the major bleeding rates between the treatment groups. However, long-term enoxaparin treatment was associated with an increase in the rate of major hemorrhage (spontaneous and instrumented; 2.9% vs. 1.5%; $p = 0.021$). At 1-year follow-up, a persistent significant benefit was associated with enoxaparin therapy (incidence of primary composite endpoint, 32.0% vs. 35.7%; $p = 0.022$; see *J Am Coll Cardiol* 2000;36:693).

Comments: When these results are pooled with the ESSENCE data, a significant reduction in death and MI is found at day 8 (4.1% vs. 5.3%), day 14 (5.2% vs. 6.5%), and day 43 (7.1% vs. 8.6%).

24. The FRAX.I.S. Study Group. Comparison of two treatment durations (6 days and 14 days) of a low molecular weight heparin with a 6-day treatment of UFH in the initial management of unstable angina or non-Q wave myocardial infarction: **FRAXIS** (FRAxiparine in Ischaemic Syndrome). *Eur Heart J* 1999;20:1553–1562.

This prospective, randomized, controlled study enrolled 3,468 patients with UA and non–Q wave MI (angina within 48 hours and ST depression, T-wave inversion, or ST elevation not justifying thrombolysis). Patients received nadroparin for a short course (6 days) or long course (14 days) or UFH (6 ± 2 days). At 14 days, the incidence of the primary composite endpoint, consisting of cardiovascular death, recurrent angina, and recurrence of UA, was similar in the three treatment groups (heparin, 18.1%; short-course fraxiparine, 17.8%; long-course fraxiparine, 20%). A higher incidence of hemorrhage was seen in the long-course fraxiparine group [at 14 days, 3.5% vs. 1.6% (UFH) and 1.5% (short-course nadroparin)].

25. Goodman SG, et al. for the Integrilin and Enoxaparin Randomized Assessment of Acute Coronary Syndrome Treatment (**INTERACT**) Trial Investigators. Randomized evaluation of the safety and efficacy of enoxaparin versus unfractionated heparin in high-risk patients with non-ST-segment elevation acute coronary syndromes receiving the glycoprotein IIb/IIIa inhibitor eptifibatide. *Circulation* 2003;107:238–244.

This prospective, randomized, open-label, multicenter trial enrolled 746 patients with ischemic chest discomfort without ST-segment elevation. Patients received UFH or enoxaparin. All aspirin (160-mg loading dose and then 80 to 325 mg/day) and the GP IIb/IIIa inhibitor eptifibatide (180-μg/kg i.v. bolus, and then 2.0 μg/kg/min for 48 hours), cardiac catheterization, and/or coronary revascularization decisions were left to the discretion of the investigator. The incidence of the primary endpoint, non-CABG TIMI major bleeding at 96 hours, occurred less frequently in the enoxaparin group than in the UFH group (1.8% vs. 4.6%; $p = 0.03$). The enoxaparin group also had a significantly lower incidence of death and nonfatal MI at 30 days (5.0% vs. 9.0%; $p = 0.031$). Limitations of this study include the open-label design and the long time to coronary revascularization (median, 101 hours vs. 21 hours in TACTICS-TIMI 18). The ongoing SYNERGY trial is examining the same issue among 8,000 patients treated with GP IIb/IIIa inhibitors.

26. **Blazing MA**, et al. For the A to Z Investigators. Safety and efficacy of enoxaparin vs unfractionated heparin in patients with non-ST-segment elevation acute coronary syndromes who receive tirofiban and aspirin: a randomized controlled trial. *JAMA* 2004;292:55–64.

This prospective, randomized, open, multicenter trial enrolled 3,987 high-risk ACS patients (ST-segment changes or positive cardiac marker). All patients received aspirin and tirofiban: 60% of patients underwent angiography; crossover from enoxaparin to UFH in the catheterization lab was allowed. Patients were randomized to enoxaparin (1 mg/kg every 12 hours) or weight-adjusted UFH. The enoxaparin had a nonsignificant 12% reduction in death, MI, or refractory ischemia compared to UFH (8.4% vs. 9.4%, $p = 0.23$); however, the trial was designed to demonstrate noninferiority and this goal was met.

27. The Fifth Organization to Assess Strategies in Acute Ischemic Syndromes Investigators. Comparison of fondaparinux and enoxaparin in acute coronary syndromes (**OASIS 5**). *N Engl J Med* 2006;354:1464–1476.

Design: Prospective, randomized, double-blind, double-dummy, multicenter, international trial. The primary endpoint was a composite of death, reinfarction, or refractory ischemia at 9 days. Patients were also followed for major bleeding and clinical outcomes out to 6 months.

Purpose: To compare efficacy and safety of fondaparinux versus enoxaparin, with regard to ischemic and bleeding outcomes, in patients with ACSs.

Population: 20,078 patients within 24 hours of symptoms of cardiac ischemia and at least two of the following—age ≤60 years, elevated troponin or CK-MG, or ECG changes indicative of ischemia.

Exclusion Criteria: Patients with contraindications to heparins, recent hemorrhagic stroke, severe renal insufficiency, or additional indications for anticoagulation.

Treatment: Fondaparinux 2.5 mg once daily (until discharge or for 8 days, whichever came first), or enoxaparin 1 mg/kg twice daily (for 2 to 8 days, or until the patient was clinically stable; enoxaparin was dose-reduced for patients with mild–moderate renal insufficiency).

Results: Similar rates of the primary endpoint were observed in each treatment group (5.8% for fondaparinux vs. 5.7% for enoxaparin; hazard ratio for fondaparinux 1.01, 95% CI, 0.90 to 1.13). This satisfied the noninferiority margin. However, rates of major bleeding at 9 days were significantly lower in the fondaparinux group (2.2% vs. 4.1%, $p < 0.001$). When bleeding was included, the composite clinical benefit endpoint of MACE and/or bleeding favored fondaparinux (7.3% vs. 9.0%, $p < 0.001$). Furthermore, mortality rates at 30 and 180 days were significantly lower in the fondaparinux group ($p = 0.02$ and 0.05, respectively).

28. **Peterson JL,** et al. Efficacy and bleeding complications among patients randomized to enoxaparin or unfractionated heparin for antithrombin therapy in non–ST-segment elevation acute coronary syndromes: a systematic overview. *JAMA* 2004;292:89–96.

The investigators combined the primary data from the ESSENCE, A to Z, SYNERGY, TIMI 11B, ACUTE II, and INTERACT trials, culminating in an analysis of 21,946 patients with NSTEMI randomized to UFH or enoxaparin, followed for clinical endpoints at 30 days. Mortality was equal between the two groups (3.0% for each); however, there was a significant reduction in the composite endpoint of death or MI at 30 days (10.1% vs. 11%; OR, 0.91; 95% CI, 0.83 to 0.99), favoring the enoxaparin group. Within 7 days, rates of major bleeding or blood transfusions were similar.

β-BLOCKERS, CALCIUM ANTAGONISTS, AND NITRATES

29. **Gibson RS,** et al. Diltiazem reinfarction study group. Diltiazem and reinfarction in patients with non–Q-wave MI. *N Engl J Med* 1986;315:423–429.

Design: Prospective, randomized, double-blind, multicenter study. Primary endpoint was reinfarction at 14 days.

Purpose: To determine whether diltiazem would reduce the incidence of early reinfarction in patients recovering from a non–Q wave MI.

Population: 576 patients with non–Q wave MI [elevated CK-MB and either ischemic pain for 30 minutes or ST-segment deviation (elevation or depression ≥1 mm or T-wave inversions in at least two leads)].

Exclusion Criteria: Included new Q waves, HR less than 50 beats/min, advanced heart block, cardiogenic shock or sustained SBP less than 100 mm Hg, coronary bypass surgery in the past 3 months, therapy with a calcium-channel blocker.

Treatment: Randomized at 24 to 72 hours to diltiazem, 90 mg every 6 hours, or placebo.

Results: Diltiazem patients had a significantly lower 14-day reinfarction rate (5.2% vs. 9.3%; $p = 0.03$) and 50% less refractory angina (3.5% vs. 6.9%; $p = 0.03$). No significant difference was observed in mortality rates (3.1% vs. 3.8%). Adverse reactions were common in the diltiazem group [overall, 24% vs. 6% (AV block, 6% vs. 2%; SBP <90 mm Hg, 8% vs. 2%)], but only 4.9% of the diltiazem patients stopped therapy because of the adverse effects.

30. Interuniversity Nifedipine/Metoprolol Trial (**HINT**) Research Group. Early treatment of unstable angina in the coronary care unit: a randomised, double blind, placebo controlled comparison of recurrent ischaemia in patients treated with nifedipine or metoprolol or both. *Br Heart J* 1986;56:400–413.

This prospective, randomized, double-blind, placebo-controlled, multicenter trial enrolled 515 patients with UA, of whom 338 were not pretreated with a β-blocker. In patients not pretreated with a β-blocker, no significant differences were found between the three groups (nifedipine, metoprolol, or both) in the incidence of recurrent ischemia or MI at 48 hours.

However, a trend was seen toward a higher incidence of MI in the nifedipine group (RR, 1.51; 95% CI, 0.87 to 2.74). In patients already taking a β-blocker, the addition of nifedipine was beneficial (RR, 0.68; 95% CI, 0.47 to 0.97). These results suggest that in patients not taking previous β-blockade, metoprolol has a beneficial short-term effect on UA, and that nifedipine alone may be detrimental.

31. **Gheorghiade M,** et al. Effects of propranolol in non–Q-wave acute MI in the β-blocker heart attack trial. *Am J Cardiol* 1990;66:129–133.

    This retrospective analysis focused on the 601 β-Blocker Heart Attack Trial patients (17%) with a non–Q wave MI. Patients in this trial were randomized to propranolol, 180 to 240 mg/day, or placebo. At follow-up (median, 24.6 months), similar mortality, sudden death, and reinfarction rates were observed.

32. **Doucet S,** et al. Randomized trial comparing intravenous nitroglycerin and heparin for treatment of unstable angina secondary to restenosis after coronary artery angioplasty. *Circulation* 2000;101:955.

    This prospective, randomized, double-blind, single-center study enrolled 200 patients hospitalized for UA within 6 months after angioplasty alone (no stenting). Patients received i.v. NTG, heparin, their combination, or placebo for 63 $\pm$ 30 hours. Recurrent angina occurred less frequently in the NTG groups [42.6% (NTG alone), 41.7% (NTG + heparin) vs. 75% (placebo and heparin-alone groups); $p < 0.003$]. Refractory angina requiring angiography occurred less often with NTG (4.3%, 4.2%, 22.9%, and 29.2%, respectively; $p < 0.002$). No deaths or MIs were found. These results suggest that smooth muscle cell proliferation and increased vasoreactivity are more important roles than thrombus formation in restenosis-related UA.

33. **Emery M,** et al. for the GRACE Investigators. Patterns of use and potential impact of early beta-blocker therapy in non-ST-elevation myocardial infarction with and without heart failure: the Global Registry of Acute Coronary Events. *Am Heart J* 2006; 152: 1015–1021. PMID: 17161045.

    In an effort to identify the benefit of β-blockers in NSTEMI, the investigators assessed data from 7,108 patients with NSTEMI in the GRACE registry. In 76% of patients without contraindications, β-blocker therapy was initiated within 24 hours of presentation (more frequently in Killip I vs. III, $p < 0.001$). In multivariable analysis, such early therapy correlated with lower in-hospital mortality for patients with NSTEMI; this benefit appeared more robust for those with Killip II/III versus those with Killip I. The lower mortality persisted for 6 months for the entire NSTEMI cohort.

34. **Ambrosio G,** et al. for the GRACE Investigators. Chronic nitrate therapy is associated with different presentation and evolution of acute coronary syndromes: insights from 52 693 patients in the Global Registry of Acute Coronary Events. *Eur Heart J* 2009;31:430–438.

    The investigators sought to assess whether prior nitrate therapy afforded protection against subsequent ischemic events in 52,693 patients with ACS (41% with STEMI, 59% with UA/NSTEMI) in the GRACE registry. In all, 2,138 (80%) were not on prior nitrates (naïve) and 10,555 (20%) had been on chronic nitrates prior to admission; after adjustment for clinical factors, chronic nitrate use significantly predicted presentation with UA/NSTEMI, as opposed to STEMI (OR, 1.36; $p < 0.0001$). Levels of cardiac biomarkers were also significantly lower in the chronic nitrate group ($p < 0.0001$ for all). The findings suggest, though observational, that chronic nitrate use may mitigate the severity of acute coronary events.

DIRECT THROMBIN INHIBITORS

35. **Topol EJ,** et al. Global Utilization of Strategies to Open Occluded Arteries **(GUSTO IIb):** a comparison of recombinant hirudin with heparin for the treatment of acute coronary syndromes. *N Engl J Med* 1996;335:775–782.

Design: Prospective, randomized, double-blind, multicenter study. Primary endpoint was death or nonfatal MI (or reinfarction) at 30 days.

Purpose: To compare the clinical effectiveness of hirudin with that of heparin in patients with all types of ACS.

Population: 12,142 patients with chest pain in the prior 12 hours accompanied by persistent ST elevation or depression ≥0.5 mm ($n \geq 4,131$) or T-wave inversion ($n \geq 8,011$).

Exclusion Criteria: Included oral anticoagulation, active bleeding, history of stroke, serum creatinine more than 2.0 mg/dL, contraindication to heparin, and SBP more than 200 mm Hg or DBP more than 110 mm Hg.

Treatment: Patients were randomized to heparin or hirudin [0.1 mg/kg i.v. bolus, and then 0.1 mg/kg/hr (vs. 0.6, and then 0.2 in GUSTO IIa)].

Results: At 30 days, the hirudin group had a nonsignificant 11% reduction in death and MI (8.9% vs. 9.8%; $p = 0.06$). Post hoc analysis showed that the hirudin group had a significant reduction in death and MI at 24 hours (1.3% vs. 2.1%; $p = 0.001$). Hirudin patients had more moderate (but not severe) bleeds (8.8% vs. 7.7%). Patients with ST elevation were younger and had fewer cardiac risk factors but a higher 30-day mortality rate (6.1% vs. 3.8%).

36. Organization to Assess Strategies for Ischemic Syndromes (**OASIS-2**) Investigators. Effects of recombinant hirudin (lepirudin) compared with heparin on death, MI, refractory angina, and revascularization procedures in patients with acute myocardial ischaemia without ST elevation: a randomised trial. *Lancet* 1999;353:429–438 (editorial, 423–424).

Design: Prospective, randomized, multicenter, double-blind, double-dummy study. Primary endpoint was cardiovascular death or new MI at 7 days.

Purpose: To evaluate whether hirudin is superior to heparin in reducing major cardiac events in patients with UA or suspected NSTEMI.

Population: 10,141 patients aged 21 to 85 years with UA (abnormal ECG required if younger than 60 years) or suspected acute MI without ST elevation.

Exclusion Criteria: Included PTCA within the prior 6 months, planned thrombolysis or primary PTCA, and history of stroke in the prior year.

Treatment: Heparin, 5,000-U bolus, and then 15 U/kg/hr for 72 hours, or hirudin, 0.4-mg/kg bolus, and then 0.15 mg/kg/hr for 72 hours.

Results: Hirudin group had a nonsignificant 16% RR reduction in cardiovascular death and MI at 7 days (3.6% vs. 4.2%; $p = 0.077$). The hirudin group also had a significant 18% RR reduction in cardiovascular death, MI, and refractory angina at 7 days (5.6% vs. 6.7%; $p = 0.0125$). Most of the differences between the groups were observed during the first 72 hours: cardiovascular death or MI RR, 0.76 ($p = 0.039$), and cardiovascular death, MI, and refractory angina RR, 0.78 ($p = 0.019$). The hirudin group had an excess of major bleeding (1.2% vs. 0.7%; $p = 0.01$) but no excess of life-threatening bleeds.

37. Stone GW, et al. for the **ACUITY** Investigators. Bivalirudin for patients with acute coronary syndromes. *N Engl J Med* 2006;355:2203–2216.

Design: Prospective, randomized, multicenter, open-label trial. Primary endpoint was cardiovascular death or new MI at 7 days. Multiple primary endpoints at 30 days included a composite of ischemic events (death, MI, or ischemia-driven revascularization), bleeding events, and net clinical benefit (a composite of ischemia and bleeding).

Purpose: To establish noninferiority (and possibly superiority, predefined) of bivalirudin as antithrombotic agent in moderate to high-risk patients with UA/NSTEMI undergoing PCI, as compared with UFH.

Population: 13,819 patients with UA/NSTEMI who had at least one of the following—significant ECG changes, elevated levels of troponin or CK-MB, known history of CAD, or all four remaining variables of the TRS (age >65, recent aspirin use in past 7 days, UA two or more times over 24 hours, and three or more cardiac risk factors).

Exclusion Criteria: STEMI, recent major bleeding.

Treatment: There were three treatment groups—heparin with GP IIb/IIIa inhibitor, bivalirudin with GP IIb/IIIa inhibitor, or bivalirudin alone.

Results: For the comparison of groups that received GP IIb/IIIa inhibitors, there was no significant difference in ischemic events (7.7% for bivalirudin plus GP IIb/IIIa vs. 7.3% for heparin plus GP IIb/IIIa), bleeding (5.3% vs. 5.7%), or net clinical events (11.8% vs. 11.7%), meeting the noninferiority margins for all three. As compared to heparin with GP IIb/IIIa inhibitor, bivalirudin alone also demonstrated noninferior rates of the composite ischemia endpoint (7.8% for bivalirudin vs. 7.3% for heparin with GP IIb/IIIa, $p = 0.32$), and significantly lower rates of bleeding (3.0% vs. 5.7%, $p < 0.001$), with significant net clinical benefit (10.1% vs. 11.7%, $p = 0.02$).

38. The Direct Thrombin Inhibitor Trialists' Collaborative Group. Direct thrombin inhibitors in acute coronary syndromes: principal results of a meta-analysis based on individual patients' data. *Lancet* 2002;359:294–302.

This meta-analysis included 35,970 patients from 11 randomized trials that enrolled 200 or more patients and assigned up to 7 days of treatment with a direct thrombin inhibitor or heparin and had a 30-day or longer follow-up. Compared with heparin, direct thrombin inhibitors were associated with a lower risk of death or MI at the end of treatment [4.3% vs. 5.1%; OR, 0.85 (95% CI, 0.77 to 0.94); $p = 0.001$] and at 30 days [7.4% vs. 8.2%; 0.91 (0.84 to 0.99); $p = 0.02$]. This was driven by fewer MIs [2.8% vs. 3.5%; 0.80 (0.71 to 0.90); $p < 0.001$]. Subgroup analyses revealed a benefit of direct thrombin inhibitors on death or MI in both ACS and PCI trials. A reduction in death or MI was evident with hirudin and bivalirudin but not with univalent agents (argatroban, efegatran, inogatran). Compared with heparin, an increased risk of major bleeding was found with hirudin, but a reduction with bivalirudin.

GLYCOPROTEIN IIB/IIIA INHIBITORS

39. Platelet Receptor Inhibition in Ischemic Syndrome Management in Patients Limited by Unstable Signs and Symptoms (**PRISM-PLUS**) Investigators. Inhibition of the platelet glycoprotein IIb/IIIa receptor with tirofiban in unstable angina and non–Q-wave myocardial infarction. *N Engl J Med* 1998;338:1488–1497 (editorial, 1539–1541).

Design: Prospective, randomized, double-blind, multicenter study. Primary endpoint was death, MI, or refractory ischemia at 7 days.

Purpose: To investigate the clinical efficacy of tirofiban, a short-acting, nonpeptide GP IIb/IIIa inhibitor, in the prevention of acute ischemic events in patients with UA and non–Q wave MI.

Population: 1,915 patients with prolonged anginal pain or repetitive episodes of angina at rest or during minimal exercise in the previous 12 hours and new ST–T changes [$\geq$1-mm elevation or depression, $\geq$3-mm T-wave inversion on at least three limb leads or precordial leads (excluding V$_1$), or pseudonormalization $\geq$1 mm] or an elevated CK or CK-MB.

Exclusion Criteria: Included ST elevation longer than 20 minutes, thrombolysis in the previous 48 hours, angioplasty in the past 6 months, or CABG surgery in the previous month, stroke in the prior year, active bleeding or high bleeding risk, history of thrombocytopenia or platelet count less than 150,000, and creatinine more than 2.5 mg/dL.

Treatment: (a) Tirofiban, 0.6 μg/kg/min for 30 minutes, and then 0.15 μg/kg/min and placebo heparin; (b) tirofiban, 0.4 μg/kg/min for 30 minutes, and then 0.1 μg/kg/min, plus heparin; or (c) heparin plus placebo tirofiban.

Results: The tirofiban-plus-heparin group had a significant reduction compared with the heparin-alone group in the 7-day composite endpoints (12.9% vs. 17.9%; RR, 0.68; $p = 0.004$). This difference persisted at 30-day and 6-month follow-up (18.5% vs. 22.3%, $p = 0.03$; 27.7% vs. 32.1%, $p = 0.02$). The tirofiban-plus-heparin group also had a significant reduction in death or MI at 7 and 30 days (4.9% vs. 8.3%, $p = 0.006$; 8.7% vs. 11.9%, $p = 0.03$).

Comments: Benefit was seen regardless of treatment strategy—medical therapy group with 25% reduction in death or MI at 30 days, PCI group with 34% reduction, and CABG group with 30% reduction. The troponin substudy also showed that the combination of tirofiban plus heparin reduced infarct size, as measured by peak troponin. Angiographic study (1,491 patients) found a lower thrombus burden with tirofiban + heparin compared with heparin alone (OR, 0.65; $p = 0.002$) and higher TIMI grade 3 flow rate (82% vs. 74%).

40. Platelet Receptor Inhibition in Ischemic Syndrome Management (**PRISM**) Study Investigators. A comparison of aspirin plus tirofiban with aspirin plus heparin for unstable angina. *N Engl J Med* 1998;338:1498–1505 (editorial, 1539–1541).

Design: Prospective, randomized, multicenter study. Primary endpoint was death, MI, and refractory ischemia at 48 hours.

Purpose: To compare i.v. tirofiban with i.v. UFH for the treatment of UA in patients receiving aspirin.

Population: 3,232 patients with rest or accelerating chest pain within 24 hours of randomization and at least one of the following criteria: (a) ST depression ≥ 1 mm in at least two contiguous leads, transient (<20 minutes) ST elevation, or T-wave inversion; (b) elevated cardiac enzymes; and (c) history of MI, revascularization more than 6 months earlier, coronary surgery more than 1 month earlier, positive exercise or pharmacologic stress test result, or more than 50% stenosis on prior angiogram.

Exclusion Criteria: Included thrombolytic therapy in previous 48 hours, creatinine greater than 2.5 mg/dL, increased bleeding risks, history of thrombocytopenia, SBP more than 180 mm Hg, and DBP more than 110 mm Hg.

Treatment: Tirofiban, 0.6 μg/kg/min for 30 minutes, and then 0.15 μg/kg/min through 48 hours, with placebo heparin, or UFH (5,000-U bolus, and then 1,000 U/hr for 48 hours, adjusted if necessary based on aPTT at 6 and 24 hours). All patients were taking aspirin, 300 to 325 mg daily.

Results: Tirofiban group had a 32% reduction in the composite primary endpoints at 48 hours— 3.8% vs. 5.6% (RR, 0.67; $p = 0.01$). At 30 days, a similar frequency of composite endpoints was observed (15.9% vs. 17.1%; $p = 0.34$). At 7 days, the tirofiban group had a significantly lower mortality rate (2.3% vs. 3.6%; $p = 0.02$) and tended toward a reduction in death and MI (5.8% vs. 7.1%; $p = 0.11$). Tirofiban was associated with increased thrombocytopenia (1.1% vs. 0.4%; $p = 0.04$). Identical major bleeding rates were observed (0.4%). At 30 days, death or MI occurred in 13.0% of troponin I–positive patients compared with 4.9% for troponin I–negative patients ($p < 0.0001$), and 13.7% compared with 3.5% for troponin T ($p < 0.001$) see Ref. 85. In troponin I–positive patients, tirofiban substantially lowered the risks of death [adjusted hazard ratio 0.25 (95% CI, 0.09 to 0.68), $p = 0.004$] and MI [hazard ratio 0.37 (0.16 to 0.84), $p = 0.01$].

41. Platelet Glycoprotein IIb/IIIa in Unstable Angina Receptor Suppression Using Integrilin Therapy (**PURSUIT**) Trial Investigators. Inhibition of platelet glycoprotein IIb/IIIa with eptifibatide in patients with acute coronary syndromes. *N Engl J Med* 1998;339: 436–443.

Design: Prospective, randomized, double-blind, placebo-controlled, multicenter study. Primary endpoint was death or nonfatal MI at 30 days.

Purpose: To determine if the addition of eptifibatide to heparin and aspirin provides additional benefit in patients with ACSs without ST elevation.

Population: 10,948 patients with ischemic chest pain lasting 10 minutes in the prior 24 hours (median, 11 hours) and ECG changes (transient or persistent ST-segment depression more than 0.5 mm, transient ST-segment elevation more than 0.5 mm, or T-wave inversion more than 1 mm within 12 hours before or after chest pain), or serum CK-MB above the ULN.

Exclusion Criteria: Included persistent ST elevation more than 1 mm, SBP more than 200 mm Hg or DBP more than 100 mm Hg, major surgery within the prior 6 weeks, nonhemorrhagic stroke in the prior 30 days, or any history of hemorrhagic stroke, renal failure, planned used of thrombolytic or GP IIb/IIIa inhibitors, and thrombolysis in the prior 24 hours.

Treatment: Eptifibatide, 180-μg/kg bolus, and then 1.3 or 2.0 μg/kg/min for 72 hours (up to 96 hours if intervention was near the end of a 72-hour period), or placebo; 1.3-μg/kg/min infusion was dropped after 3,218 patients enrolled. No protocol-mandated strategy of catheterization and revascularization was undertaken.

Results: Eptifibatide was associated with a 9.6% relative reduction in death or MI at 30 days (14.2% vs. 15.7%; $p = 0.04$); this effect was apparent by 72 hours. Among patients undergoing early (<72 hours) PCI, eptifibatide was associated with a 32% benefit. Eptifibatide was associated with increased major bleeding (10.6% vs. 9.1%; $p = 0.02$) and higher transfusion rates (11.6% vs. 9.2%; RR, 1.3; 95% CI, 1.1 to 1.4). The eptifibatide group also had more cases of profound thrombocytopenia (platelet count <20,000): RR, 5.0 (nine vs. two patients; 95% CI, 1.3 to 32.4). Eptifibatide was not associated with increased incidence of bleeding in those undergoing CABG surgery. Stroke occurred in 79 (0.7%) patients, 66 of whom were nonhemorrhagic, and no significant differences in stroke rates were found between patients who received placebo and those assigned high-dose eptifibatide.

42. **Cannon CP,** et al. Oral glycoprotein IIb/IIIa inhibition with orbofiban in patients with unstable coronary syndromes (**OPUS-TIMI 16**) trial. *Circulation* 2000;102:149–156.

Design: Prospective, randomized, double-blind, multicenter study. Primary endpoint was death, MI, recurrent ischemia requiring rehospitalization, urgent revascularization, or stroke.

Purpose: To determine whether prolonged oral GP IIb/IIIa inhibition with orbofiban provides additional reduction in recurrent ischemic events.

Population: 10,288 patients with ACS defined as ischemic rest pain within 72 hours and one or more of the following—new ST-segment deviation of 0.5 mm or more, T-wave inversion of 3 mm or more in three leads or LBBB, positive cardiac markers, or (for the first 3,000 patients only) history of MI, PCI, CABG surgery, coronary stenosis of 50% or more, age 65 years or older, and a history of angina or positive stress test, prior peripheral arterial or cerebrovascular disease, or diabetes mellitus.

Exclusion Criteria: Included increased bleeding risks [prior intracranial hemorrhage (ICH), peptic ulcer within 6 months, etc.].

Treatment: Orbofiban, 50 mg twice daily (50/50 group); orbofiban, 50 mg twice daily for 30 days followed by 30 mg orbofiban twice daily (50/30 group), or placebo.

Results: Trial was terminated early because of increased 30-day mortality in the 50/30 orbofiban group. At 10 months, mortality was 3.7% in the placebo group versus 5.1% in the 50/30 group ($p = 0.008$) and 4.5% in the 50/50 group ($p = 0.11$). No differences were found between the three groups in the incidence of the primary composite endpoint (22.9%, 23.1%, and 22.8%, for the placebo, 50/30, and 50/50 groups, respectively). The orbofiban groups had a significantly higher incidence of major or severe bleeding (but not ICH) compared with placebo [3.7% (50/30) and 4.5% (50/50) vs. 2.0%)].

43. Sibrafiban versus aspirin to yield maximum protection from ischemic heart events post-acute coronary syndromes (SYMPHONY) Investigators. Comparison of sibrafiban with aspirin for prevention of cardiovascular events after acute coronary syndromes: a randomised trial. *Lancet* 2000;355:337–345.

Design: Prospective, randomized, double-blind, multicenter study. Primary endpoint was death, MI, or severe recurrent ischemia at 90 days.

Purpose: To compare the efficacy, safety, and tolerability of long-term administration of the oral GP IIb/IIIa inhibitor sibrafiban with aspirin in ACS.

Population: 9,233 patients seen within 7 days of an ACS, clinically stable for 12 hours or more, and Killip class 1 or 2.

Exclusion Criteria: Serious illness, predisposition to bleeding, major surgery, previous stroke or ICH, thrombocytopenia, renal failure, treatment with oral anticoagulants, antiplatelet agents, or NSAIDs.

Treatment: Aspirin, 80 mg, low-dose sibrafiban (LDS; 4.5 or 3 mg, depending on creatinine and body weight), high-dose oral sibrafiban (6, 4.5, or 3 mg depending on creatinine and body weight). All were taken every 12 hours.

Results: No differences were found between the three groups in the incidence of the primary composite endpoint [9.8% (aspirin), 10.1% (LDS), 10.1% (high-dose sibrafiban, HDS); OR for aspirin vs. both the LDS and HDS, 1.03; 95% CI, 0.87 to 1.21]. Death or MI rates also were similar (7.0%, 7.4%, and 7.9%, respectively). Large MIs (CK-MB more than five times the ULN) occurred less frequently in the aspirin group (37.4%) than in the sibrafiban groups [45.3% (low dose), 49.7% (high dose)]. The aspirin group had a significantly lower incidence of bleeding (13.0% vs. 18.7% and 25.4%), whereas major bleeding occurred in 3.9%, 5.2%, and 5.7%, respectively.

44. **SYMPHONY II** Investigators. Randomized trial of aspirin, sibrafiban, or both for secondary prevention after acute coronary syndromes. *Circulation* 2001;103:1727–1733.

Design: Prospective, randomized, double-blind, multicenter study. Primary endpoint was death, MI, and severe recurrent ischemia.

Purpose: To assess whether longer treatment (12 to 18 months) with LDS in combination with aspirin or HDS alone was more effective for secondary prevention than is aspirin alone.

Population: Same inclusion criteria as SYMPHONY I; 6,671 patients completed a median of 90 days of follow-up (original design, 8,400 patients).

Exclusion Criteria: See SYMPHONY I.

Treatment: Aspirin alone (80 mg twice daily), LDS + aspirin, or HDS. Average time from qualifying event to first dose was 94 hours (range, 63 to 132 hours).

Results: Study terminated after SYMPHONY I results were reported. No difference was noted between the three groups in the incidence of the primary composite endpoint (aspirin, 9.3%; LDS + aspirin, 9.2%; HDS, 10.5%). The HDS group had a higher incidence of death or MI compared with the aspirin-alone group (6.1% vs. 8.6%), whereas major bleeding occurred more frequently in the LDS + aspirin group compared with the aspirin-alone group (5.7% vs. 4.0%).

Comments: Some evidence suggests that the increased thrombosis seen with oral GP IIb/IIIa inhibitors is due to enhanced receptor activity during the hours when the drugs are less active or not available.

45. **Simoons ML,** GUSTO IV-ACS Investigators. Effect of glycoprotein IIb/IIIa receptor blocker abciximab on outcome in patients with acute coronary syndromes without early coronary revascularisation: the GUSTO IV-ACS randomised trial. *Lancet* 2001;357:1915–1924.

Design: Prospective, randomized, open, multicenter study. Primary endpoint was death or MI at 30 days.

Purpose: To study the effect of the GP IIb/IIIa blocker abciximab in ACS patients not undergoing early revascularization.

Population: 7,800 patients with UA or NSTEMI. Eligible if chest pain longer than 5 minutes within the last 24 hours, 0.5-mm or more ST-segment depression, OR positive troponin T or I.

Exclusion Criteria: Included ST elevation or new LBBB, PCI within the past 2 weeks, planned PCI/CABG in the next 30 days, active bleeding or bleeding disorder, or other risk factor for bleeding.

Treatment: Abciximab for 24 hours, or abciximab for 48 hours, or placebo. All received aspirin and either UFH or LMWH.

Results: No significant differences were observed between the groups in the incidence of death or MI at 30 days (abciximab for 24 hours, 8.2%; abciximab for 48 hours, 9.1%; placebo, 8.0%; p = NS). No differences were noted among those with a positive troponin or in any other subgroups. The mortality rate was actually higher in first 48 hours in both abciximab groups compared with the placebo group [0.7% and 0.9% vs. 0.3%; ORs, 2.3 (p = 0.048) and 2.9 (p = 0.007)]. In particular, no benefit was seen in patients with increased cardiac troponin T or I concentrations at enrollment, although these patients had a strongly increased risk of subsequent events. Bleeding rates were low but were higher with abciximab, particularly in the 48-hour group. Thrombocytopenia also was more common in the abciximab groups.

46. **Kastrati A,** et al. Abciximab in patients with acute coronary syndromes undergoing percutaneous coronary intervention after clopidogrel pretreatment: the ISAR-REACT 2 randomized trial. *JAMA* 2006;295(13):1531–1538.

Design: Prospective, randomized, placebo-controlled, international, multicenter trial. Primary endpoint was death, MI, or urgent TVR at 30 days.
Purpose: To study the effect of the GP IIb/IIIa blocker abciximab in UA/NSTEMI patients undergoing PCI with clopidogrel adjunctive therapy.
Population: 2,022 patients with UA or NSTEMI (roughly 50% with elevated troponin) who received aspirin and clopidogrel prior to undergoing PCI (roughly half received DES).
Exclusion Criteria: Included ST elevation or new LBBB, hemodynamic instability, increased risk of bleeding (e.g., recent stroke), and concomitant malignancy shortening life expectancy.
Treatment: Abciximab infusion for 12 hours or placebo; both groups received heparin infusion.
Results: There was a significant reduction in the primary endpoint in the abciximab group (8.9% vs. 11.9%, $p = 0.03$); however, this difference was absent in patients without elevated troponin levels. Major bleeding, minor bleeding, and need for transfusion did not differ between the two groups.

47. **Roffi M,** et al. Platelet glycoprotein IIb/IIIa inhibitors reduce mortality in diabetic patients with non-ST-segment-elevation acute coronary syndromes. *Circulation* 2001;104:2767–2771.

This meta-analysis examined patients enrolled in six large GP IIb/IIIa inhibitor trials (PRISM, PRISM-PLUS, PARAGON A, PARAGON B, PURSUIT, GUSTO IV). Among the 6,458 diabetic patients, GP IIb/IIIa inhibitor use was associated with a significantly lower 30-day mortality compared with no GP inhibition (4.6% vs. 6.2%; OR, 0.74; 95% CI, 0.59 to 0.92; $p = 0.007$). The largest benefit was seen in the subgroup of 1,279 diabetic patients who underwent PCI during the index hospitalization; they had a 70% lower mortality with GP inhibitor use (1.2% vs. 4.0%; OR, 0.30; 95% CI, 0.14 to 0.69; $p = 0.002$). In contrast, among the 23,072 nondiabetic patients, no survival benefit was associated with GP inhibitor use (3.0% in both groups). The interaction between GP IIb/IIIa inhibition and diabetic status was statistically significant ($p = 0.036$).

48. **Boersma E,** et al. Platelet glycoprotein IIb/IIIa inhibitors in acute coronary syndromes: a meta-analysis of all major randomised clinical trials. *Lancet* 2002;359:189–198.

This meta-analysis examined the same six trials (see preceding) that randomized 31,402 ACS patients to various GP IIb/IIIa inhibitors versus placebo or control. The meta-analysis of all endpoints was performed by using Cochrane–Mantel–Haenszel, Breslow–Day, and Kaplan–Meier methods. The 30-day pooled incidence of death or MI showed a significant absolute reduction of 1% with GP inhibitor use [10.8% vs. 11.8% (placebo or control); OR, 0.91; $p = 0.015$). A significant benefit also was seen at 5 days (5.7% vs. 6.9%; OR, 0.84; $p = 0.0003$). The benefits were seen in all important subgroups, such as age, diabetics, and prior cardiac history. GP IIb/IIIa inhibitor use was associated with an increased risk of bleeding (OR, 1.62), but no increased rate of ICH or stroke was seen. Gender difference favored treatment of men with GP IIb/IIIa inhibitors, but women benefited when controlled for baseline troponin. No benefit is apparent with GP inhibitor use when patients do not have a positive troponin test.

49. **Giugliano RP,** et al. for the EARLY-ACS Investigators. Early versus delayed, provisional eptifibatide in acute coronary syndromes. *N Engl J Med* 2009;360(21):2176–2190.

Design: Prospective, randomized, placebo-controlled, international, multicenter trial. Primary endpoint was death, myocardial infarction, urgent TVR, or the requirement of bolus "thrombotic bailout" therapy during PCI at 96 hours.
Purpose: To study the effect of early versus provisional GP IIb/IIIa blocker administration in patients with UA/NSTEMI undergoing PCI.
Population: 9,492 patients with high-risk UA/NSTEMI undergoing PCI within 1 calendar day of randomization. Patients were high risk if they had at least two of the following: significant ECG changes, elevated troponin or CK-MB, and age greater than 60 years.

Exclusion Criteria: Increased bleeding risk.

Treatment: Early, routine treatment with eptifibatide or placebo; following angiography, provisional administration of eptifibatide at the investigator's discretion (those who previously received eptifibatide got placebo bolus, and then open-label infusion; those who received placebo early got eptifibatide bolus, and then open-label infusion). If no provisional therapy was requested prior to PCI, and the operator detected a thrombotic complication of PCI after the guidewire crossed the lesion, they could request a "bailout" kit containing study drug assignment opposite that of the initial assignment (if the "bailout" kit was requested for any of the seven predefined thrombotic complications, this was considered a primary endpoint event by the Clinical Events Committee).

Results: There was no significant difference in rates of the primary endpoint at 96 hours, between patients receiving early routine eptifibatide (9.6%) and delayed, provisional administration (10.0%, $p = 0.23$). At 30 days, rates of death or MI were also similar, though with a trend toward the "early" group (11.2% for early eptifibatide vs. 12.3% for delayed, $p = 0.08$). TIMI major hemorrhage was 2.6% versus 1.8% (OR, 1.42; $p = 0.02$) and bleeding defined according to the Global Utilization of Streptokinase and Tissue Plasminogen Activator for Occluded Coronary Arteries (GUSTO) criteria, moderate bleeding was 6.8% in the early eptifibatide group versus 4.3% in the provisional eptifibatide group OR 1.60 ($p < 0.001$). GUSTO severe bleeding rates were similar but minor bleeding and red cell transfusions were higher in the "early" group.

Conclusion: Early, routine administration of eptifibatide, as compared with provisional usage, in patients with UA/NSTEMI going to PCI did not significantly improve outcomes at 96 hours or 30 days, and there was a significant increase in major bleeding.

THROMBOLYTICS

50. **Bar FW,** et al. Unstable Angina Study Using Eminase **(UNASEM).** Thrombolysis in patients with unstable angina improves the angiographic but not clinical outcome: results of UNASEM, a multicenter, randomized, placebo-controlled, clinical trial with anistreplase. *Circulation* 1992;86:131–137.

Prospective, randomized, double-blind, placebo-controlled, multicenter study of 159 patients aged 30 to 70 years with angina of recent onset (<4 weeks) or of the crescendo type with the last episode within 12 hours of admission and ischemic ST changes (ST depression, ≥1 mm; T-wave inversion, ≥2 mm). After coronary angiography, patients were randomized to anistreplase, 30 U over 5 minutes, or placebo; repeated angiography was performed at 12 to 28 hours. All patients were given heparin and aspirin, 300 mg/day (started after second catheterization). Anistreplase group had a significant decrease in stenosis diameter between the first and second angiograms [11% (from 70% to 59%) vs. 3% (from 66% to 63%); $p = 0.008$]. No difference was observed in clinical outcome between the groups (e.g., infarct size, MI rate), but more bleeding complications occurred with anistreplase (32% vs. 11%; $p = 0.001$).

51. Thrombolysis in Myocardial Ischemia **(TIMI 3A)** Investigators. Early effects of tissue-type plasminogen activator added to conventional therapy on the culprit coronary lesion in patients presenting with ischemic cardiac pain at rest: results of the TIMI 3A trial. *Circulation* 1993;87:38–52.

Design: Prospective, randomized, open, parallel-group, multicenter study. Primary endpoint was 10% reduction of stenosis and improvement of two TIMI flow grades.

Purpose: To evaluate the effects of tissue-type plasminogen activator (tPA) added to conventional therapy on the culprit coronary lesion in patients with UA or non–Q wave MI.

Population: 306 patients aged 22 to 75 years with chest pain at rest lasting 5 minutes to 6 hours and accompanied by ECG changes or documented CAD.

Exclusion Criteria: Included CABG surgery, MI in the prior 21 days, PTCA in the prior 6 months, cardiogenic shock, and oral anticoagulation requirement.

Treatment: Front-loaded tPA (maximum, 80 mg) or placebo plus conventional antianginal therapy. All patients received heparin (5,000-U bolus and infusion for 18 to 48 hours) and aspirin, 325 mg daily.

Results: The tPA group had more frequent improvement of TIMI flow by two grades or reduction of stenosis by 20% on repeated angiography at 18 to 48 hours (15% vs. 5%; $p = 0.003$). The tPA benefit was most marked in patients with thrombus-containing lesions (36% vs. 15%; $p < 0.01$) and non–Q wave MI (33% vs. 8%; $p < 0.005$).

Comments: Only modest angiographic improvement was observed.

52. **Ambrose JA,** et al. Thrombolysis and Angioplasty in Unstable Angina **(TAUSA).** Adjunctive thrombolytic therapy during PTCA for ischemic rest angina. *Circulation* 1994;90:69–77.

Design: Prospective, randomized, double-blind, multicenter study.

Purpose: To assess the role of intracoronary urokinase during angioplasty for UA or postin-farction rest angina.

Population: 469 patients aged ≤80 years with ischemic rest pain accompanied by ST-segment or T-wave changes and an angiogram demonstrating 70% stenosis.

Exclusion Criteria: Included normal baseline ECG, blood pressure greater than 180/110, prior stroke, recent (within fewer than 10 days) major surgery, bleeding diathesis, and active GI or GU bleeding.

Treatment: Intracoronary urokinase (250,000 or 500,000 U) or placebo. All patients received aspirin and heparin.

Results: No significant differences in incidence of post-PTCA thrombi were observed [13.8% (urokinase) vs. 18%; $p = $ NS], but the urokinase group had a higher acute closure rate (10.2% vs. 4.3%, $p < 0.02$; most of difference was in the in 500,000-U group) and more adverse outcomes (ischemia, MI, CABG surgery; 6.3% vs. 2.9%, $p < 0.02$).

Comments: Possible explanations of adverse effects of urokinase include increased hemor-rhagic dissection, lack of intimal sealing, and procoagulant or platelet-activating effects.

53. Thrombolysis in MI **(TIMI 3B).** Effects of tissue plasminogen activator and a compari-son of early invasive and conservative strategies in unstable angina and non–Q-wave MI. *Circulation* 1994;89:1545–1556.

Design: Prospective, randomized (2 × 2 factorial design), double-blind, placebo-controlled, multicenter study. Primary endpoint was death, MI, or failure of treatment at 6 weeks (for tPA comparison), and death, MI, or positive ETT (for strategy comparison).

Purpose: To evaluate the use of thrombolytic therapy in UA and non–Q wave MI and to com-pare an early invasive with a conservative strategy.

Population: 1,473 patients aged 21 to 76 years within 24 hours of ischemic discomfort at rest consistent with UA or non–Q wave MI.

Exclusion Criteria: Included treatable cause of UA, MI in the prior 21 days, coronary angiog-raphy in the prior 30 days, PTCA within 6 months, history of CABG, SBP higher than 180 mm Hg or DBP higher than 100 mm Hg, and contraindication to thrombolysis.

Treatment: tPA, 0.8 mg/kg over a 90-minute period (maximum, 80 mg; mean, 63 mg), includ-ing one-third of dose as an i.v. bolus (up to 20 mg); or placebo. The early invasive strategy involved catheterization 18 to 48 hours after randomization, and revascularization, if feasi-ble. Conservative strategy allowed catheterization for recurrent ischemia at rest with ECG changes or other failure of medical therapy.

Results: No difference was observed between invasive and conservative strategies in combined primary endpoints (16.2% vs. 18.1%), but the early invasive strategy was associated with a shorter hospital stay and lower incidence of rehospitalization. tPA was not shown to be ben-eficial and may be harmful (e.g., four ICHs vs. none with placebo; $p = 0.06$).

Comments: One-year results showed similar death and nonfatal reinfarction rates between tPA and placebo (12.4% vs. 10.6%; $p = 0.24$) and early invasive versus early conservative groups (10.8% vs. 12.2%; $p = 0.42$). The early invasive group had a higher revascularization rate (64% vs. 58%; $p < 0.001$), primarily because of more PTCAs (39% vs. 32%), but fewer readmissions (26% vs. 33%; $p < 0.001$).

Invasive versus Conservative Management

(See Also Ref. 52)

54. **Boden WE,** et al. for the Veteran Affairs Non–Q-Wave Infarction Strategies in Hospital (**VANQWISH**) Trial Investigators. Outcomes in patients with acute non–Q-wave MI randomly assigned to an invasive as compared with a conservative strategy. *N Engl J Med* 1998;338:1785–1792 (editorial, 1838–1839).

Design: Prospective, randomized, controlled, multicenter study. Primary endpoint was death or MI.

Purpose: To compare a conservative with an invasive strategy on the incidence of clinical outcomes in non–Q wave MI.

Population: 920 patients with an evolving MI characterized by no Q waves on serial ECGs and CK-MB more than 1.5 times the ULN.

Exclusion Criteria: Persistent or recurrent ischemia at rest despite intensive medical therapy, severe heart failure despite i.v. diuretics and/or vasodilators, and serious coexisting conditions.

Treatment: Patients were assigned within 24 to 72 hours to invasive strategy (routine angiography followed by revascularization, if feasible) or conservative strategy [medical therapy, noninvasive testing (radionuclide left ventriculography and symptom-limited ETT with thallium scintigraphy), and invasive procedures only in a setting of spontaneous or inducible ischemia]. All patients received aspirin (325 mg daily) and diltiazem (180 to 300 mg/day).

Results: Only 9% were excluded secondary to high-risk ischemic complications. Only 29% of the conservative group (vs. 64% in TIMI 3B) underwent catheterization within 30 days. At follow-up (average, 23 months), the two groups had a similar incidence of death and MI [152 events (invasive, 32.9%) vs. 139 (conservative, 30.3%); $p = 0.35$]. The conservative group showed a nonsignificant trend toward lower mortality (hazard ratio, 0.72; 95% CI, 0.51 to 1.01). Fewer patients treated conservatively had death plus MI or death at hospital discharge (36 vs. 15 patients; $p = 0.004$; 21 vs. 6; $p = 0.007$), at 1 month (48 vs. 26; $p = 0.012$; 23 vs. 9; $p = 0.021$), and at 1 year (111 vs. 85; $p = 0.05$; 58 vs. 36; $p = 0.025$). The invasive group had a higher CABG surgery mortality rate [11.6% vs. 3.4% (11 vs. 3 patients in the conservative group)].

55. **McCullough PA,** et al. Medicine vs. Angioplasty in Thrombolytic Exclusion (**MATE**). A prospective, randomized trial of triage angiography in acute coronary syndromes ineligible for thrombolytic therapy. *J Am Coll Cardiol* 1998;32:596–605.

Design: Prospective, randomized, controlled, multicenter study. Primary composite endpoint was death and recurrent ischemic events.

Purpose: To determine whether early triage with revascularization, if indicated, favorably affects clinical outcomes in patients with suspected acute MI who are ineligible for thrombolysis.

Population: 201 patients seen within 24 hours with an acute chest syndrome consistent with acute MI (high clinical suspicion with or without immediate enzymatic confirmation) and considered ineligible for thrombolysis because of lack of ECG changes (68% without ST elevation), symptoms for more than 6 hours, or increased bleeding or stroke risks.

Exclusion Criteria: Included symptoms for more than 24 hours or an absolute indication or contraindication to cardiac catheterization.

Treatment: Early triage angiography and subsequent therapies based on the angiogram versus conventional medical therapy consisting of aspirin, i.v. heparin, NTG, β-blockers, and analgesics.

Results: Acute MI was confirmed in 51% and 54% of triage angiography and conservative patients, respectively. The triage angiography group had a significant reduction in the primary endpoints of recurrent ischemic events and death (13% vs. 34%; RR, 45%; 95% CI, 27% to 59%; $p = 0.0002$). In the triage angiography group, 58% received revascularization, whereas in the conservative group, 60% subsequently underwent nonprotocol angiography because of recurrent ischemia, and 37% received revascularization ($p = 0.004$). The mean time to revascularization was substantially shorter in the triage angiography group (27 vs. 98 hours; $p = 0.0001$). No differences were seen in length of stay or hospital costs. At long-term follow-up (median, 21 months), no significant differences in late revascularization, recurrent MI, or all-cause mortality were observed.

56. FRagmin and Fast Revascularization during InStability in coronary artery disease (**FRISC II**) Investigators. Invasive compared with noninvasive treatment in unstable coronary artery disease: FRISC II prospective randomized multicenter study. *Lancet* 1999;354:708–715.

Design: Prospective, randomized, partially open (strategy assignment), multicenter study. Primary endpoint was death or MI at 6 months.

Purpose: To compare an early invasive with a noninvasive strategy in patients with unstable coronary disease in addition to optimal background antithrombotic medication.

Population: 2,457 patients with ischemic symptoms in the previous 48 hours accompanied by ECG changes (ST depression or T-wave inversion ≥0.1 mV) or elevated markers (e.g., CK-MB >6 mg/L; troponin T >0.10 mg/dL).

Exclusion Criteria: See Ref. 22.

Treatment: Early invasive or noninvasive treatment strategy (coronary angiography within 7 days performed in 96% and 10%, and revascularization in first 10 days, in 71% and 9%). Patients also received dalteparin or placebo for 3 months.

Results: The invasive group had a significantly lower incidence of death or MI at 6 months [9.4% vs. 12.1% (noninvasive group); $p = 0.031$]. A significant decrease in MI alone was noted (7.8% vs. 10.1%; $p = 0.045$), whereas the reduction in mortality was nonsignificant (1.9% vs. 2.9%; $p = 0.10$). Subgroup analysis showed that these benefits were restricted to men (RRs of death or MI at 6 months, 0.64 and 1.26 in men and women, respectively). Invasive strategy also was associated with 50% lower recurrent angina and hospital readmission rates. At 1-year follow-up, a persistent reduction in the incidence of death or MI was seen in the invasive group (10.4% vs. 14.1%; RR, 0.74; $p = 0.005$); 52% of the noninvasive group had undergone coronary angiography (see *Lancet* 2000;354:9).

57. **Cannon CP**, et al. for the Treat Angina with Aggrastat and Determine Cost of Therapy with an Invasive or Conservative Strategy (**TACTICS**)-**TIMI 18** Investigators. Comparison of early invasive versus early conservative strategies in patients with unstable angina and non-ST elevation myocardial infarction treated with early glycoprotein IIb/IIIa inhibition. *N Engl J Med* 2001;344:1879–1887.

Design: Prospective, randomized, multicenter study. Primary endpoint composite of death, nonfatal MI, and rehospitalization for an ACS at 6 months.

Purpose: To compare an early invasive strategy with an early conservative strategy in patients with UA and NSTEMI treated with early GP IIb/IIIa inhibition.

Population: 2,220 patients with UA and NSTEMI who had one of more of the following— ECG changes, elevated levels of cardiac markers, or a history of CAD (prior cardiac catheterization, revascularization, or MI).

Exclusion Criteria: Included persistent ST elevation, secondary angina, PTCA or CABG within 6 months, history of GI bleeding, platelet disorder, thrombocytopenia or hemorrhagic cerebrovascular disease, nonhemorrhagic stroke or transient ischemic attack (TIA) within 1 year, severe CHF or cardiogenic shock, serum creatinine greater than 2.5 mg/dL, treatment with abciximab within 96 hours, or current long-term treatment with ticlopidine, clopidogrel, or warfarin.

Treatment: Early invasive strategy (routine catheterization within 4 to 48 hours and revascularization as appropriate), or more conservative strategy [catheterization only if patient had objective evidence of recurrent ischemia (ECG changes, positive markers) or an abnormal stress test]. All patients were treated with aspirin, heparin, and tirofiban, 0.4 μg/kg/min for 30 minutes.

Results: At 6 months, the early invasive strategy had a significantly lower incidence of the primary endpoint compared with the conservative strategy (15.9% vs. 19.4%; OR, 0.78; $p = 0.025$). The early invasive group also had a lower rate of death or nonfatal MI at 6 months (7.3% vs. 9.5%; OR, 0.74; $p < 0.05$). The invasive strategy provided a significantly greater benefit in the patients with baseline ST-segment changes (p for interaction ≥ 0.006). In patients with a troponin T level greater than 0.01 ng/mL, a 39% relative reduction in the primary endpoint with the invasive strategy was noted, compared with the conservative strategy ($p < 0.001$), whereas patients with a troponin T level of 0.01 ng/mL or more had similar outcomes with either strategy. In a prespecified analysis that used the TRS (see *JAMA* 2000;284:835), the benefits of the invasive strategy were observed in intermediate- and high-risk patients (75% of the study population).

58. **Fox KAA,** et al. for the Randomized Intervention Trial of unstable Angina (RITA) Investigators. Interventional versus conservative treatment for patients with unstable angina or non–ST-elevation myocardial infarction: the British Foundation **RITA 3** randomised trial. *Lancet* 2002;360:743–751.

Design: Prospective, randomized, open, multicenter trial. Co-primary endpoints were death, MI, or refractory angina at 4 months and death or MI at 1 year. Median follow-up was 2.0 years.
Purpose: To determine whether routine early angiography with myocardial revascularization (as clinically indicated) is better than a conservative strategy in UA/NSTEMI patients.
Population: 1,810 patients with non–ST elevation ACS.
Exclusion Criteria: Included probable evolving MI, CK or CK-MB twice the ULN before randomization, planned PCI within 72 hours, MI in the previous month, PCI in the previous year, or CABG at any time.
Treatment: Early intervention (angiography with PCI if indicated) or conservative strategy [ischemia- or symptom-driven angiography (performed in 48% at 1 year)]. Antithrombin agent in both groups was enoxaparin. Approximately 25% received a GP IIb/IIIa inhibitor.
Results: At 4 months, the early intervention group had a 34% lower incidence of death, MI, or refractory angina compared with the conservative strategy group (9.6% vs. 14.5%; $p = 0.001$). This benefit was primarily driven by a 53% reduction in refractory angina in the intervention group. Refractory angina required occurrence of ischemic pain, at rest or with minimal exertion, despite maximal medical treatment, associated with ECG changes, and prompting revascularization within 24 hours. At 1 year, the incidence of death or MI was similar in both groups (7.6% vs. 8.3%; $p = 0.58$). Using the ESC/ACC MI definition, death or MI at 1 year was reduced (12.5% vs. 17.1%, $p = 0.007$). The interventional group had a significant reduction in symptoms of angina and use of antianginal medications ($p < 0.0001$).

59. **Neumann F-J,** et al. Evaluation of prolonged antithrombotic pretreatment ("cooling-off" strategy) before intervention in patients with unstable coronary syndromes. A randomized controlled trial (ISAR-COOL). *JAMA* 2003;290:1593–1599.

Design: Prospective, randomized, controlled trial. Primary endpoint was a composite of death or MI at 30 days.
Purpose: To determine whether prolonged antithrombotic treatment prior to PCI is beneficial in patients undergoing PCI for UA/NSTEMI.
Population: 410 patients with UA/NSTEMI with *either* ST-segment depression or elevated levels of troponin.
Treatment: All patients received the same antithrombotic regimen—heparin infusion (with bolus), aspirin, clopidogrel (with load), and tirofiban infusion (with bolus). Patients in the immediate-intervention group went to PCI within 6 hours, whereas the prolonged group went to PCI at 3 to 5 days following presentation (unless they exhibited refractory ischemia, hemodynamic instability, or met the primary endpoint).
Results: Patients in the prolonged pretreatment group had significantly higher rates of the primary endpoint at 30 days (11.6% vs. 5.9%, $p = 0.04$). The surplus of events occurred prior to catheterization, as there was no difference in the rates of events following catheterization.

Delay of intervention for antithrombotic pretreatment is not beneficial in patients with moderate-risk UA/NSTEMI.

60. **de Winter RJ**, et al. for the Invasive versus Conservative Treatment in Unstable Coronary Syndromes (ICTUS) Investigators. Early invasive versus selectively invasive management for acute coronary syndromes. *N Engl J Med* 2005;353:1095–1104.

Design: Prospective, randomized, multicenter, controlled trials. Primary endpoint was death, MI, or rehospitalization for angina.

Purpose: To identify the reduction in mortality, if any, of an early invasive strategy (compared with a "selectively" invasive strategy) for patients with UA/NSTEMI at moderate risk.

Population: 1,200 patients with UA/NSTEMI including elevated troponin levels and *either* significant ECG changes or known history of CAD.

Treatment: All patients received aspirin, enoxaparin, and abciximab (at the time of PCI). Clopidogrel and aggressive lipid-lowering therapy was recommended. Randomization was to either early invasive strategy of angiography within 24 to 48 hours or "selectively" invasive strategy where patients were treated medically and underwent angiography *only* if they had refractory symptoms, hemodynamic or ECG instability, or clinically significant ischemia on the predischarge stress test.

Results: There was no difference in rates of the primary endpoint between the early and selectively invasive groups (22.7% for early vs. 21.2% for selective, $p = 0.33$). Importantly, 53% of patients assigned to the selectively invasive strategy underwent catheterization during the index hospitalization. One-year mortality was identical between the two groups (2.5%), but rates of recurrent MI favored the selectively invasive group (15% for early vs. 10.0% for selective, $p = 0.005$). Patients in the selectively invasive group had a higher rate of rehospitalization (7.4% vs. 10.9%, $p = 0.04$).

61. **O'Donaghue M**, et al. Early invasive vs. conservative treatment strategies in women and men with unstable angina and non–ST-segment elevation myocardial infarction: a meta-analysis. *JAMA* 2008;300(1):71–80.

The authors combined data from eight trials (TIMI 3B, MATE, VANQWISH, FRISC II, TACTICS-TIMI 18, VINO, RITA 3, ICTUS) of invasive versus conservative strategies in patients with UA/NSTEMI (including 3,075 women and 7,075 men), and compiled patient-level data for rates of death, MI, or rehospitalization for ACS at 12 months. The benefit of invasive strategy was not significant in women (21.1% vs. 25.0%; OR, 0.81; 95% CI, 0.65 to 1.01), but did reach significance for men (21.2% vs. 26.3%; OR, 0.73; 95% CI, 0.55 to 0.98), without significant heterogeneity between sexes ($p_{interaction} = 0.26$). However, when restricted to women with elevated troponin or CK-MB, the benefit of invasive strategy was statistically significant (OR, 0.67; 95% CI, 0.50 to 0.88). The authors conclude that the data support the most recent guideline recommendations for consideration of a conservative strategy in low-risk women.

62. **Montalescot G**, et al. for the ABOARD Investigators. Immediate vs. delayed intervention for acute coronary syndromes: a randomized clinical trial. *JAMA* 2009;302(9):947–954.

Design: Prospective, randomized, multicenter trial. Primary endpoint was the peak troponin I during hospitalization. Secondary endpoint was a composite of death, MI, or urgent revascularization at 1 month.

Purpose: To identify the optimal timing of intervention in patients with UA/NSTEMI.

Population: 352 patients with UA/NSTEMI and a TRS of 3 or more.

Treatment: Invasive strategy undergoing intervention either immediately or the next business day (between 8 and 60 hours after enrollment).

Results: The groups differed in time from randomization to sheath insertion by approximately 20 hours (70 minutes for immediate intervention vs. 21 hours for delayed intervention), and roughly half of patients who underwent PCI received DES. There was no significant difference in the primary endpoint of peak troponin I (median 2.1 for immediate vs. 1.7 for delayed, $p = 0.70$). Clinical events of the composite secondary endpoint also were not statistically different (13.7% vs. 10.2%, $p = 0.31$). Individual rates of death, MI, urgent revascularization, recurrent ischemia, or major bleeding at 1 month all were similar in the two groups.

63. **Gluckman TJ,** et al. A simplified approach to the management of non–ST-segment elevation acute coronary syndromes. *JAMA* 2005;293:349–357.

The authors performed a review of the literature and guidelines for the management of UA/NSTEMI, and then refined a simplified approach to each patient. They base their approach on the initial risk stratification of patients to identify those most likely to benefit from an early invasive strategy, and then use the "ABCDE" mnemonic for subsequent therapies: "A" for antiplatelet therapy, anticoagulation, and ACE-I/ARB; "B" for β-blockade and blood pressure control; "C" for cholesterol treatment and cigarette smoking cessation; "D" for diabetes management and diet; and "E" for exercise.

Miscellaneous

64. **Schwartz GG,** et al. Myocardial Ischemia Reduction with Aggressive Cholesterol Lowering (**MIRACL**) Study Investigators. Effects of atorvastatin on early recurrent ischemic events in acute coronary syndromes: the MIRACL study: a randomized controlled trial. *JAMA* 2001;285:1711–1718.

Design: Prospective, randomized, double-blind, placebo-controlled, multicenter trial. Primary composite endpoint was death, nonfatal acute MI, cardiac arrest with resuscitation, or recurrent symptomatic MI with objective evidence and requiring emergency rehospitalization.

Purpose: To determine whether treatment with high-dose atorvastatin initiated 24 to 96 hours after an ACS reduces death and nonfatal ischemic events.

Population: 3,086 conservatively managed patients with UA/NSTEMI. Patients had chest pain for more than 15 minutes at rest or with minimal exertion in the previous 24 hours and a change from a previous pattern of angina, new or dynamic ST- or T-wave changes, or new wall-motion abnormality, or positive noninvasive test; troponin or CK-MB less than twice the ULN for UA, or more than twice the ULN for non–Q wave MI.

Exclusion Criteria: Included serum cholesterol more than 270, Q-wave MI in the prior 4 weeks, CABG surgery in the prior 3 months, PCI in the prior 6 months, LBBB or paced rhythm, lipid-lowering drugs other than niacin at doses greater than 500 mg daily, vitamin E unless at doses of less than 400 IU daily, liver dysfunction [alanine aminotransferase (ALT) greater than twice the ULN], and insulin-dependent diabetes.

Treatment: Atorvastatin, 80 mg once daily, or matching placebo, in addition to standard therapy.

Results: The atorvastatin group had a significantly lower incidence of the composite primary endpoint compared with the placebo group (14.8% vs. 17.4%; RR, 0.84; $p = 0.048$). No significant differences were found between the groups in death, nonfatal MI, or cardiac arrest, although the atorvastatin group had less symptomatic recurrent ischemia with objective evidence and requiring emergency rehospitalization (6.2% vs. 8.4%; $p = 0.02$) and fewer strokes (12 vs. 24 events; $p = 0.045$). In the atorvastatin group, mean LDL cholesterol level decreased from 124 mg/dL (3.2 m*M*) to 72 mg/dL (1.9 m*M*). Abnormal liver transaminases (more than three times ULN) were more common in the atorvastatin group than in the placebo group (2.5% vs. 0.6%; $p < 0.001$); no cases of rhabdomyolysis were observed.

Prognosis and Assessment
CLINICAL OR GENERAL ANALYSES

65. **Scirica BM,** et al. for the Thrombolysis in Myocardial Ischemia III Registry Investigators. Prognosis in the thrombolysis in myocardial ischemia III registry according to the Braunwald unstable angina pectoris classification. *Am J Cardiol* 2002;90:821–826.

The Braunwald classification of UA was prospectively validated in the TIMI 3 Registry. Of 3,318 patients, rates of death or MI at 1 year were lowest in those with "primary" UA, 9.7%, versus 16.7% for those with "secondary" UA and 19.7% for those with post-MI UA ($p < 0.001$). Patients with "secondary" UA had similar extent of disease at angiography as primary UAP. Patients with class I (nonrest pain) UA had lower rates of death on MI at 1 year than patients with UAP at rest (8.2% vs. 12.5%, $p = 0.004$). Patients with ST-segment duration and those already receiving antianginal medication had worse outcomes. Thus, the Braunwald UA classification was well correlated with prognosis; patients with secondary UA, post-MI UA, and patients with pain at rest, who have higher risk for death or recurrent cardiac events, and thus deserve aggressive treatment.

66. **Armstrong PW,** et al. Acute coronary syndromes in the GUSTO-IIb trial: prognostic insights and impact of recurrent ischemia. *Circulation* 1998;98:1860–1868.

   Recurrent ischemia was approximately 50% more common in non–ST elevation patients than in ST-elevation patients (35% vs. 23%; $p < 0.001$). This may explain why the non–ST elevation group had a lower mortality rate at 30 days (3.8% vs. 6.1%; $p < 0.001$) but a similar rate by 1 year (8.8% vs. 9.6%). Compared with UA patients, NSTEMI patients had higher rates of reinfarction at 6 months (9.8% vs. 6.2%) and higher 6-month and 1-year mortality rates (8.8% vs. 5.0%; 11.1% vs. 7.0%).

67. **Farkouh ME,** et al. A clinical trial of a chest-pain observation unit for patients with unstable angina. *N Engl J Med* 1998;339:1882–1888.

   This community-based, prospective study of 424 UA patients showed that a chest pain observation unit located in the emergency department can be safe, effective, and result in cost savings. Patients with rest angina lasting longer than 20 minutes, new-onset angina on exertion (CCS class 3 or higher), and postinfarction angina were eligible. High-risk patients were excluded (e.g., ST-segment depression in several ECG leads). Eligible patients were randomized to routine hospital admission (monitored bed on cardiology service) or admission to the chest pain observation unit. No significant difference was found in the rate of cardiac events between the two groups (OR for chest pain observation unit group, 0.50; 95% CI, 0.20 to 1.24). At 6 months, chest pain observation unit patients had used less resources ($p = 0.003$ by rank-sum test).

68. **Hoffmann U,** et al. Coronary computed tomography angiography for early triage of patients with acute chest pain: the **ROMICAT** (Rule Out Myocardial Infarction using Computer Assisted Tomography) trial. *J Am Coll Cardiol* 2009;53:1642–1650.

   In 368 patients in the emergency department with chest pain of low risk (negative troponin, nonischemic ECG), the investigators performed 64-slice coronary CTA prior to admission. Results were not disclosed, and they were subsequently treated as per routine and followed up for outcomes of ACS during index hospitalization or MACEs at 6 months. Freedom from CAD on CTA was highly and negatively predictive of events, with both sensitivity and negative predictive values for AS of 100%. They found that coronary plaque and stenosis on CTA not only independently predicted ACS, but also predicted ACS incrementally over the TRS ($p < 0.0001$).

69. **Stone PH,** et al. Influence of race, sex and age of management of unstable angina and non–Q-wave MI (TIMI 3 registry). *JAMA* 1996;275:1104–1112.

   This prospective analysis of 3,318 patients showed disparities in care among blacks, women, and the elderly. Compared with non-blacks, blacks were less likely to be treated with intensive anti-ischemic therapy and to undergo invasive procedures (RR, 0.65; $p < 0.001$). However, of those who had angiography (45% of blacks and 61% of non-blacks), blacks had less extensive and severe coronary stenoses. Blacks also had less recurrent ischemia. Women also were less likely to receive intensive anti-ischemic therapy and to undergo angiography (RR, 0.71; $p < 0.001$) and had less severe and extensive coronary disease; however, they had a similar risk of experiencing an adverse cardiac event by 6 weeks. Elderly patients (older than

75 years) received less aggressive therapy and had less-frequent angiography (RR, 0.65; $p <$ 0.001) and fewer revascularization procedures (RR, 0.79; $p = 0.002$) despite having more extensive disease. At 6 weeks, the elderly had a higher incidence of adverse cardiac events (RR, 1.91; $p < 0.001$).

70. **Vaccarino V**, et al. Sex and racial differences in the management of acute myocardial infarction, 1994 through 2002. *N Engl J Med* 2005;353:671–682.

In the National Registry of Myocardial Infarction from 1994 to 2002, investigators reviewed 598,911 patients with acute MI. After multivariable adjustment, significant differences persisted in rates of reperfusion therapy (RR for white women 0.97, black men 0.91, black women 0.89, compared with white men) and angiography (0.91, 0.82, 0.76, respectively). Significant differences for use of aspirin and β-blockers in unadjusted rates were no longer significant in multivariable analysis. The only significant difference in mortality was for the comparison of black women to white men (RR 1.11). These results were unchanged over the time period studied.

71. **Popescu I**, et al. Differences in mortality and use of revascularization in black and white patients with acute MI admitted to hospitals with and without revascularization services. *JAMA* 2007;297:2489–2495.

In a study of 1,215,924 Medicare beneficiaries admitted with acute MI, the authors analyzed outcomes by race, including adjusted rates of revascularization at 30 days, mortality at 1 year, and transfer to a hospital with revascularization services (for patients presenting to hospitals without revascularization services). In adjusted analyses, the investigators found that black patients admitted with acute MI were less likely to be transferred for revascularization (hazard ratio 0.78, $p < 0.001$) and less likely to undergo revascularization in hospitals with (hazard ratio 0.71, $p < 0.001$) and without revascularization available (hazard ratio 0.68, $p < 0.001$). In the first 30 days, adjusted rates of mortality were lower for black patients ($p < 0.001$), but were higher in intervals up to 1 year ($p < 0.001$).

72. **Berger JS**, et al. Sex differences in mortality following acute coronary syndromes. *JAMA* 2009;302(8):874–882.

In a pooled sample of 11 randomized, clinical trials of ACS, the investigators assessed 30-day mortality rates of 136,247 patients by gender. Overall, 38,048 (28%) were women; 102,004 (26% women) had STEMI, 14,466 (29% women) had NSTEMI; and 19,777 (40% women) had UA. Overall, unadjusted 30-day mortality rates were 9.6% for women and 5.3% for men (OR, 1.91; 95% CI, 1.83 to 2.00). After multivariable analyses, this difference was no longer significant (OR, 1.06; 95% CI, 0.99 to 1.15). There was a significant interacting between gender and type of ACS ($p < 0.001$): in adjusted analyses, STEMI mortality rates were higher for women (OR, 1.15; 95% CI, 1.06 to 1.24), whereas NSTEMI and UA mortality rates were lower for women (OR, 0.77; 95% CI, 0.63 to 0.95 and OR, 0.55; 95% CI, 0.43 to 0.70, respectively). In further analyses of angiographic data in a subset of 35,128 patients, there were no significant differences in mortality between sexes or interaction with ACS type after multivariable analyses with adjustment for angiographic variables included. The authors conclude to suggest that angiographic differences in presentation between men and women could likely explain differences in mortality rates after ACS.

73. **Alexander JH**, et al. Prior aspirin use predicts worse outcomes in patients with non-ST elevation acute coronary syndromes. *Am J Cardiol* 1999;83:1147–1151.

This analysis of 9,461 PURSUIT trial patients found that prior aspirin users had a higher rate of death or MI at 30 days and 6 months (16.1% vs. 13.0%, $p = 0.001$; 19.9% vs. 15.9%, $p = 0.001$) despite a lower incidence of an index MI (vs. UA; 43.9% vs. 48.8%, $p = 0.001$). After adjustment for all significant, independent baseline predictors, prior aspirin users remained less likely to have an index MI (OR, 0.88; 95% CI, 0.79 to 0.97) and more likely to have MI or death at 30 days (OR, 1.16; 95% CI, 1.00 to 1.33) but not at 6 months (OR, 1.14; 95% CI, 0.98 to 1.33).

74. **Donahoe SM**, et al. Diabetes and mortality following acute coronary syndromes. *JAMA* 2007;298(7):765–775.

The investigators pooled 11 randomized trials of ACS from 1997 to 2006, to analyze outcomes in 62,036 patients with and without diabetes. In all, 46,577 had STEMI, 15,459 had UA/NSTEMI, and 10,613 (17.1%) had diabetes. Outcomes included mortality at 30 days and 1 year. After adjustment for other characteristics, diabetes predicted significantly higher 30-day mortality from UA/NSTEMI (OR, 1.78; 95% CI, 1.24 to 2.56) and STEMI (OR, 1.40; 95% CI, 1.24 to 1.57). Patients with diabetes at initial presentation also had higher 1-year mortality for both UA/NSTEMI (hazard ratio, 1.65; 95% CI, 1.30 to 2.10) and STEMI (hazard ratio, 1.22, 95% CI, 1.08 to 1.38). An interesting finding when comparing mortality rates is that diabetes associated with UA/NSTEMI appeared to portend a similar 1-year prognosis as STEMI without diabetes.

75. **Antman EM**, et al. The **TIMI Risk Score** for unstable angina/non–ST elevation MI. A method for prognostication and therapeutic decision making. *JAMA* 2000;284:835–842.

This retrospective analysis of the TIMI IIB and ESSENCE trials (see references) developed a simple risk score that has broad applicability, is easily calculated, and identifies patients with different responses to treatments for UA/NSTEMI. The test cohort was the 1,957 TIMI IIB patients who received UFH, whereas the three validation cohorts were the UFH group from ESSENCE and both enoxaparin groups. Outcomes were TRS for developing at least one component of the primary endpoint (all-cause mortality, new or recurrent MI, or ischemia requiring urgent revascularization at 14 days). The seven TRS predictor variables were age older than 65 years, more than three CAD risk factors, prior coronary stenosis of more than 50%, ST-segment deviation on initial ECG, more than two anginal events in the prior 24 hours, use of aspirin in the prior 7 days, and elevated serum cardiac markers. As the TRS increased in the test cohort, event rates increased: 4.7% for a score of 0/1; 8.3% for 2; 13.2% for 3; 19.9% for 4; 26.2% for 5; and 40.9% for 6/7 ($p < 0.001$ by χ^2 for trend). The pattern of increasing event rates with increasing TRS was confirmed in all three validation groups ($p < 0.001$). The enoxaparin groups had a slower rate of increase in event rates with an increasing TRS.

76. **Budaj A**, et al. for the CURE Trial Investigators. Benefit of clopidogrel in patients with acute coronary syndromes without ST-segment elevation in various risk groups. *Circulation* 2002;106:1622–1626.

The investigators stratified 12,562 patients in the CURE trial by TRS stratum (0–2, 3–4, or 5–7), and assessed outcomes from NSTEMI. The risk score was validated in the CURE cohort (c statistic 0.634), and use of clopidogrel significantly benefited patients at all levels of risk, for the endpoint of death, MI, or stroke: 4.1% for placebo versus 5.7% for clopidogrel in TRS 0–2 ($p < 0.04$), 9.8% versus 11.4% in TRS 3–4 ($p < 0.03$), and 15.9% versus 20.7% in TRS 5–7 ($p < 0.004$). There was no heterogeneity among the groups.

77. **Eagle KA**, et al. for the GRACE Investigators. A validated prediction model for all forms of acute coronary syndrome: estimating the risk of 6-month postdischarge death in an international registry. *JAMA* 2004;291:2727–2733.

In 17,142 patients with ACS enrolled in the GRACE registry from 1999 to 2002, investigators developed a simple regression model for mortality at 6 months. For all forms of ACS, the model included nine characteristics of presentation: age, history of MI, history of CHF, increased pulse, decreased SBP, elevated serum creatinine, elevated cardiac biomarkers, ST-segment depression on electrocardiogram, and not having in-hospital PCI. The c statistic for the development model was 0.81. It was subsequently validated in another GRACE cohort of 7,638 patients admitted from 2002 to 2003 (c statistic 0.75). Six-month mortality rates between the two cohorts were similar (4.8% in development cohort vs. 4.7% in validation cohort). Additionally, the GRACE score was also validated in a Canadian cohort, which implemented it to predict in-hospital mortality in patients with ACS (see *Am Heart J* 2009;158:392–399).

78. **Yan AT**, et al. Risk scores for risk stratification in acute coronary syndromes: useful but simpler is not necessarily better. *Eur Heart J* 2007;28:1072–1078.

In a prospective Canadian registry of 1,728 patients with UA/NSTEMI, the investigators calculated for each patient their PURSUIT risk score, TRS, and GRACE risk score. Each demonstrated decent predictive value for the endpoint of in-hospital mortality (c statistics 0.68 for TIMI, 0.80 for PURSUIT, and 0.81 for GRACE, all $p < 0.001$), as well as 1-year mortality (c statistics 0.69, 0.77, 0.79, respectively, all $p < 0.0001$). Significant predictive advantage was identified for the PURSUIT and GRACE risk scores over the TRS ($p < 0.04$ for each comparison to the TRS for both in-hospital and 1-year mortality rates).

Biomarkers

REVIEW ARTICLES AND MULTIMARKER STUDIES

79. **Sabatine MS**, et al. Multimarker approach to risk stratification in non-ST elevation acute coronary syndromes: simultaneous assessment of troponin I, C-reactive protein, and B-type natriuretic peptide. *Circulation* 2002;105:1760–1763.

In analysis of 450 patients with ACS in the OPUS-TIMI 16 trial, the investigators measured troponin I, CRP, and BNP. With each additional biomarker elevation, they identified significant increases in the risk of the composite endpoint of death, MI, or CHF ($p = 0.01$ for the trend). This was consistent up to 10 months. The assessment of risk by these three biomarkers was then validated with similar results in 1,635 patients in the TACTICS-TIMI 18 trial.

80. **Morrow DA**, Braunwald E. Future of biomarkers in acute coronary syndromes moving toward a multimarker strategy. *Circulation* 2003;108:250–252.

The authors address the evolution of multiple biomarkers in ACS, their role in relation to the pathophysiology of ACS, as well as their clinical utility for risk stratification and prognostication.

81. **Eggers KM**, et al. Prognostic value of biomarkers during and after non-ST-segment elevation acute coronary syndrome. *J Am Coll Cardiol* 2009;54:357–364.

In 877 patients with UA/NSTEMI in the FRISC study, the authors measured CRP, BNP, and troponin I, and estimated glomerular filtration rate (GFR) at randomization, 6 weeks, and 6 months. At randomization, BNP was the strongest predictor of mortality at 5 years (adjusted hazard ratio 1.7, $p < 0.001$). Predictive value of CRP was increased later in follow-up.

TROPONINS

82. **Hamm CW**, et al. The prognostic value of serum troponin T in unstable angina. *N Engl J Med* 1992;327:146–150 (editorial, 192–194).

This prospective, multicenter analysis focused on 109 consecutive UA patients (84 with rest angina and 25 with accelerated or subacute angina) who had CK, CK-MB, and troponin T sampled every 8 hours for 2 days after hospital admission. Troponin T was detected (range, 0.20 to 3.64 μg/L) in 39% of the 84 patients with rest angina; only 3 of these patients had an elevated CK-MB (1 of the 3 with negative troponin T). Positive troponin-T patients had high event rates, with MI occurring in 30%, and in-hospital death in 15%. In contrast, only 1 of the 51 patients with rest angina and a negative troponin T had an MI ($p < 0.001$), and this patient died ($p = 0.03$). Troponin T was not detected in any of the 25 patients with accelerated or subacute angina.

83. **Lindahl B,** et al. Relation between troponin T and the risk of subsequent cardiac events in unstable coronary artery disease. *Circulation* 1996;93:1651–1657.

This prospective analysis of 976 FRISC patients showed that 5-month rates of cardiac death and MI correlate with troponin T. In the first quintile (maximum troponin T in first 24 hours <0.06 μg/L), the incidence of death and MI was 4.3%; the second quintile (0.06 to 0.18 μg/L), 10.5%; the top three quintiles, 16.1%. In multivariate analysis, independent predictors of death and MI included troponin T (other predictors were age, hypertension, number of antianginal drugs, and rest ECG changes). A subsequent analysis showed that the dalteparin group had a lower rate of death and MI only if troponin T was ≥0.1 μg/L (7.4% vs. 14.2%; $p < 0.01$).

84. **Antman E,** et al. Cardiac-specific troponin I levels to predict the risk of mortality in patients with acute coronary syndromes. *N Engl J Med* 1996;335:1342–1349 (editorial, 1388–1389).

This analysis focused on 1,404 TIMI 3B patients. Troponin I was elevated (≥0.4 ng/mL) in 573 patients and associated with a significantly increased 42-day mortality rate (3.7% vs. 1.0%; $p < 0.001$). Each 1-ng/mL increase in troponin I was associated with a mortality increase: ≤0.4, 1%; 0.4 to 0.9, 1.7%; 1 to 1.9, 3.4%; 2 to 4.9, 3.7%; 5 to 8.9, 6%; and ≥9, 7.5%. If no CK-MB elevation was present (948 patients), a troponin I elevation was still associated with increased mortality: 2.5% vs. 0.8% (RR, 3.0; 95% CI, 0.97 to 9.2).

85. **Hamm CW,** et al. Benefit of abciximab in patients with refractory unstable angina in relation to serum troponin T levels. *N Engl J Med* 1999;340:1623–1629.

This analysis focused on 890 CAPTURE trial patients with UA who had serum samples drawn at the time of randomization to abciximab or placebo. Patients with postinfarction angina were excluded. Among placebo-treated patients, the incidence of death or nonfatal MI at 6 months was threefold higher in patients with elevated troponin-T levels (more than 0.1 ng/mL; 23.9% vs. 7.5%; $p < 0.001$), whereas no difference was found among abciximab-treated patients (9.5% vs. 9.4%). The lower incidence of death or MI in elevated troponin-T patients receiving abciximab compared with placebo (RR, 0.32; $p = 0.002$) was owing to the significant reduction in MI rate (OR, 0.23; $p < 0.001$). In patients without elevated troponin-T levels, no significant benefit was associated with abciximab treatment.

86. **Heescham C,** et al. Troponin concentrations for stratification of patients with acute coronary syndromes in relation to therapeutic efficacy of tirofiban: PRISM Study Investigators. Platelet Receptor Inhibition in Ischemic Syndrome Management. *Lancet* 1999;354:1757–1762.

A total of 629 (28.3%) patients had troponin-I concentrations higher than the diagnostic threshold of 1.0 μg/L, and 644 (29.0%) had troponin-T concentrations higher than 0.1 μg/L. At 30 days, death or MI occurred in 13.0% of troponin I–positive patients compared with 4.9% for troponin I–negative patients ($p < 0.0001$), and 13.7% compared with 3.5% for troponin T ($p < 0.001$). At 30 days, in troponin I–positive patients, tirofiban lowered the risk of death [adjusted hazard ratio, 0.25 (95% CI, 0.09 to 0.68); $p = 0.004$] and MI [hazard ratio, 0.37 (0.16 to 0.84); $p = 0.01$). By contrast, no treatment effect was seen for troponin I–negative patients. Similar benefits were seen for troponin T–positive patients.

87. **Morrow DA,** et al. for the TACTICS-TIMI 18 Investigators. Ability of minor elevations of troponin I and T to predict benefit from an early invasive strategy in patients with unstable angina and non-ST elevation myocardial infarction: results from a randomized trial. *JAMA* 2001;286:2405–2412.

This prospective study obtained baseline troponin-level data in 1,821 ACS patients (of 2,220 total). An elevated cTnI level (0.1 ng/mL or greater; $n \geq 1,087$) was associated with a significant reduction in death, MI, or rehospitalization for ACS at 6 months with the invasive versus conservative strategy (15.3% vs. 25.0%; OR, 0.54; 95% CI, 0.40 to 0.73). Low-level cTnI elevations (0.1 to 0.4 ng/mL) also were associated with a benefit of an invasive strategy (30-day incidence of composite endpoint, 4.4% vs. 16.5%; OR, 0.24; 95% CI, 0.08 to 0.69). Patients with cTnI levels less than 0.1 ng/mL had no significant benefit from an early invasive strategy (16.0% vs. 12.4%; OR, 1.4; 95% CI, 0.89 to 2.05; $p < 0.001$ for interaction). Similar results were observed with cTnT. Furthermore, even in patients without significant CAD on angiography, elevated troponin in patients presenting with ACS predicted a high risk for death or reinfarction (see *J Am Coll Cardiol* 2005;45:19–24).

INFLAMMATORY MARKERS

88. **Haverkate F,** et al. Production of C-reactive protein and risk of coronary events in stable and unstable angina. *Lancet* 1997;349:362–366.

This analysis focused on 2,121 outpatients with angina (1,030 unstable, 743 stable, 348 atypical); all had baseline angiography. At 2-year follow-up, patients with CRP in the fifth quintile (more than 3.6 mg/L) had a twofold higher risk of a coronary event. Thus, acute-phase responses are probably not due to myocardial necrosis.

89. **Toss H,** et al. Prognostic influence of increased fibrinogen and C-reactive protein levels in unstable coronary artery disease. *Circulation* 1997;96:4204–4210.

This analysis of 965 FRISC study patients with UA or non–Q wave MI showed the independent predictive value of fibrinogen and CRP. Fibrinogen and CRP were measured at inclusion and related to outcomes at 5 months. Fibrinogen by tertiles (<3.38, 3.38 to 3.99, and more than 4.0 g/L) was associated with death in 1.6%, 4.6%, and 6.9% ($p = 0.005$) and death and MI in 9.3%, 14.2%, and 19.1% of patients ($p = 0.002$). CRP by tertiles (<2, 2 to 10, and more than 10 mg/L) was associated with death in 2.2%, 3.6%, and 7.5% of patients ($p = 0.003$). In multiple logistic regression analysis, increased fibrinogen levels were independently associated with death and death and/or MI ($p = 0.013$), and CRP was independently associated with death ($p = 0.012$).

90. **Morrow DA,** et al. C-reactive protein is a potent predictor of mortality independent of and in combination with troponin T in acute coronary syndromes: a TIMI-11 substudy. *J Am Coll Cardiol* 1998;31:1460–1465.

A total of 437 UA/non–Q wave MI patients had quantitative CRP and rapid troponin-T assays performed. CRP was higher among patients who died than in survivors (7.2 vs. 1.3 mg/dL; $p = 0.0038$). Patients with CRP = 1.55 mg/dL and an early positive troponin-T assay result (≥ 10 minutes) had the highest mortality rates, followed by those with either CRP = 1.55 or early positive troponin-T assay results, whereas those with a low CRP and negative troponin-T assay results were at very low risk (9.10% vs. 4.65% vs. 0.36%; $p = 0.0003$).

91. **James SK,** et al. for GUSTO-IV-ACS Investigators. Troponin and C-reactive protein have different relations to subsequent mortality and myocardial infarction after acute coronary syndrome: a GUSTO-IV substudy. *J Am Coll Cardiol* 2003;41:916–924.

The investigators measured baseline levels of troponin T and CRP in 7,108 patients in the GUSTO IV trial, and assessed outcomes at 30 days. Both biomarkers significantly and independently predicted mortality in multivariable analysis. Troponin T elevation also helped predict recurrent MI, whereas CRP did not.

92. **Blake GJ,** Ridker PM. C-reactive protein and other inflammatory risk markers in acute coronary syndromes. *J Am Coll Cardiol* 2003;41(4 suppl S):37S–42S.

The authors review the additional prognostic benefit of CRP in patients with ACS. In contrast to those markers of acute myocardial necrosis, they offer CRP as a longer term prognostic tool, as well as a marker of which patients might be most likely to benefit from additional pharmacologic therapy, as well as lifestyle modifications.

93. **Schiele F**, et al. C-reactive protein improves risk prediction in patients with acute coronary syndromes. *Eur Heart J* 2009;31:290–297.

The investigators measured the GRACE risk score in 1,408 patients with ACS, and then added CRP to the prediction model for the outcome of 30-day mortality. CRP significantly improved the GRACE risk score model (c statistic from 0.795 to 0.823), and was an independent predictor of mortality.

94. **Morrow DA**, et al. Concurrent evaluation of novel cardiac biomarkers in acute coronary syndrome: myeloperoxidase and soluble CD40 ligand and the risk of recurrent ischaemic events in TACTICS-TIMI 18. *Eur Heart J* 2008;29:1096–1102.

In the TACTICS-TIMI 18 trial, the investigators measured novel biomarkers MPO and soluble CD40 ligand (sCD40L). When added to BNP and troponin I, they found MPO independently added to short-term prediction of recurrent ischemic events; however, sCD40L did not.

B-TYPE NATRIURETIC PEPTIDE

95. **de Lemos JA,** et al. The prognostic value of B-type natriuretic peptide in patients with acute coronary syndromes. *N Engl J Med* 2001;345:1014–1021.

This substudy of 2,525 ACS patients in the OPUS-TIMI 16 trial measured BNP in plasma samples obtained at mean of 40 ± 20 hours after the onset of symptoms. Baseline BNP level was significantly correlated with the risk of death, heart failure, and new or recurrent MI at 30 days and 10 months. The unadjusted rate of death increased in a stepwise fashion among patients in increasing quartiles of baseline BNP levels ($p < 0.001$). This mortality association was significant in the major patient subgroups [STEMI ($p = 0.02$), NSTEMI ($p < 0.001$), and UA ($p < 0.001$)]. After risk-factor adjustment, the ORs for death at 10 months in the second, third, and fourth quartiles of BNP were 3.8 (95% CI, 1.1 to 13.3), 4.0 (95% CI, 1.2 to 13.7), and 5.8 (95% CI, 1.7 to 19.7).

96. **Morrow DA**, et al. Evaluation of B-type natriuretic peptide for risk assessment in unstable angina/non-ST-elevation myocardial infarction: B-type natriuretic peptide and prognosis in TACTICS-TIMI 18. *J Am Coll Cardiol* 2003;41:1264–1272.

The investigators measured BNP, in addition to troponin I, in 1,676 patients with UA/NSTEMI in the TACTICS-TIMI 18 trial. At a cutoff of 80 pg/mL, patients with elevated BNP above that threshold had a higher rate of death at 7 days (2.5% vs. 0.7%, $p = 0.006$). At 6 months, elevated BNP predicted mortality (8.4% vs. 1.8%, $p < 0.0001$), and this remained significant in multivariable analysis including clinical predictors, as well as troponin I level. Risk of developing CHF was also significantly higher in the elevated BNP at 30 days (5.9% vs. 1.0%, $p < 0.0001$).

97. **Morrow DA**, et al. for the A to Z Investigators. Prognostic value of serial B-type natriuretic peptide testing during follow-up of patients with unstable coronary artery disease. *JAMA* 2005;294:2866–2871.

In a substudy of the A to Z trial, the investigators sought to identify the utility of serial measurements of BNP in patients following any ACS. In 4,497 patients with UA/NSTEMI or STEMI, they measured BNP prior to discharge, at 4 months, and at 12 months to assess its prognostic significance for death or new CHF at 2 years. At each time period, elevated BNP (>80 pg/mL) was significantly associated with elevated risk of death or new CHF. Patients with newly elevated BNP at 4 months were at increased risk of the primary outcome, whereas those whose BNP levels normalized from discharge to 4 months had only modestly increased risk (compared with patients that had normal BNP at both visits). The authors conclude that serial measurements of BNP could provide improved prognostic ability, as well as potentially facilitate clinical decision-making.

SPECIFIC TESTS: ANGIOGRAPHY, ECG, AND HOLTER

98. **Dewood MA,** et al. Coronary arteriographic findings soon after non-Q wave MI. *N Engl J Med* 1986;315:417–423.

   In this angiography study, 341 non–Q wave MI patients were divided into three groups: angiography at $\leq$24, 24 to 72, and more than 72 hours for 7 days. Frequency of total occlusion and visible collateral vessels both increased with time [26% at $\leq$24 hours vs. 42% at $\geq$72 hours ($p < 0.05$); 27% vs. 42% ($p < 0.05$)]. The subtotal occlusion rate decreased with time.

99. **Cannon CP,** et al. The electrocardiogram predicts one year outcome of patients with unstable angina and non–Q-wave MI: results of TIMI 3 Registry Ancillary Study. *J Am Coll Cardiol* 1997;30:133–140.

   This prospective study focused on 1,416 patients, 14.3% with new ST deviation $\geq$1 mm; 21.9% had isolated T-wave inversion, and 9% had LBBB. The incidence of death and MI at 1 year was 11% in the group with ST changes [$p < 0.001$ (vs. no ST deviation)], 6.8% with T-wave inversion, and 8.2% without ECG changes. Two high-risk groups were identified: one with LBBB [22.9%; RR, 2.80 (multivariate analysis)] and the other with 0.5-mm ST changes (16.3%; RR, 2.45).

100. **Al-Khatib SM,** et al. Sustained ventricular arrhythmias among patients with acute coronary syndromes with no ST-segment elevation. *Circulation* 2002;106:309–312.

   Data analyzed from 26,416 patients in GUSTO-IIb, PURSUIT, PARAGON-A, and PARAGON-B trials. Independent predictors of in-hospital ventricular fibrillation included prior MI, prior hypertension, chronic obstructive pulmonary disease, and ST-segment changes at presentation. In-hospital VT was predicted by prior MI, COPD, and ST changes. In Cox proportional-hazards modeling, in-hospital VF and VT were independently associated with markedly higher rates of 30-day mortality (hazard ratio, 23.2; 95% CI, 18.1 to 29.8, for VF; and hazard ratio, 7.6; 95% CI, 5.5 to 10.4, for VT) and 6-month mortality (hazard ratio, 14.8; 95% CI, 12.1 to 18.3, for VF; and hazard ratio, 5.0; 95% CI, 3.8 to 6.5, for VT). After exclusion of heart failure patients, those in cardiogenic shock, and those who died within 24 hours of enrollment, these differences remained significant.

CHAPTER 4

ST-Elevation Myocardial Infarction

Christopher P. Cannon and Benjamin A. Steinberg

EPIDEMIOLOGY

In the United States, in approximately 1.2 million patients, an acute myocardial infarction (AMI) develops each year; 40% to 50% are accompanied by ST-segment elevation. Between 25% and 30% of nonfatal MIs are unrecognized by the patient and are discovered by routine electrocardiogram (ECG) or at postmortem examination. The overall associated early mortality rate ranges from 5% to 30%, depending on patient characteristics, with half of the deaths [most of them due to ventricular fibrillation (VF)] occurring before the patient receives medical attention. Among those who arrive at a hospital, approximately 25% of deaths occur in the first 48 hours. Men typically experience the first MI 10 years earlier in life than do women.

PATHOGENESIS

ST-elevation MI (STEMI) is the result of thrombotic coronary artery occlusion in more than 90% of patients. Nonatherosclerotic causes include emboli (atrial fibrillation, endocarditis), cocaine, trauma/contusion, arteritis, spasm, and dissection. Non-STEMIs are typically the result of nonocclusive thrombus over an underlying stenosis (see Chapter 3). Approximately two thirds of MIs occur in plaques with less than 50% underlying stenosis. Inflammation appears to play a role in plaque rupture. Extent of damage is related to the site and duration of occlusion and the presence or absence of adequate collateral supply (see *Circulation* 2001;104;365–372).

DIAGNOSIS

Even with a strong clinical suspicion of MI based on history and physical examination, MI is subsequently confirmed in only 85% to 90% of patients. The revised 2007 joint ESC/ACCF/AHA/WHF criteria require detection of a rise and/or fall in cardiac biomarkers (including at least one value over the upper reference limit of normal), as well as at least one of the following: symptoms of ischemia, serial ECG changes, or imaging suggestive of new loss of viable myocardial tissue. Alternatively, sudden, unexpected cardiac death accompanied by either significant ECG changes [new ST elevation or left bundle branch block (LBBB)] or thrombotic coronary occlusion on angiography or autopsy can also define an MI. Separate definitions for periprocedural MI [for percutaneous coronary intervention (PCI), coronary artery bypass graft (CABG)] have also been formally outlined (see *J Am Coll Cardiol* 2000;36:959; *Eur Heart J* 2007;28:2525–2538).

Pain

The pain of MI is often described as pressure and typically lasts for more than 30 minutes. In one study, the probability of MI (or unstable angina) was very low if (a) the pain was sharp or stabbing, (b) the pain was reproducible by palpation or was pleuritic or positional, and (c) the patient had no history of angina or MI.

Electrocardiography

Early ECG may show only hyperacute T waves. ST elevation 1 mm or more in two contiguous leads is highly sensitive, but also can be seen in left ventricular (LV) hypertrophy, early repolarization, and pericarditis. New LBBB should raise strong clinical suspicion of MI. Approximately 75% of STEMIs evolve Q waves.

With right ventricular (RV) infarction, ST elevation is seen in the V_4R lead with a sensitivity of approximately 90% and specificity of approximately 80% (212). With posterior infarction, precordial ST-segment depression is seen in leads V_1 and V_2 and/or ST elevation in leads V_7 to V_9 (see also *N Engl J Med* 2003;348:933–940) (9,218).

Echocardiography

Echocardiography is useful if the ECG results have been nondiagnostic and in those with suspected aortic dissection. Areas of abnormal wall motion are typically observed in patients with AMI, especially those with transmural involvement.

Serum Markers

Creatine kinase (CK)-MB and troponin I (TnI) and troponin T (TnT) exceed normal ranges within 4 to 8 hours, and levels peak at 24 hours (CK-MB peak occurs sooner with successful thrombolysis). CK-MB levels normalize by 48 to 72 hours, whereas TnI remains elevated for up to 7 to 10 days, and TnT for up to 14 days, allowing detection of MI days before, but reducing their value in the diagnosis of recurrent MI within this time frame. TnI and TnT are cardiac specific, and levels strongly correlate with mortality (15). Myoglobin peak levels are reached earlier (within 1 to 4 hours), with a rapid increase indicative of successful reperfusion (17). Myoglobin also has an excellent negative predictive value (12), yet is less specific for cardiac injury than troponin.

TREATMENT

Aspirin

In the second International Study of Infarct Survival (ISIS-2) (25), aspirin (162 mg chewed, to ensure rapid therapeutic blood levels) use was associated with a 23% lower mortality rate, as well as significantly fewer reinfarctions and strokes (see Table 4.1). Aspirin and thrombolytic therapy have an additive benefit (42% lower mortality rate in ISIS-2). If a patient has an aspirin allergy, clopidogrel (75 mg daily) can be substituted because it showed a slight benefit compared with aspirin in more than 8,000 patients with a recent MI (CAPRIE trial; see Chapter 1).

Clopidogrel

A novel antiplatelet agent, clopidogrel blocks platelet activation by inhibiting the ADP receptor. Its efficacy in STEMI was demonstrated in the Clopidogrel as Adjunctive Reperfusion Therapy (CLARITY)–Thrombolysis in Myocardial Infarction (TIMI) 28 study, in which 3,491 patients with STEMI were randomized to clopidogrel or placebo, in addition to fibrinolysis and contemporary therapies (28). Patients receiving clopidogrel had a significantly lower rate of the composite endpoint of infarct-artery occlusion on angiography (within 48 to 192 hours), or death or recurrent MI before angiography (15.0% vs. 21.7%; $p < 0.001$). At 30 days, there was also a significant 20% reduction in adverse clinical events without a significant increase in bleeding events. Data from the ClOpidogrel and Metoprolol in Myocardial Infarction Trial (COMMIT) confirmed these findings, with a significant

TABLE 4.1 Treatment of ST-Elevation Myocardial Infarction

Beneficial	Limited Data or No Benefit	Special Situations	Harmful
Aspirin		Coumadin	Nifedipine
β-Blockers	Nitrates	Vasopressors	Lidocaine
Thrombolytics	Magnesium	Diuretics	
Primary PCI	Verapamil	Insulin	
ACE inhibitors		Intra-aortic balloon pump	
GP IIb/IIIa inhibitors	Amiodarone	Surgery	
Anticoagulants	Adenosine		

PCI, percutaneous coronary intervention; ACE, angiotensin-converting enzyme; GP, glycoprotein.

reduction in total mortality seen as well, thus expanding clopidogrel's application to patients who received either fibrinolysis or no reperfusion therapy (29).

The 2007 update to the guidelines subsequently made clopidogrel treatment a class I recommendation for all patients with STEMI, regardless of reperfusion strategy (if any).

A second thienopyridine, prasugrel, is the latest to be approved; however, its indication is only for use during PCI in the setting of acute coronary syndromes (30; see also Chapter 3). A reversible inhibitor of the P2Y12 receptor, ticagrelor, also has been shown to be beneficial in ACS patients, including patients with STEMI undergoing primary PCI. in the PLATO trial (see chapter 3).

β-Blockers

Metoprolol, 5 mg intravenously (i.v.), may be given every 2 to 5 minutes for three doses along with 25 mg orally, and then, if tolerated, up to 50 mg every 6 hours (ultimately converted to twice-daily dosing). Alternatively, atenolol, 5 to 10 mg, may be administered i.v., and then 100 mg/day orally; or carvedilol can be started, initially 6.25 mg once daily, and titrated up to 25 mg twice daily over a 4- to 6-week period.

Contraindications to the use of β-blockers include hypotension [systolic blood pressure (SBP) < 100 mm Hg], bradycardia [heart rate (HR) < 60 beats/min], severe LV failure, PR interval greater than 0.24 seconds, second- or third-degree heart block, severe chronic obstructive pulmonary disease (COPD), asthma, and insulin-dependent diabetes with frequent hypoglycemia. If β-blockade is still desired, the clinician should consider using esmolol (500 μg/kg/min for 1 minute, and then 50 to 200 μg/kg/min).

Early randomized trials showed mortality benefits with timolol, propranolol, and metoprolol (70,71,77). In the large ISIS-1 trial (73), use of atenolol (5 to 10 mg i.v., and then 100 mg/day orally) was associated with a 15% mortality benefit. In the TIMI IIB trial (74), immediate initiation of β-blockade was shown to be superior to delayed initiation (at 6 to 8 days). A meta-analysis of randomized trials (most completed before the widespread use of thrombolysis and aspirin) showed a 13% mortality reduction with early initiation of a β-blocker agent. However, even delayed therapy provides substantial benefit, as shown in the early placebo-controlled trials (70,71). β-Blockade also was associated with a decreased incidence of cardiac rupture and VF (78). One analysis showed that the benefits of β-blockade are independent of thrombolytic and angiotensin-converting enzyme (ACE) inhibitor use.

However, in the latest and largest trial of early β-blockade in acute MI, the COMMIT enrolled 45,852 patients within 24 hours of suspected acute MI and randomized to early metoprolol (intravenously then oral) or placebo (there was also an antiplatelet agent randomization in the trial, as discussed later). β-Blockade did not reduce the incidence of the primary endpoint, a composite of death, reinfarction, or cardiac arrest; however, it did reduce the rates of reinfarction and VF at the expense of increased risk of cardiogenic shock. The trial underscored the need for attentive hemodynamic evaluation and monitoring prior to the use of β-blockade in patients with acute MI, and this impact was highlighted in the most recent guidelines (79). In 2007, the ACC/AHA guidelines added a class III recommendation that "It may be harmful to administer intravenously beta blockers to UA/NSTEMI patients who have contraindications to beta blockade (as noted above), signs of heart failure or low-output state, or other risk factors for cardiogenic shock, which include age greater than 70 years, systolic blood pressure less than 120 mmHg, sinus tachycardia greater than 110 or heart rate less than 60, presentation more than 6 hour after symptom onset."

The newer agent carvedilol, which is both a β and an α antagonist, has shown significant promise in AMI patients and is now indicated for use in post-MI patients with LV dysfunction. In the CAPRICORN trial (76), which enrolled 1,959 patients with an ejection fraction (EF) of 40% or less, long-term use of carvedilol was associated with a 23% relative reduction in all-cause mortality compared with placebo. These beneficial effects are additive to those provided by ACE inhibitors. Additional agents new to the market, including nebivolol (Bystolic), are primarily approved for hypertension and have not been sufficiently evaluated in the treatment of acute MI.

Angiotensin-converting Enzyme Inhibitors

Captopril, 6.25 to 50 mg, three times daily (rapidly titrated); lisinopril, 5 to 20 mg daily; and ramipril, 2.5 to 5 mg twice daily are used most commonly. Early initiation of ACE inhibition was found to decrease mortality in two large placebo-controlled trials. In Gruppo Italiano per lo Studio della Sopravvivenza nell' Infarto Miocardico (GISSI-3) (168), use of lisinopril (5 to 10 mg daily) was associated with a 12% mortality reduction, whereas in ISIS-4 (170), use of captopril (initially 6.25 mg, titrated to maximum 50 mg) was associated with a 7% mortality reduction (greatest benefit in those with anterior MI). Among patients with LV dysfunction, mortality was reduced by approximately 20% to 30% by oral ACE inhibition [Survival and Ventricular Enlargement (SAVE), Acute Infarction Ramipril Efficacy (AIRE), and Trandolapril Cardiac Evaluation (TRACE) trials (165,167)]. Intravenously administration was used in the Cooperative New Scandinavian Enalapril Survival Study (CONSENSUS II) and was deemed harmful (166). A meta-analysis of 15 trials with more than 100,000 patients showed a 7% relative risk reduction (RRR), with the majority of benefit seen in anterior MIs (1.2% absolute mortality benefit vs. 0.1% for inferior MIs) (164). Approximately one third of the benefit of ACE inhibition is seen in the first few days after MI. Based on these data, current class I indications are as follows: (a) within 24 hours with anterior ST elevation or evidence of congestive heart failure (CHF) and (b) left ventricular ejection fraction (LVEF) less than 40% or evidence of CHF during or after recovery.

Results from trials of angiotensin II receptor blockers (ARBs) confirm that ACE inhibitors should remain first-line therapy in high-risk AMI patients. For example, in the OPTIMAAL study (172), losartan was compared with captopril in 5,477 MI patients within 10 days of presentation, and a nonsignificant trend toward an increased incidence of mortality was found with losartan (18.2% vs.

16.4%; $p = 0.069$). In patients who cannot tolerate ACE inhibitors, ARBs appear beneficial. The large VALIANT study evaluated valsartan compared with or in addition to captopril in 14,703 post-MI patients complicated by heart failure and/or LV dysfunction. There was no difference among all three groups (valsartan alone, captopril alone, or valsartan and captopril) in the primary endpoint of death from any cause at median follow-up of 2 years. The combination of valsartan and captopril did increase the rates of adverse events (173). This finding, combined with other trials showing parity of ARB with ACE inhibitors, has led the 2009 ACC/AHA STEMI guideline focused update to add ARB as an equally suitable choice as ACE inhibitor for STEMI patients (2).

Thrombolytic Therapy

Thrombolytic therapy confers a 20% to 25% mortality benefit. Time to treatment is important: a 6.5% absolute mortality benefit if given in the first hour versus 2% to 3% if given after 1 to 6 hours (**Fig. 4.1**) (82). No benefit results if thrombolytic therapy is given after 12 hours (104). The largest absolute benefit is seen in those with LBBB and anterior MI (**Fig. 4.2**).

Figure 4.1 • Absolute 35-day mortality reduction versus treatment delay. ●, Information from trials included in Fibrinolytic Therapy Trialists (FTT) analysis, which found a linear relation between treatment delay and absolute mortality benefit (*dotted line*). ○, Information from additional trials. □, Data beyond scale of *x/y* cross. ■, Average effects in six time-to-treatment groups. (Areas of squares are inversely proportional to variance of absolute benefit described.) Analysis by Boersma et al., of randomized trials with 100 or more patients (50,246 patients), yielded a nonlinear regression curve (*solid line*), suggesting greatest benefit with time saved early after symptom onset. (Reprinted from Boersma E, Maas A, Deckers J, et al. Early thrombolytic treatment in acute myocardial infarction: reappraisal of the golden hour. *Lancet* 1996;348(9030):771–775, with permission from Elsevier.)

Figure 4.2 • Mortality differences during days 0 to 35 subdivided by presentation features in a collaborative overview of nine thrombolytic trials. Absolute mortality rates are shown for the fibrinolytic and control groups in the center portion of the figure for each of the clinical features at presentation listed on the left side of the figure. The ratio of the odds of death in the fibrinolytic group to that in the control group is shown for each subdivision (■), along with its 99% confidence interval (*horizontal line*). The summary OR at the bottom of the figure corresponds to an 18% proportional reduction in 35-day mortality and is highly statistically significant. The absolute reduction is nine deaths per 1,000 patients treated with thrombolytic agents. (Reprinted from Fibrinolytic Therapy Trialists' (FTT) Collaborative Group. Indications for fibrinolytic therapy in suspected acute myocardial infarction: collaborative overview of early mortality and major morbidity results from all randomised trials of more than 1000 patients. *Lancet* 1994;343(8893):311, with permission from Elsevier.)

INDICATIONS FOR THROMBOLYSIS

Thrombolysis should be considered if symptoms have been present for 12 hours or less (3 hours or less preferred) and ST elevation is 1 mm or more in contiguous precordial leads in anatomically related limb leads, or if new LBBB is present. Thrombolysis is underused, given to only 65% to 70% of eligible patients (83).

CONTRAINDICATIONS

Contraindications include substantial gastrointestinal (GI) bleeding, aortic dissection (known or suspected), intracranial neoplasm/aneurysm/arteriovenous malformation, trauma or surgery in the prior 2 weeks, pregnancy, prior hemorrhagic stroke, or any stroke within the prior year.

Relative contraindications include nonhemorrhagic stroke more than 1 year earlier, active peptic ulcer disease, coumadin use, bleeding diathesis, prolonged cardiopulmonary resuscitation (CPR), SBP 180 mm Hg or higher, or diastolic BP 110 mm Hg or higher.

Advanced age is not a contraindication (class IIa if older than 75 years). These patients have increased complications (especially intracranial hemorrhage) but a substantial absolute mortality reduction.

Prehospital administration has been shown to confer a benefit in several trials (103,105). A systematic overview showed a significant 17% mortality reduction. The magnitude of benefit correlates with time saved; in the ER-TIMI 19 trial, the median time saved was 32 minutes (107).

COMMON AGENTS

Streptokinase

Intravenously streptokinase (SK) regimens proved superior to placebo in the trial of the GISSI-1 (18% lower mortality) (98) and ISIS-2 (25% lower mortality) (see Table 4.2) (99). SK was comparable with tissue plasminogen activator (tPA) in GISSI-2 and ISIS-3 (87,88), but was inferior to it in the Global Utilization of Strategies to Open Occluded Arteries (GUSTO I) study (see the section "Tissue Plasminogen Activator") (89). This agent is routinely used in certain parts of the world because of its lower cost.

Tissue Plasminogen Activator

A clear mortality benefit with tPA compared with placebo was shown in the Anglo-Scandinavian Study of Early Thrombolysis (ASSET) (101). When compared with SK in the large GISSI-2 and ISIS-3 trials, mortality rates were similar. However, the front-loaded tPA regimen was not used, and tPA was given without heparin or with subcutaneous (s.c.) heparin. The now standard front-loaded regimen (15-mg bolus, and then 50 mg over a 30-minute period, and 35 mg over the final 60 minutes) was shown to achieve earlier patency with better TIMI grade 3 flow at 60 and 90 minutes. This also was demonstrated in TIMI-4 (91) and the GUSTO Angiography substudy (90).

In the GUSTO I trial (89), the tPA and Intravenously heparin group had the best outcome: 6.3% 30-day mortality versus 7.2% and 7.4% in the SK groups ($p <$ 0.001). The greatest benefit was seen in those patients with large anterior MIs.

Reteplase

A double-bolus regimen of reteplase (rPA) was approved for use by the U.S. Food and Drug Administration (FDA) based on demonstrated equivalence to SK in the

TABLE 4.2 Characteristics of Commonly Used Fibrinolytic Agents

Agent	Dosage	90-Minute TIMI Grade 3 Flow	Heparin	Allergy	Cost
SK	1.5 million U over 60 min	30–35%	No	Yes	Low
tPA	15-mg bolus, 0.75 mg/kg over 30 min, and then 0.5 mg/kg over 60 min (maximum, 100 mg)	54–60%	Yes	No	High
TNK	Bolus over 5–10 min (30 mg if <60 kg, 35 mg if 60–69 kg, 40 mg if 70–79 kg, 45 mg if 80–89 kg, 50 mg if ≥90 kg)	~60%	Yes	No	High
rPA	10 + 10 U given 30 min apart	~60%	Yes	No	High

TIMI, Thrombolysis in Myocardial Infarction; tPA, tissue plasminogen activator; TNK, tenecteplase; rPA, reteplase. (From Refs. 87, 88, and 91.)

International Joint Efficacy Comparison of Thrombolytics (INJECT) trial (92). In the RAPID II angiographic trial (93), rPA showed better TIMI grade 3 flow at 90 minutes compared with front-loaded tPA (60% vs. 45%; $p = 0.01$); however, mortality was similar to that with tPA in the large GUSTO-III study (94).

Tenecteplase

Tenecteplase (TNK) is a single-bolus thrombolytic that achieves TIMI grade 3 flow similar to or slightly higher than that of tPA alone. The Assessment of the

Safety and Efficacy of a New Thrombolytic: TNK (ASSENT-2) trial enrolled 16,949 patients and showed TNK to be statistically equivalent to tPA alone (30-day mortality rates, 6.17% and 6.15%) (96). A potential benefit of bolus administration is ease of administration. [In GUSTO I, incorrect dosing of tPA was associated with higher mortality (7.7% vs. 5.5% for correct dosing; $p < 0.0001$).] Intracranial hemorrhage rates were similar, whereas noncerebral bleeding occurred less frequently with TNK (26.4% vs. 29.0%).

Reduced-dose Thrombolysis in Conjunction with Glycoprotein IIb/IIIa Inhibitors

See the section "Intravenous Glycoprotein IIb/IIIa Inhibitors."

PROGNOSTIC INDICATORS

1. Early infarct-related artery (IRA) patency. Ninety-minute patency (TIMI grade 2 or 3 flow) correlates strongly with outcome: greater than twofold higher 1-year mortality rate in those with persistent occlusion at 90 minutes in TIMI 1 and similar findings in subsequent studies (251). Subsequent analyses showed TIMI grade 3 flow to be associated with significantly better outcomes than TIMI grade 2 flow (251,252,255). The corrected TIMI frame count (CTFC), which treats flow as a continuous variable, appears to provide an even more accurate prognostic assessment (257).

2. Microvascular reperfusion. The TIMI myocardial perfusion (TMP) grade classification is as follows: TMP grade (TMPG) 1 indicates presence of myocardial blush but no clearance from the microvasculature (blush or a stain was present on the next injection); TMPG 2 blush clears slowly (blush is strongly persistent and diminishes minimally or not at all during three cardiac cycles of the washout phase); and TMPG 3 indicates that blush begins to clear during washout (blush is minimally persistent after three cardiac cycles of washout). Analyses of angiographic cinefilms from the TIMI 10B (thrombolysis) (258) and ESPRIT trials (PCI trial, see Chapter 2) demonstrate that a TMPG 0/1 is associated with frequent adverse outcomes even in patients with optimal epicardial flow (TIMI grade 3), whereas the lowest mortality is seen in patients with both TMPG 3 and TIMI 3 flow. In a multivariate model, TIMI flow, TMPG, and TIMI frame count were all predictors of mortality (259).

3. Time to treatment. Lower mortality is achieved with early administration of thrombolytic agents, especially within the first "golden" hour (74).

4. Reocclusion. A 4% to 10% incidence is observed at 2 to 4 weeks. Although approximately 50% of cases are not accompanied by clinical reinfarction or ischemia (i.e., silent), reocclusion is associated with a more than twofold higher mortality rate (289). Revascularization appears to be helpful.

5. Reinfarction is associated with a two- to threefold higher mortality rate.

Percutaneous Coronary Intervention

PRIMARY ANGIOPLASTY

The 2007 updated AHA/ACC class I indications for primary PCI are as follows: (a) within 12 hours or after 12 hours if ischemic symptoms persist, and when performed within 90 minutes of presentation by an experienced operator (>75 PCI cases/year) and supported by experienced personnel in an appropriate laboratory environment (>200 procedures/year and cardiac surgical capability); (b) within 36 hours if shock, younger than 75 years, and in whom PCI can be done within 18 hours of onset of shock (see the section "Cardiogenic Shock") (see **Fig. 4.3**). The 2005 ACC/AHA/SCAI PCI guidelines have a class IIb recommendation for primary PCI without surgical backup.

Procedural Volume Studies

Substantial data on operator and hospital volume have now been accumulated. An analysis of New York State data found that primary PCI performed by a high-volume operator (11 or more cases/year) was associated with a 57% lower in-hospital mortality compared with those treated by low-volume operators (1 to 10 cases/year) (110). Primary PTCA performed in high-volume hospitals (57 or more cases/year) was associated with a 44% lower in-hospital mortality reduction compared with that in low-volume hospitals. As for hospital volume, one large analysis of 62,299 patients found that primary PCI was superior to thrombolytic therapy for treatment of acute STEMI at hospitals with intermediate (17 to 48 procedures/year) and high volume (>49 per year), whereas no significant mortality difference was found between the treatments at low-volume hospitals (109). Another analysis of 98,898 Medicare patients found that those admitted to hospitals in the lowest quartile of volume of invasive procedures had a 17% higher in-hospital mortality rate compared with patients at highest-volume-quartile hospitals [hazard ratio, 1.17; 95% confidence interval (CI), 1.09 to 1.26; $p < 0.001$] (108).

Primary Angioplasty versus Thrombolysis

A meta-analysis of 10 trials through 1997 showed a significant mortality benefit of primary angioplasty compared with thrombolysis: odds ratio (OR), 0.66 (95% CI, 0.46 to 0.94) (112). An updated meta-analysis of 23 studies published in 2003 confirmed primary PCI had lower short-term mortality than thrombolytic therapy (7% vs. 9%) (113).

PCI had a lower associated mortality rate in the Primary Angioplasty in MI (PAMI) trial (2.6% vs. 6.5%) (109), and a nonsignificant trend toward lower mortality was observed in the larger GUSTO-IIb trial (119). However, no mortality difference was found in a subsequent study of 19 Seattle hospitals (118).

More recent studies compared primary PCI with thrombolysis, including two that included facilities without PCI capability (i.e., transfer required for the PCI group). In the second Danish Trial in Acute MI (DANAMI-2), primary PCI was

Figure 4.3 • Options for transportation of STEMI patients and initial reperfusion treatment goals.
(Adapted from ACC/AHA Task Force on Practice Guidelines. STEMI Focused Update. 2007 Focused Update of the ACC/AHA 2004 Guidelines for the Management of Patients with ST-Elevation Myocardial Infarction. *J Am Coll Cardiol* 2008;51;210–247.

associated with a 45% lower incidence of death, reinfarction, or disabling stroke, primarily because of less reinfarction [1.6% vs. 6.3% (tPA)] (122). In PRAGUE-2, primary PCI was associated with a nonsignificant mortality reduction compared with SK (6.8% vs. 10%); however, a significant mortality reduction was seen in those seen at 3 to 12 hours (6% vs. 15.3%) (123). The rapid transfer and door-to-balloon times in these two trials are likely not typical of the usual community setting. In the Air PAMI study, all enrolled patients arrived in hospitals without on-site PCI; despite long transfer delays, the emergency transfer for the primary PCI group had a nonsignificant 38% reduction in major events compared with on-site thrombolysis (120). Finally, in the Atlantic Cardiovascular Patient Outcomes Research team (C-PORT) study, sites without a de novo primary PCI program had one developed (without on-site surgery) and involved high-volume, experienced operators and catheterization teams. The primary PCI group had significantly lower incidence of death, recurrent MI, or disabling stroke compared with those given tPA (121).

In summary, primary PCI is superior to thrombolysis for STEMI when performed at experienced centers that can achieve a short door-to-balloon time.

Rescue Angioplasty

Rescue angioplasty has been defined as PCI carried out very early (1 to 2 hours) after failed thrombolytic therapy—that is, in patients who have evidence of not achieving reperfusion of the IRA usually diagnosed by persistent ST elevation and chest pain. Several trials have shown that rescue PCI is superior to conservative therapy or repeat thrombolysis (142,145,146). The ACC/AHA 2007 guidelines giving a class IIa recommendation with level of evidence B for a strategy of coronary angiography with intent to perform rescue PCI is reasonable for patients in whom fibrinolytic therapy has failed (ST-segment elevation < 50% resolved after 90 minutes following initiation of fibrinolytic therapy in the lead showing the worst initial elevation) and a moderate or large area of myocardium at risk (anterior MI, inferior MI with RV involvement or precordial ST-segment depression). A class IIb recommendation was given for lower risk patients.

Routine Percutaneous Coronary Intervention (After Thrombolysis) versus Delayed or Conservative Management

A significant evolution of interventional approaches has led to changes in recommendations for early PCI following fibrinolysis. Early trials performed in the mid-1980s showed immediate PCI to be associated with increased bleeding and an overall trend toward increased mortality [Thrombolysis and Angioplasty in MI (TAMI), TIMI-2A, and European Cooperative Study Group (ECSG-4)] (126,127). In addition, routine *delayed* angioplasty following fibrinolysis was not seen to improve mortality or reinfarction rates in older studies [TIMI IIB and the Should We Intervene Following Thrombolysis (SWIFT) study] (74,129).

However, given the advances in interventional approaches and antithrombotic therapy, revisiting these issues was needed. Observational data from recent trials suggested a potential benefit of early PCI (138). Now several randomized trials have shown benefit of early PCI: The GRACIA trial compared routine angiography within 24 hours of thrombolysis with an ischemia-guided approach (137) and showed that the routine invasive group had a significantly lower incidence of death, reinfarction, or revascularization (0.8% vs. 3.7%; $p = 0.003$). The CARESS-in-AMI trial also found benefit of early transfer in high-risk STEMI patients (139,140), as did the Trial of Routine Angioplasty and Stenting after Fibrinolysis to Enhance Reperfusion in Acute Myocardial Infarction (TRANSFER-AMI). Approximately 1,000 patients with STEMI who received fibrinolytic therapy and were then transferred for PCI within 6 hours had a significant reduction in the composite endpoint of death, reinfarction, recurrent ischemia, new/worsening CHF, or cardiogenic shock at 30 days, when compared to patients who received fibrinolytic therapy alone (11.0% vs. 17.2%, relative risk (RR) RR 0.64; $p = 0.0004$) (139). No mortality benefit was seen, but a reduction in recurrent MI and ischemia was seen—and this strategy of early transfer and PCI for high-risk patients with STEMI has now been added to the 2009 focused update of the ACC/AHA guidelines.

"Facilitated" Percutaneous Coronary Intervention

Given the benefit of primary PCI, the concept of combining fibrinolysis and immediate PCI was pursued as a way to achieve earlier reperfusion but retain the benefits of primary PCI. Following small observational analyses, several randomized trials were conducted comparing facilitated PCI to *primary PCI*. (The section above showed that early PCI following fibrinolysis was superior to fibrinolysis.)

In 2006, the Assessment of the Safety and Efficacy of a New Treatment Strategy with Percutaneous Coronary Intervention (ASSENT-4 PCI) trial patients were randomized to receive TNK and immediate PCI (approximately 1 hour) versus primary PCI. Despite a planned enrollment of 4,000 patients for the primary endpoint of death, CHF, or shock within 90 days, the trial was stopped early due to a higher in-hospital mortality in the facilitated PCI group (6% vs. 3%; $p = 0.0105$) (132). A meta-analysis published simultaneously, and including this trial, combined 17 trials and 4,504 patients and concluded that there was no benefit to facilitated PCI compared with primary PCI, and that such regimens including full-dose thrombolytics should not be used. (134).

However, additional data on alternative regimens for facilitated PCI came from the Facilitated Intervention with Enhanced Reperfusion Speed to Stop Events (FINESSE) study, randomizing patients with STEMI to primary PCI versus PCI facilitated with either abciximab only or abciximab in combination with half-dose reteplase. Neither of the comparator regimens demonstrated any improvement in rates of the primary outcome, a composite of death, VF (>48 hours from randomization), cardiogenic shock, or CHF within 90 days (9.8% vs. 10.5% vs. 10.7% in the combination-facilitated, PCI group, abciximab-facilitated group, and primary PCI group, respectively; $p = 0.55$) (see also *Eur Heart J* 2007;28:1545–1553) (133). As such, the current guidelines recommend against use of a strategy of immediate PCI (<1 hour).

Cardiogenic Shock

The Should We Emergently Revascularize Occluded Coronaries for Cardiogenic Shock (SHOCK) trial found that emergency revascularization (ERV; balloon angioplasty or bypass surgery) did not result in improved 30-day survival (primary endpoint) compared with aggressive medical management [e.g., thrombolysis, intraaortic balloon pump (IABP)] (148). However, at 6 months, mortality was lower with ERV (50.3% vs. 63.1%; $p = 0.027$). Among patients younger than 75 years, ERV was significantly better than medical therapy (30-day mortality, 41% vs. 57%, $p < 0.01$; 6 months, 48% vs. 69%, $p < 0.01$). Based on these results, the 2004 ACC/AHA guidelines consider primary PCI a class I indication in those within 36 hours of symptom onset in whom cardiogenic shock develops, are younger than 75 years, and in whom revascularization can be performed within 18 hours of onset of shock.

STENTING

Before the identification of an effective antiplatelet regimen to prevent stent thrombosis, stent use was typically avoided in the patients with AMI. However, several studies then showed that stenting in the AMI was safe and efficacious (149,150). The STAT and STOPAMI-2 trials demonstrated superior outcomes with stenting compared with fibrinolytic therapy (152,153). The larger Stent PAMI study compared primary PTCA alone with heparin-coated Palmaz–Schatz stenting in 900 patients (151). At 6 months, stenting was associated with a significant reduction in the 6-month composite primary endpoint (12.6% vs. 20.1%; $p < 0.01$), primarily because of a lower rate of ischemia-driven target vessel revascularization (TVR; 7.7% vs. 17%; $p < 0.001$). The Controlled Abciximab and Device Investigation to Lower Late Angioplasty Complications (CADILLAC) trial enrolled 2,082 patients and compared PTCA alone, PTCA plus abciximab, stenting alone, and stenting plus abciximab in 2,082 patients (54). At 6 months, the stent groups had a lower incidence of death, reinfarction, disabling stroke, and ischemia-driven TVR [11.5% (stent alone) and 10.2% vs. 20% (PTCA alone) and 16.5% (PTCA plus abciximab)]. As in Stent PAMI, the benefit was owing to a lower TVR-rate benefit, whereas no difference in mortality rates was found. These lower TVR rates are the result of the lower restenosis rates seen with PTCA compared with angioplasty alone.

The 2003 meta-analysis of 23 intervention trials (a minority of the trials did not use stents) identified a significant, absolute 2% reduction in short-term death for patients receiving primary PCI (7% vs. 9%; $p = 0.0002$) (113). Subsequent analysis of data from the National Registry of Myocardial Infarction (NRMI) demonstrated significantly improved outcomes in patients treated at hospitals with greater specialization of primary PCI. In summary, these data demonstrate that in experienced centers, stent implantation should be considered the preferred reperfusion strategy (see *N Engl J Med* 2007;356:47–54.)

The release in 2004 of the first drug-eluting stents (DES) saw a significant increase in their use for STEMI, despite an indication limited to elective, nonurgent PCI (see Chapter 2 for more detailed information). Thus, while multiple retrospective and observational studies of off-label DES use in acute MI have yielded mixed results, randomized trials have demonstrated noninferior short-term outcomes with DES and potentially fewer repeat procedures over the long term (156,157). The 2009 Updated ACC/AHA guidelines now indicate it is reasonable to use a DES as an alternative to a bare-metal stent (BMS) for primary PCI in STEMI.

Antithrombotic/Antiplatelet Agents

HEPARIN

Intravenously heparin should be used in conjunction with tPA, or rPA or TNK [GUSTO data show the optimal partial thromboplastin time (PTT) range to be 50 to 70 seconds]. Heparin is optimal if the patient is not also receiving a thrombolytic agent. A meta-analysis of prethrombolytic trials showed an approximately 20% mortality benefit (24). Another meta-analysis of trials comprising approximately 70,000 patients showed borderline benefit when used with thrombolytics (6% lower mortality; $p = 0.03$). Subcutaneous administration showed no benefit in reducing death or reinfarction (ISIS-3 and GISSI-2) (87,88).

Given the effectiveness of contemporary therapies, the true benefit of heparin as adjunctive therapy to thrombolysis and aspirin is unclear; however, it remains a class I recommendation, particularly for patients at high risk of systemic emboli. However, newer and potentially more efficacious agents are now acceptable alternatives and may eventually become the standard of care (see below).

ENOXAPARIN

Low-molecular-weight heparins have now been evaluated in several studies and appear safe and efficacious in the acute STEMI setting. In the Assessment of the Safety and Efficacy of a New Thrombolytic Regimen (ASSENT)-3 trial, those treated with enoxaparin and TNK had significantly fewer major events compared with the unfractionated heparin (UFH) and TNK group (11.4% vs. 15.4%; $p < 0.001$); bleeding events were similar in both groups. In the smaller ENTIRE-TIMI 23 trial, TIMI grade 3 flow rates were similar between enoxaparin- and UFH-treated patients (33). However, among patients receiving full-dose TNK, the enoxaparin group had a lower incidence of death or recurrent MI at 30 days (4.4% vs. 15.9%; $p = 0.005$). The Enoxaparin and Thrombolysis Reperfusion for Acute Myocardial Infarction Treatment (ExTRACT)–TIMI 25 study compared enoxaparin to UFH in 25,056 patients with STEMI who received thrombolytics. There was a significant, absolute 2.1% reduction in the primary endpoint of death or non-fatal, recurrent MI at 30 days (12.0% vs. 9.9%; $p < 0.001$) (34).

FONDAPARINUX

Fondaparinux is a newer, synthetic pentasaccharide antithrombin, which selectively inhibits factor Xa. The Organization for the Assessment of Strategies for Ischemic Syndromes (OASIS) 6 trial randomized 12,092 patients with STEMI to either fondaparinux or control (either placebo or UFH depending on whether UFH was contraindicated). At 30 days, the composite primary endpoint of death or reinfarction was significantly reduced in the fondaparinux group (11.2% vs. 9.7%; $p = 0.008$), a finding that later was isolated to only those patients who did not undergo PCI. Patients who received PCI derived no benefit from fondaparinux. Based on these studies, use of fondaparinux is an acceptable class IIa recommended alternative for patients with STEMI not receiving reperfusion therapy. However, currently this is an off-label use in the United States; the drug's Canadian label does provide an indication for STEMI, as well as UA/NSTEMI.

DIRECT THROMBIN INHIBITORS

Trials using hirudin showed no significant advantage [TIMI-5, TIMI-9B (38), GUSTO-IIb (119)]. In the Hirulog Early Perfusion/Occlusion (HERO) trial (39), hirulog showed better TIMI grade 3 flow compared with SK. In the larger HERO-2 trial (17,073 patients), bivalirudin was compared with UFH in patients receiving SK (40). No mortality difference occurred between the two groups. The bivalirudin group had a 30% reduction in the reinfarction rate, but it also was associated with an increased bleeding rate. In the Harmonizing Outcomes with Revascularization and Stents in Acute Myocardial Infarction (HORIZONS-AMI) trial, bivalirudin, as compared with heparin plus glycoprotein IIb/IIIA inhibitors, reduced net clinical events at 30 days, including major bleeding and ischemic cardiovascular events (43).

WARFARIN

In the Aspirin/Anticoagulants Following Thrombolysis with Eminase in Recurrent Infarction (AFTER) trial, patients treated with warfarin had similar cardiac outcomes compared with aspirin-treated patients, but warfarin was associated with an increased incidence of bleeding (46). In the Warfarin, Aspirin, Reinfarction Study (WARIS), a 24% lower mortality rate versus placebo was observed (15.5% vs. 20.3%; $p = 0.03$) (44). Based on these data, it was recommended that warfarin could be used in aspirin-intolerant patients. It also should be considered in those at high risk of LV thrombus formation (large anterior MI, EF <20%), or with atrial fibrillation. In one analysis of 11 studies, anticoagulation was associated with 68% lower rate of embolization (297).

Several recent studies examined warfarin plus aspirin with various intensities of anticoagulation. In the large Combination Hemotherapy and Mortality Prevention (CHAMP) study, lower intensity anticoagulation [international normalized ratio (INR), 1.5 to 2.5] plus aspirin had outcomes similar to those with aspirin alone, whereas major bleeding occurred more frequently with combination therapy (48). In the Antithrombotics in the Prevention of Reocclusion in Coronary Thrombolysis (APRICOT)-2 trial, aspirin plus moderate-intensity warfarin (goal INR, 2.0 to 3.0) was associated with less reocclusion compared with aspirin alone (15% vs. 28%; $p = 0.02$), as well as a lower incidence of death, reinfarction, or revascularization (14% vs. 34%; $p < 0.01$) (51). No increased incidence of bleeding events was observed. In the Antithrombotics in the Secondary Prevention of Events in Coronary Thrombosis-2 (ASPECT-2) study, high-dose oral anticoagulation alone (target INR, 3.0 to 4.0) and the combination of aspirin and moderate-dose anticoagulation (target INR, 2.0 to 3.0) resulted in a lower incidence of death, MI, or stroke compared with low-dose aspirin (80 mg once daily) (49). Bleeding rates were similar in all groups. The Warfarin, Aspirin, Reinfarction Study-2 (WARIS-2) examined high-intensity anticoagulation (INR, 2.8 to 4.2) as well as moderate-dose anticoagulation (INR, 2.0 to 2.5) plus low-dose aspirin and low-dose aspirin alone (75 mg/day) (50). Both warfarin groups had a lower incidence of death, nonfatal MI, and stroke compared with aspirin alone. The warfarin plus aspirin group also had a significantly lower mortality than did aspirin alone ($p = 0.003$). However, the warfarin groups had more major bleeding, but these rates were relatively low (0.58/100 and 0.52/100 patient years vs. 0.15/100 patient years for aspirin).

In summary, these data suggest that with careful monitoring of INR, the combination of warfarin (INR, 2.0 to 3.0) plus low-dose aspirin or warfarin alone (INR, 2.5 to 3.5) reduces major events compared with aspirin alone. However, given the slight increased bleeding risk and frequent monitoring required, the routine use of long-term warfarin will not likely supplant the current antiplatelet therapy regimen. These studies did not evaluate long-term warfarin regimens compared with dual antiplatelet therapy (e.g., aspirin and clopidogrel).

Intravenously Glycoprotein IIb/IIIa Inhibitors

USE IN PRIMARY PCI The ReoPro and Primary PTCA Organization and Randomized Trial (RAPPORT) showed that abciximab use in conjunction with primary PTCA resulted in a significant reduction in death, MI, and urgent revascularization at 30 days. (See also EPIC and GUSTO-III subgroup analyses.) The Abciximab before Direct Angiography and Stenting in MI Regarding Acute and Long-term Follow-up (ADMIRAL) trial showed that abciximab use in conjunction with stenting resulted in a nearly 50% reduction in the incidence of death, MI, and urgent revascularization (53). The larger CADILLAC trial compared PTCA alone, PTCA plus abciximab, stenting alone, or stenting plus abciximab (54). At 6 months, death, reinfarction, disabling stroke, and ischemia-driven TVR occurred in 20.0% of the PTCA-alone group, 16.5% with PTCA plus abciximab, 11.5% with stenting, and 10.2% with stenting plus abciximab (p , 0.001). The differences in the incidence of this composite endpoint were primarily owing to varying TVR rates (15.7% with PTCA alone, 13.8% with PTCA 1 abciximab, 8.3% with stenting, and only 5.2% with stenting 1 abciximab; p , 0.001).

A 2007 meta-analysis of the ISAR-2, ADMIRAL, and ACE studies combined 1,101 patients with STEMI undergoing primary PCI and randomized to abciximab or placebo, for a primary endpoint of death or reinfarction at 3 years of follow-up (57). The abciximab group had a significantly lower event rate at 3 years (12.9% vs. 19.0%; $p = 0.008$), without significant increasing in bleeding.

However, data comparing abciximab to the small-molecule IIb/IIIa inhibitors have been less definitive. Several studies comparing these agents have failed to demonstrate a significant difference in outcomes (58–61). Subsequent meta-analyses have also failed to demonstrated significant differences among the agents. Thus, the newest guidelines support the use of any IIb/IIIa inhibitor in certain settings of STEMI, with a level of evidence of "A" for abciximab, and "B" for both tirofiban and eptifibatide.

GLYCOPROTEIN IIB/IIIA INHIBITION PLUS REDUCED-DOSE THROMBOLYSIS
Reduced-dose thrombolysis in conjunction with i.v. glycoprotein IIb/IIIa administration has been intensely evaluated. TIMI-14 found that a combination of abciximab and tPA (15-mg bolus and then 35 mg over a 60-minute period) resulted in better TIMI grade 3 flow at 60 and 90 minutes compared with tPA alone (72% vs. 43%, p 5 0.0009; 77% vs. 62%, p 5 0.02) (65). The Strategies for Patency Enhancement in the Emergency Department (SPEED) trial evaluated a regimen of abciximab plus reteplase (66). TIMI grade 3 flow rates were 54% with abciximab and reteplase, 5 1 5 U, compared with 47% reteplase only (10 1 10 U; p 5 0.32).

In IMPACT-AMI, eptifibatide (180 μg/kg i.v. bolus and then 0.75 μg/kg/min) with full-dose tPA was associated with better TIMI grade 3 flow at 90 minutes compared with full-dose tPA alone; no significant difference was seen between the groups in major in-hospital events. However, the planned pivotal trial ADVANCE MI was prematurely terminated due to poor enrollment, and demonstrated significantly higher adverse clinical event rates (both bleeding and ischemic), despite better angiographic outcomes in patients receiving eptifibatide plus half-dose TNK (in addition to enoxaparin or UFH) (see *Am Heart J* 2005;150:116–122).

The ASSENT-3 trial evaluated abciximab and TNK as well as comparing UFH and enoxaparin (97). The half-dose TNK and abciximab group had a lower incidence of death, in-hospital MI, or in-hospital refractory ischemia compared with full-dose TNK and UFH (11.1% vs. 15.4%) and similar to TNK and enoxaparin (11.4%). Of concern, the abciximab group had nearly twice the risk of major hemorrhage compared with the UFH group (4.3% vs. 2.2%, $p = 0.0002$; enoxaparin group, 3.0%, $p =$ NS vs. UFH).

The 16,558-patient GUSTO-V trial (67) compared standard-dose reteplase (two 10-U boluses, 30 minutes apart) with half-dose reteplase (two 5-U boluses) and full-dose abciximab. No significant differences were seen between the two groups in 30-day mortality. The combination-therapy group had significantly lower rates of death and reinfarction (7.4% vs. 8.8%; $p = 0.0011$) and reinfarction (at 7 days, 2.3% vs. 3.5%) but was associated with higher rate of nonintracranial bleeding complications.

Combination therapy of abciximab and half-dose reteplase or TNK is currently not used although it is a class IIb recommendation, to prevent complications in selected patients, less than 75 years old. Due to the unacceptably high risk of intracranial hemorrhage, the combination is not recommended for patients over the age of 75.

Nitrates

Nitrates are indicated for relief of persistent pain and treatment of heart failure or hypertension [sublingual nitroglycerin (NTG), 0.4 mg every 5 minutes for three doses, or i.v. NTG, 10 to 200 μg/min]. A meta-analysis of data on approximately 2,000 patients treated in the prereperfusion era demonstrated a 35% mortality reduction with nitrate use. However, in the large GISSI-3, ISIS-4, and CCS-1 trials (168,170,171), routine use of i.v. and oral nitrates after MI conferred no mortality benefit. As such, current recommendations are for use of nitrates to relieve symptoms of ischemia and treat hypertension (class I); their use should not supersede that of agents proven to improve clinical outcomes, such as β-blockers and ACE inhibitors.

Nitrates should not be used in patients with inferior MI complicated by RV involvement (reduces preload).

Calcium-Channel Blockers

Nifedipine has been associated with increased mortality [Trial of Early Nifedipine in Acute MI (TRENT), and Secondary Prevention Reinfarction Israel Nifedipine Trials I and II (SPRINT-I and -II)] (177,180). In the Multicenter Diltiazem Postinfarction Trial (MDPIT) (178), diltiazem was deemed harmful in those with pulmonary congestion and low EF (41% increase in cardiac events). A meta-analysis performed in 1993 of 24 trials of all types of calcium-channel blockers showed a nonsignificant 4% increase in mortality (191). Verapamil appears to be safe; a meta-analysis of verapamil studies showed a significant 19% lower reinfarction rate and nonsignificant 7% mortality reduction (181). These agents should be considered only in patients with clear contraindication(s) to β-blockade and with good LV function. They are not routinely used for the acute treatment of STEMI.

Antiarrhythmics

Prophylactic use of lidocaine appears to be harmful, with a meta-analysis showing a 12% higher mortality rate (192). However, lidocaine (1 to 3 mg/min) can be used in patients who have had ventricular tachycardia (VT) or VF.

In the Cardiac Arrhythmia Suppression Trials (CAST I and II) (187), the routine use of type I agents (e.g., encainide, flecainide, moricizine) was associated with significantly higher all-cause mortality rates.

In the Basel Antiarrhythmic Study of Infarct Survival (BASIS) (186), amiodarone (1 g for 5 days, and then 200 mg daily) in patients with complex ventricular ectopy was associated with 61% lower 1-year mortality rates ($p < 0.05$). However, in two large trials [the European MI Amiodarone Trial (EMIAT) and Canadian Amiodarone MI Arrhythmia Trial (CAMIAT) (189,190)], when given to patients with frequent ventricular ectopy and LV dysfunction, amiodarone (vs. placebo) showed no overall mortality benefit, although arrhythmic deaths were decreased. The Survival with Oral D-sotalol (SWORD) trial showed 65% increased mortality with D-sotalol (188).

Magnesium

Initial studies suggested a mortality benefit [second Leicester Intravenous Magnesium Intervention Trial (LIMIT-2) (183)], and an early meta-analysis showed 54% lower mortality. However, in the ISIS-4 megatrial (184), magnesium had no mortality benefit and was associated with excess hypotension. Proponents of magnesium argued that it could be beneficial in high-risk patients and perhaps when given before thrombolytic therapy to prevent reperfusion injury. However, the large 6,213-patient National Heart, Lung, and Blood Institute (NHLBI)-sponsored MAGIC trial examined these hypotheses and found no benefit associated with magnesium administration (185). Thus, current guidelines recommend *against* the routine use of intravenously magnesium in STEMI patients, *without* significant electrolyte abnormalities or ventricular arrhythmias.

Adenosine

Results with this agent have been mixed. In the Acute Myocardial Infarction Study of Adenosine (AMISTAD) trial, 236 patients were enrolled, and adenosine-treated patients were found to have reduced infarct size (203). In the larger AMISTAD II trial (2,118 patients), adenosine was associated with a nonsignificant trend toward a reduction in death and CHF at 6 months (204).

Glucose–Insulin–Potassium

Results with this combination therapy have been promising, but further study is needed to clearly identify the subgroups of patients in which it provides benefit. A meta-analysis performed several years ago of nine randomized, placebo-controlled, prethrombolytic era trials with 1,932 patients (all prethrombolytic era) found that glucose–insulin–potassium (GIK) was associated with lower hospital mortality (16.1% vs. 21%; OR, 0.72; $p = 0.004$). A 48% reduction was seen in the four trials using high-dose GIK (to suppress free fatty acid levels maximally). The OASIS-6 GIK trial of 2,748 STEMI patients found no benefit to GIK (overall mortality 10.8% for GIK vs. 10.4% controls at 6 months, $p = 0.72$). When combined with the CREATE-ECLA trial, there was a nonsignificant trend toward *harm* in the GIK group (9.7% mortality in GIK vs. 9.3% in the control at 30 days, $p = 0.33$). Thus, GIK infusions are not routinely used for care of STEMI.

OTHER MODES OF TREATMENT

Analgesia

Morphine sulfate may be administered, 2 to 5 mg i.v., repeated every 5 to 15 minutes (some patients require up to 30 mg for adequate pain relief). It is particularly helpful in patients with pulmonary edema due to vasodilatory effect.

Diuretics

Intravenously furosemide (Lasix) is indicated in severe CHF but should be avoided in an inferior MI complicated by RV infarction (RVI).

Vasopressors/Inotropes

Vasopressors/inotropes are useful in the treatment of cardiogenic shock (SBP, <90 mm Hg; cardiac index, 2.2 L/kg/m^2 or less). Initial choices include dopamine (5 to 20 μg/kg/min) and dobutamine (2.5 to 20 μg/kg/min; an ideal agent if BP is adequate but cardiac output is poor). If SBP is less than 60 mm Hg, norepinephrine should be considered.

Temporary Pacing

Class I indications are as follows: (a) asystole; (b) symptomatic bradycardia including sinus block with hypotension and Mobitz type I second-degree block with hypotension unresponsive to atropine; (c) bilateral BBB (alternating BBB or RBBB with alternating left anterior fascicular block/left posterior fascicular block); (d) new or indeterminate-age bifascicular block with first-degree atrioventricular (AV) block; or (e) Mobitz-type II second-degree block.

Insulin

Aggressive serum glucose control in diabetics with insulin drip resulted in a significant mortality benefit in the Diabetic Insulin–Glucose Infusion in Acute MI (DIGAMI) trial (200). Follow-up studies such as the GIK studies noted aove however, have not confirmed this benefit.

Intra-aortic Balloon Pump

A balloon pump appears useful in the treatment of cardiogenic shock (trend toward lower mortality in GUSTO I) (189) and after emergency catheterization [IABP Trial (194)]. Contraindications include the presence of aortic regurgitation, thoracic or abdominal aortic pathology (aneurysm, dissection), and severe peripheral vascular disease. Vascular complications occur in 5% to 20% of cases (194–196).

Emergency Coronary Artery Bypass Graft Surgery

Emergency CABG surgery should be considered if PCI fails and results in persistent pain or hemodynamic instability, or left main disease is present. Acute mitral regurgitation and ventricular septal defect typically require immediate surgical intervention.

SPECIAL CASE

Right Ventricular Infarction

RVI is typically caused by right coronary artery occlusion proximal to the acute marginal branch and is associated with 20% to 50% of inferior MIs (212–217). If the right coronary artery is occluded, RVI is six times more likely in the absence of pre-infarction angina (217).

DIAGNOSIS

1. Triad of hypotension, clear lung fields, and elevated jugular venous pressure is highly specific, but only 25% sensitive.
2. Hemodynamics: Right atrial pressure is more than 10 mm Hg and within 1 to 5 mm Hg of pulmonary capillary wedge pressure (73% sensitivity, 100% specificity).
3. ECG: ST elevation is present in lead V_4R (80% to 100% sensitivity, 80% to 100% specificity) and resolves quickly. In one study, ST elevation resolved in 48% of patients within 10 hours. RBBB and complete heart block may be observed.
4. Echocardiography: Typical features are RV dilatation, RV wall asynergy, and abnormal interventricular septal motion. Tricuspid regurgitation, ventricular septal defect, and/or early pulmonary valve opening also may be seen.

COMPLICATIONS

High-degree AV block is present in up to 50% of patients, and atrial fibrillation in up to one third. A high incidence of pericarditis is seen, mostly because of transmural involvement of the thin-walled right ventricle. Less common complications include rupture of the interventricular septum, RV free-wall rupture (FWR), pulmonary embolism, right atrial infarction, and right-to-left shunting across a patent foramen ovale.

TREATMENT

Diuretics and nitrates should be avoided (i.e., to not decrease preload). Beneficial measures include:

1. Volume loading (2 to 4 L of normal saline is commonly needed).
2. Inotropic support (dobutamine) if volume does not improve cardiac output.
3. Temporary wire placement if complete heart block develops and AV sequential pacing if hemodynamics are poor.
4. Cardioversion if atrial fibrillation is present.
5. Thrombolysis significantly reduces mortality (214).

   Unsuccessful PCI is associated with high mortality [58% vs. 2% in one study (215)].

COMPLICATIONS

Early

1. Pump failure/cardiogenic shock: incidence, 3% to 7%; most common if more than 40% of myocardium involved; hospital mortality is very high: 50% to 70%; prompt IABP insertion can be useful as a bridge to revascularization.
2. Postinfarct angina: more frequent after thrombolysis than after primary PCI.

3. Reinfarction: more frequent after thrombolysis, and if non–Q wave MI; should be treated as initial MI with medical therapy and intervention.

4. Arrhythmias:
   a. VT: incidence, 5%; associated with larger infarcts/LV dysfunction; nonsustained VT (NSVT) occurring beyond 24 to 48 hours after MI portends poorer prognosis (235) and is an indication for an EP study and implantable cardioverter defibrillator (ICD) implantation.
   b. VF: declining incidence (now <1%); primary VF occurs in 85% to 90% of cases in the first 24 hours, 60% in the first 6 hours; secondary VF: occurs at 1 to 4 days, often associated with pump failure/shock; poor prognosis (40% to 60% in-hospital mortality).
   c. Asystole: associated with high mortality; transcutaneous or transvenous pacing is indicated.
   d. Atrial fibrillation (275): incidence, 5% to 15%; treated with anticoagulation, rate control (β-blockers, calcium-channel blockers, digoxin), cardioversion if hemodynamically unstable, or amiodarone if multiple episodes occur.
   e. Heart block: common with inferior MI (increased vagal tone, AV node ischemia)—first-degree heart block typically progresses to Mobitz I and then to third degree; anterior MI (His–Purkinje system affected)—BBB progresses to Mobitz II and then third degree (advanced block associated with mortality rate of >40%); temporary pacer indicated for high-degree block that develops via Mobitz II mechanism or bifascicular block.
   f. Accelerated idioventricular rhythm: occurs more frequently in patients with early reperfusion; temporary pacing is not indicated.
   g. Premature ventricular contractions: incidence approximately 75%; routine suppression with lidocaine associated with increased mortality.
   h. Sinus tachycardia: if it persists, may signify evolving CHF.

5. Cholesterol embolization: more common with thrombolytic therapy.

Intermediate

1. LV thrombus: incidence, 4% to 20%; most common in anterior MI; treatment: anticoagulation (usually warfarin for 3 to 12 months); decreases the risk of embolization (296); primary prevention: consider anticoagulation if EF is less than 30% to 35%.

2. Myocardial rupture: causes a higher percentage of deaths in patients undergoing thrombolysis [12% vs. 6% (276)]; risk factors include first MI, female gender, age older than 60 years, no LV hypertrophy, hypertension, and possibly thrombolysis after 12 hours [while primary PTCA appears protective (280)]:
   a. Free wall: incidence approximately 5%; lower risk after thrombolysis and with use of β-blockers; although most die immediately, treatment includes emergency pericardiocentesis and fluids, followed by immediate surgical repair.

b. Septum: incidence, 0.5% to 2.0%; new murmur with palpable thrill in up to 90%; surgical mortality, 20% to 30% (higher if inferior MI and/or cardiogenic shock) versus 80% to 90% with medical therapy (300).

c. Papillary muscle: incidence approximately 1%; murmur is only 50%; occurs primarily with inferior MIs; posteromedial papillary muscle affected more often (six times) than anterolateral; best treatment is surgery (mortality, approximately 10%).

3. Fibrinous pericarditis: most common after Q-wave MI; treated with aspirin and analgesics [avoid nonsteroidal anti-inflammatory drugs (NSAIDs) and steroids; both may impair healing].

Late

1. Ventricular aneurysm: usually do not rupture, but often complicated by mural thrombi and severe CHF; treated with surgical resection if complicated by CHF, severe arrhythmias, and thromboemboli; primary prevention is early ACE inhibition.

2. Pseudoaneurysm: contained rupture of myocardium; surgical resection usually recommended.

3. Dressler syndrome (late pericarditis): usually occurs at 4 to 6 weeks; incidence, approximately 1%; treated with NSAIDs (if they fail, steroids).

4. Sudden cardiac death is increased in patients with reduced EF. The MAD IT 2 Trial showed a 31% reduced mortality at 2 years with prophylactic ICD implantations in patients with EF <30%.

PROGNOSIS AND RISK STRATIFICATION AFTER MYOCARDIAL INFARCTION

The majority of hospitalized patients with MI are at low risk for adverse outcomes. Age is a strong predictor of outcome. In a multivariate analysis of GUSTO I data, mortality ranged from 1.1% in those younger than 45 years to 20.5% in those older than 75 (264). Other factors associated with mortality included lower SBP, higher Killip class, elevated HR, and anterior infarct. These five factors contributed to approximately 90% of prognostic information (**Fig. 4.4**). Another analysis of 3,339 TIMI-2 patients identified a low-risk group (26%; none of eight risk factors) that had a 6-week mortality rate of 1.5%. Patients with one risk factor (age 70 years, female gender, diabetes, prior MI, anterior MI, atrial fibrillation, SBP < 100 mm Hg, HR > 100 beats/min) had a 6-week mortality rate of 5.3% ($p < 0.001$), whereas those with four risk factors had a 17.2% mortality rate (**Fig. 4.5**).

Psychosocial predictors of adverse outcomes include depression (267) and living alone (266). Finally, an analysis of more than 8,000 Medicare patients showed that MI patients treated by cardiologists fared better than those treated by other types of physicians (269).

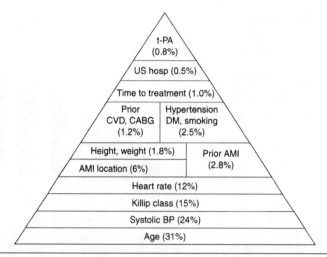

Figure 4.4 • Influence of clinical characteristics on 30-day mortality after myocardial infarction (MI) in patients treated with thrombolytic agents based on GUSTO I data. Although much attention has been paid to optimizing thrombolytic regimens, the choice of the agent is far less important than are certain clinical variables with respect to mortality. This pyramid depicts the importance of such clinical characteristics, as calculated from a regression analysis in the GUSTO trial. Numbers in parentheses represent the proportion of risk for 30-day mortality associated with the particular characteristics. AMI, acute myocardial infarction; BP, blood pressure; CVD, cardiovascular disease; DM, diabetes mellitus; tPA, tissue-type plasminogen activator; US hosp, patients treated in a U.S. hospital. A more recently developed clinical score, the TIMI risk score, was derived based on an analysis of 11,114 patients from the InTIME II trial (224). Ten baseline variables accounted for 97% of the predictive capacity of the model. These included age older than 75 years (3 points); age 65 to 74 years (2 points); diabetes, hypertension, or angina (1 point); SBP less than 100 mm Hg (3 points); heart rate more than 100 beats/min (2 points); Killip class II to IV (2 points); weight less than 67 kg (1 point); anterior STEMI or LBBB (1 point); and time to treatment more than 4 hours (1 point). The risk score showed a more than 40-fold graded increase in mortality ($<$1% with a score of 0 vs. 35.9% for score more than 8) (see **Fig. 4.5**). This scoring system was then applied to 84,029 STEMI patients in NRMI-3, and it showed a similar strong prognostic capacity with a graded increase in mortality with increasing TIMI risk score (range, 1.1% to 30.0%; $p < 0.001$ for trend) (225). The risk score was equally predictive in those treated with thrombolytic therapy or primary PCI. (Modified from Braunwald EB. *Heart Disease*. Philadelphia, PA: WB Saunders, 1997:1218, with permission.)

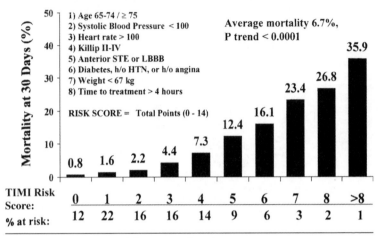

Figure 4.5 • TIMI risk score for STEMI. Derivation set based on InTIME II data. Ten baseline variables accounted for 97% of the predictive capacity of the model and compose the TIMI risk score. These included age older than 75 years (3 points); age 65 to 74 years (2 points); diabetes, hypertension, or angina (1 point); systolic blood pressure, <100 mm Hg (3 points); heart rate, >100 (2 points); Killip class II to IV (2 points); weight, <67 kg (1 point); anterior ST-elevation myocardial infarction or left bundle branch block (1 point); and time to treatment, >4 hours (1 point). The risk score showed a >40-fold graded increase in mortality (<1% with a score of 0 vs. 35.9% for score >8). (Adapted from Morrow DA, et al. Evaluation of the time saved by pre-hospital initiation of reteplase for ST-elevation myocardial infarction: results of the Early Retavase-Thrombolysis in Myocardial Infarction (ER-TIMI) 19 trial. *J Am Coll Cardiol.* 2002;40:71–77.)

Uncomplicated Course

In patients treated with primary PCI, early hospital discharge has been shown to be safe and more cost effective. For a large STEMI not treated with PCI, the clinician should consider obtaining an echocardiogram, especially with a high clinical suspicion of LV dysfunction. Catheterization should be considered if the EF is less than 40%. If the EF is 40% or higher, the TIMI IIB study observed no difference in outcome between an early conservative approach when the patient undergoes an exercise treadmill test (ETT) and an early invasive approach with routine angiography. Accordingly, the ACC/AHA guidelines recommend an early conservative approach. If the result of the ETT is positive for ischemia, or patient has rest pain, the patient should undergo cardiac catheterization.

For a small MI, the patient should usually have a submaximal predischarge ETT. If results of this test are negative, medical therapy should be continued, with repeated symptom-limited ETT after several weeks. If the results are positive, catheterization is usually warranted (130).

Complicated Course

Examples of a complicated course include severe heart failure, cardiogenic shock, failed thrombolysis, recurrent ischemia, and VT or VF after 48 hours.

Treatment is composed of catheterization and PCI or CABG surgery, as indicated; for late VT/VF, electrophysiologic testing with possible defibrillator implantation should be considered.

Specific Tests

1. ETT: submaximal test (70% predicted maximal HR or 5 to 6 METS) can be performed at days 3 to 5, or a symptom-limited test can be performed at days 14 to 21 (often as a prelude to initiation of rehabilitation program). This test has an excellent safety record: 0.03% mortality in one review of 151,949 tests (237). The strongest predictors of poor outcome are limited exercise duration and hypotension. ST depression was predictive of death in only 43% of studies in one large overview. If no predischarge ETT is performed, it is associated with a poor prognosis (238). An ETT is not required if complete revascularization has been performed (i.e., successful PCI).
2. ETT with nuclear imaging may be used in patients who have baseline ECG abnormalities or who require localization of ischemia to guide planned PCI. Positive test results lead to angiography and revascularization, which reduce the future cardiac event rate.
3. Pharmacologic stress imaging is indicated in those who cannot exercise. It also is preferred to dobutamine stress echocardiography in those who had significant arrhythmia(s) (especially VT) and/or with marked hypertension.
4. Echocardiography is useful in the assessment of LV function (242), which often guides decisions about the need for catheterization, coronary bypass surgery (mortality benefit if EF <35%, and three-vessel disease is present), prolonged ACE-inhibition therapy, and long-term anticoagulation. End-systolic volume may be a stronger predictor of survival than is LVEF (243).
5. Pharmacologic stress echocardiography is performed by using agents such as dobutamine, adenosine, and dipyridamole and typically is performed in higher risk patients (243,244). Even a negative test result has been associated with subsequent moderate event rate.

REFERENCES

General Review Articles and Guidelines

1. **Antman EM,** et al. **ACC/AHA guidelines for the management of patients with ST-elevation myocardial.** *Circulation* 2004;110:82–292 (focused update: *J Am Coll Cardiol* 2008;51;210–247).

2. **Kushner FG**, et al. 2009 focused updates: ACC/AHA guidelines for the management of patients with ST-elevation myocardial infarction (updating the 2004 guideline and 2007 focused update) and ACC/AHA/SCAI guidelines on PCI (updating the 2005 guideline and 2007 focused update): a report of the American College of Cardiology Foundation/American Heart Association Task Force on Practice Guidelines. *J Am Coll Cardiol* 2009;54:2205–2241.

This focused update to the STEMI guidelines largely addressed the timing of and role for GP IIb/IIIa inhibitors in patients with STEMI undergoing primary PCI. The committee also includes recommendations for the newest thienopyridine, prasugrel, and the anticoagulant bivalirudin.

Diagnosis

CHEST PAIN AND SYMPTOMS

3. **Edmondstone WM.** Cardiac chest pain: does body language help the diagnosis? *BMJ* 1995;311:1660–1661.

This study was composed of 203 consecutive patients with chest pain. Among the patients in whom a cardiac etiology was established (68%), 80% used three types of hand movements—Levine sign (clenched fist to middle of chest), flat hand to center of chest, and both hands placed flat in middle of chest and drawn outward—versus only 51% with noncardiac etiology ($p < 0.01$). Overall, sensitivity was 80%; specificity, 49%; positive predictive value, 77%; and negative predictive value, 53%.

4. **Douglas PS,** Ginsburg GS. The evaluation of chest pain in women. *N Engl J Med* 1996;334:1311–1315.

This review article discusses the major determinants of coronary artery disease (CAD) in women [chest pain (quality and incidence), hormonal status, diabetes, peripheral vascular disease], as well as intermediate determinants (hypertension, smoking, lipoproteins) and minor determinants (age older than 65 years, obesity, sedentary lifestyle, family history). The review concludes with a discussion of diagnostic testing.

5. **Goldman L,** et al. Prediction of the need for intensive care in patients who come to emergency departments with chest pain. *N Engl J Med* 1996;334:1498–1504.

This study was composed, in part, of a derivation set (10,682 patients) used to identify clinical predictors of major complications: ST elevation or Q waves, other ECG changes indicating myocardial ischemia, low SBP, pulmonary rales above bases, or an exacerbation of known ischemic heart disease. The validation set (4,676 patients) stratified patients into four groups with risk of major complications ranging from 0.15% to 8%. After 12 hours, the probability was updated based on whether the patient had a complication or confirmed MI. Patients with intermediate events (e.g., heart block, pulmonary edema without hypotension, recurrent ischemia not requiring CABG or PTCA within 72 hours) or confirmed MI had 3.5% to 7.5% risk of a major event per 24-hour period. Authors recommended intensive care unit (ICU) admission in this group. Echocardiographic, serum marker, or stress imaging data were not incorporated into this risk-stratification algorithm.

6. **Panju AA,** et al. Is this patient having a myocardial infarction? *JAMA* 1998;280:1256–1263.

Case-based discussion of history, physical, and ECG findings that are suggestive of the diagnosis of MI. Likelihood ratios are provided for these features; the most powerful predictors (or nonpredictors) of MI include new ST elevation (likelihood ratio range, 5.7 to 53.9), new Q wave (5.3 to 24.8), chest pain radiating to both arms simultaneously (7.1), positional chest pain (0.3), chest pain reproduced by palpation (0.2 to 0.4), pleuritic chest pain (0.2), and a normal ECG (0.1 to 0.3).

7. **Lee TH,** Goldman L. Evaluation of the patient with acute chest pain. *N Engl J Med* 2000;342(16):1187–1195.

This review focuses on the evaluation of chest pain related to cardiac ischemia, highlighting the most useful tests, expected cardiac marker trends, and emergent management. Algorithms are provided for the safe "rule-out" of patients without immediate evidence of cardiac injury, as well as helpful aids and guidelines for admitting such patients and identifying those at high risk for short-term morbidity and mortality.

ELECTROCARDIOGRAPHY

8. **Sgarbossa EB,** et al. Electrocardiographic diagnosis of evolving acute MI in the presence of left bundle branch block. *N Engl J Med* 1996;334:481–487 (editorial, 528–529).

Three ECG criteria were derived from an analysis of 131 GUSTO patients: (a) ST elevation of 1 mm concordant with QRS complex; (b) ST depression of 1 mm in V_1, V_2, or V_3; and (c) ST elevation of 5 mm discordant with QRS. ORs for confirmed MI were 25.2, 6.0, and 4.3. If the index score was 3 (a, $n = 5$ patients; b, $n = 3$ patients; c, $n = 2$ patients), sensitivity was 78%, and specificity 90%. However, sensitivity was only 36% in the validation group of 45 patients. The authors assert that the low sensitivity is an intrinsic property of ST elevation. The reported sensitivity and specificity depend on a 50% prevalence of MI (i.e., high index of suspicion of MI necessary). A retrospective cohort analysis of 83 patients with LBBB and symptoms suggestive of MI found that the sensitivity of this algorithm was only 10%.

9. **Casas RE,** et al. Value of leads V_7–V_9 in diagnosing posterior wall acute MI and other causes of tall R waves in V_1–V_2. *Am J Cardiol* 1997;80:508–509.

This large retrospective analysis found that 250 of approximately 17,000 hospital patients had leads V_7 to V_9 assessed because of a tall R in V_1 and/or suspicion of posterior MI. Among this selected group, 110 patients had evidence of new or old posterior MI, and in 25% of cases, V_7 to V_9 were the only leads diagnostic of MI.

10. **Zimetbaum PJ,** Josephson ME. Use of the electrocardiogram in acute myocardial infarction. *N Engl J Med* 2003;348:933–940.

This review mainly focuses on the identification of ST elevations, the common distributions, and their anatomically correlating infarct territories. Prognostic signs on the ECG are reviewed, as are the common conduction diseases and sequelae of acute MI. The guidelines for temporary and permanent pacing, as well as a review of tachyarrhythmias, are also discussed.

11. **Wang K,** et al. ST-segment elevation in conditions other than acute myocardial infarction. *N Engl J Med* 2003;349:2128–2135.

The article discusses first the features of ST-segment elevation that are both typical and atypical for ischemia versus normal variants in healthy patients. The authors go on to discuss such identification in LBBB, as well as alternative causes of ST-segment elevation, such as pericarditis, myocarditis, hyperkalemia, Brugada syndrome, arrhythmogenic RV cardiomyopathy, pulmonary embolus, Prinzmetal angina, and post-cardioversion ST-segment elevation. Examples of ECGs are provided.

SERUM MARKERS

12. **deWinter RJ,** et al. Value of myoglobin, troponin T and CK-MB in ruling out an acute MI in the emergency room. *Circulation* 1995;92:3401–3407.

This prospective analysis focused on 309 consecutive patients with chest pain. At 3 to 6 hours after symptoms, myoglobin yielded the best negative predictive value (89% at 4 hours).

The negative predictive value of CK-MB reached 95% at 7 hours. The markers were found to increase fastest with large MIs.

13. **Stubbs P,** et al. Prognostic significance of admission troponin T concentration in patients with MI. *Circulation* 1996;94:1291–1297.

This prospective study was composed of 240 patients showing any detectable TnT on admission associated with worse prognosis (median follow-up, 3 years). Admission TnT of 0.2 ng/mL was associated with a higher risk of subsequent cardiac death ($p = 0.0002$) and death plus MI ($p = 0.00006$). Most of this excess risk was confined to those with ST-segment elevation on admission ECG.

14. **Ohman EM,** et al. Cardiac troponin T levels for risk stratification in acute myocardial ischemia. *N Engl J Med* 1996;335:1333–1341.

This analysis focused on 801 GUSTO-IIa patients, of whom 72% had an MI. An elevated TnT (>1 ng/mL) was associated with a threefold higher 30-day mortality rate (11.9% vs. 3.9%; $p < 0.001$). Overall, the top mortality predictors were an elevated TnT (χ^2, 21; $p < 0.001$), ECG category (ST change or T-wave inversion; χ^2, 14; $p = 0.003$), and CK-MB (χ^2, 11; $p = 0.004$). TnT was still predictive in a model incorporating all three of these factors (χ^2, 9.2; $p = 0.027$). Proposed explanations of the increased mortality with elevated TnT included (a) later presentation; (b) higher cases of reocclusion, which is known to be associated with increased mortality; and (c) larger infarcts (also earlier release) in patients who died. TnT also had predictive prognostic value, even in patients with ST elevation.

15. **Antman E,** et al. Cardiac-specific TnI levels to predict the risk of mortality in patients with acute coronary syndromes. *N Engl J Med* 1996;335:1342–1349.

This analysis focused on 1,404 TIMI IIIB patients. TnI was elevated (0.4 ng/mL or more) in 573 patients and associated with a significantly increased 42-day mortality rate (3.7% vs. 1.0%; $p < 0.001$). Even after adjustments for ST depression and age 65 years or older (the two independent mortality predictors), each 1-ng/mL increase in TnI was associated with a mortality increase: 0.4 or less, 1%; 0.4 to 0.9, 1.7%; 1 to 1.9, 3.4%; 2 to 4.9, 3.7%; 5 to 8.9, 6%; and 9, 7.5%. TnI provided more prognostic information in patients with a late presentation (>6 to 24 hours): mortality 4% (TnI, 0.4 ng/mL or more) vs. 0.4% (relative risk, 9.5). In contrast, in patients seen early, the relative risk was only 1.8 (3.1% vs. 1.7%; $p = $ NS). If no CK-MB elevation was present (948 patients), a TnI elevation was still associated with increased mortality: 2.5% versus 0.8% (relative risk, 3.0; 95% CI, 0.97 to 9.2). The elevated TnI group had more ST deviation and less stenosis on angiography at 18 to 48 hours after symptom onset. However, few had angiography within hours of symptom onset.

16. **Newby LK,** et al. Value of serial TnT measures for early and late risk stratification in patients with acute coronary syndromes. *Circulation* 1998;98:1853–1859.

This GUSTO-IIa substudy of 734 patients showed the usefulness of the addition of later cardiac TnT (cTnT) samples. All patients had cTnT samples drawn at baseline, 8 hours, and 16 hours. At baseline, 260 patients were cTnT positive (>0.01 ng/mL), 323 became positive later, and 151 remained negative. The mortality rates were 10% in the baseline-positive group, 5% in the late positive group, and none in negative patients; thus, late-positive patients are at intermediate risk. After adjustment for baseline characteristics, any positive cTnT result predicted 30-day mortality. Only age and ST-segment elevation were stronger predictors than baseline cTnT. Most of the mortality difference between cTnT-positive and -negative patients occurred in the first 30 days.

17. **Tanasijevic MJ,** et al. Myoglobin, creatine-kinase-MB and cardiac troponin I 60-minute ratios predict infarct-related artery patency after thrombolysis for acute MI: results from TIMI 10B. *J Am Coll Cardiol* 1999;34:739–747.

This study was composed of 442 TIMI 10B patients who had CK-MB and cTnI measured immediately before and 60 minutes after TNK administration. Patent IRA (TIMI grade 2 or 3 flow) at 60 minutes was demonstrated in 77.8%. The diagnostic performance of the three assays was similar: area under receiver operating characteristic (ROC) curve for diagnosis of occlusion was 0.71, 0.70, and 0.71 for myoglobin, cTnI, and CK-MB. Sixty-minute ratios (concentration at 60 minutes/concentration at baseline) of 4.0 or more for myoglobin, 3.3 or more for CK-MB, and more than 2.0 for cTnI yielded probabilities of patency of 90%, 88%, and 87%, respectively. Authors assert that early invasive interventions to establish IRA patency may not be needed in these patients with high 60-minute ratios.

18. **Steen H,** et al. Cardiac troponin T at 96 hours after acute myocardial infarction correlates with infarct size and cardiac function. *J Am Coll Cardiol* 2006;48:2192–2194.

The authors correlate a single measurement of TnT 96 hours after STEMI/NSTEMI (23 STEMI, 21 NSTEMI) with contrast-enhanced magnetic resonance imaging (CE-MRI) of myocardial scar. Linear regression correlation coefficients were excellent for STEMI ($r = 0.910$), and less so, but still significant, for NSTEMI ($r = 0.575$).

EMERGENCY DEPARTMENT EVALUATION

19. **Gibler WB,** et al. A rapid diagnostic and treatment center for patients with chest pain in the emergency department. *Ann Emerg Med* 1995;25:1–8.

This analysis focused on 1,010 patients with possible acute ischemic heart disease (patients directly admitted if known CAD, hemodynamic instability, ST-segment changes > 1 mm, or ongoing chest pain). Serial CK-MB sampling was done at 0, 3, 6, and 9 hours, and continuous ECG monitoring was done for 9 hours. Two-dimensional echocardiography was performed at 9 hours if these tests were negative. If the echocardiogram was negative, the patient underwent a graded exercise test. Overall, 82% of patients were discharged from the emergency room Of the admitted patients, a substantial portion (34%) was found to have cardiac causes.

20. **Gomez MA,** et al. For the Rapid Rule-Out of Myocardial Ischemia Observation (**ROMIO**) study group. An emergency department-based on protocol for rapidly ruling out myocardial ischemia reduces hospital time and expense: result of a randomized study (ROMIO). *J Am Coll Cardiol* 1996;28:25–33.

This study randomized 100 low-risk patients to ED rule-out or hospital care. The ED protocol consisted of enzyme tests at 0, 3, 6, and 9 hours, serial ECGs with continuous ST-segment monitoring, and, if results were negative, predischarge exercise testing. The protocol group had a shorter hospital stay and incurred fewer costs. The routine care group included more MI and unstable angina patients, but among patients ruled out, the protocol still was associated with decreased stay and cost (12 hours vs. 23 hours; $p = 0.0001$; initial stay, $890 vs. $1,350; 30 days, $900 vs. $1,520; $p < 0.0001$).

21. **Kontos MC,** et al. Comparison of myocardial perfusion imaging and cardiac troponin I in patients admitted to the emergency department with chest pain. *Circulation* 1999;99: 2073–2078.

This study was composed of 620 patients considered at low to moderate risk for acute coronary syndromes who underwent gated single-photon emission Tc sestamibi imaging and serial measurements of CK, CK-MB, and TnI over an 8-hour period. The incidence of MI was 9%, significant CAD was demonstrated in 13%, and revascularization was performed in 9%. Perfusion imaging was more sensitive but less specific than TnI in identifying patients who were revascularized [sensitivity, 81% vs. 26% (TnI, 1.0 ng/mL); specificity, 74% vs. 96%].

22. **Carstensen S,** et al. Field triage to primary angioplasty combined with emergency department bypass reduces treatment delays and is associated with improved outcome. *Eur Heart J* 2007;28:2313–2319.

The investigators randomized 301 Australian patients with STEMI to either ECG and triage in the field by emergency medical services (EMSs) (with then the option of going to a center offering primary PCI) or ECG and triage at the nearest emergency department. Not only did patients triaged in the field have lower symptom-to-balloon times (154 minutes vs. 249 minutes; $p < 0.001$) and peak creatinine kinase levels (in early presenting patients only, 1,435 vs. 2,320; $p = 0.009$), but also overall in-hospital mortality was significantly reduced for patients triaged in the field (1.9% vs. 7.3%; $p = 0.046$).

23. **LeMay MR,** et al. A citywide protocol for primary PCI in ST-segment elevation myocardial infarction. *N Engl J Med* 2008;358:231–240.

The authors demonstrate the results of a citywide, integrated system by which all patients with STEMI are referred from the field to specialized centers for primary PCI in the city of Ottawa. Compared with patients referred from emergency departments for primary PCI at another institution, those referred from the field had lower door-to-balloon times (median 69 minutes vs. 123 minutes; $p < 0.01$) and more commonly achieved door-to-balloon times of less than 90 minutes (79.7% vs. 11.9%; $p < 0.001$). While this was not a randomized trial (and the populations were not equivalent), clinical outcomes were similar with a trend toward lower in-hospital mortality for those referred directly from the field (3.0% vs. 5.7%; $p = 0.30$).

Treatment

GENERAL META-ANALYSIS

24. **Lau JL,** et al. Cumulative meta-analysis of therapeutic trials for MI. *N Engl J Med* 1992;327:248–254.

This overview showed that significant mortality reduction was associated with aspirin (19,077 patients; OR, 0.77; $p < 0.001$), β-blockers (31,669 patients; OR, 0.88; $p = 0.024$), thrombolytics (OR, 0.75; $p < 0.001$), intravenously vasodilators (2,170 patients; OR, 0.57; $p < 0.001$), magnesium (only 1,304 patients; OR, 0.44; $p < 0.001$), and anticoagulation (4,975 patients; OR, 0.78; $p < 0.001$). Calcium-channel blockers and prophylactic lidocaine were both associated with a nonsignificant increase in mortality (6,420 patients; OR, 1.12; 8,745 patients; OR, 1.15). For secondary prevention, a protective effect was seen with β-blockers (20,138 patients; OR, 0.81; $p < 0.001$), anticoagulation (4,975 patients; OR, 0.78; $p < 0.001$), cholesterol-lowering drugs (10,775 patients; OR, 0.86; $p < 0.001$), and antiplatelet agents (18,411 patients; OR, 0.90; $p = 0.051$). Rehabilitation programs were beneficial (5,022 patients; OR, 0.80; $p = 0.012$). No benefit was seen with calcium-channel blockers (13,114 patients; OR, 1.10), and class I antiarrhythmics were harmful (4,336 patients; OR, 1.28; $p = 0.03$).

Antithrombotic Agents

ASPIRIN

25. **Second International Study of Infarct Survival (ISIS-2).** Randomised trial of intravenously streptokinase, oral, both, or neither among 17,187 cases of suspected acute MI. *Lancet* 1988;332:349–360.

This large trial clearly demonstrated the additive benefit of thrombolytic therapy and aspirin administration. Patients were randomized to SK, 1.5 million U over 60 minutes; and/or aspirin, 162.5 mg; or placebo. The SK and aspirin-alone groups had 25% and 23% lower 5-week vascular mortality, respectively [9.2% vs. 12.0% (placebo); $p < 0.00001$; 9.4% vs. 11.8%; $p < 0.00001$]. The SK and aspirin groups had a larger 42% mortality reduction (8% vs. 13.2%). Combination therapy also was effective in patients with LBBB (mortality, 14% vs. 27.7%). Aspirin reduced nonfatal reinfarction and stroke rates (1.0% vs. 2.0%; 0.3% vs. 0.6%).

26. **Roux S,** et al. Effect of aspirin on coronary reocclusion and recurrent ischemia after thrombolysis: a meta-analysis. *J Am Coll Cardiol* 1992;19:671–677.

    This analysis of 32 studies (19 randomized, 13 nonrandomized) from 1980 to 1990 showed the impressive benefits of aspirin. In these studies, 3,209 of 4,930 patients were treated with aspirin. Among the 1,022 patients who underwent angiography, aspirin use was associated with a 56% lower reocclusion rate (11% vs. 25%; $p < 0.001$) and fewer recurrent ischemic events (25% vs. 41%; $p < 0.001$). This protective effect of aspirin was similar in trials with either SK or recombinant tPA (rtPA).

27. **Berger JS,** et al. Initial aspirin dose and outcome among ST-elevation myocardial infarction patients treated with fibrinolytic therapy. *Circulation* 2008;117:192–199.

    Combining data from the Global Utilization of Streptokinase and Tissue Plasminogen Activator for Occluded Coronary Arteries (GUSTO I) and Global Use of Strategies to Open Occluded Coronary Arteries (GUSTO III) trials ($n = 48,422$ STEMI patients), the investigators assessed both ischemic and bleeding events in patients, stratified by aspirin dose, and adjusted for previously identified risk factors for morbidity and mortality. In adjusted analyses, mortality did not differ between patients receiving 162 mg aspirin versus 325 mg aspirin. However, after adjustment, 325-mg dosing was associated with significantly more moderate/severe bleeding (OR 1.14; $p = 0.003$). Importantly, this was limited to patients receiving lysis; no primary PCI patients were included.

THIENOPYRIDINES

28. **Sabatine MS,** et al. For the CLARITY-TIMI 28 Investigators. Addition of clopidogrel to aspirin and fibrinolytic therapy for myocardial infarction with ST-segment elevation. *N Engl J Med* 2005;352:1179–1189.

Design: Prospective, randomized, double-blind, international, multicenter study. Primary endpoint was a composite of occluded IRA on angiography or death or recurrent MI before angiography (at 48 to 192 hours).

Purpose: To determine the effect of clopidogrel on infarct-artery reperfusion in patients with STEMI receiving fibrinolysis.

Population: 3,491 patients aged 18 to 75 years old, with STEMI, presenting with 12 hours of symptom onset, treated with fibrinolytic therapy.

Exclusion Criteria: Use of clopidogrel within the last 7 days, any contraindication to fibrinolytic therapy, prior CABG.

Treatment: Clopidogrel (300-mg load, followed by 75 mg daily), or placebo.

Results: Clopidogrel reduced the incidence of the primary endpoint (15.0% vs. 21.7%; $p < 0.001$). At 30 days rates of clinical adverse events (a composite of cardiovascular death, recurrent MI, or urgent recurrent revascularization) were also reduced in the clopidogrel group (11.6% vs. 14.1%; $p = 0.03$). There was no increase in major bleeding.

29. COMMIT (Cl Opidogrel and Metoprolol in Myocardial Infarction Trial) Collaborative Group. Addition of clopidogrel to aspirin in 45 852 patients with acute myocardial infarction: randomized placebo-controlled trial. *Lancet* 2005;366:1607–1621.

Design: Prospective, randomized, placebo-controlled, multicenter study. There were two pre-specified co-primary endpoints at discharge or over a treatment period of 4 weeks (whichever came sooner): (1) a composite of death, reinfarction, or stroke, and (2) death from any cause.

Purpose: To determine the benefit, if any, of adding clopidogrel to aspirin in the treatment of STEMI.

Population: 45,852 patients admitted within 24 hours of acute MI, with ST elevation, LBBB, or ST depression (7% of the trial population) on ECG.

Exclusion Criteria: Patients scheduled for primary PCI (clopidogrel would be indicated).

Treatment: Clopidogrel 75 mg daily, or placebo.

Results: Clopidogrel reduced the incidence of the composite primary endpoint (9.2% vs. 10.1%; $p = 0.002$), as well as overall mortality (7.5% vs. 8.1%; $p = 0.03$). There was no increase in overall bleeding detected (0.58% vs. 0.55%; $p = 0.59$), or in the subgroups of those who received fibrinolytic therapy or older than 70 years of age. Importantly, these results were consistent across a wide and diverse range of subgroups analyzed, without any heterogeneity.

Comment: There was also a β-blocker arm of this study, reported below.

30. **Montalescot G**, et al. for the TRITON-TIMI 38 Investigators. Prasugrel compared with clopidogrel in patients undergoing percutaneous coronary intervention for ST-elevation myocardial infarction (TRITON-TIMI 38): double-blind, randomised controlled trial. *Lancet* 2009;373:723–731.

The authors examine the subset of patients with STEMI from the TRITON-TIMI 38 trial, which included all spectra of ACS (see Chapter 3 for the complete trial details). Briefly, the trial compared the newest thienopyridine, prasugrel, with clopidogrel in 13,608 patients with ACS. Of these, 3,534 patients presented with STEMI (approximately 26%), the vast majority of whom underwent primary PCI (>95%). Roughly one third received a DES. The primary endpoint of a composite of cardiovascular death, MI, or stroke at 15 months was significantly lower in the prasugrel group (6.5% vs. 9.5%; $p = 0.0017$), compared to clopidogrel. Consistently, the composite outcome of cardiovascular death, MI, or urgent TVR was also reduced at 30 days ($p = 0.0205$) and 15 months ($p = 0.025$). Overall, bleeding rates were similar, with the exception being patients who subsequently underwent CABG and had higher bleeding in the prasugrel group ($p = 0.0033$).

HEPARIN

31. **Hsia J**, et al. for the Heparin Aspirin Reperfusion Trial (**HART**) Investigators. A comparison between heparin and low-dose aspirin as adjunctive therapy with tissue plasminogen activator for acute MI. *N Engl J Med* 1990;323:1433–1437.

Design: Prospective, randomized, open-label, multicenter study. Primary endpoint was IRA patency at 7 to 24 hours and 7 days.

Purpose: To compare the effects of heparin with aspirin after rtPA in patients with acute MI.

Population: 205 patients aged 75 years and older with acute STEMI (0.1 mm or more in at least two contiguous leads).

Exclusion Criteria: Severe hypotension, cerebrovascular disease, bleeding disorders, LBBB, prior CABG, recent surgery, and prolonged CPR.

Treatment: rtPA, 100 mg i.v. over a 6-hour period (6-mg bolus, 54 mg during hour 1, 20 mg in hour 2, 5 mg/hr for 4 hours) plus either aspirin, 80 mg/day, or heparin, 5,000 U i.v. bolus, and then 1,000 U/hr [adjusted to keep activated partial thromboplastin time (aPTT) within 1.5 to 2.0 times control]. Coronary angiography was performed 7 to 24 hours after rtPA infusion was started and again at 7 days.

Results: Heparin group had higher patency (TIMI grade 2 or 3 flow) at initial angiography (82% vs. 52%; $p < 0.0001$), but no significant difference was seen by the time of the second angiograms (88% vs. 95%). No significant differences were seen in hemorrhagic or recurrent ischemic events.

Comments: A retrospective analysis showed that patients with open arteries at early angiography had a higher mean PTT (81 seconds vs. 54 seconds; $p < 0.02$). However, patients with a PTT of more than 100 at 8 hours had a higher rate of access-related hemorrhage.

LOW-MOLECULAR-WEIGHT HEPARINS

32. **Ross AM,** et al. Randomized comparison of enoxaparin, a low-molecular-weight heparin with unfractionated heparin adjunctive to recombinant tissue plasminogen activator

thrombolysis and aspirin: second trial of Heparin and Aspirin Reperfusion Therapy (**HART II**). *Circulation* 2001;104:648–652.

Design: Prospective, randomized, open-label, parallel-group, international trial. Primary endpoint was IRA patency (TIMI grade 2 or 3 flow) at 90 minutes.

Purpose: To demonstrate noninferiority of enoxaparin compared with UFH as an adjunctive therapy during thrombolytic treatment for acute MI.

Population: 400 patients seen within 12 hours and with ST elevation 0.1 mV or more in two or more limb leads or ST elevation of 0.2 mV or more in two or more contiguous precordial leads.

Exclusion Criteria: Contraindications to thrombolysis and serum creatinine more than 2 mg/dL.

Treatment: Enoxaparin or UFH for at least 3 days. All received accelerated tPA regimen and aspirin.

Results: Patency rates at 90 minutes were 80.1% and 75.1% in the enoxaparin and UFH groups, respectively. TIMI grade 3 flow was observed in 52.9% and 47.6%, respectively. Reocclusion at 5 to 7 days from TIMI grade 2 or 3 to TIMI 0 or 1 flow and TIMI grade 3 to TIMI 0 or 1 flow, respectively, occurred in 5.9% and 3.1% of the enoxaparin group versus 9.8% and 9.1% in the UFH group. Bleeding and 30-day mortality rates were similar in both groups.

Comments: The results of this study complement the findings of the larger ASSENT-3 trial (98).

33. **Antman EM,** et al. Enoxaparin as adjunctive antithrombin therapy for ST-elevation myocardial infarction: results of the ENTIRE-Thrombolysis in Myocardial Infarction (**TIMI) 23** trial. *Circulation* 2002;105:1642–1649.

Design: Prospective, randomized, open, 2 × 2 factorial, multicenter trial. Primary endpoint: TIMI grade 3 flow at 60 minutes.

Purpose: To evaluate enoxaparin with full-dose TNK and half-dose TNK plus abciximab.

Population: 483 patients with STEMI seen less than 6 hours from symptom onset.

Exclusion Criteria: Included contraindications to thrombolysis, abciximab within the prior 7 days or eptifibatide or tirofiban within the prior 24 hours; treatment with any LMWH or UFH within 24 hours.

Treatment: Full-dose TNK and either UFH (60-U/kg bolus and then 12 U/kg/hr) or enoxaparin (1.0 mg/kg s.c. every 12 hours ± initial 30-mg i.v. bolus) or half-dose TNK plus abciximab and either UFH (40-U/kg bolus and then 7 U/kg/hr) or enoxaparin (0.3 to 0.75 mg/kg s.c. every 12 hours ± initial i.v. bolus of 30 mg).

Results: With full-dose TNK and UFH, TIMI grade 3 flow at 60 minutes was 52%, and was 48% to 51% with enoxaparin. With combination therapy, the TIMI 3 flow was achieved in 48% with UFH and 47% to 58% with enoxaparin. The rate of TIMI 3 flow among all UFH patients was 50% compared with 51% among enoxaparin patients. At 30 days, death or recurrent MI occurred with the full-dose TNK group in 15.9% of patients with UFH compared with only 4.4% with enoxaparin (*p* = 0.005). With combination therapy, the rates were 6.5% with UFH and 5.5% with enoxaparin. Major hemorrhage with full-dose TNK occurred in 2.4% with UFH and 1.9% with enoxaparin; with combination therapy, 5.2% with UFH and 8.5% with enoxaparin.

Comments: Major finding is that in patients receiving full-dose TNK, enoxaparin was associated with similar TIMI 3 flow rates but fewer ischemic events at 30 days compared with UFH.

34. **Antman EM,** et al. for the ExTRACT-TIMI 25 Investigators. Enoxaparin versus unfractionated heparin with fibrinolysis for ST-elevation myocardial infarction. *N Engl J Med* 2006;354:1477–1488.

Design: Prospective, randomized, double-blind, international, multicenter trial. Primary endpoint: death or nonfatal recurrent MI at 30 days.

Purpose: To compare efficacy and safety of enoxaparin versus UFH in patients with STEMI receiving fibrinolytic therapy.

Population: 20,056 patients with STEMI seen less than 6 hours from symptom onset and eligible for fibrinolysis.

Exclusion Criteria: Included cardiogenic shock, pericarditis, symptoms of aortic dissection, contraindications to fibrinolysis, receipt of a low-molecular-weight heparin within the prior eight hours, known renal insufficiency (serum creatinine > 2.5 mg/dL for men, 2.0 mg/dL for women), or life expectancy less than 12 months.

Treatment: UFH for at least 48 hours versus enoxaparin throughout hospitalization (or 8 days, whichever was shorter). Enoxaparin dosing was reduced in patients 75 years of age or older. All patients received aspirin and fibrinolysis (the agent at the physician's discretion), and clopidogrel was given at the physician's discretion.

Results: Enoxaparin significantly reduced the primary endpoint (9.9% vs. 12.0%; $p < 0.001$), with the majority of the benefit in reduction of reinfarction. Major bleeding was significantly higher in the enoxaparin group (2.1% vs. 1.4%; $p < 0.001$). When ischemic and bleeding events were combined (death, reinfarction, intracranial hemorrhage), this net clinical effect favored enoxaparin (10.1% vs. 12.2%; $p < 0.001$).

Comments: The superiority of enoxaparin over UFH was subsequently verified in multiple prespecified, post hoc analyses of different subgroups of the trial, including by age stratification (*Eur Heart J* 2007;28:1066–1071), in patients with impaired renal function (*J Am Coll Cardiol* 2007;49:2249–2255), in patients who did and did **not** receive clopidogrel (*J Am Coll Cardiol* 2007;49:2256–2263), in each type of fibrinolytic agent (*Eur Heart J* 2007;28:1566–1573), and also in those patients in the ExTRACT-TIMI 25 trial who subsequently underwent PCI as a "rescue" strategy or for recurrent symptoms (*J Am Coll Cardiol* 2007;49:2238–2246).

35. **Murphy SA**, et al. Efficacy and safety of the low-molecular weight heparin enoxaparin compared with unfractionated heparin across the acute coronary syndrome spectrum: a meta-analysis. *Eur Heart J* 2007;28:2077–2086.

The investigators combined patient-level data from 12 randomized studies (6 each of both STEMI and UA/NSTEMI), including 49,088 patients. The net clinical events endpoint was a composite of death, MI, or major bleeding at 30 days. Across the spectrum of ACS, enoxaparin proved superior to UFH for ischemic events (9.8% vs. 11.4% for death or MI; $p < 0.001$), and reduced the net clinical event rate nonsignificantly (12.5% vs. 13.5%; $p = 0.051$). Major bleeding remained higher in the enoxaparin group (4.3% vs. 3.4%; $p = 0.019$). When isolated to STEMI patients only, the net clinical events endpoint significantly favored enoxaparin (OR 0.94; $p = 0.015$).

36. **Yusuf S**, et al. for the CREATE Trial Group Investigators. Effects of reviparin, a low-molecular weight heparin, on mortality, reinfarction, and strokes in patients with acute myocardial infarction presenting with ST-segment elevation. *JAMA* 2005;293:427–435.

Design: Prospective, randomized, double-blind, placebo-controlled, multicenter, international trial. Primary endpoint was a composite of death, reinfarction, or stoke at 7 and 30 days.

Purpose: To compare the effects of reviparin versus placebo, in addition to standard therapy, for patients with STEMI.

Population: 15,570 patients with STEMI presenting within 12 hours of symptoms.

Treatment: Reviparin twice daily or placebo for 7 days.

Results: Reviparin significantly reduced the primary outcome at 7 days (9.6% vs. 11%; $p = 0.005$), and the effect persisted at 30 days (11.8% vs. 13.6%; $p = 0.001$). Overall mortality at 30 days was also significantly reduced in the reviparin group (9.8% vs. 11.3%; $p = 0.005$), as well as reinfarction (2.0% vs. 2.6%; $p = 0.01$) without a change in stroke rate (1.0% vs. 0.8%; $p = 0.19$). There was a significant time-to-benefit effect with reviparin ($p = 0.04$ for trend to increased benefit for every 2 hours sooner it was given). Life-threatening bleeding occurred at a higher, albeit nonsignificant, rate in the reviparin group at 7 days (0.2% vs. 0.1%; $p = 0.07$).

FONDAPARINUX

37. **The OASIS-6 Trial Group**. Effects of fondaparinux on mortality and reinfarction in patients with acute ST-segment elevation myocardial infarction: the OASIS-6 randomized trial. *JAMA* 2006;295:1519–1530.

Design: Prospective, randomized, double-blind, multicenter, international trial. The primary endpoint was a composite of death or reinfarction at 30 days. Additional secondary analyses at 9 days, 3 months, and 6 months.

Purpose: To compare efficacy and safety of fondaparinux versus control (either placebo or UFH) for treatment in patients with STEMI in whom UFH is indicated and in patients in whom it is not indicated.

Population: 12,092 patients with STEMI, presenting within 12 to 24 hours of symptom onset; enrollment was stratified by whether the clinician-investigator felt UFH was indicated.

Treatment: Patients in whom UFH was not indicated (stratum 1) were randomized to either fondaparinux or placebo (control group); patients in whom UFH was indicated (stratum 2) were randomized to either fondaparinux or UFH. If patients went for PCI, blinded study drug was maintained, with dosing adjusted depending on whether they received UFH and/or glycoprotein IIb/IIIa inhibitors prior to randomization. Both strata were combined [comparing fondaparinux vs. control (placebo or UFH)] for reporting of the primary outcome.

Results: The primary endpoint was significantly decreased in the fondaparinux group, compared to control (9.7% vs. 11.2%; $p = 0.008$). This benefit was significant at 9 days ($p = 0.003$). In patients in stratum 2 not undergoing PCI, fondaparinux nonsignificantly reduced rates of death and reinfarction at 30 days, compared with UFH (hazard ratio 0.82; $p = 0.08$). For patients undergoing primary PCI, there was no difference in outcomes between fondaparinux and either control. With respect to the primary outcome, fondaparinux proved superior to control in patients receiving thrombolytic therapy (hazard ratio 0.79; $p = 0.003$), and among those receiving no reperfusion therapy (hazard ratio 0.80; $p = 0.03$).

DIRECT THROMBIN INHIBITORS

38. **Antman EM,** et al. for the **TIMI-9B** Investigators. Hirudin in AMI. *Circulation* 1996;94:911–921.

Design: Prospective, randomized, double-blind, parallel-group, multicenter study. Primary endpoint was 30-day incidence of death, nonfatal MI, severe CHF, and cardiogenic shock.

Purpose: To compare the safety and effectiveness of hirudin with heparin in patients undergoing thrombolysis for acute MI.

Population: 3,002 patients within 12 hours of onset of symptoms and with greater than 1-mm ST elevation in at least two contiguous ECG leads; mean age, 60 ± 12 years.

Exclusion Criteria: Contraindications to thrombolytic therapy, creatinine more than 2.0 mg/dL, cardiogenic shock, and therapeutic anticoagulation (PT, 14 seconds; aPTT, 60 seconds).

Treatment: Heparin, 5,000-U i.v. bolus, and then 1,000 U/hr, or hirudin, 0.1-mg/kg i.v. bolus, and then 0.1 mg/kg/hr (maximum, 15 mg/hr) for 96 hours. Infusions were started before or immediately after thrombolysis (front-loaded tPA or SK) and adjusted to keep aPTT at 55 to 85 seconds. All patients were given thrombolysis.

Results: No significant difference in primary endpoints was observed—12.9% (hirudin) versus 11.9%, nor were any differences observed in hemorrhage and intracranial hemorrhage rates (4.6% vs. 5.3; 0.4% vs. 0.9%). Target aPTT was achieved more frequently with hirudin.

39. **White HD,** et al. on behalf of the Hirulog Early Perfusion/Occlusion (**HERO**) Trial Investigators. Randomized, double-blind comparison of hirulog versus heparin in patients receiving streptokinase and aspirin for acute MI (HERO). *Circulation* 1997;96:2155–2161 (editorial, 2118–2120).

Design: Prospective, randomized, double-blind, multicenter study. Primary outcome was TIMI grade flow at 90 to 120 minutes.

Purpose: To evaluate and compare the safety and efficacy of two hirulog regimens with heparin in acute MI patients receiving SK.

Population: 412 patients seen within 12 hours of symptom onset and with 1-mm ST elevation or greater in at least two contiguous limb leads and/or V_4 to V_6 or 2 mm or more in V_1 to V_3.

Exclusion Criteria: Prior SK, cardiogenic shock, and contraindications to thrombolysis.

Treatment: Heparin, 5,000-U i.v. bolus, and then 1,000 to 1,200 U/hr, low-dose hirulog (0.125 mg/kg i.v. bolus, 0.25 mg/kg/hr for 12 hours, and then 0.125 mg/kg/hr), or high-dose hirulog (0.25-mg/kg intravenously bolus, 0.5 mg/kg/hr for 12 hours, and then 0.25 mg/kg/hr).

Results: Hirulog groups had better TIMI grade 3 flow at 90 to 120 minutes (primary outcome)—46% and 48% versus 35% (heparin vs. hirulog, $p = 0.023$; heparin vs. high-dose hirulog, $p = 0.03$). However, no significant difference in rates of reocclusion was observed at 48 hours (5% and 1% vs. 7%) or death, shock, and reinfarction at 35 days (14% and 12.5% vs. 17.9%). Hirulog also was associated with less major bleeding: 14% and 19% versus 28% (low-dose hirulog vs. heparin, $p < 0.01$).

40. **Behar S,** et al. Argatroban versus heparin as adjuvant therapy for thrombolysis for acute myocardial infarction: safety considerations **ARGAMI-2** study [abstract]. *Circulation* 1998;98(1 Suppl):I453–I454.

This prospective, randomized, placebo-controlled study was composed of 1,200 patients seen within 6 hours and with ST elevation in two or more leads. Exclusion criteria included CNS events, elevated creatinine, and increased bleeding risk(s). Patients were randomized to argatroban (60 μg + 2 μg/kg/min or 120 μg + 4 μg/kg/min for 72 hours) or heparin (5,000 IU + 1,000 IU/hr for 72 hours) with dose adjustment(s) to achieve aPTT of 55 to 85 seconds. All received aspirin and tPA or SK. Low-dose argatroban arm was closed after interim analysis of first 609 patients. At 30 days, no difference was found between the high-dose argatroban and heparin groups in total cardiovascular events, mortality, recurrent MI, heart failure/ cardiogenic shock, need for revascularization, or stroke. The argatroban group had a lower incidence of major bleeding, intracranial hemorrhage, and stroke. Maintaining aPTT was easier with argatroban, with only 35% of having an aPTT value less than 55 seconds at 24 hours compared with 68% in the heparin group.

41. **The Hirulog and Early Reperfusion or Occlusion (HERO)-2** Trial Investigators. Thrombin-specific anticoagulation with bivalirudin versus heparin in patients receiving fibrinolytic therapy for acute myocardial infarction: the HERO-2 randomized trial. *Lancet* 2001;358:1855–1863.

Design: Prospective, randomized, open, multicenter study. Primary endpoint: 30-day mortality.

Purpose: To evaluate the effect on 30-day mortality of bivalirudin versus UFH in acute MI patients treated with SK.

Population: 17,073 patients with acute STEMI seen within 6 hours of symptom onset and with 1 mm or more of ST elevation in two limb leads or 2 mm or more in two contiguous precordial leads or presumed new LBBB.

Exclusion Criteria: Included contraindications to thrombolysis, LMWH therapy within 12 hours, and previous SK therapy.

Treatment: Bivalirudin (0.25-mg/kg bolus, and then 0.5 mg/kg/hr for 12 hours, and then 0.25 mg/kg/hr for 36 hours) or UFH. All received SK, 1.5 MU over a 30- to 60-minute period, and aspirin, 150 to 325 mg once daily.

Results: At 30 days, no significant difference appeared between the two groups in unadjusted mortality (bivalirudin, 10.8%; heparin, 10.9%) and adjusted mortality (10.5% vs. 10.9%). At 96 hours, the bivalirudin group had a 30% reduction in reinfarction compared with the heparin group (1.6% vs. 2.3%; $p = 0.001$). Nonsignificant trends were seen toward increased severe bleeding and intracerebral bleeding with bivalirudin (0.7% vs. 0.5%, $p = 0.07$; 0.6% vs. 0.4%, $p = 0.09$), whereas significant increased risks of both moderate and mild bleeding were noted (1.4% vs. 1.1%, $p = 0.05$; 12.8% vs. 9.0%, $p < 0.001$).

42. The **Direct Thrombin Inhibitor** Trialists' Collaborative Group. Direct thrombin inhibitors in acute coronary syndromes: principal results of a meta-analysis based on individual patients' data. *Lancet* 2002;359:294–302.

This meta-analysis examined 11 randomized trials (35,970 total patients) comparing a direct thrombin inhibitor (DTI; hirudin, bivalirudin, argatroban, efegatran, or inogatran) with heparin. Compared with heparin, DTIs were associated with a lower risk of death or MI at the end of treatment [4.3% vs. 5.1%; OR, 0.85 (95% CI, 0.77 to 0.94); $p = 0.001$] and at 30 days [7.4% vs. 8.2%; OR, 0.91 (95% CI, 0.84 to 0.99); $p = 0.02$]. This was due primarily to a reduction in MI [2.8% vs. 3.5%; OR, 0.80 (95% CI, 0.71 to 0.90); $p < 0.001$] with no significant effect on mortality [1.9% vs. 2.0%; OR, 0.97 (95% CI, 0.83 to 1.13); $p = 0.69$]. Subgroup analyses suggested a benefit of DTIs on death or MI in trials of both acute coronary syndromes and PCIs. Compared with heparin, an increased risk of major bleeding with hirudin was seen, but a reduction with bivalirudin. No increased incidence of intracranial hemorrhage was found with DTIs.

43. **Stone GW,** et al. for the HORIZONS-AMI Trial Investigators. Bivalirudin during primary PCI in acute myocardial infarction. *N Engl J Med* 2008;358:2218–2230.

Design: Prospective, randomized, open-label, multicenter study. Two co-primary endpoints: (1) major bleeding and (2) combined adverse clinical events (major bleeding, death, reinfarction, TVR for ischemia, or stroke), both at 30 days.

Purpose: To evaluate the strategy of bivalirudin as anticoagulation for patients undergoing primary PCI for STEMI, as compared with a combination of UFH and glycoprotein IIb/IIIa inhibitor.

Population: 3,602 patients with STEMI, presenting within 12 hours of symptom onset, undergoing primary PCI.

Treatment: Bivalirudin alone versus UFH plus a glycoprotein IIb/IIIa inhibitor.

Results: Treatment with bivalirudin resulted in decreased rates of clinical adverse events (9.2% vs. 12.1%; $p = 0.005$), mainly driven by reduced rates of major bleeding (4.9% vs. 8.3%; $p < 0.001$). However, there was a significant increase in acute stent thrombosis in the bivalirudin group at 24 hours (1.3% vs. 0.3%; $p < 0.001$). Despite this, 30-day rates of stent thrombosis (1.7% vs. 1.2%; $p = 0.28$) were similar, and cardiac mortality (1.8% vs. 2.9%; $p = -0.03$) and overall mortality (2.1% vs. 3.1%; $p = 0.047$) were both reduced at 30 days.

WARFARIN

44. **Smith P,** et al. Warfarin Reinfarction Study (**WARIS**). The effect of warfarin on mortality and reinfarction after MI. *N Engl J Med* 1990;323:147–152.

Design: Prospective, randomized, double-blind, placebo-controlled, multicenter study. Mean follow-up period was 37 months. Primary endpoint was all-cause mortality and reinfarction.

Purpose: To evaluate the effects of warfarin on mortality, reinfarction, and cerebrovascular events in post-MI patients.

Population: 1,214 patients aged 75 years or younger; mean time since index MI, 27 days.

Exclusion Criteria: Required anticoagulant use and significant bleeding risk.

Treatment: Warfarin dose adjusted to achieve target INR of 2.8 to 4.8, or placebo.

Results: Warfarin group had 24% lower all-cause mortality (15.5% vs. 20.3%; $p = 0.03$), 34% fewer reinfarctions (13.5% vs. 20.4%; $p < 0.001$), and 55% fewer cerebrovascular accidents (CVAs; 3.3% vs. 7.2%; $p = 0.0015$). Serious bleeding rate in the warfarin group was 0.6% per year (intracranial hemorrhage rate, 0.2% per year).

45. **Anticoagulants in Secondary Prevention of Events in Coronary Thrombosis (ASPECT)** Research Group. Effect of long-term anticoagulant treatment on mortality and cardiovascular morbidity after MI. *Lancet* 1994;343:499–503.

Design: Prospective, randomized, double-blind, placebo-controlled, multicenter study. Mean follow-up period was 37 months. Primary endpoint was all-cause mortality.

Purpose: To evaluate the impact of long-term anticoagulation in the secondary prevention of morbidity and mortality after acute MI.

Population: 3,404 patients with cardiac serum marker evidence of an acute MI (2× or more the upper limit of normal).

Exclusion Criteria: Need for long-term anticoagulation, anticoagulation therapy in the prior 6 months, increased bleeding tendency, and anticipated coronary revascularization procedure.

Treatment: Phenprocoumon or nicoumalone started within 6 weeks of hospital discharge to achieve an INR of 2.8 to 4.8, or placebo.

Results: No significant mortality difference was observed between groups [10% (anticoagulation) vs. 11.1%]. Anticoagulation was associated with a reduction in two secondary endpoints: more than 50% fewer recurrent MIs (6.7% vs. 14.2%) and approximately 40% fewer cerebrovascular events (2.2% vs. 3.6%). The anticoagulation group had more major bleeding complications (4.3% vs. 1.1%).

Comments: A post hoc analysis showed that the optimal INR was 3 to 4. The rate of major bleeding plus thromboembolic complications was 3.2 per 100 patient years (INR, <2, 8.0; 2 to 3, 3.9; 4 to 5, 6.6; >5, 7.7).

46. **Julian DG,** et al. for the Aspirin/Anticoagulants Following Thrombolysis with Eminase in Recurrent infarction (**AFTER**) Study Group. A comparison of aspirin and anticoagulation following thrombolysis for MI (the AFTER study): a multicentre unblinded randomised clinical trial. *BMJ* 1996;313:1429–1431.

Design: Prospective, randomized, unblinded, multicenter study. Follow-up period was 1 year. Primary endpoint was cardiac death and nonfatal MI at 30 days.

Purpose: To compare aspirin with heparin followed by oral anticoagulation therapy in MI patients undergoing thrombolysis with anistreplase.

Population: 1,036 patients treated with anistreplase within 6 hours of onset of symptoms (ECG criteria, 2 mm or more ST elevation in at least two adjacent precordial leads or 1 mm or more in at least two limb leads).

Treatment: Aspirin, 150 mg/day, or heparin, 1,000 U/hr for 24 hours (started 6 hours after anistreplase, 30 U) followed by oral anticoagulation to achieve a target INR of 2.0 to 2.5. Therapy was discontinued after 3 months.

Results: Similar 30-day incidences of cardiac death and reinfarction were observed [11.2% (aspirin) vs. 11%]. The anticoagulation group had more severe bleeding and strokes: at 3 months, 3.9% vs. 1.7% ($p = 0.04$).

47. **Coumadin Aspirin Reinfarction Study (CARS) Investigators**. Randomised double-blind trial of fixed low-dose warfarin with aspirin after MI. *Lancet* 1997;350:389–396.

Design: Prospective, randomized, double-blind, multicenter study. Median follow-up period was 14 months. Primary endpoint was MI, stroke, and cardiovascular death.

Purpose: To compare long-term administration of aspirin alone with lower dose aspirin in combination with fixed low-dose regimens of oral anticoagulation in acute MI patients.

Population: 8,803 patients aged 21 to 85 years with a documented MI 3 to 21 days before enrollment.

Treatment: Aspirin, 160 mg/day; aspirin, 80 mg/day; and warfarin, 1 mg/day; or aspirin, 80 mg/day; and warfarin, 3 mg/day.

Results: Average measured INRs at week 4 were 1.02 (aspirin alone), 1.05 (aspirin and warfarin, 1 mg/day), and 1.27 (aspirin and warfarin, 3 mg/day). No significant difference in primary endpoints (MI, stroke, or cardiovascular death) was observed [1-year rates, 8.6% (aspirin), 8.8% (aspirin and warfarin, 1 mg/day), 8.4% (aspirin and warfarin, 3 mg/day)]. However, the warfarin, 3 mg/day, group had a higher rate of spontaneous major hemorrhage versus aspirin alone: 0.74% per year versus 1.4% per year ($p = 0.014$).

48. **Fiore LD,** et al. for the Combination Hemotherapy and Mortality Prevention (**CHAMP**) Study. Department of Veterans Affairs Cooperative Studies Program clinical trial comparing

combined warfarin and aspirin with aspirin alone in survivors of acute myocardial infarction: primary results of the CHAMP Study. *Circulation* 2002;105:557–563.

Design: Prospective, randomized, open-label, multicenter. Primary endpoint was all-cause mortality. Median follow-up was 2.7 years.

Purpose: To determine if the combination of aspirin and warfarin is more effective than aspirin monotherapy in the secondary prevention of vascular events and death after AMI.

Population: 5,059 patients with AMI within 14 days. Diagnosis of AMI as defined by the presence of two of the following: (a) chest discomfort typical of AMI, (b) ECG changes typical of AMI, and (c) blood enzyme changes typical of AMI.

Exclusion Criteria: Included more than 14 days after MI, ongoing bleeding or bleeding risk, alternative indication for anticoagulant therapy, treatment with high-dose aspirin or NSAID, and hypersensitivity to aspirin or warfarin.

Treatment: Warfarin (target INR, 1.5 to 2.5) plus aspirin (81 mg once daily) or aspirin alone (162 mg once daily).

Results: At follow-up, all-cause mortality was similar in the two groups [17.6% (combination group) vs. 17.3% (aspirin only)]. No significant difference was seen between the groups in recurrent MI (13.3% vs. 13.1%, respectively; log-rank $p = 0.78$) or stroke (3.1% vs. 3.5%, respectively; log-rank $p = 0.52$). Major bleeding, primarily GI, occurred more often in the combination-therapy group than in the aspirin group (1.28 events per 100 patient years vs. 0.72 events per 100 patient years, respectively; $p < 0.001$).

49. **van Es RF,** et al. for the Antithrombotics in the Secondary Prevention of Events in Coronary Thrombosis-2 (ASPECT-2) Research Group. Aspirin and coumadin after acute coronary syndromes (the ASPECT-2 study): a randomised controlled trial. *Lancet* 2002;360:109–113.

Design: Prospective, randomized, open-label, multicenter trial. The primary composite endpoint was MI, stroke, or death.

Purpose: To determine whether the combination of aspirin and oral anticoagulants provides a greater benefit than either of these agents alone, without excessive risk of bleeding.

Population: 999 patients with AMI or unstable in previous 8 weeks.

Exclusion Criteria: Included established indication(s) for oral anticoagulation or platelet inhibitors, planned revascularization, increased risk of bleeding, bleeding diathesis, history of stroke, and pregnancy.

Treatment: Low-dose aspirin (80 mg), high-intensity oral anticoagulation (target INR, 3.0 to 4.0), or combined low-dose aspirin and moderate-intensity oral anticoagulation (target INR, 2.0 to 2.5).

Results: The anticoagulant and combination-therapy groups had a significantly lower incidence of the primary composite endpoint compared with the aspirin group [hazard ratio, 0.55 (95% CI, 0.30 to 1.00); $p = 0.0479$; hazard ratio, 0.50 (0.27 to 0.92); $p = 0.03$], respectively. Major bleeding was similar in the three groups (1% to 2%). Frequency of minor bleeding was 5%, 8% [1.68 (0.92 to 3.07); $p = 0.20$], and 15% [3.13 (1.82 to 5.37); $p \leq 0.0001$], in the aspirin, anticoagulant, and combination groups, respectively.

50. **Hureln M,** et al. Warfarin, aspirin, or both after myocardial infarction: **WARIS-II** (Warfarin–Aspirin Reinfarction Study). *N Engl J Med* 2002;347:969–974.

Design: Prospective, randomized, open-label, multicenter trial. Primary endpoint: death, nonfatal MI, and stroke. Mean follow-up, 4 years.

Purpose: To compare the efficacy and safety of long-term treatment with warfarin alone, aspirin alone, or the two combined in survivors of AMI.

Population: 3,630 patients aged 20 to 74 years with two or more of following—ischemic chest pain, ECG changes typical of AMI, CK greater than 250 U/L, and/or aspartate aminotransferase greater than 50 U/L of probable cardiac origin.

Exclusion Criteria: Included history of serious bleeding or bleeding diathesis, spontaneous bleeding with aspirin or warfarin, and any contraindication to or indication for aspirin or warfarin.

Treatment: Randomized on hospital discharge to warfarin (target INR, 2.8 to 4.2) or aspirin (160 mg/day) or warfarin (target INR, 2.0 to 2.5) and aspirin (75 mg/day). The average INR was 2.8 in the warfarin-alone group and 2.2 in the warfarin + aspirin group; however, measured INRs were below target one third of the time.

Results: The incidence of death, nonfatal MI, and stroke was 20.0% in the aspirin-alone group compared with 16.7% in warfarin-alone group [relative risk ratio compared with aspirin, 0.81 (95% CI, 0.67 to 0.98); $p = 0.028$] and 15.0% in the aspirin + warfarin group [relative risk ratio compared with aspirin, 0.71 (95% CI, 0.58 to 0.86); $p = 0.0005$]. The aspirin + warfarin group had a significantly higher cumulative probability of survival compared with the aspirin-alone group ($p = 0.0033$), whereas no significant difference was seen between the warfarin-alone and the warfarin + aspirin groups. However, major bleeding rates (bleeding requiring transfusion or surgical intervention) were higher in the warfarin groups (0.58/100 patient years with warfarin alone and 0.52/100 patient years in the warfarin + aspirin group) compared with aspirin alone (0.15/100 patient years in the aspirin group). Minor bleeding rates were 0.81, 2.16, and 2.75/100 patient years, respectively.

Comments: The exclusion of patients 75 years or older likely attenuated the excess warfarin-associated bleeding risk. Only 35% of patients underwent revascularization (PCI or CABG). The efficacy of warfarin as part of an early revascularization strategy and in conjunction with thienopyridine therapy is unknown.

51. **Brouwer MA,** et al. Aspirin plus coumarin versus aspirin alone in the prevention of reocclusion after fibrinolysis for acute myocardial infarction: results of the Antithrombotics in the Prevention of Reocclusion in Coronary Thrombolysis (**APRICOT**)-2 trial. *Circulation* 2002;106:659–665.

Design: Prospective, randomized, open, multicenter trial. Primary endpoint was angiographic reocclusion at 3 months.

Purpose: To evaluate a prolonged anticoagulation regimen as an adjunct to aspirin in the prevention of reocclusion and recurrent ischemic events after fibrinolysis for STEMI.

Population: 308 STEMI patients receiving aspirin and IVH and angiography within 48 hours showing TIMI grade 3 flow in IRA.

Treatment: Standard in-hospital heparinization and aspirin, or aspirin and coumarin for 3 months (target INR, 2.0 to 3.0; median achieved INR, 2.6).

Results: The incidence of reocclusion (TIMI grade 2 flow or less) at 3 months was significantly lower in aspirin and coumarin compared with aspirin alone (15% vs. 28%; RR, 0.55; 95% CI, 0.33 to 0.90; $p < 0.02$). TIMI grade 0 to 1 flow rates were 9% and 20%, respectively (RR, 0.46; 95% CI, 0.24 to 0.89; $p < 0.02$). Aspirin and coumarin were also associated with lower rate of death, reinfarction, and revascularization (14% vs. 34%; $p < 0.01$). Bleeding rates (TIMI major and minor) were similar (5% vs. 3%; $p =$ NS).

GLYCOPROTEIN IIB/IIIA INHIBITORS

52. **Brener SJ,** et al. on behalf of the Reopro and Primary PTCA Organization and Randomized Trial (**RAPPORT**) Investigators. Randomized, placebo-controlled trial of primary glycoprotein IIb/IIIa blockade with primary angioplasty for acute MI. *Circulation* 1998;98:734–741.

Design: Prospective, randomized, double-blind, placebo-controlled, multicenter study. Primary endpoint (at 6 months) was death, MI, and any TVR.

Purpose: To evaluate whether platelet IIb/IIIa-receptor blockade with abciximab reduces ischemic events in AMI patients undergoing primary angioplasty.

Population: 483 patients seen within 12 hours of onset of symptoms with ischemic chest pain lasting more than 20 minutes accompanied by significant ST elevation in at least two contiguous leads or new LBBB.

Exclusion Criteria: Included severe thrombocytopenia, baseline PTT greater than 1.2× control, previous stroke, severe uncontrolled hypertension, PTCA of IRA in prior 3 months, cardiogenic shock, and prior abciximab or thrombolytic therapy.

Treatment: Abciximab, 0.25-mg/kg bolus, and then 0.125 μg/kg/min (maximum, 10 μg/min) for 12 hours. All patients received aspirin and heparin, 100-U/kg bolus before PTCA [with further boluses as needed to keep activated clotting time (ACT) longer than 300 seconds]. Stenting was discouraged but was allowed for residual dissection with more than 50% restenosis and for abrupt or threatened closure.

Results: No difference was observed between the two groups in incidence of 6-month primary endpoints (28.1% vs. 28.2%). However, the abciximab group had lower rates of death, MI, and urgent TVR at 7 days (3.3% vs. 9.9%; $p = 0.003$), 30 days (5.8% vs. 11.2%; $p = 0.03$), and 6 months (11.6% vs. 17.8%; $p = 0.05$). The abciximab group had 42% less bailout stenting (11.9% vs. 20.4%; $p = 0.008$). Abciximab was associated with increased major bleeding (defined as hematocrit decrease of >5; 16.6% vs. 9.5%; $p = 0.02$), mostly at the arterial access site. On-treatment analysis showed that abciximab was associated with decreased death and MI at 7 days (1.4% vs. 4.7%; $p = 0.047$) with a trend at 6 months (6.9% vs. 12%; $p = 0.07$).

Comments: Increased bleeding with abciximab was likely due to double-blind design, as the investigators were unwilling to discontinue heparin immediately after procedure(s) for early sheath removal.

53. **Montalescot G,** et al. for the **ADMIRAL** Investigators. Platelet glycoprotein IIb/IIIa inhibition with coronary stenting for acute myocardial infarction. *N Engl J Med* 2001;344: 1895–1903.

Design: Prospective, randomized, multicenter, double-blind, placebo-controlled trial. Primary composite endpoint at 30 days: death, reinfarction, or urgent TVR.

Purpose: To compare the combination of primary stenting and platelet glycoprotein IIb/IIIa receptor inhibition with primary stenting alone in AMI.

Population: 300 patients seen within 12 hours of onset of symptoms with 1 mm or more ST elevation in two or more contiguous leads.

Exclusion Criteria: Included bleeding diathesis, thrombolytic administration for current episode, recent stroke, uncontrolled hypertension, recent surgery, oral anticoagulant therapy, and known contraindications to aspirin, ticlopidine, or heparin.

Treatment: Abciximab (0.25-mg/kg bolus and then 0.125 μg/kg/min for 12 hours) plus stent implantation or primary stenting alone. Therapy was initiated before sheath insertion and coronary angiography. Follow-up angiography at 24 hours and 6 months.

Results: Abciximab group had a significantly higher initial TIMI grade 3 flow compared with placebo (16.8% vs. 5.4%, $p = 0.01$; grade 2 or 3, 25.8% vs. 10.8%, $p = 0.006$). TIMI grade 3 flow after procedure and at 6 months also was higher in the abciximab group (95.1% vs. 86.7%, $p = 0.04$; 94.3% vs. 82.8%, $p = 0.04$). At 30 days, the abciximab group had a nearly 60% lower incidence of the primary endpoint (6.0% vs. 14.6%, $p = 0.01$; at 6 months, 7.4% vs. 15.9%). Much of this benefit was from a lower rate of urgent TVR with abciximab (at 30 days, 1.3% vs. 6.6%; $p = 0.02$), although mortality also trended lower (at 30 days, 3.4% vs. 6.6%; $p = 0.19$). The abciximab group had a significantly higher LVEF at 24 hours (57.0% vs. 53.9%; $p < 0.05$) and at 6 months (61.1% vs. 57.0%; $p = 0.05$).

54. **Stone GW,** et al. for the Controlled Abciximab and Device Investigation to Lower Late Angioplasty Complications (**CADILLAC**) Investigators. Comparison of angioplasty with stenting, with or without abciximab, in acute myocardial infarction. *N Engl J Med* 2002;346:957–966.

Design: Prospective, randomized, open, 2 × 2 factorial, multicenter trial. Primary endpoint at 6 months: death, reinfarction, disabling stroke, and ischemia-driven TVR.

Purpose: To determine whether used in combination with PTCA, coronary stenting and platelet glycoprotein IIb/IIIa inhibitors can further improve outcomes in AMI patients.

Population: 2,082 patients seen within 6 hours who underwent urgent cardiac catheterization and were eligible for stent placement.

Exclusion Criteria: Included cardiogenic shock, bleeding diathesis, CVA in previous 2 years, history of leukopenia, thrombocytopenia, or hepatic or renal dysfunction.

Treatment: PTCA alone, PTCA plus abciximab, stenting alone (Multilink stent), or stenting plus abciximab.

Results: TIMI grade 3 flow rates were similar in the four groups (95% to 97%). At 6 months, the primary composite endpoint occurred in 20.0% of the PTCA-alone group, 16.5% with PTCA plus abciximab, 11.5% with stenting, and 10.2% with stenting plus abciximab ($p < 0.001$). No significant differences were found in 6-month mortality between the four groups (PTCA alone, 4.5%; PTCA + abciximab, 2.5%; stenting, 3.0%; stenting + abciximab, 4.2%). Stroke and reinfarction rates also were similar. The difference in the incidence of the primary endpoint was owing to differences in the rates of TVR (15.7% with PTCA alone, 13.8% with PTCA + abciximab, 8.3% with stenting, and only 5.2% with stenting + abciximab; $p < 0.001$). Follow-up angiography demonstrated a lower restenosis rate with stenting compared with PTCA (22.2% vs. 40.8%; $p < 0.001$). Reocclusion rates of the IRA were 11.3% and 5.7% ($p = 0.01$), respectively, and both were independent of abciximab use.

Comments: Inclusion criteria were "soft" because patients with infarct suspicion and angiographic evidence were enrolled; as a result, fewer than 90% had ST elevation or new LBBB.

55. **Neumann FJ,** et al. Effect of glycoprotein IIb/IIIa receptor blockade with abciximab on clinical and angiographic restenosis rate after the placement of coronary stents following acute myocardial infarction. *J Am Coll Cardiol* 2000;35:915–921 [the Intracoronary Stenting and Antithrombotic Regimen-2 trial (ISAR-2)].

Design: Prospective, randomized, single-blind study. Primary endpoint was a composite of death, reinfarction, or TLR at 30 days. Follow-up angiography at 6 months was performed in patients who had not had a primary event.

Purpose: To determine the effect of abciximab on clinical and angiographic endpoints in STEMI patients undergoing PCI.

Population: 401 patients undergoing PCI within 48 hours of acute STEMI.

Exclusion Criteria: Any contraindication to the study drugs.

Treatment: Standard-dose heparin versus abciximab plus reduced-dose heparin.

Results: At 30 days, patients in the abciximab group had a significantly lower rate of the composite primary endpoint (5.0% vs. 10.5%; $p = 0.038$). The absolute difference persisted for 1 year, though without statistical significance. However, rates of TLR at 1 year were similar in the two groups.

56. **Antoniucci D**, et al. A randomized trial comparing primary infarct artery stenting with or without abciximab in acute myocardial infarction. *J Am Coll Cardiol* 2003;42:1879–1885 [also called the Abciximab and Carbostent Evaluation (ACE) trial].

Design: Prospective, randomized, open-label trial study. Primary endpoint was a composite of death, reinfarction, TVR, or stroke at 1 month.

Purpose: To determine the effect of abciximab on clinical endpoints in STEMI patients undergoing PCI.

Population: 400 patients undergoing PCI for STEMI, presenting with 6 hours of symptoms.

Treatment: Stenting of IRA with abciximab or alone. Patients not receiving abciximab had a higher target ACT for heparin dosing.

Results: After 1 month of follow-up, patients in the abciximab group had a significantly lower rate of the primary endpoint (4.5% vs. 10.5%; $p = 0.023$). Patients in the abciximab group also experience sooner ST-segment resolution. Rates of mortality or reinfarction at 6 months were also lower in the abciximab group (5.5% vs. 13.5%; $p = 0.006$).

57. **Montalescot G**, et al. Abciximab in primary coronary stenting of ST-elevation myocardial infarction: a European meta-analysis on individual patients' data with long-term follow-up. *Eur Heart J* 2007;28:443–449.

The authors combined patient-level data from the ISAR-2, ACE, and ADMIRAL trials, comparing clinical outcomes in patients receiving primary PCI for STEMI between those who received abciximab adjunctive therapy with stenting and those who received standard heparin only. The primary endpoint was a composite of death or reinfarction at 3 years of follow-up. The total population summed to 1,101, and patients in the abciximab group had significantly fewer primary events (hazard ratio 12.9% vs. 19.0%; $p = 0.008$), as well as a nonsignificant trend toward lower overall mortality (10.9% vs. 14.3%; $p = 0.052$). Major bleeding episodes were similar (2.5% for the abciximab group, vs. 2.0% without abciximab, $p = $ NS).

58. **Zeymer U**. et al. Randomized comparison of eptifibatide versus abciximab in primary percutaneous coronary intervention in patients with acute ST-segment elevation myocardial infarction: results of the EVA-AMI trial. *J Am Coll Cardiol* 2010;56:463–469.

Preliminary data were presented at AHA, with 400 patients with STEMI presenting within 12 hours of symptoms randomized to either double-bolus plus infusion eptifibatide or abciximab with single-bolus infusion. Across a spectrum of in-hospital events, eptifibatide proved noninferior: death (3.5% vs. 3.5%), reinfarction (0% for abciximab vs. 1.5% for eptifibatide), TVR (4% vs. 2.7%), and CABG (0.5% vs. 0.9%). These were the first data of a head-to-head comparison of abciximab and eptifibatide in primary PCI for STEMI.

59. **De Lusa G**, et al. Benefits from small molecule administration as compared with abciximab among patients with ST-segment elevation myocardial infarction treated with primary angioplasty: a meta analysis. *J Am Coll Cardiol* 2009;53:1668–1673.

The authors combined six randomized trials comparing abciximab to small-molecule glycoprotein IIb/IIIa inhibitors (high-dose tirofiban in five trials, eptifibatide in one) in primary PCI, including a total of 2,197 patients. For all outcomes, abciximab was *not* superior to small-molecule inhibitors; this included postprocedural TIMI flow grade 3 (89.8% vs. 89.1%; $p = 0.72$), ST-segment resolution (67.8% vs. 68.2%; $p = 0.66$), 30-day mortality (2.2% vs. 2.0%; $p = 0.66$), and reinfarction (1.2% vs. 1.2%; $p = 0.88$).

60. **Van't Hof AW**, et al. Prehospital initiation of tirofiban in patients with ST-elevation myocardial infarction undergoing primary angioplasty (**On-TIME 2**): a multicentre, double-blind, randomised controlled trial. *Lancet* 2008;372:537–546.

Design: Double-blind, randomized, placebo-controlled, multicenter, international trial. Primary endpoint was residual ST-segment elevation 1 hour after PCI.
Purpose: To identify the benefit, if any, of early, high-dose tirofiban (compared with placebo), in addition to aspirin, heparin, and clopidogrel in patients with STEMI undergoing PCI.
Population: 984 patients with STEMI undergoing PCI.
Treatment: High-dose, bolus tirofiban or placebo, randomized in the ambulance.
Results: Patients who received tirofiban had significantly lower residual ST-segment elevation at 1 hour ($p = 0.003$), without higher bleeding rates.

61. **Mehilli J**, et al. for the Bavarian Reperfusion Alternatives Evaluation-3 (**BRAVE-3**) Study Investigators. Abciximab in patients with acute ST-segment-elevation myocardial infarction undergoing primary percutaneous coronary intervention after clopidogrel loading: a randomized double-blind trial. *Circulation*. 2009;119:1933–1940.

Design: Randomized, double-blind, placebo-controlled trial. Primary endpoint was infarct size, as measured by sestamibi, at discharge.
Purpose: To identify the benefit, if any, of abciximab added to clopidogrel in patients with STEMI undergoing primary PCI.
Population: 800 patients with STEMI undergoing primary PCI.

Treatment: Abciximab or placebo prior to transfer to the catheterization laboratory.

Results: There was no significant difference in infarct size between the two groups (15.7% for abciximab vs. 16.6% for placebo; $p = 0.47$). Bleeding complications occurred at equal rates between the two groups. At 30 days, rates of the composite of death, recurrent MI, stroke, or urgent TVR were similar (5.0% for abciximab vs. 3.8% for placebo; $p = 0.40$).

META-ANALYSES

62. **Pannu R**, Andraws R. Effects of glycoprotein IIb/IIIa inhibitors in patients undergoing percutaneous coronary intervention after pretreatment with clopidogrel: a meta-analysis of randomized trials. *Crit Pathways Cardiol* 2008;7:5–10.

The authors combined data from five trials of IIb/IIIa inhibitors—two trials in the setting of ACS, and three trials of patients undergoing elective PCI. The objective of this meta-analysis was to assess the benefit, if any, of IIb/IIIa inhibitor addition to clopidogrel in these 5,303 patients undergoing PCI. Compared with placebo, IIb/IIIa inhibition did not reduce the rates of death (OR 0.84; $p = 0.35$), MI (OR 0.86; $p = 0.19$), or TVR (OR 0.96; $p = 0.68$) at the end of follow-up for each study (ranging from 30 days to 1 year). When restricted to patients undergoing PCI for ACS, results did not vary. However, rates of bleeding were higher in the IIb/IIIa inhibitor group (OR 1.35; $p = 0.02$).

63. **Gurm H**, et al. A comparison of abciximab and small molecule glycoprotein IIb/IIIa inhibitors in patients undergoing primary percutaneous coronary intervention: a meta-analysis of contemporary randomized controlled trials. *Circ Cardiovasc Intervent* 2009;2:230–236.

Investigators combined data from five randomized trials, including 2,138 patients with STEMI, comparing abciximab to small-molecule IIb/IIIa inhibitors (tirofiban and eptifibatide) as adjunctive therapy for primary PCI. Rates of death (1.9% for small molecules vs. 2.3% for abciximab; $p = 0.58$), recurrent MI (1.3% vs. 1.2%; $p = 0.69$), or major bleeding (1.7% vs. 1.3%; $p = 0.61$) did not differ at 30 days. These findings persisted to follow-up of 8 months for rates of death or recurrent MI.

64. **De Luca G**, et al. Benefits from small molecule administration as compared with abciximab among patients with ST-segment elevation myocardial infarction treated with primary angioplasty: a meta-analysis. *J Am Coll Cardiol* 2009;53:1668–1673.

Six trials comparing abciximab with small-molecule IIb/IIIa inhibitors in a total of 2,197 patients undergoing primary PCI for STEMI were combined in this analysis. Angiographic and clinical outcomes were available: there was no difference in rates of postprocedural TIMI 3 flow (89.8% for abciximab vs. 89.1% for small molecules; $p = 0.72$) or ST-segment resolution ($p = 0.66$). Mortality at 30 days was not different (2.2% vs. 2.0%; $p = 0.66$), nor were reinfarction rates (1.2% vs. 1.2%; $p = 0.88$) or bleeding rates (1.3% vs. 1.9%; $p = 0.27$).

Glycoprotein IIb/IIIa Inhibitors and Reduced-dose Thrombolysis

65. **Antman EM,** et al. for the **TIMI-14** Investigators. Abciximab facilitates the rate and extent of thrombolysis. *Circulation* 1999;99:2720–2732 (editorial, 2714–2716).

Design: Prospective, randomized, dose-ranging, multicenter study. Primary endpoint was IRA TIMI grade 3 flow at 90 minutes (also see ASSENT-3, Ref. 97).

Purpose: To determine whether abciximab is an effective and safe addition to reduced-dose thrombolytic regimens for STEMI.

Population: 888 patients aged 18 to 75 years seen within 12 hours of symptom onset with 1 mm or greater ST elevation in at least two contiguous ECG leads.

Exclusion Criteria: LBBB, 6,000-U heparin in the hour before randomization, prior CABG surgery, PCI or thrombolytic therapy in prior 7 days, and history of stroke or transient ischemic attack (TIA).

Treatment: (a) 100 mg of accelerated-dose alteplase (control); (b) abciximab (0.25-mg/kg bolus, and then 0.125 μg/kg/min for 12 hours) plus reduced-dose SK (500,000 to 1.5 million U); (c) abciximab plus reduced-dose alteplase (20 to 65 mg); (d) abciximab alone. All patients received aspirin. Control patients received standard weight–based heparin (70-U/kg bolus; initial infusion, 15 U/kg/hr), whereas the abciximab groups received low-dose heparin (60-U/kg bolus, and then 7 U/kg/hr). Very low-dose heparin also was tested in the dose-confirmation phase (30-U/kg bolus, and then 4 U/kg/hr).

Results: Abciximab alone achieved TIMI grade 3 flow at 90 minutes in only 32%, and abciximab plus SK, 500,000 to 1.25 million U in only 34% to 46%. Higher rates of TIMI grade 3 flow at 60 and 90 minutes were seen with increasing duration of alteplase infusion, progressing from bolus alone to bolus and 30- or 60-minute infusion ($p < 0.02$). Best regimen was abciximab and alteplase, 50 mg (15-mg bolus, 35 mg over 60 minutes), which produced TIMI 3 flow in 77% at 90 minutes (vs. 62% with alteplase alone; $p = 0.02$). TIMI 3 flow at 60 minutes also was significantly better with this regimen [72% vs. 43% (alteplase alone); $p = 0.0009$]. Major hemorrhage occurred in 3% receiving abciximab alone, 6% with alteplase alone, 10% with SK plus abciximab, 7% with 50-mg alteplase plus abciximab plus low-dose heparin, and 1% with 50-mg alteplase plus abciximab plus very low-dose heparin.

66. **Strategies for Patency Enhancement in the Emergency Department (SPEED)** Group. Trial of abciximab with and without low-dose reteplase for acute myocardial infarction. *Circulation* 2000;101:2788–2794.

This prospective, randomized, open-label, multicenter, phase II study enrolled 528 patients with STEMI within 6 hours of chest pain onset. Patients were randomized in a 4:1 fashion to abciximab alone ($n = 63$) or with 5, 7.5, 10, 5 + 2.5, or 5 + 5 U of reteplase ($n = 241$). Phase B tested the best phase A strategy (abciximab plus 5 + 5 U reteplase, $n = 115$) against 10 + 10 U reteplase alone ($n = 109$). Initial angiography was performed at a median of 63 minutes from the beginning of reperfusion therapy. In phase A, 62% of the abciximab–reteplase 5 + 5 U group had TIMI grade 3 flow (primary endpoint) versus 27% of the abciximab-only patients ($p = 0.001$). In phase B, 54% of the abciximab–reteplase 5 + 5 U group had grade 3 flow versus 47% of the reteplase-only patients ($p = 0.32$). TIMI grade 3 flow rates were 61% for a 60-U/kg heparin bolus and abciximab–reteplase 5 + 5 U, 51% for a 40-U/kg heparin bolus and abciximab–reteplase 5 + 5 U ($p = 0.22$), and 47% for reteplase alone ($p = 0.05$ vs. the 60-U/kg heparin group). Major bleeding rates in phase A were 3.3% for abciximab alone and 5.3% for abciximab–reteplase 5 + 5 U; rates in phase B were 9.8% for abciximab–reteplase 5 + 5 U and 3.7% for reteplase alone. Major bleeding rates were not significantly different with standard- or low-dose heparin (6.3% vs. 10.5%; $p = 0.30$). An analysis of the 323 (61%) patients who underwent early PCI found that it was used more frequently in patients with initial TIMI flow grade 0 or 1 versus flow grade 2 or 3 (83% vs. 60%; $p < 0.0001$) (see *J Am Coll Cardiol* 2000;36:1489). The early PCI group had a significantly lower incidence of reinfarction [1.2% vs. 4.9% (no early PCI); $p = 0.03$], urgent revascularization (1.6% vs. 9.3%; $p = 0.001$), transfusion requirement (9.0% vs. 16%; $p = 0.02$), and a significantly higher freedom from death, reinfarction, urgent revascularization, major bleeding, or transfusion at 30 days (85.4% vs. 70.4%; $p < 0.001$).

67. **Topol EJ.** The **GUSTO-V** Investigators. Reperfusion therapy for acute myocardial infarction with fibrinolytic therapy or combination reduced fibrinolytic therapy and platelet glycoprotein IIb/IIIa inhibition: the GUSTO-V randomised trial. *Lancet* 2001;357:1905–1914.

Design: Prospective, randomized, open, multicenter trial. Primary endpoint was 30-day mortality, and secondary endpoints included various complications of MI.

Purpose: To compare the effect of reteplase alone with reteplase plus abciximab in patients with AMI.

Population: 16,588 patients seen within 6 hours of symptom onset with ST elevation.

Exclusion Criteria: Included planned PCI and contraindications to thrombolysis.

Treatment: Standard-dose reteplase (two 10-U boluses, 30 minutes apart) or half-dose reteplase (two 5-U boluses) and full-dose abciximab.

Results: No significant differences were seen between the two groups in 30-day mortality [5.9% (reteplase) vs. 5.6% (OR, 0.95); $p = 0.43$]; the 0.3% absolute decrease with combination therapy fulfilled the criteria of noninferiority. At 1 year, mortality rates were identical (8.38% in both groups) (*JAMA* 2002;288:2130). The combination-therapy group had significantly lower rates of death and reinfarction (7.4% vs. 8.8%; $p = 0.0011$) and reinfarction (at 7 days: 2.3% vs. 3.5%). Reinfarction was associated with much higher 1-year mortality (22.6% vs. 8.0%). However, more nonintracranial bleeding complications were seen in the combination group (4.6% vs. 2.3%). The rates of intracranial hemorrhage and nonfatal disabling stroke were similar.

68. **Brenner SJ**, et al. for the **INTRO AMI** Investigators. Eptifibatide and low-dose tissue plasminogen activator in acute myocardial infarction: the Integrelin and Low-dose Thrombolysis in Acute MI (INTRO AMI) trial. *J Am Coll Cardiol* 2002;39:277–286.

This prospective, randomized, open-label, multicenter trial enrolled 649 patients with acute STEMI seen within 6 hours of symptom onset. In phase A, patients were randomized to eptifibatide, single or double bolus (30 minutes apart) of 180, 180/90, or 180/180 μg/kg, followed by infusion of 1.33 or 2.0 μg/kg/min (sequentially added to 25 or 50 mg of tPA). In phase B, patients were randomized to (a) double-bolus eptifibatide, 180/90 (30 minutes apart) and 1.33 μg/kg/min infusion with 50-mg tPA (group I); (b) 180/90 (10 minutes apart) and 2.0 g/kg/min with 50-mg tPA (group II); or (c) full-dose, weight-adjusted tPA (group III). In phase A, the highest rate of TIMI flow grade 3 (primary endpoint) was seen with eptifibatide 180/90/1.33 and 50-mg tPA (65% and 78% at 60 and 90 minutes, respectively). In phase B, the incidence of TIMI grade 3 flow at 60 minutes was 42%, 56%, and 40%, for groups I through III, respectively ($p = 0.04$, group II vs. group III). The median CTFCs were 38, 33, and 50, respectively ($p = 0.02$). No differences were found between the three groups in TIMI major bleeding or intracranial hemorrhage. Mortality, reinfarction, and revascularization rates at 30 days also were similar.

69. **Giugliano RP**, et al. on behalf of the **INTEGRETI** Investigators. Combination reperfusion therapy with eptifibatide and reduced dose tenecteplase for ST-elevation myocardial infarction: results of the Integrelin and Tenecteplase in Acute Myocardial Infarction (INTEGRETI) phase II angiographic trial. *J Am Coll Cardiol* 2003;41:1251–1260.

This prospective, randomized, open-label, multicenter trial enrolled 438 STEMI patients seen within 6 hours.

In the dose-finding phase, 189 patients were randomized to different combinations of double-bolus eptifibatide and reduced-dose TNK. In dose confirmation, 249 patients were randomized to eptifibatide, 180-μg/kg boluses, 2-μg/kg/min infusion, and a second bolus 10 minutes later (180/2/180) plus half-dose TNK (0.37 mg/kg), or standard-dose (0.53 mg/kg) TNK monotherapy. All received aspirin and UFH [60-U/kg bolus and then 7 U/kg/hr (combination therapy) or 12 U/kg/hr (monotherapy)]. In dose finding, TIMI grade 3 flow rates at 60 minutes (primary endpoint) were similar across groups (64% to 68%). Arterial patency (TIMI grade 2 or 3 flow) was highest for eptifibatide, 180/2/180, plus TNK (96%; $p = 0.02$) vs. eptifibatide, 180/2/90, plus half-dose TNK. In dose confirmation, this combination, compared with TNK monotherapy, tended to achieve better TIMI 3 flow (59% vs. 49%; $p = 0.15$), arterial patency (85% vs. 77%; $p = 0.17$), and ST resolution (71% vs. 61%; $p = 0.08$). However, it was associated with increased rates of noncerebral major bleeding (7.6% vs. 2.5%; $p = 0.14$) and transfusion (13.4% vs. 4.2%; $p = 0.02$).

β-BLOCKERS

70. **Norwegian Multicenter Group.** Timolol-induced reduction in mortality and reinfarction in patients surviving acute MI. *N Engl J Med* 1981;304:801–807.

Design: Prospective, randomized, double-blind, placebo-controlled, multicenter study. Mean follow-up period was 17 months. Primary endpoint was all-cause mortality.

Purpose: To evaluate the efficacy of long-term β-blockade after MI.

Population: 1,884 patients randomized at 7 to 28 days after AMI meeting at least two of the following criteria: (a) chest pain longer than 15 minutes, acute pulmonary edema, or cardiogenic shock; (b) pathologic Q waves and/or ST elevation followed by T-wave inversion in at least two leads; or (c) elevated serum markers.

Exclusion Criteria: HR, less than 50 beats/min; severe CHF; second- or third-degree AV block; SBP less than 100 mm Hg.

Treatment: Timolol, 10 mg twice daily, or placebo.

Results: Timolol group had a 39% lower mortality rate (13.3% vs. 21.9%; $p < 0.001$) and a 28% lower reinfarction rate (14.4% vs. 20.1%; $p < 0.001$).

Comments: Six-year follow-up showed a persistent mortality benefit of timolol (26.4% vs. 32.3%; $p = 0.003$).

71. **β-Blocker Heart Attack Trial (BHAT)** Research Group. A randomized trial of propranolol in patients with acute MI. *JAMA* 1982;247:1707–1714.

Design: Prospective, randomized, double-blind, placebo-controlled, multicenter study. Mean follow-up period was 25 months. Primary endpoint was all-cause mortality.

Purpose: To evaluate if long-term propranolol administration after MI reduces mortality.

Population: 3,837 patients younger than 70 years enrolled 5 to 21 days after an AMI.

Exclusion Criteria: Marked bradycardia, current β-blocker therapy, history of severe heart failure or asthma, and planned cardiac surgery.

Treatment: Propranolol, 60 to 80 mg, three times daily, or placebo.

Results: Propranolol group had 26.5% lower mortality (7.2% vs. 9.8%; $p < 0.005$), 28% fewer sudden cardiac deaths (3.3% vs. 4.6%; $p < 0.05$), and 23% fewer major cardiac events (nonfatal MI plus fatal coronary disease). Serious side effects were infrequent.

Comments: Post hoc analysis showed that the benefit of propranolol was restricted to a high-risk group of 383 patients—43% mortality reduction ($p < 0.01$).

72. **The Metoprolol in Acute MI (MIAMI)** Trial Research Group. Metoprolol in Acute MI (MIAMI): a randomised placebo-controlled international trial. *Eur Heart J* 1985;6:199–226.

Design: Prospective, randomized, double-blind, placebo-controlled, multicenter study. Primary endpoint was all-cause mortality.

Purpose: To evaluate whether metoprolol administration after MI reduces mortality.

Population: 5,728 patients younger than 75 years, seen within 24 hours of onset of symptoms (average, 7 hours).

Exclusion Criteria: Current treatment with β-blockers or calcium antagonists, and HR 65 beats/min or less.

Treatment: Metoprolol, 15 mg i.v., and then 200 mg/day orally, or placebo.

Results: Metoprolol group had a nonsignificant 13% mortality reduction at 15 days (4.3% vs. 4.9%). The high-risk subgroup (meeting at least three of the following criteria: older than 60 years, prior MI, ECG consistent with MI, previous angina, CHF, diabetes, taking digoxin or diuretics) had 29% lower mortality.

73. **ISIS-1** Collaborative Group. Randomised trial of intravenous atenolol among 16,107 cases of suspected acute MI. *Lancet* 1986;328:57–65.

Design: Prospective, randomized, open, parallel-group, multicenter study. Primary endpoint was vascular mortality at 7 days.

Purpose: To determine the effects of atenolol in MI patients on 7-day vascular mortality.

Population: 16,107 patients seen within 12 hours (average, 5 hours) of an AMI who were not taking a β-blocker or verapamil.

Exclusion Criteria: HR less than 50 beats/min, SBP less than 100 mm Hg, second- or third-degree heart block, severe heart failure, and bronchospasm.

Treatment: Atenolol, 5 to 10 mg i.v., over a 5-minute period, followed by 100 mg/day orally for 7 days. No placebo was given to controls.

Results: Atenolol group had a 15% lower 7-day vascular mortality rate (3.89% vs. 4.57%; $p < 0.04$). Most of mortality difference occurred in the first 24 hours. At 1 year, the benefit persisted, with an 11% vascular mortality reduction (10.7% vs. 12.0%; $p < 0.01$). After year 1, nonsignificant excess of vascular deaths was found in the atenolol group (179 vs. 145; $p = 0.07$).

Comments: A later analysis showed that the benefit of atenolol in the first 24 hours was primarily owing to a lower rate of pulseless electrical activity (PEA), reflecting less cardiac rupture.

74. **Roberts R,** et al. for the **TIMI-IIB** Investigators. Immediate vs. deferred beta-blockade following thrombolytic therapy in patients with acute MI: results of TIMI II-B. *Circulation* 1991;83:422–437.

Design: Prospective, randomized, open, parallel-group, multicenter study. Primary endpoint was predischarge LVEF.

Purpose: To compare immediate intravenously versus deferred (started on day 6) β-blocker in AMI patients treated with rtPA.

Population: 1,434 patients aged 75 years or younger seen within 4 hours of chest pain and with 1 mm or greater ST elevation in at least two contiguous ECG leads and having no contraindications to β-blockade. Low-risk subgroup is defined as an absence of all the following: history of MI, anterior ST elevation, rates greater than one-third up lung fields, SBP less than 100 mm Hg or cardiogenic shock, HR more than 100 beats/min, atrial fibrillation or flutter, and age 70 years or older.

Exclusion Criteria: HR less than 55 beats/min, SBP consistently less than 100 mm Hg, severe first-degree or advanced heart block, and wheezing or significant COPD.

Treatment: Immediate β-blockade group received metoprolol, 5 mg i.v., for three doses (given within 2 hours of rtPA), and then 50 to 100 mg twice daily. The deferred β-blockade group received metoprolol, 50 mg twice daily on day 6, followed by 100 mg twice daily. All patients received aspirin, heparin (i.v. for 5 days, and then s.c. every 12 hours), and lidocaine (1.0 to 1.5 mg/kg, and then 2.0 to 4.0 mg/min for 24 hours).

Results: No significant differences in mortality or LVEF were observed at discharge, but the subgroup of low-risk patients receiving β-blockade had a lower rate of death and nonfatal reinfarction (5.4% vs. 13.7%; $p = 0.01$), as well as less recurrent chest pain (18.8% vs. 24.1%; $p < 0.02$).

75. **Gottlieb SS,** et al. Cooperative Cardiovascular Project. Effect of beta-blockade on mortality among high-risk and low-risk patients after MI. *N Engl J Med* 1998;339:489–497.

Design: Retrospective, observational study. Primary efficacy endpoint was 2-year mortality rate.

Purpose: To compare the mortality rates of patients in high- and low-risk subgroups who were treated with β-blockers with rates among those not receiving these agents.

Population: 201,752 patients from the Cooperative Cardiovascular Project database (most discharges occurred between February 1994 and July 1995) with a principal diagnosis of AMI. Approximately two thirds of patients had relative contraindications to β-blocker administration (per ACC/AHA guidelines). Only 8,464 patients were not followed up for 24 months.

Treatment: Of patients, 34.3% received β-blockers (based on discharge prescription data).

Results: Patients with the following characteristics received β-blockers less frequently—very elderly, blacks, low EF, heart failure, COPD, elevated creatinine, or type 1 diabetes mellitus. However, mortality was lower in all of these subgroups of patients who were treated with β-blockers. Overall, 2-year mortality was 40% lower among patients without complications. Mortality also was 40% lower with β-blockers in patients with a non–Q wave MI or COPD, whereas slightly smaller reductions (28% to 35%) were seen in those with an EF less than 20%, blacks, age older than 80 years, creatinine greater than 1.4 mg/dL, and diabetes. However, absolute mortality reduction in these latter groups was similar to or greater than that among patients with no risk factors.

76. **Dargie HJ.** Effect of carvedilol on outcome after myocardial infarction in patients with left-ventricular dysfunction: the **CAPRICORN** randomised trial. *Lancet* 2001;357: 1385–1390.

Design: Prospective, randomized, placebo-controlled, multicenter trial. The primary endpoint was all-cause mortality or CV-related hospital admission.

Purpose: To investigate the long-term efficacy of carvedilol on morbidity and mortality in patients with LV dysfunction treated according to current evidence-based practice.

Population: 1,959 patients with AMI and a LVEF of 40% or less.

Treatment: Carvedilol (6.25 mg once daily titrated to 25 mg twice daily over 4 to 6 weeks), or placebo.

Results: No significant difference was observed between the carvedilol and placebo groups in the incidence of primary endpoint [35% vs. 37%; hazard ratio, 0.92 (95% CI, 0.80 to 1.07)]. However, all-cause mortality was significantly lower in the carvedilol group [12% vs. 15%; hazard ratio, 0.77 (95% CI, 0.60 to 0.98); $p = 0.03$]. The carvedilol group also had lower rates of cardiovascular mortality, nonfatal MI, and all-cause mortality or nonfatal MI.

77. **Hjalmarson A,** et al. Effect on mortality of metoprolol in acute MI. *Lancet* 1981;2: 823–827.

A total of 1,395 patients with chest pain lasting 30 minutes or longer and ECG changes were randomized at an average of 11 hours from onset of symptoms to 15 mg i.v. and then 100 mg twice daily or placebo. MI was confirmed in 69.6% of patients. The metoprolol group had a 36% lower 90-day mortality rate (5.7% vs. 8.9%; $p < 0.03$).

78. **Ryden L,** et al. A double-blind trial of metoprolol in acute MI: effects on ventricular arrhythmias. *N Engl J Med* 1983;308:614–618.

A total of 1,395 patients with suspected MI were given metoprolol, 15 mg i.v., 50 mg every 6 hours for 2 days, and then 100 mg twice daily for 3 months. Antiarrhythmic drugs were given only for VF and sustained VT. Only 58% of patients had a definite MI. The metoprolol group had less VF (0.9% vs. 2.4%; $p < 0.05$) and less lidocaine use ($p < 0.01$).

79. **COMMIT (ClOpidogrel and Metoprolol in Myocardial Infarction Trial) Collaborative Group.** Early intravenous then oral metoprolol in 45 852 patients with acute myocardial infarction: randomised placebo-controlled trial. *Lancet* 2005;366:1622–1632.

Design: Prospective, randomized, placebo-controlled, multicenter study. There were two pre-specified co-primary endpoints at discharge or over a treatment period of 4 weeks (whichever came sooner): (1) a composite of death, reinfarction, or cardiac arrest and (2) death from any cause.

Purpose: To determine the benefit, if any, of adding β-blockade (metoprolol) to contemporary regimens for acute MI.

Population: 45,852 patients admitted within 24 hours of acute MI, with ST elevation, LBBB, or ST depression (7% of the trial population) on ECG.

Treatment: Metoprolol (up to 15 mg intravenously then 200 mg oral daily), or placebo.

Results: Similar rates of primary outcome events were observed in the metoprolol and placebo groups (9.4% for metoprolol vs. 9.9% for placebo; $p = 0.1$). While metoprolol did reduce rates of reinfarction (2.0% vs. 2.5%; $p = 0.001$) and VF (2.5% vs. 3.0%; $p = 0.001$), more patients in the metoprolol group developed cardiogenic shock (5.0% vs. 3.9%; $p < 0.00001$), predominantly in the first 24 hours of hospitalization.

Comment: The benefits of metoprolol were observed in hemodynamically stable patients, later in their course, while the adverse effects of metoprolol were seen early in the course of patients who were unstable hemodynamically. Thus, the trial highlighted the benefits, and more importantly, the pitfalls of β-blockade in acute MI in patients with evidence of heart failure or hemodynamic instability at presentation. See above for results of the clopidogrel arm of this trial.

THROMBOLYTIC THERAPY

Review Articles, Meta-analyses, and Miscellaneous

80. **White HD.** Thrombolytic therapy for patients with MI presenting after six hours. *Lancet* 1992;340:221–222.

This analysis of trials with late thrombolytic administration showed a significant 12% reduction in 35-day mortality with treatment at 7 to 12 hours. A nonsignificant 6% reduction was seen with treatment at 13 to 24 hours.

81. **Fibrinolytic Therapy Trialists (FTT)** Collaborative Group. Indications for fibrinolytic therapy in suspected acute MI: collaborative overview of early mortality and major morbidity results from all randomised trials of >1000 patients. *Lancet* 1994;343:311–322.

This analysis focused on nine studies (GISSI-1, ISAM, AIMS, ISIS-2 and ISIS-3, ASSET, USIM, EMERAS, and LATE) with more than 1,000 patients (58,600 total). During days 0 and 1, the use of thrombolytics was associated with a higher mortality rate, especially in the elderly and those treated more than 12 hours after symptom onset. However, much greater benefit was seen on days 2 to 35. Thrombolytic-treated patients with ST-segment elevation or BBB had a 3% lower mortality rate when treated from 0 to 6 hours versus 2% lower at 7 to 12 hours and only 1% lower (p = NS) at 13 to 18 hours.

82. **Boersma E,** et al. Early thrombolytic therapy in acute MI: reappraisal of the golden hour. *Lancet* 1996;348:771–775.

This analysis focused on 22 randomized trials enrolling 100 or more patients (total, 50,246 patients). Substantial mortality benefit (6.5% absolute reduction) was seen when a thrombolytic was given within 1 hour of onset of symptoms (vs. 2.6% at 1 to 2 hours, 2.6% at 2 to 3 hours, and 2.9% at 3 to 6 hours). Comparing those treated within 2 hours with those treated after 2 hours, the proportional mortality reduction was −44% versus –20% (p = 0.001). These data fit a nonlinear regression equation (i.e., most benefit early). In contrast, a similar prior analysis by the Fibrinolytic Therapy Trialists (FTT) Collaborative Group had generated a linear model (1.6 additional lives per 1,000 treated patients for each hour of delay). However, their analysis included data from 4,250 patients who had unstable angina (USIM trial) and minimal or no ST elevation (ISIS-3).

83. **Eagle KA,** et al. Practice variation and missed opportunities for reperfusion in ST-segment-elevation myocardial infarction: findings from the Global Registry of Acute Coronary Events (**GRACE**). *Lancet* 2002;359:373–377.

This study assessed current treatment practices of STEMI from prospectively collected data in the multinational (14 countries) Global Registry of Acute Coronary Events. Of 9,251 patients enrolled, 1,763 were seen within 12 hours of symptom onset with STEMI; of these, 30% did not receive reperfusion therapy. Patients less likely to receive reperfusion therapy were elderly patients (aged 75 years or older), those seen without chest pain, and those with a history of diabetes, CHF, MI, or coronary bypass surgery. A substantial percentage of eligible patients failed to receive reperfusion treatment. The United States had the highest rate of primary PCI. The rate at sites with a catheterization laboratory was only 19%.

84. **de Belder MA**. Acute myocardial infarction: failed thrombolysis. *Heart* 2001;85:104–112.

This review highlights the risk of failed thrombolysis in acute MI—the incidence, potential mechanisms, and means of diagnosis. It finishes with a discussion of potential management options.

85. **Llevadot J,** et al. Bolus fibrinolytic therapy in acute myocardial infarction. *JAMA* 2001;286:442–449.

The authors review studies that evaluated the newest fibrinolytic agents, reteplase, lanoteplase, and TNK; specifically, they assessed pharmacokinetics, pharmacodynamics, as well as angiographic and clinical outcomes. They found an overall similarity in rates of efficacy and mortality among the four agents (they compared all three to tPA). However, lanoteplase and heparin bolus plus infusion increased the rate of intracranial hemorrhage significantly.

Thrombolytic Comparative Studies

86. **TIMI-1,** The Thrombolysis in MI (TIMI) Trial. Phase I findings. *N Engl J Med* 1985;312:932–936.

Design: Prospective, randomized, double-blind, placebo-controlled, multicenter study. Primary endpoint was IRA patency at 90 minutes.

Purpose: To evaluate the efficacy of intravenously administered thrombolytic therapy and to compare the effects of tPA and SK.

Population: 316 patients younger than 76 years seen 7 hours or less from onset of symptoms with chest pain lasting 30 minutes or longer and ST-segment elevation in at least two ECG leads.

Treatment: SK, 1.5 million U over a 60-minute period and a 3-hour infusion of tPA placebo, or a 3-hour infusion of plasminogen activator [80 mg (40 mg in the first hour, and then 20 mg for 2 hours)] and a 1-hour infusion of SK placebo.

Results: The 290 patients received treatment; 26 had a less than 50% reduction in the diameter of the IRA not treated. Among the 214 patients with total baseline occlusion, tPA achieved better reperfusion at 90 minutes: 60% versus 35% (TIMI grade 2 or 3 flow; $p < 0.001$). No significant differences in rates of bleeding events were observed.

87. **Gruppo Italiano per lo Studio della Streptochinasi nell'Infarto Miocardico (GISSI-2).** GISSI-2: a factorial randomised trial of alteplase vs. streptokinase and heparin vs. no heparin among 12,490 patients with acute MI. *Lancet* 1990;336:65–71.

Design: Prospective, randomized, open, parallel-group, 2×2 factorial, multicenter study. Primary endpoint was death, clinical heart failure, and EF 35% or less.

Purpose: To compare the efficacy of i.v. SK and tPA for the treatment of suspected acute STEMI and to study the effects of heparin on the incidence of recurrent ischemia.

Population: 12,490 patients seen within 6 hours of onset of symptoms with chest pain and 1 mm or more ST elevation in any limb lead or 2 mm or more in any precordial lead.

Treatment: (a) SK, 1.5 million U over a 30- to 60-minute period, and heparin, 12,500 U s.c. twice daily (starting 12 hours after initiation of the thrombolytic and continued through hospital discharge); (b) tPA, 10-mg bolus, and then 50 mg over 1 hour, and then 40 mg over 2 hours, and heparin, 12,500 U s.c. twice daily; (c) SK, 1.5 million U over 30 to 60 minutes without heparin; or (d) tPA, 10-mg bolus, and then 50 mg over 1 hour, and then 40 mg over 2 hours without heparin.

Results: No significant difference was observed in combined endpoints between SK and tPA [22.5% vs. 23.1% (mortality, 8.6% vs. 9.0%)]. No difference was observed in the rates of recurrent infarction, postinfarction angina, stroke, or bleeding. No differences were observed between heparin and no heparin, except for increased bleeding with heparin (1.0% vs. 0.6%; RR, 1.64; 95% CI, 1.09 to 2.45).

Comments: The International Study Group recruited an additional 8,401 patients. Among these 20,891 patients, no difference was seen in in-hospital mortality rates (tPA, 8.9%; SK, 8.5%), but tPA was associated with a significantly higher stroke rate (1.33% vs. 0.94%).

88. **ISIS-3** Collaborative Group. A randomised comparison of streptokinase versus tissue plasminogen activator versus anistreplase and of aspirin and heparin versus aspirin alone among 41,299 cases of suspected acute MI. *Lancet* 1992;339:753–770.

Design: Prospective, randomized, double-blind (thrombolytic agents) and open-label (heparin), 3×2 factorial, multicenter study. Primary endpoint was 35-day mortality rate.

Purpose: To compare the effects on mortality of tPA, SK, and acylated plasminogen–streptokinase activator complex (APSAC) and to compare aspirin alone with aspirin plus s.c. administered heparin.

Population: 41,299 patients with suspected MI seen within 24 hours of onset of symptoms (no ECG criteria).

Exclusion Criteria (suggested): Recent severe trauma, stroke, GI bleeding or ulcer, and SK allergy.

Treatment: (a) SK, 1.5 million U over 60 minutes; (b) rtPA, 0.6 million U/kg over 4 hours (0.04 million U/kg as a bolus, 0.36 million U/kg over 1 hour, and then 0.067 million U/kg/hr for 3 hours); or (c) APSAC 30 U over 3 minutes. All patients received aspirin (162.5 mg daily), and half of the patients also received heparin, 12,500 U twice daily s.c. for 7 days (started 4 hours after initiation of thrombolytic therapy).

Results: No differences in 35-day mortality rate were seen between the three thrombolytic groups—SK, 10.6%; tPA, 10.3%; APSAC, 10.5%. The SK group did have fewer strokes (1.04% vs. 1.39% for tPA; $p < 0.01$), whereas tPA was associated with fewer reinfarctions [2.9% vs. 3.5% (SK)]. A trend toward a lower mortality difference was seen with heparin while it was being administered [7-day mortality rate, 7.4% vs. 7.9% (aspirin alone); $p = 0.06$], but this disappeared at 35-day and 6-month follow-ups. Heparin was associated with an excess of major noncerebral and cerebral hemorrhages (1.0% vs. 0.8%; $p < 0.01$; 0.56% vs. 0.40%; $p < 0.05$), but no difference was seen in the total stroke rate (1.28% vs. 1.18%).

Comments: No difference in mortality seen with tPA and SK, but questions remained because of the suboptimal heparin regimen (i.e., delayed and subcutaneous).

89. **GUSTO I.** The Global Utilization of Streptokinase and tPA for Occluded Coronary Arteries Study (**GUSTO**) Investigators. An international randomized trial comparing four thrombolytic strategies for acute MI. *N Engl J Med* 1993;329:673–682.

Design: Prospective, randomized, open-label, multicenter study. Primary endpoint was 30-day all-cause mortality rate.

Purpose: To compare the effects of four thrombolytic regimens using SK and/or tPA.

Population: 41,021 patients seen less than 6 hours from onset of symptoms with chest pain lasting more than 20 minutes and ST elevation 1 mm or more in at least two limb leads or 2 mm or more in at least two precordial leads.

Exclusion Criteria: Prior stroke, active bleeding, prior treatment with SK or anistreplase, and recent trauma or major surgery; relative contraindication was SBP 180 or greater unresponsive to therapy.

Treatment: (a) SK, 1.5 million U over 60 minutes, with s.c. heparin, 12,500 U twice daily; (b) SK, 1.5 million U over 60 minutes and i.v. heparin (5,000-U bolus and then 1,000 U/hr); (c) accelerated tPA [15-mg bolus, and then 0.75 mg/kg (maximum, 50 mg) over 30 minutes, and then 0.5 mg/kg (maximum, 35 mg) over 60 minutes] with i.v. heparin (5,000-U bolus and then 1,000 U/hr); or (d) tPA, 1.0 mg/kg over 60 minutes (10% given as a bolus; maximum dose, 90 mg), and SK, 1 million U over 60 minutes with i.v. heparin (5,000-U bolus and then 1,000 U/hr).

Results: Accelerated tPA with i.v. heparin (c) was associated with the lowest 30-day mortality rate—6.3% (vs. 7.2%, 7.4%, and 7.0% for regimens a, b, and c), which corresponds to a 14% reduction compared with the SK-only regimens ($p = 0.001$). Despite an increased intracranial hemorrhage risk seen with tPA (0.72% vs. 0.49%, 0.54%, and 94%), tPA still was associated with a significant reduction in the combined endpoint of death or disabling stroke (6.9% vs. 7.8% in SK-only groups; $p = 0.006$). tPA appeared to confer a greater benefit in patients with anterior MI (8.6% vs. 10.5% mortality). A mortality benefit similar to that of tPA overall was seen in patients older than 75 years (1.3% vs. 1.1%), although limited numbers prevented the subgroup analysis from having the power to achieve statistical significance.

Comments: The mortality rate was only 4.3% in patients treated within 2 hours versus 5.5% at 2 to 4 hours and 8.9% at 4 to 6 hours. Thus, time to therapy also is an important factor. A secondary analysis showed age to be a powerful mortality predictor: 3% if younger than 65 years old versus 9.5%, 19.6%, and 30.3% if 65 to 74, 75 to 85, and older than 85 years, respectively. One-year follow-up showed a persistent benefit of tPA with an increase in mortality of only 1.4% from 30 days to 1 year. Another secondary analysis showed the optimal PTT range to be 50 to 70 seconds (lowest 30-day mortality, stroke, and bleeding rates) with a clustering of reinfarctions in the first 10 hours after discontinuation of heparin. Finally, a cost-effectiveness analysis showed that tPA costs $32,678 per year of life saved.

90. The **GUSTO Angiographic** Investigators. The effects of tissue plasminogen activator, streptokinase, or both on coronary artery patency, ventricular function and survival after acute MI. *N Engl J Med* 1993;329:1615–1622.

Design: Prospective, randomized, open-label, multicenter study. Primary endpoint was TIMI grade 2 or 3 flow at 90 minutes.

Purpose: To compare the patency rates and the effect on LV function of tPA and SK.

Population: 2,431 patients seen less than 6 hours from onset of symptoms with chest pain lasting more than 20 minutes and ST elevation 1 mm or more in at least two limb leads or 2 mm or more in at least two precordial leads.

Exclusion Criteria: See GUSTO I trial summary.

Treatment: Four thrombolytic regimens (see GUSTO I trial summary). Patients were then randomized to cardiac catheterization at 90 minutes, 180 minutes, 24 hours, or 5 to 7 days. The 90-minute group underwent repeated catheterization at 5 to 7 days.

Results: Highest patency (TIMI grade 2 or 3 flow) at 90 minutes was seen with tPA and intravenously heparin—81% versus 54% with SK and s.c. heparin, 60% with SK and i.v. heparin, and 73% with combination therapy ($p < 0.001$ for tPA vs. SK groups). Normal flow (TIMI grade 3) was seen in 54% of the tPA patients versus 29%, 32%, and 38% in the other three groups. Surprisingly, the differences between the tPA and SK groups disappeared at 180 minutes. The reocclusion rate was low and similar in all four groups (4.9% to 6.4%). LV function paralleled patency at 90 minutes, with the tPA group having better regional wall motion. Mortality also was strongly correlated with 90-minute patency: a low 4.4% with TIMI grade 3 flow versus 8.9% with grade 1 flow ($p = 0.009$).

Comments: Results support the open-artery theory asserting that early reperfusion of the IRA results in improved outcome (see accompanying editorial). A subsequent analysis of the 559 patients who underwent catheterization twice (at 90 minutes and 5 to 7 days) showed that early patency results were not predictive of reocclusion. Another analysis showed that the mortality benefit of achieving 90-minute TIMI grade 3 flow was amplified beyond the initial 30 days: unadjusted mortality hazard ratio (TIMI grade 3 vs. 2 or less) from 30 to 688 days was only 0.39 (vs. 0.57 at 30 days).

91. **Cannon CP**, et al. **TIMI-4**. Comparison of front-loaded recombinant tissue plasminogen activator, anistreplase and combination thrombolytic therapy for acute MI. *J Am Coll Cardiol* 1994;24:1602–1610.

This prospective, double-blind, multicenter study randomized 382 patients seen within 6 hours of symptom onset to front-loaded rtPA [15-mg bolus, and then 0.75 mg/kg (maximum, 50 mg) over a 30-minute period, and then 0.50 mg/kg (maximum, 35 mg) over a 30-minute period]; or anistreplase, 30-U bolus over 2 to 5 minutes; or rtPA [15-mg bolus, and then 0.75 mg/kg (maximum, 50 mg) over 30 minutes] and anistreplase, 20-U bolus. All received i.v. heparin and aspirin. The rtPA group had higher patency (TIMI grade 2 or 3 flow) at 60 minutes: 78% versus 59% for two other groups ($p = 0.02$). Similar results were observed at 90 minutes [TIMI grade 3 flow in 60%, 43% (anistreplase only), and 44% (combination)]. No significant differences were seen in the composite primary endpoint, consisting of in-hospital death, severe CHF or cardiogenic shock, low EF, reinfarction, TIMI grade flow less than 2 at 90 minutes or 18 to 36 hours, reocclusion (on sestamibi imaging), major spontaneous hemorrhage, and severe anaphylaxis (rtPA, 41.3%; anistreplase, 49%; combination, 53.6%). However, the 6-week mortality rate was lowest in the rtPA group: 2.2% versus 8.8% with anistreplase ($p = 0.02$) and 7.2% with combination therapy ($p = 0.06$).

92. **International Joint Efficacy Comparison of Thrombolytics (INJECT).** Randomized, double-blind comparison of reteplase double-bolus administration with streptokinase in acute MI: trial to investigate equivalence. *Lancet* 1995;346:329–336.

Design: Prospective, randomized, double-blind, double-dummy, multicenter study. Primary endpoint was 35-day mortality rate.

Purpose: To determine whether the effect of reteplase on 35-day mortality is at least equivalent to that of SK.

Population: 6,010 patients seen within 12 hours of onset of symptoms with chest pain lasting 30 minutes or longer and ST elevation 1 mm or more in at least two of the three inferior leads or leads I and aVL, 2 mm or more in at least two contiguous precordial leads, or new LBBB.

Treatment: SK, 1.5 million U over a 60-minute period, or reteplase, 10 million U bolus, and repeated 30 minutes later. All patients received heparin for 24 hours.

Results: The 35-day mortality rates were similar—9.0% (reteplase) and 9.5% (SK). Results show that reteplase is at least as effective as SK. Reinfarction and bleeding rates also were similar (5.0% vs. 5.4%; 0.7% vs. 1.0%), whereas the reteplase group had less atrial fibrillation (7.2% vs. 8.8%; $p < 0.05$), cardiogenic shock (4.7% vs. 6.0%; $p < 0.05$), heart failure (23.6% vs. 26.3%; $p < 0.05$), and hypotension (15.5% vs. 17.6%; $p < 0.05$).

93. **Bode C,** et al. for the **RAPID II** Investigators. Randomized comparison of coronary thrombolysis achieved with double-bolus reteplase (recombinant plasminogen activator) and front-loaded, accelerated alteplase (recombinant tissue plasminogen activator) in patients with acute MI. *Circulation* 1996;94:891–898.

Design: Prospective, randomized, open-label, parallel-group, multicenter study.

Purpose: To compare the bolus-administered thrombolytic reteplase with an accelerated infusion of alteplase on infarct-related patency and major events.

Population: 324 patients aged 18 to 75 years seen within 12 hours (from onset of symptoms to planned administration of treatment) with chest pain lasting 30 minutes or longer and ST elevation 1 mm or more in at least two of the three inferior leads or lateral leads or 2 mm or more in at least two contiguous leads, or LBBB.

Treatment: Reteplase, 10 million U, over 2 to 3 minutes, and then 10 million U repeated 30 minutes later, or front-loaded alteplase. All patients received aspirin and i.v. heparin.

Results: The reteplase group had better TIMI grade 3 flow at 90 minutes (60% vs. 45%; $p = 0.01$) and 51% fewer coronary interventions (13.6% vs. 26.5%; $p < 0.01$); a greater than 50% statistically nonsignificant mortality reduction (4.1% vs. 8.4%) also was observed, as were similar rates of transfusion, hemorrhage, and stroke.

94. **GUSTO III** Investigators. A comparison of reteplase with alteplase for acute MI. *N Engl J Med* 1997;337:1118–1123 (editorial, 1159–1161).

Design: Prospective, randomized (2:1), open-label, parallel-group, multicenter study. Primary endpoint was 30-day mortality rate.

Purpose: To determine whether reteplase is superior to alteplase in reducing mortality in AMI.

Population: 15,059 patients seen with 30 minutes or more of continuous symptoms and within 6 hours of their onset and 1 mm or more ST elevation in at least two limb leads or 2 mm or more in precordial leads, or BBB.

Exclusion Criteria: Active bleeding, history of stroke, recent major surgery, SBP 200 mm Hg or higher or DBP 110 mm Hg or higher, and requirement for oral anticoagulation.

Treatment: Reteplase given as two 10 million U boluses 30 minutes apart or an accelerated infusion of alteplase [15-mg bolus, and then 0.75 mg/kg (maximum, 50 mg) over a 30-minute period, and then 0.50 mg/kg (maximum, 35 mg) over 60 minutes].

Results: Reteplase and alteplase groups had similar 30-day mortality rates: 7.47% versus 7.24% ($p = 0.54$; 95% CI for absolute difference in mortality rates was -1.1% to 0.66%). Stroke rate and combined endpoints of death or nonfatal, disabling stroke were both similar (1.64% vs. 1.79%; 7.89% vs. 7.91%).

Comments: Although this trial was designed as a superiority trial, the accompanying editorial points out that these results do not demonstrate equivalence according to the GUSTO trial margin of benefit. Nonetheless, clinical equivalence of reteplase was observed in this large trial.

95. **Cannon CP,** et al. for the **TIMI-10B** Investigators. TNK-tissue plasminogen activator compared with front-loaded alteplase in acute MI. *Circulation* 1998;98:2805–2814.

This prospective, randomized, multicenter trial was composed of 886 acute STEMI patients seen within 12 hours of onset of symptoms. Patients received TNK, 30 or 50 mg, or front-loaded tPA. All patients underwent immediate angiography. The 50-mg dose of TNK was discontinued early because of an increased rate of intracranial hemorrhage and was replaced by a 40-mg dose, and heparin doses were decreased. TNK, 40 mg, and tPA produced similar rates of TIMI grade 3 flow at 90 minutes (62.8% vs. 62.7%; p = NS; TNK, 30 mg, 54.3%, p = 0.035). TNK doses of 0.5 mg/kg resulted in higher TIMI grade 3 flow and lower median CTFCs (i.e., faster flow) than did lower doses. Lower rates of major bleeding and intracranial hemorrhage were observed after the heparin doses were lowered and titration of heparin was begun at 6 hours.

96. **Assessment of the Safety and Efficacy of a New Thrombolytic: TNK-tPA (ASSENT-2).** Single-bolus tenecteplase compared with front-loaded alteplase in acute MI: the ASSENT-2 double-blind randomized trial. *Lancet* 1999;354:716–722.

Design: Prospective, randomized, open-label, multicenter study. Primary endpoint was all-cause mortality at 30 days.
Purpose: To assess the efficacy and safety of TNK compared with alteplase (tPA).
Population: 16,949 patients seen within 6 hours of symptom onset with ST-segment elevations of 1 mm or more in two or more limb leads or 2 mm or more in two or more contiguous precordial leads; or new LBBB.
Treatment: TNK administered over 5 to 10 seconds (30 mg if >60 kg; 35 mg if 60 to 60.9 kg; 40 mg if 70 to 79.9 kg; 45 mg if 80 to 89.9 kg; 50 mg if 90 kg or more) or accelerated infusion of tPA over a 90-minute period (100 mg or less).
Results: All-cause mortality rate at 30 days was nearly identical in the two groups: 6.18% (TNK) and 6.15% (tPA). Intracranial hemorrhage rates also were similar [0.43% (TNK), 0.44% (tPA)], but fewer noncerebral bleeding complications (26.4% vs. 29.0%; p = 0.0003) and less need for blood transfusion (4.3% vs. 5.5%; p = 0.0002) were observed with TNK. Subgroup analysis showed that the mortality rate among patients treated more than 4 hours after the onset of symptoms was significantly lower with TNK (7.1% vs. 9.2%; p = 0.018). This finding may be owing to the increased fibrin specificity of TNK.

97. **The Assessment of the Safety and Efficacy of a New Thrombolytic Regimen (ASSENT-3)** Investigators. Efficacy and safety of tenecteplase in combination with enoxaparin, abciximab, or unfractionated heparin: the ASSENT-3 randomized trial in acute myocardial infarction. *Lancet* 2001;358:605–613.

Design: Prospective, randomized, open-label, multicenter trial. Primary composite endpoint at 30 days: death, in-hospital MI, or in-hospital refractory ischemia.
Purpose: To evaluate whether the combination of TNK plus enoxaparin or abciximab is safe and efficacious compared with TNK and UFH in AMI patients.
Population: 6,095 AMI patients seen within 6 hours of symptom onset.
Treatment: Three groups: (a) full-dose TNK and enoxaparin for a maximum of 7 days; (b) half-dose TNK with weight-adjusted low-dose UFH and a 12-hour infusion of abciximab; or (c) full-dose TNK with weight-adjusted UFH for 48 hours.
Results: The enoxaparin and abciximab groups had a lower incidence of the primary efficacy endpoint compared with the UFH group (11.4% and 11.1% vs. 15.4%, respectively; RR, 0.74 and 0.72; both p < 0.001). Similarly, the efficacy plus safety endpoint (in-hospital intracranial hemorrhage or in-hospital major bleeding complications) was significantly lower for the enoxaparin group [13.7% vs. 17.0% (UFH); p = 0.0146] and trended to be lower in the

abciximab group (14.2% vs. 17.0%; $p = 0.057$). Among patients older than 75 years, the incidence of efficacy or safety events was *higher* in the abciximab group compared with the UFH group (36.9% vs. 28.0%; $p = 0.001$); a similar finding was seen among diabetic patients (22.3% vs. 16.5%; $p = 0.0007$). Overall, the abciximab group had nearly twice the risk of major hemorrhage compared with the UFH group (4.3% vs. 2.2%; $p = 0.0002$; enoxaparin group, 3.0%; $p = $ NS vs. UFH).

Placebo-controlled Studies

98. **GISSI-1.** Effectiveness of intravenous thrombolytic treatment in acute MI. *Lancet* 1986;327:397–401.

Design: Prospective, randomized, open, parallel-group, multicenter study. Primary endpoint was 21-day mortality rate.

Purpose: To evaluate the safety and efficacy of i.v. SK in AMI and to determine whether any effect is dependent on the interval between onset of pain and treatment.

Population: 11,806 patients seen within 12 hours of onset of symptoms with chest pain and ST elevation or depression 1 mm or more in any limb lead or 2 mm or more in any precordial lead.

Treatment: SK, 1.5 million U over a 60-minute period.

Results: SK-treated patients had a 21-day mortality rate that was 18% lower than that of controls (10.7% vs. 13.0%; $p = 0.0002$). The largest mortality advantage [23% ($p = 0.0005$)] was associated with administration to those seen within 3 hours of onset of symptoms (RR, 0.74 vs. 1.19 for 9 to 12 hours). At 1 year, the mortality benefit persisted (17.2% vs. 19.0%; $p = 0.0008$).

Comments: The 10-year follow-up showed that the mortality benefit was still significant, with 19 lives saved/1,000 patients ($p = 0.02$).

99. **ISIS-2** Collaborative Group. Randomised trial of intravenous streptokinase, oral, both, or neither among 17,187 cases of suspected acute MI. *Lancet* 1988;332:349–360.

Design: Prospective, randomized, double-blind, placebo-controlled, multicenter study. Primary endpoint was vascular mortality.

Purpose: To assess the separate and combined effects on mortality of i.v. SK and oral aspirin in patients with suspected AMI.

Population: 17,187 patients with suspected MI seen within 24 hours (median, 5 hours) of onset of symptoms.

Exclusion Criteria: Any history of stroke, GI hemorrhage, or ulcer. Possible contraindications included recent trauma, severe persistent hypertension (not defined), and allergy to SK or aspirin.

Treatment: SK, 1.5 million U over a 60-minute period, and/or aspirin, 162.5 mg daily; or placebo.

Results: SK and aspirin-alone groups had 25% and 23% lower 5-week vascular mortality rates, respectively [9.2% vs. 12.0% (placebo), $p < 0.00001$; 9.4% vs. 11.8%, $p < 0.00001$]. The SK-and-aspirin group had an even larger 42% mortality reduction (8% vs. 13.2%). Combination therapy also was effective in patients with LBBB (mortality, 14% vs. 27.7%). SK was associated with hypotension in 10% and more bleeds requiring transfusion (0.5% vs. 0.2%), but fewer strokes (0.6% vs. 0.8%). Aspirin reduced nonfatal reinfarction and stroke rates (1.0% vs. 2.0%; 0.3% vs. 0.6%).

100. Intravenous Streptokinase in Acute MI (**ISAM**) Study Group. A prospective trial of intravenous streptokinase in acute MI: mortality, morbidity and infarct size at 21 days. *N Engl J Med* 1986;314:1465–1471.

Design: Prospective, randomized, double-blind, placebo-controlled, multicenter study. Primary endpoint was 21-day mortality rate.

Purpose: To assess the effects of i.v. SK on 21-day mortality and to compare results in those treated within 3 hours with those treated at 3 to 6 hours.

Population: 1,741 patients aged 75 years or younger seen within 6 hours of onset of symptoms.

Treatment: SK, 1.5 million U over a 60-minute period, or placebo. All patients received heparin for 72 to 96 hours and coumadin for 3 weeks.

Results: The SK group had nonsignificant reduction in 21-day mortality (6.3% vs. 7.1%), significantly higher LVEF (56.8% vs. 53.9%), and an earlier CK-MB peak (13.9 vs. 19.2 hours). Among those treated within 3 hours, the mortality rates were lower [5.2% (SK) vs. 6.5%; p = NS].

Comments: A subsequent report determined that anterior MI patients treated with SK had higher EFs (50% vs. 42%; p = 0.013), especially those treated within 3 hours (p = 0.004). These differences persisted through 3-year follow-up.

101. **Wilcox RG**, et al. Anglo-Scandinavian Study of Early Thrombolysis (**ASSET**). Trial of tissue plasminogen activator for mortality reduction in acute MI. *Lancet* 1988;332: 525–530.

Design: Prospective, randomized, double-blind, placebo-controlled, multicenter study. Primary endpoint was mortality at 1 month.

Purpose: To evaluate the effects of tPA on mortality after AMI.

Population: 5,013 patients aged 18 to 75 years with suspected AMI who were treated within 5 hours of onset of symptoms.

Treatment: tPA, 10-mg bolus, followed by 50 mg over a 1-hour period, and then 20 mg/hr for 2 hours (100 mg total), or placebo.

Results: The tPA group had a 26% lower 1-month mortality rate—7.2% vs. 9.8% [26% hazard ratio (95% CI, 11% to 39%)]. This benefit persisted at 6 months: 10.4% vs. 13.1%. Among patients with proven MI, the mortality difference was more impressive: 12.6% versus 17.1%. The tPA group had more bleeding and more frequent bradycardia (27 patients vs. 5 patients).

102. **Topol EJ**, et al. and the Thrombolysis and Angioplasty in MI (**TAMI-6**) Study Group. A randomized trial of late reperfusion therapy for acute MI. *Circulation* 1992;85: 2090–2099.

This prospective, randomized, double-blind, placebo-controlled, multicenter study enrolled 197 patients aged 75 years or younger seen 6 to 24 hours after onset of symptoms with 1 mm or more ST elevation in at least two contiguous leads. Patients received tPA over a 2-hour period [1 mg/kg over the first 60 minutes (10% as bolus; maximum, 80 mg), and then 20 mg over the second hour], or placebo. Angiography was performed within 24 hours; 71 patients had persistent IRA occlusion and met eligibility criteria for randomization to PTCA or no PTCA. Better early patency (TIMI grade 2 or 3 flow) was achieved with tPA [65% vs. 27% (placebo)], but similar rates were observed for late (6-month) patency (both 59%), in-hospital mortality, and LVEF. At 6 months, the tPA group had no increase in LV end-diastolic volume (vs. approximately 25% increase in the placebo group). PTCA patients had an 81% initial recanalization rate and improved ventricular function at 1 month, but no advantage was evident at late follow-up (the non-PTCA group had a 38% spontaneous recanalization rate).

103. **The European MI Project (EMIP)** Group. Prehospital thrombolytic therapy in patients with suspected MI. *N Engl J Med* 1993;329:383–389.

Prospective, randomized, double-blind, crossover, multicenter study of 5,469 patients seen within 6 hours with 1 mm or greater ST elevation in two or more limb leads or 2 mm or more in two or more precordial leads. Patients received anistreplase, 30 U, before hospitalization, followed by placebo in hospital or placebo followed by anistreplase. Trial was terminated early because of failure to reach target of 10,000 patients in a 2-year period. Patients in the prehospital group received anistreplase 55 minutes earlier on average than did those in the hospital group. Prehospital anistreplase was associated with a nonsignificant 13% overall mortality reduction (9.7% vs. 11.1%; p = 0.08) and a significant 16% cardiac mortality reduction (8.3% vs. 9.8%; p = 0.049). More adverse events [VF (p = 0.02), shock (p < 0.001), symptomatic hypotension (p < 0.001), bradycardia (p = 0.001)] occurred in the prehospital group before hospitalization, but this was offset by a higher incidence during the hospital period in the hospital group.

104. **Late Assessment of Thrombolytic Efficacy (LATE)** Study Group. Late assessment of thrombolytic efficacy study with alteplase 6–24 hours after onset of MI. *Lancet* 1993; 342:759–766.

Design: Prospective, randomized, double-blind, placebo-controlled, multicenter study. Primary endpoint was 35-day mortality rate.

Purpose: To compare administration of alteplase with placebo in AMI patients seen at 6 to 24 hours.

Population: 5,711 patients seen 6 to 24 hours after onset of symptoms with 1 mm or more ST elevation in at least two limb leads, 2 mm or more ST elevation in at least two precordial leads, ST depression 2 mm or more in at least two leads, pathologic Q waves, or abnormal T-wave inversion in at least two leads thought to represent a non–Q wave infarct.

Treatment: Alteplase, 100 mg over a 3-hour period (10-mg bolus, 50 mg for 1 hour, 20 mg/hr for 2 hours), or placebo.

Results: Intention-to-treat analysis showed a nonsignificant 14% thirty–five–day mortality reduction in the alteplase group (8.9% vs. 10.3%). However, prespecified survival analysis according to treatment within 12 hours showed that the alteplase group had a 25.6% mortality reduction (8.9% vs. 11.9%; $p = 0.023$). Treatment for 12 to 24 hours was associated with a nonsignificant 5% mortality reduction (8.7% vs. 9.2%). Alteplase was not associated with a higher cardiac rupture rate, but rather earlier occurrence of rupture (within 24 hours after thrombolysis).

Prehospital Thrombolysis Studies

105. **Weaver WD,** et al. MI Triage and Intervention (**MITI**). Pre-hospital versus hospital-initiated thrombolytic therapy. *JAMA* 1993;270:1211–1216.

Design: Prospective, randomized, open, parallel-group study. Primary endpoint was a composite score that combined death, stroke, major bleeding, and infarct size.

Purpose: To compare prehospital and hospital initiation of thrombolytic therapy in patients with chest pain and ST-segment elevation.

Population: 360 patients aged 75 years or younger seen within 6 hours of onset of symptoms with ST elevation.

Exclusion Criteria: History of stroke, recent bleeding or surgery, and SBP less than 180 mm Hg or DBP greater than 120 mm Hg.

Treatment: Prehospital or hospital administration of alteplase (100 mg over a 3-hour period) plus aspirin (325 mg).

Results: Despite earlier time to treatment in the prehospital-initiated group (77 minutes vs. 110 minutes), no significant differences were seen in primary composite endpoint score ($p = 0.64$), mortality rate (5.7% vs. 8.1%; $p = 0.49$), EF, or infarct size. A secondary analysis showed that when treatment was initiated at sooner than 70 minutes, prehospital therapy was associated with a lower mortality rate (1.2% vs. 8.7%) and better EF (53% vs. 49%; $p = 0.03$). However, at 2-year follow-up, the mortality benefit in this subgroup was no longer statistically significant [2% (<70 minutes) vs. 12%; $p = 0.12$].

106. **Rawles J,** et al. on behalf of the Grampian Region Early Anistreplase Trial (**GREAT**) Group. Halving of mortality at one year by domiciliary thrombolysis in the GREAT. *J Am Coll Cardiol* 1994;23:1–5.

Design: Prospective, randomized, double-blind, parallel-group, multicenter study.

Purpose: To evaluate the feasibility, safety, and efficacy of home-administered thrombolysis by general practitioners compared with hospital thrombolysis.

Population: 311 patients with suspected MI seen by their general practitioners within 4 hours of symptom onset (ECG recordings required but not reported).

Treatment: Anistreplase, 30 U, at home or in hospital.

Results: Home-administered anistreplase was given more than 2 hours sooner, at a median 101 minutes versus 240 minutes. The home-treated group had a 52% lower 1-year mortality rate (10.4% vs. 21.6%; p = 0.007).

107. **Morrow DA,** et al. Evaluation of the time saved by prehospital initiation of reteplase for ST-elevation myocardial infarction: results of the Early Retavase-Thrombolysis in Myocardial Infarction **(ER-TIMI 19)** trial. *J Am Coll Cardiol* 2002;40:71–77.

Design: Prospective, randomized, controlled, open, multicenter trial. Time from EMS arrival to fibrinolytic administration was compared between study patients receiving prehospital rPA and sequential control patients from 6 to 12 months before the study who received a fibrinolytic in the hospital.

Purpose: To test the feasibility of prehospital initiation of the bolus fibrinolytic reteplase and determine the time saved by prehospital rPA in the setting of contemporary emergency cardiac care.

Population: 315 patients with STEMI at 20 North American emergency medical systems; 630 controls were treated in-hospital with fibrinolytic therapy.

Treatment: Prehospital administration of reteplase (10 U over a 2-minute period followed by second bolus 30 minutes later, either in ambulance or in ED). All received aspirin and i.v. UFH [60-U/kg bolus (maximum, 4,000 U), and then 12 U/kg/hr (maximum, 800 U/hr)].

Results: AMI was verified in 98%. The median time from EMS arrival to initiation of reteplase was 31 minutes. The time from EMS arrival to in-hospital fibrinolytic for 630 control patients was 63 minutes, resulting in a time saved of 32 minutes (p < 0.0001). By 30 minutes after first medical contact, 49% of study patients had received the first bolus of fibrinolytic compared with only 5% of controls (p < 0.0001). In-hospital mortality was 4.7%. Intracranial hemorrhage occurred in 1.0%.

PERCUTANEOUS CORONARY INTERVENTION

Operator and Hospital Volume Studies

108. **Thiemann DR,** et al. The association between hospital volume and survival after acute myocardial infarction in elderly patients. *N Engl J Med* 1999;340:1640.

This retrospective cohort analysis focused on 98,898 Medicare patients aged 65 years or older with a principal discharge diagnosis of AMI. Patients admitted to hospitals in the lowest quartile of volume of invasive procedures had a 17% higher in-hospital mortality rate compared with patients at highest-volume-quartile hospitals (hazard ratio, 1.17; 95% CI, 1.09 to 1.26; p < 0.001).

109. **Magid DJ,** et al. Relation between hospital primary angioplasty volume and mortality for patients with acute MI treated with primary angioplasty vs thrombolytic therapy. *JAMA* 2000;284:3131–3138.

This retrospective cohort study analyzed 62,299 AMI patients at 446 acute care hospitals treated with primary angioplasty or thrombolytic therapy from June 1994 to July 1999. At hospitals with intermediate volume (17 to 48 procedures/year) and high volume (>49 procedures), mortality was significantly lower among patients undergoing angioplasty compared with thrombolysis (4.5% vs. 5.9%, p < 0.001; 3.4% vs. 5.4%, p < 0.001). At low-volume hospitals, no significant difference in mortality was found between the two treatment modalities (6.2% vs. 5.9%; p = 0.58).

110. **Vakili BA,** et al. Volume–outcome relation for physicians and hospitals performing angioplasty for acute myocardial infarction in New York state. *Circulation* 2001;104:2171–2176.

This analysis examined 1,342 patients who underwent angioplasty procedures within 23 hours of onset of AMI without preceding thrombolytic therapy. Primary PTCA performed by a high-volume operator (11 or more cases/year) was associated with a 57% lower in-hospital mortality compared with those treated by low-volume operators (1 to 10 cases/year; adjusted RR, 0.43; 95% CI, 0.21 to 0.83). Primary PTCA performed in high-volume hospitals (57 or more cases/year) resulted in a 44% in-hospital mortality reduction compared with that in low-volume hospitals (adjusted RR, 0.56; 95% CI, 0.29 to 1.1).

111. **Srinivas VS,** et al. Effect of physician volume on the relationship between hospital volume and mortality during primary angioplasty. *J Am Coll Cardiol* 2009;53:574–579.

This, the most contemporary analysis of the New York State PCI registry, looked at 7,321 patients receiving primary PCI for acute MI. It compared risk-adjusted in-hospital mortality between high-volume hospitals (>50 cases/year) and high-volume operators (>10 cases/year) versus lower volume centers and physicians. ORs for in-hospital mortality in high-volume hospitals (0.58; 95% CI, 0.38 to 0.88) and high-volume operators (OR, 0.66; 95% CI, 0.48 to 0.92) were significantly lower than those for their lower volume counterparts. Furthermore, physician volume modified hospital outcome as well—low-volume physicians had higher mortality outcomes in both low- and high-volume hospitals. The absolute difference was highest in low-volume hospitals (8.4% in-hospital mortality for low-volume physicians vs. 4.8% for high-volume physicians; OR, 1.44; 95% CI, 0.68 to 3.03). The difference was significant in high-volume hospitals (3.8% for high-volume physicians vs. 6.5% for low-volume physicians; OR, 0.58; 95% CI, 0.39 to 0.86).

Meta-analyses of Percutaneous Transluminal Coronary Angioplasty versus Thrombolysis

112. **Weaver WD,** et al. Comparison of primary coronary angioplasty and intravenous thrombolytic therapy for acute MI: a quantitative review. *JAMA* 1997;278:2093–2098.

Data analysis from 10 randomized trials with a total of 2,606 patients. Mortality at 30 days or less was significantly lower in patients treated with primary PTCA compared with thrombolysis (4.4% vs. 6.5%; OR, 0.66; 95% CI, 0.46 to 0.94; $p = 0.02$). Primary PTCA also was associated with lower rates of reinfarction [7.2% vs. 11.9%, or 0.58% (95% CI, 0.44 to 0.75); $p < 0.001$]. Authors point out that the primary angioplasty results were primarily achieved in specialized, high-volume centers.

113. **Keeley EC,** et al. Primary angioplasty versus intravenous thrombolytic therapy for acute myocardial infarction: a quantitative review of 23 randomised trials. *Lancet* 2003; 361:13–20.

This analysis identified 23 studies with a total of 7,739 patients. SK was used in 8 trials ($n = 1,837$), and fibrin-specific agents in 15 ($n = 5,902$). Stents were used in 12 trials. Primary PTCA had lower short-term mortality compared with thrombolytic therapy (7% vs. 9%; $p = 0.0002$), nonfatal MI (3% vs. 7%; $p < 0.0001$), and stroke (1% vs. 2%; $p = 0.0004$). Results with primary PTCA remained better during long-term follow-up.

114. **Dalby M,** et al. Transfer for primary angioplasty versus immediate thrombolysis in acute myocardial infarction: a meta-analysis. *Circulation* 2003;108:1809–1814.

To further identify the best strategy for patients with acute MI presenting to hospitals without catheterization services, the authors analyzed six trials including 3,750 patients comparing immediate thrombolysis with transfer for primary PCI (within 3 hours). For the combined primary endpoint of death, reinfarction, or stroke, there was a significant 42% reduction ($p < 0.001$) in the group transferred for primary PCI, compared with immediate thrombolysis. This was primarily driven by significant reductions in reinfarction (68%, $p < 0.001$) and stroke (56%, $p = 0.015$), with a nonsignificant trend for overall mortality favoring PCI (19% reduction, $p = 0.08$).

Primary Angioplasty Reviews

115. **Keeley EC,** Hillis LD. Primary PCI for myocardial infarction with ST-segment elevation. *N Engl J Med* 2007;356:47–54.

The authors present a case vignette, and then review the pathophysiology and treatment effect for primary PCI in STEMI. They discuss the clinical evidence for such a strategy, indications for PCI versus fibrinolysis, as well as potential adverse events. The manuscript concludes with a discussion of still uncertain areas, as well as a review of the current guidelines.

116. **Nallamothu BK,** et al. Time to treatment in primary percutaneous coronary intervention. *N Engl J Med* 2007;357:1631–1638.

In light of guidelines to reduce door-to-balloon times, the authors review the pathophysiology of MI, use of fibrinolysis, as well as primary PCI. The evidence and rationale behind expediting reperfusion time is discussed, as well as guidance on selecting the most appropriate reperfusion strategy. Helpful strategies for reducing door-to-balloon times are presented, and the manuscript concludes with future challenges to meeting such goals and improving care.

Primary Angioplasty Trials

117. **Grines CL,** et al. Primary Angioplasty in MI (**PAMI**). A comparison of immediate angioplasty with thrombolytic therapy for acute MI. *N Engl J Med* 1993;328:673–679.

Design: Prospective, randomized, open, multicenter study. Endpoints included in-hospital death, reinfarction, and intracranial bleeding and EF at 6 weeks.
Purpose: To compare immediate PTCA with thrombolytic therapy in AMI.
Population: 395 patients seen within 12 hours of ischemic pain with 1 mm or more ST elevation in at least two contiguous ECG leads.
Exclusion Criteria: Complete LBBB, cardiogenic shock, and increased bleeding risk.
Treatment: tPA, 100 mg i.v. (or 1.25 mg/kg if patient weighed <65 kg) over a 3-hour period; or immediate PTCA. All patients received i.v. heparin for 3 to 5 days.
Results: A 97% PTCA success rate was observed. The PTCA group had a 60% lower in-hospital mortality rate (2.6% vs. 6.5%; $p = 0.06$) and a significant 58% reduction in in-hospital death or reinfarction (5.1% vs. 12.0%; $p = 0.02$). The PTCA group also had less intracranial bleeding (none vs. 2.0%; $p = 0.05$). No difference was seen between groups in EF at 6 weeks (both at rest and during exercise). The benefits of primary angioplasty were maintained at 2-year follow-up: lower incidence of death or MI (14.9% vs. 23%; $p = 0.034$), less recurrent ischemia (36.4% vs. 48%; $p = 0.026$), lower reintervention rates (27.2% vs. 46.5%; $p < 0.0001$), and lower rehospitalization rates (58.5% vs. 69.0%; $p = 0.035$).
Comments: A short randomization to balloon time was observed (average, 60 minutes vs. 42 minutes for door-to-thrombolysis time). Editorial asserts that high-risk patients are most likely to benefit from immediate PTCA (e.g., older than 75 years, anterior MI, cardiogenic shock).

118. **Every NR,** et al. for the MI Triage and Intervention (**MITI**) Investigators. A comparison of thrombolytic therapy with primary coronary angioplasty for acute MI. *N Engl J Med* 1996;335:1253–1260.

Design: Retrospective cohort analysis of MITI Registry (19 Seattle-area hospitals, 10 with primary angioplasty capability).
Purpose: To compare outcomes in AMI patients receiving thrombolytic therapy and primary angioplasty.
Population: 3,145 MITI patients (thrombolytic group, $n = 2,095$; PTCA group, $n = 1,050$) treated between 1988 and 1994.
Exclusion Criteria: Lack of ECG data and angioplasty more than 6 hours after admission.

Treatment: Thrombolysis with alteplase (65%), SK (32%), or urokinase (3%; 8% were treated before hospitalization); or coronary angiography within 6 hours of admission followed by angioplasty if indicated.

Results: No significant differences were observed between thrombolysis and PTCA in the in-hospital [5.6% (thrombolytic) vs. 5.5%] or 3-year mortality rates. At 3-year follow-up, the thrombolysis group had 30% less coronary angiography, 15% fewer coronary angioplasties, and 13% lower costs. Thrombolysis patients were treated faster (1 hour vs. 1.7 hours after arrival) and sooner after chest pain than the PAMI thrombolysis group (198 minutes vs. 230 minutes). Low-volume-PTCA hospitals did provide later treatment (2.3 hours vs. 1.5 hours) and had higher in-hospital mortality rates (8.1% vs. 4.5%).

119. **GUSTO IIb** Angioplasty Substudy. The global use of strategies to open occluded arteries in acute coronary syndromes: Angioplasty Substudy Investigators. *N Engl J Med* 1997;336:1621–1628.

Design: Prospective, randomized, open, multicenter substudy (57 sites; all performed 200 angioplasties/year, with one operator doing 50 per year). Thirty-day primary endpoint was death, MI, and stroke.

Purpose: To compare thrombolytic therapy with primary angioplasty in patients with acute STEMI.

Population: 1,138 patients seen within 12 hours of STEMI.

Exclusion Criteria: Same as main GUSTO-IIb trial.

Treatment: Accelerated tPA [15-mg i.v. bolus, and then 0.75 mg/kg over a 30-minute period (maximum, 50 mg), 0.50 mg/kg over a 60-minute period (maximum, 35 mg)] or primary angioplasty (average door-to-balloon time, 1.9 hours).

Results: PTCA group had one-third lower rate of death, MI, and stroke (OR, 0.67; 9.6% vs. 13.7%; $p = 0.033$). Most of the observed benefit occurred from days 5 to 10. By 6 months, the difference was no longer significant (14% vs. 16%). Breakdown by endpoint (at 30 days): death, 5.7% versus 7% ($p = 0.37$); MI, 4.5% versus 6.5% ($p = 0.13$); stroke, 0.2% versus 0.9% ($p = 0.11$). PTCA was not associated with any extra benefit in high-risk groups. PTCA achieved TIMI grade 3 flow in a surprisingly low 73% of cases (technical success rate, 93%), which was associated with a 1.6% mortality rate (vs. 21.4%, 14.3%, 19.9% for TIMI flow grades 0 to 2).

120. **Grines CL**, et al. A randomized trial of transfer for primary angioplasty vs. on-site thrombolysis in patients with high risk myocardial infarction: the **Air PAMI** Study. *J Am Coll Cardiol* 2002;39:1713–1719.

Design: Prospective, randomized, open, multicenter study. Primary endpoint was a 30-day composite of death, recurrent MI, and disabling stroke.

Purpose: To evaluate whether early transfer for primary PTCA of AMI results in better outcomes than on-site thrombolysis.

Population: High-risk MI patients (older than 70 years, anterior MI, Killip class II/III, HR >100 beats/min, or SBP <100 mm Hg) who were eligible for thrombolytic therapy and seen in hospitals without on-site PCI.

Treatment: On-site thrombolysis or emergency transfer for primary PCI.

Results: Because of slow recruitment, the study was terminated after 138 patients enrolled (32% of the projected sample size). Median door-to-therapy time was 51 minutes in the thrombolytic group and 155 minutes in the transfer group. The long delay in the transfer group was mostly due to initiation of transfer (43 minutes) and transport time (26 minutes), as time from arrival in hospital to catheterization laboratory was 11 minutes, and catheterization laboratory arrival to treatment was only 14 minutes. No deaths occurred during transfer. In the transfer group, all patients underwent catheterization, and 89% had primary PCI. At 30-day follow-up, a nonsignificant 38% reduction in the primary composite endpoint in the transfer group was found compared with the thrombolytic group (8.4% vs. 13.6%; $p = 0.331$). Multivariate logistic regression analysis identified randomization to transfer as independent predictor of a reduction in the primary endpoint (OR, 0.159; 95% CI, 0.031 to 0.820; $p = 0.028$). The transfer group had a reduced hospital stay (6.1 days vs. 7.5 days; $p = 0.015$) and less ischemia (12.7% vs. 31.8%; $p = 0.007$).

121. **Aversano T,** et al. Atlantic Cardiovascular Patient Outcomes Research Team **(C-PORT).** Thrombolytic therapy vs primary percutaneous coronary intervention for myocardial infarction in patients presenting to hospitals without on-site cardiac surgery: a randomized controlled trial. *JAMA* 2002;287:1943–1951.

Design: Prospective, randomized trial conducted from July 1996 to December 1999 at 11 community hospitals without on-site cardiac surgery or existing PCI programs. Primary endpoint at 6 months was death, recurrent MI, or stroke.

Purpose: To determine whether treatment of acute MI with primary PCI is superior to thrombolytic therapy at hospitals without on-site cardiac surgery.

Population: 451 thrombolytic-eligible patients with acute STEMI seen within 12 hours of symptom onset.

Exclusion Criteria: Included those ineligible for thrombolytic therapy.

Treatment: Primary PCI program was developed at all sites. Patients were randomized to receive primary PCI or accelerated tPA.

Results: The primary PCI group had a significantly lower incidence of the primary composite endpoint at 6 weeks (10.7% vs. 17.7%; $p = 0.03$) and 6 months (12.4% vs. 19.9%; $p = 0.03$). The benefit was primarily driven by a lower incidence of recurrent MI (at 6 months: 5.3% vs. 10.6%; $p = 0.04$). Mortality rates were similar (6.2% vs. 7.1%; $p = 0.72$), whereas stroke occurred in 2.2% and 4.0%, respectively ($p = 0.28$). The primary PCI group also had a shorter median length of stay (4.5 days vs. 6.0 days; $p = 0.02$).

122. **Andersen HR,** et al. for the DANAMI-2 Investigators. A comparison of coronary angioplasty with fibrinolytic therapy in acute myocardial infarction. *N Engl J Med* 2003;349:733–742.

Design: Prospective, randomized, open, multicenter trial. Primary endpoint at 30 days: death, clinical reinfarction, or significant disabling stroke.

Purpose: To demonstrate that a primary PCI strategy will be superior in both patients seen at on-site interventional facilities (no transfer of patient required) and without (transfer of patient required).

Population: 1,572 patients seen within 12 hours with a sum of greater than 4-mm ST elevation in all leads.

Exclusion Criteria: Included contraindications to thrombolytic therapy; expected time between randomization and arrival in catheterization laboratory longer than 3 hours for patients randomized in referral hospitals, and more than 2 hours in invasive-equipped hospitals.

Treatment: Primary PCI or front-loaded tPA. PCI patients were transferred to referring center if catheterization laboratory facilities were not available on-site. All received aspirin (300 mg, and then 75 to 150 mg daily) and heparin (5,000 U bolus + 1,000 U/hr infusion for at least 48 hours in patients randomized to tPA; 10,000-U initial bolus + additional heparin to keep the ACT between 350 and 450 seconds during the procedure in patients randomized to PCI).

Results: The trial was terminated early because of a clear benefit for PCI. The PCI group had 40% reduction in the primary composite endpoint compared with the fibrinolytic group (8.5% vs. 14.2%; $p = 0.002$), primarily because of a lower incidence of recurrent MI (6.3% vs. 1.6%; $p < 0.001$). The 30-day mortality was 7.8% in the fibrinolysis group versus 6.6% in the PCI group ($p = 0.35$), and disabling stroke occurred in 2.0% and 1.1% ($p = 0.15$), respectively. A similar benefit with PCI was seen in patients who were transferred and those who were not transferred (time difference to balloon inflation between the referred and on-site patients was only 10 minutes).

123. **PRAGUE-2** Widimsky P, et al. Long distance transport for primary angioplasty vs immediate thrombolysis in acute myocardial infarction. *Eur Heart J* 2003;24:94–104.

This prospective, randomized trial enrolled 850 patients with acute STEMI seen within 12 hours in a community hospital and compared on-site thrombolysis (SK) with transfer for primary PCI. Exclusion criteria included contraindications to thrombolytic therapy and failure to initiate transfer within 30 minutes. Routine glycoprotein IIb/IIIa receptor antagonists before planned PCI were not used. At 30 days, mortality rates were not significantly different [10.4% (thrombolysis) vs. 6.0% (PCI); $p < 0.05$]. However, among those seen at 3 to 12 hours (vs. <3 hours), the PCI group had a stronger relative mortality reduction (6% vs. 15.3%; $p < 0.02$). The incidence of death, MI, and stroke also was significantly lower in the PCI group (8.4% vs. 15.2%; $p < 0.003$).

124. **O'Neill W,** et al. A prospective randomized clinical trial of intracoronary streptokinase versus coronary angioplasty for acute MI. *N Engl J Med* 1986;314:812–818.

In this first randomized trial of angioplasty versus thrombolysis (albeit intracoronary), only 56 patients were enrolled, all younger than 75 years and with symptoms for less than 12 hours. No differences were seen in the recanalization rate (83% vs. 85%), but the angioplasty group had decreased residual stenosis (43% vs. 83%) and significant EF improvement (+8% vs. +1%; $p < 0.001$).

125. **Gibbons RJ,** et al. Immediate angioplasty compared with the administration of a thrombolytic agent followed by conservative treatment for MI. *N Engl J Med* 1993;328:685–691.

In this small randomized trial of 108 patients seen within 12 hours of chest pain, the PTCA group did not have better myocardial salvage (by technetium-99m scan) nor were any differences in EF or mortality rate observed. However, PTCA patients did have a shorter stay (7.7 days vs. 10.6 days; $p = 0.01$) and less rehospitalization (in the first 6 months, 4% vs. 18%).

Percutaneous Coronary Intervention After Thrombolysis

126. **Topol EJ,** et al. and the Thrombolysis and Angioplasty in MI (**TAMI**) Study Group. A randomized trial of immediate versus delayed elective angioplasty after intravenous tissue plasminogen activator in acute MI. *N Engl J Med* 1987;317:581–588 (editorial, 624–626).

Design: Prospective, randomized, multicenter study. Primary endpoint was infarct-related vessel patency and global LV function.

Purpose: To compare immediate with delayed elective angioplasty in patients undergoing thrombolysis for AMI.

Population: 386 patients met initial criteria (75 years or younger, within 6 hours of onset of symptoms, and 1 mm or more ST elevation in at least two contiguous leads); 197 patients had appropriate catheterization findings (i.e., lesions amenable to angioplasty) and were randomized to immediate or delayed angioplasty.

Exclusion Criteria: Contraindications related to angiographic findings included more than 50% left main stenosis, severe/diffuse disease, and infarct-related vessel unidentifiable.

Treatment: Predominantly single-chain tPA, 150 mg i.v. over a 6- to 8-hour period followed by angiography with either immediate angioplasty or deferred angioplasty (latter performed at 7 to 10 days and if indicated). The immediate group also had angiography at 7 to 10 days to assess for reocclusion and LV function.

Results: Immediate PTCA success rate was 86%. Similar reocclusion rates were observed [11% (immediate) vs. 13%]. Neither group had an improvement in global LV function. In the delayed group, 14% did not require angioplasty (residual stenosis <50%), but a higher crossover rate was found to emergency angioplasty (16% vs. 5%). Immediate angioplasty had its own risks: Seven of nine patients with abrupt closure required emergency CABG surgery.

127. **Rogers WJ,** et al. for the **TIMI-IIA** Investigators. Comparison of immediate invasive, delayed invasive and conservative strategies after tissue-type plasminogen activator. *Circulation* 1990;81:1457–1476.

Design: Prospective, randomized, open, multicenter study. Primary endpoint was predischarge LVEF.

Purpose: To compare immediate versus delayed (at 18 to 48 hours) PTCA or CABG versus conservative treatment in AMI patients treated with tPA.

Population: 586 patients 75 years or younger seen within 4 hours of chest pain and with 1 mm or more ST elevation in at least two contiguous ECG leads.

Treatment: All patients received tPA [first 195 patients, 150 mg over a 6-hour period; next 391 patients, 100 mg over a 6-hour period (6-mg bolus, and then 54 mg over the first hour, 20 mg in the second hour, and 5 mg/hr for 4 hours)]; 195 underwent immediate invasive treatment, 194 delayed invasive treatment, and 197 conservative treatment [angiography ± angioplasty allowed with ischemic symptoms (spontaneous or provoked with testing)]. All patients received heparin for 5 days.

Results: All groups had similar predischarge LVEF (average, 49.3%) and IRA patency (TIMI grade 2 or 3 flow; mean, 83.7%). The immediate invasive group had a significantly higher CABG rate [7.7% vs. 2.1% (delayed invasive) vs. 2.5% (conservative); $p < 0.01$], and more transfusions were required among non-CABG patients (13.8% vs. 3.1% vs. 2.0%). Similar 1-year mortality rates were observed despite higher PTCA rates in immediate and delayed invasive groups (76% vs. 64% vs. 24%).

128. **Califf RM,** et al. for the **TAMI** Study Group. Evaluation of combination thrombolytic therapy and timing of cardiac catheterization in acute MI. *Circulation* 1991;83: 1543–1556.

Design: Prospective, randomized, open, parallel-group, factorial (3 × 2), multicenter study. Primary endpoint was global LVEF.

Purpose: To evaluate combination thrombolytic therapy by comparison with monotherapy and to compare an aggressive with a deferred angiography strategy.

Population: 575 patients aged 75 years or younger seen within 6 hours of symptoms and with greater than 1-mm ST elevation in at least two contiguous ECG leads.

Treatment: Urokinase (1.5 million U i.v. bolus, and then 1.5 million U over a 60-minute period), rtPA [100 mg over a 3-hour period (6-mg i.v. bolus, 60 mg over a 1-hour period, 20 mg/hr for 2 hours)], or combination therapy [urokinase, 1.5 million U over a 1-hour period and rtPA, 1 mg/kg, over a 1-hour period (10% as i.v. bolus; maximum dose, 90 mg)]. Aggressive strategy consisted of immediate angiography, whereas deferred strategy involved angiography before discharge (days 5 to 10).

Results: Global LVEF was well preserved and nearly identical at predischarge angiography (54%), regardless of thrombolytic or catheterization strategy. Combination thrombolysis resulted in higher 90-minute patency: TIMI grade 2 or 3 flow in 76% [tPA, 71% (p = NS); urokinase, 62% (p = 0.049)]. Less reocclusion [2% vs. 12% (p = 0.04) and 7% (p = NS)] and recurrent ischemia (25% vs. 31% vs. 35%) were observed. An aggressive strategy yielded better results with fewer adverse outcomes: death, stroke, reinfarction, heart failure, or recurrent ischemia in 55% versus 67% (p = 0.004), as well as a trend toward a higher predischarge patency rate (94% vs. 90%; p = 0.065).

129. **Should We Intervene Following Thrombolysis (SWIFT)** Trial Study Group. SWIFT trial of delayed elective intervention vs conservative treatment after thrombolysis with anistreplase in acute MI. *BMJ* 1991;302:555–560.

In this prospective, multicenter (n = 21) trial of 800 patients younger than 70 years, patients randomized to early angiography and appropriate intervention (PTCA, 43%; CABG, 15%) or conservative care [PTCA, 2.5%; CABG, 1.7% (initial admission)]. All patients were treated with anistreplase, 30 U over a 5-minute period. No differences in 1-year mortality

(5.8% vs. 5%) and reinfarction rates (15% vs. 13%) were observed. Intervention group did have longer stay (11 days vs. 10 days).

130. **Madsen JK,** et al. Danish Trial in Acute MI **(DANAMI).** Danish multicenter randomized study of invasive vs. conservative treatment in patients with inducible ischemia after thrombolysis in acute MI (DANAMI). *Circulation* 1997;96:748–755.

Design: Prospective, randomized, open, multicenter study. Median follow-up period was 2.4 years. Primary endpoint was death, AMI, and admission with unstable angina.

Purpose: To compare an invasive strategy of PTCA or CABG with a conservative strategy in patients with inducible ischemia after thrombolysis for MI.

Population: 1,008 patients younger than 70 years with a first MI and inducible ischemia [spontaneous ischemia 36 hours or less after admission or positive bicycle exercise tolerance test result (0.1 mm or more ST depression, 0.2 mm or more ST elevation)].

Exclusion Criteria: Prior MI, PTCA, or CABG; incomplete thrombolysis; BP decrease during exercise; significant noncoronary disease; ECG abnormalities precluding ST-segment evaluation during exercise (e.g., LBBB).

Treatment: Invasive therapy group received angiography within 2 weeks, PTCA and CABG if significant disease (50% or greater stenosis). In the conservative arm, angiography was allowed if severe angina developed (e.g., Canadian Cardiovascular Society class 3 or 4).

Results: In the invasive group, PTCA was performed in 52.9%, and CABG in 29.2% (at 2 to 10 weeks). In the conservative group, at 2 months, only 1.6% had undergone revascularization (at 1 year, 15%). At follow-up, no significant mortality difference was observed [3.6% (invasive) vs. 4.4%], but the invasive group had 47% fewer MIs (5.6% vs. 10.5%; $p = 0.0038$) and fewer unstable angina admissions (17.9% vs. 29.5%; $p < 0.00001$). Overall, the invasive group had 36% fewer primary endpoints (death, MI, and unstable angina) at 2 years (23.5% vs. 36.6%; $p < 0.0001$).

Comments: Editorial points out that few U.S. cardiologists follow ACC/AHA guidelines that recommend stress testing before invasive testing, and propose performing angiography for medium or large MIs, and revascularization if evidence of an incomplete infarct is present (e.g., lower than expected CK peak, ECG evolution, preserved wall motion of infarct zone), and stress testing first those with only small MIs (e.g., leads II, III, aVF only).

131. **Ross AM,** et al. A randomized trial comparing primary angioplasty with a strategy of short-acting thrombolysis and immediate planned rescue angioplasty in acute myocardial infarction: the **PACT** trial. *J Am Coll Cardiol* 1999;34:1954–1962.

Design: Prospective, randomized, open, multicenter trial. Primary endpoint: predischarge EF. Follow-up, 1 year.

Purpose: To evaluate the effectiveness and safety of a "facilitated" PCI approach to AMI management.

Population: 606 patients seen 6 hours or less after symptom onset with ST 0.1 mV or more in two or more limb leads or 0.2 mV or more in two or more contiguous leads.

Treatment: Precatheterization thrombolysis (tPA, 50-mg bolus) or placebo followed by immediate angiography. If TIMI grade 3 flow present, second bolus of tPA, 50 mg, administered. If TIMI grade 0 to 2 flow, PCI performed.

Results: Initial angiography demonstrated that the tPA group had higher TIMI grade 3 flow (32.8% vs. 14.8%) and patency (TIMI grade 2 or 3; 61% vs. 34%; $p = 0.001$). After angioplasty, TIMI flow grade was similar between the two groups [TIMI grade 3 flow in 77% (rescue) and 79% (primary)], indicating that tPA administration did not adversely affect procedural outcomes. No significant difference was noted between the groups in predischarge EF (primary endpoint), but the EF was higher in those with TIMI 3 flow on catheterization laboratory arrival (62.4%). The small group of patients (12%) who had PTCA performed less than 1 hour after the tPA bolus also had better EFs (62.5% vs. 57.3%). No significant differences were found in bleeding rates, suggesting that immediate angioplasty could be performed safely after reduced-dose tPA.

132. Assessment of the Safety and Efficacy of a New Treatment Strategy with Percutaneous Coronary Intervention (**ASSENT-4 PCI**) Investigators. Primary versus tenecteplase-facilitated percutaneous coronary intervention in patients with ST-segment elevation acute myocardial infarction (ASSENT-4 PCI): randomized trial. *Lancet* 2006;367: 569–578.

Design: Prospective, randomized, open, multicenter trial. Primary endpoint was death, CHF, or shock within 90 days.

Purpose: To evaluate the effectiveness of full-dose TNK to facilitate delayed PCI, in cases of acute STEMI.

Population: 1,667 (4,000 planned) patients with STEMI, symptom duration of less than 6 hours, and scheduled to undergo primary PCI with an anticipated delay of 1 to 3 hours.

Treatment: Standard primary PCI, or PCI preceded by full-dose TNK ("facilitated" PCI). All patients received aspirin and only a bolus of UFH (no infusion).

Results: The trial was stopped early, as recommended by the Data and Safety Monitoring Board, due to higher mortality in the facilitated PCI group (6% vs. 3%; $p = 0.01$). There was a higher rate of the primary endpoint in the facilitated PCI group (19% vs. 13%; $p = 0.0045$), as well as significantly more strokes (1.8% vs. 0%; $p < 0.0001$). Median time from TNK to balloon inflation was 104 minutes. Major, noncerebral bleeding was similar (6% for facilitated vs. 4% in the standard PCI group; $p = 0.3118$), yet there were higher rates of reinfarction (6% vs. 4%; $p = 0.0279$) and repeat TVR (7% vs. 3%; $p = 0.0041$).

133. **Ellis SG**, et al. for the FINESSE Investigators. Facilitated PCI in patients with ST-elevation myocardial infarction. *N Engl J Med* 2008;358:2205–2217.

Design: Prospective, randomized, double-blind, placebo-controlled, international, multicenter trial. Primary endpoint was a composite of death, VF (>48 hours after randomization), cardiogenic shock, or CHF within 90 days.

Purpose: To evaluate strategy of early abciximab, or abciximab plus half-dose reteplase to facilitate primary PCI in patients with STEMI.

Population: 2,452 patients with STEMI who presented within 6 hours of symptoms.

Treatment: Standard primary PCI, abciximab-facilitated PCI, or combination-facilitated PCI (with abciximab and half-dose reteplase). All patients received UFH or enoxaparin prior to PCI, as well as a 12-hour infusion of abciximab after PCI.

Results: The rates of primary events were 9.8%, 10.5%, and 10.7% in the combination-facilitated, abciximab-facilitated, and standard PCI groups, respectively ($p = 0.55$), with 90-day mortality rates 5.2%, 5.5%, and 4.5%, respectively ($p = 0.49$). However, patients in the combination-facilitated group were significantly more likely to have early ST-segment resolution (43.9%), compared with abciximab-facilitated (33.1%), or standard PCI (31.0%, $p = 0.01$ and 0.003, respectively).

134. **Keeley EC**, et al. Comparison of primary and facilitated percutaneous coronary interventions for ST-elevation myocardial infarction: quantitative review of randomised trials. *Lancet* 2006;367:579–588.

The authors identified 17 trials of facilitated versus primary PCI for STEMI, including a total of 4,504 patients. Primary endpoints were short-term outcomes of death, stroke, reinfarction, urgent TVR, and major bleeding at 6 weeks. While early TIMI grade 3 flow favored the facilitated approach (37% vs. 15%; OR, 3.18; 95% CI, 2.22 to 4.55), final TIMI grade 3 flow rates were similar (89% vs. 88%; OR, 1.19; 95% CI, 0.86 to 1.64). However, worse outcomes in the facilitated PCI group were observed for death (5% vs. 3%; OR, 1.38; 95% CI, 1.01 to 1.87), reinfarction (3% vs. 2%; OR, 1.71; 95% CI, 1.16 to 2.51), and urgent TVR (4% vs. 1%; OR, 2.39; 95% CI, 1.23 to 4.66), as well as major bleeding (7% vs. 5%; OR, 1.51; 95% CI, 1.10 to 2.08). The authors note that the majority of adverse events were observed in the thrombolytic-based facilitated PCI groups.

135. **Di Mario C**, et al. on behalf of the CARESS-in-AMI Investigators. Immediate angioplasty versus standard therapy with rescue angioplasty after thrombolysis in the Combined Abciximab Reteplase Stent Study in Acute Myocardial Infarction (CARESS-in-AMI): an open, prospective, randomised, multicentre trial. *Lancet* 2008;371: 559–568.

Design: Prospective, randomized, open, multicenter trial. Primary endpoint was a composite of death, reinfarction, or refractory ischemia at 30 days.

Purpose: To identify the best subsequent management of patients with STEMI who receive thrombolytic therapy.

Population: 600 patients less than 76 years old with acute MI with one or more high-risk features (ST-segment elevation, new LBBB, previous MI, Killip class >2, or LVEF ≤35%).

Treatment: All patients received half-dose reteplase, abciximab, heparin, and aspirin and were either managed conservatively locally or transferred to another center for PCI.

Results: Rates of events in the primary endpoint were significantly lower in the group receiving PCI (4.4% vs. 10.7%; $p = 0.004$), and 30.3% of patients in the conservative therapy arm underwent rescue PCI. Rates of major bleeding were not significantly different (3.4% in the conservative group vs. 2.3% in the PCI group, $p = 0.47$), and neither were rates of strokes (0.7% vs. 1.3%; $p = 0.50$).

136. **Bonnefoy E**, et al. on behalf of the Comparison of Angioplasty and prehospital Thrombolysis in Acute Myocardial infarction **(CAPTIM)** Study Group. Primary angioplasty versus prehospital fibrinolysis. *Lancet* 2002;360:825–829.

Design: Prospective, randomized, open, multicenter trial. Primary endpoint: death, nonfatal reinfarction, and nonfatal disabling stroke at 30 days.

Purpose: To determine whether primary angioplasty is better than prehospital fibrinolysis followed by transfer to an interventional facility for possible rescue PTCA.

Population: 840 patients seen within 6 hours of symptom onset with 2 mm or more ST elevation in at least two contiguous leads or LBBB.

Treatment: Prehospital fibrinolysis (accelerated alteplase) with angiography only for ongoing chest pain or ECG signs of continuing ischemia OR primary angioplasty. Each ambulance was staffed with a physician.

Results: The median delay between onset of symptoms and treatment was 130 minutes in the fibrinolysis group and 190 minutes (time to first balloon inflation) in the primary PTCA group. Rescue angioplasty was performed in 26% of fibrinolysis patients. No significant differences were seen between the groups in the incidence of the primary composite endpoint (primary PTCA, 6.2%; fibrinolysis, 8.2%; $p = 0.29$).

Comments: Study was underpowered—planned enrollment was 1,200 patients, which would have allowed a detection of a 40% relative reduction in incidence of primary endpoint.

137. **Fernandez-Avilés F**, et al. on behalf of the GRACIA Group. Routine invasive strategy within 24 hours of thrombolysis versus ischaemia-guided conservative approach for acute myocardial infarction with ST-segment elevation (GRACIA-1): a randomised controlled trial. *Lancet* 2004;364:1045–1053.

Design: Prospective, randomized, open, multicenter, international trial. Primary endpoint was a composite of death, nonfatal reinfarction, or revascularization at 12 months.

Purpose: To determine the role for early, post-thrombolysis PCI in patients with STEMI, in the era of contemporary therapies.

Population: 500 patients with STEMI who received thrombolytics.

Treatment: Early angiography within 24 hours, with intervention if indicated versus conservative, ischemia-guided interventional approach.

Results: At 1 year, the interventional group had a significantly lower incidence of primary endpoint events (9% vs. 21%; $p = 0.0008$). Rates of death or reinfarction were also nonsignificantly reduced in the early interventional group (7% vs. 12%, $p = 0.07$). Importantly, rates of major bleeding were similar, and length of hospitalization was shorter in the early intervention group.

138. **Schweiger MJ,** et al. for the TIMI 10B and TIMI 14 Investigators. Early coronary intervention following pharmacologic therapy for acute myocardial infarction (the combined TIMI 10B-TIMI 14 experience). *Am J Cardiol* 2001;88:831–836.

This study analyzed 1,938 AMI patients from TIMI 10B (tPA vs. TNK) and TIMI 14 (thrombolytic therapy with or without abciximab). All patients underwent angiography at 90 minutes. Patients who underwent PCI were described as having a rescue procedure (TIMI 0 or 1 flow at 90 minutes), an adjunctive procedure (TIMI 2 or 3 flow at 90 minutes), or a delayed procedure [performed >150 minutes after symptom onset (median, 2.8 days)]. Among patients with TIMI 0 or 1 flow, a trend was found toward lower 30-day mortality with rescue PCI compared with no PCI (6% vs. 17%; $p = 0.01$, adjusted $p = 0.28$). Patients who underwent adjunctive PCI had 30-day mortality and/or reinfarction rates similar to those who underwent delayed PCI. In a multivariate model, adjunctive and delayed PCI patients had lower 30-day mortality and/or reinfarction rates ($p = 0.02$) than did patients with "successful thrombolysis" (i.e., TIMI 3 flow at 90 minutes) who did not undergo revascularization. Thus, early PCI after AMI is associated with favorable outcomes. Randomized trials of an early invasive strategy after thrombolysis are warranted.

139. **Cantor WJ,** et al. for the TRANSFER-AMI Trial Investigators. Routine early angioplasty after fibrinolysis for acute myocardial infarction. *N Engl J Med* 2009;360:2705–2718.

Design: Prospective, randomized, open, multicenter, trial. Primary endpoint was a composite of death, reinfarction, recurrent ischemia, new or worsening CHF, or cardiogenic shock at 30 days.
Purpose: To identify the optimal timing of routine PCI following thrombolysis for acute STEMI.
Population: 1,059 patients with STEMI who received fibrinolytics at a center without PCI capability.
Treatment: Early angiography within 6 hours requiring transfer to another institution, or routine conservative therapy (including rescue PCI if necessary, or delayed angiography).
Results: In the early invasive group, median time to PCI was 2.8 hours; for the standard-therapy group 88.7% of patients underwent PCI at a median time of 32.5 hours after randomization. Incidence of primary endpoint events occurred in 11.0% of patients in the early invasive group versus 17.2% in the standard-therapy group ($p = 0.004$). Rates of major bleeding were similar in the two groups.

140. **Kiernan TJ,** et al. Facilitated percutaneous coronary intervention: current concepts, promises, and pitfalls. *Eur Heart J* 2007;28:1545–1553.

In this review, the authors highlight the therapeutic options facing physicians following administration of fibrinolytics for STEMI. They review the rationale, data, benefits, and risks for facilitated PCI, the pharmacoinvasive approach (delayed, routine PCI following lytics), and the ischemia-driven or "watchful waiting" pathway. The authors also demonstrate the evidence for why they believe there is no role for facilitated PCI (with any combination of fibrinolytic and/or glycoprotein IIb/IIIa inhibitor). The article concludes with a discussion of areas for future investigation.

Rescue Percutaneous Transluminal Coronary Angioplasty

141. **Ellis SG,** et al. Present status of rescue coronary angioplasty: current polarization of opinion and randomized trials. *J Am Coll Cardiol* 1992;19:681–686.

This overview of 12 trials (only 1 randomized) included a total of 560 patients. The average success rate of rescue PTCA was 80%. Reocclusion occurred in 18%. The overall mortality rate was 10.6%, but it was much higher (up to 39%) in those for whom rescue failed.

142. **Ellis SG,** et al. **RESCUE.** Randomized comparison of rescue angioplasty with conservative management of patients with early failure of thrombolysis for acute anterior MI. *Circulation* 1994;90:2280–2284.

Design: Prospective, randomized, multicenter study. Primary endpoint was LVEF at 25 to 35 days.
Purpose: To assess the clinical benefit of rescue angioplasty in a relatively high-risk population.
Population: 151 patients aged 21 to 79 years seen with ST elevation 2 mm or more in at least two precordial leads.
Exclusion Criteria: Cardiogenic shock, prior MI, and left main stenosis 50% or more.
Treatment: Thrombolysis followed by PTCA or aspirin, heparin, and vasodilators.
Results: Rescue PTCA was successful in 92%. The rescue PTCA group had less death and severe heart failure (6% vs. 17%; $p = 0.05$) and better exercise (but not rest) EFs (43% vs. 38%; $p = 0.04$).

143. **Gibson CM,** et al. Rescue angioplasty in the thrombolysis in MI **(TIMI)** 4 trial. *Am J Cardiol* 1997;80:21–26.

This retrospective analysis focused on 402 TIMI-4 patients with either successful rescue angioplasty (PTCA) or successful thrombolysis. The successful PTCA group had better 90-minute TIMI grade 3 flow (87% vs. 65%; $p = 0.002$) and a lower TIMI frame count (27 vs. 39; $p < 0.001$). The successful versus failed rescue PTCA group had fewer in-hospital adverse endpoints, consisting of death, MI, severe CHF/shock, and EF 40% or less (29% vs. 83%; $p = 0.01$). The rescue PTCA (all) versus other groups had similar event rates (both with adverse outcomes in 35%).

144. **Ross AM,** et al. Rescue angioplasty after failed thrombolysis: technical and clinical outcomes in a large thrombolysis trial. *J Am Coll Cardiol* 1998;31:1511–1517.

This retrospective analysis focused on GUSTO I angiographic substudy data. Rescue PTCA was performed in 198 patients; the artery was successfully opened in 88.4%, with 68% achieving TIMI grade 3 flow. Successful rescue PTCA resulted in better LV function and 30-day mortality than did failed rescue, comparable with outcomes in those with closed infarct arteries managed conservatively (266 patients), but less favorable than those with successful thrombolysis (1,058 patients). Failed rescue was associated with high 30.4% mortality (multivariate analysis predictor, severe heart failure).

145. **Gershlick AH,** et al. for the REACT Trial Investigators. Rescue angioplasty after failed thrombolytic therapy for acute myocardial infarction. *N Engl J Med* 2005;353:2758–2768.

Design: Prospective, randomized, multicenter study. Primary endpoint was a composite of death, reinfarction, stroke, or severe CHF at 6 months.
Purpose: To compare emergent PCI with repeated thrombolysis in patients with STEMI who fail to reperfuse following initial thrombolysis.
Population: 427 patients with STEMI had less than 50% ST-segment resolution 90 minutes after thrombolytic therapy.
Exclusion Criteria: Any contraindication to thrombolysis and cardiogenic shock.
Treatment: Conservative treatment (no intervention or further lysis), repeat thrombolysis, or emergent, rescue PCI.
Results: More patients in the rescue PCI group were event free (84.6%), compared with conservative therapy (70.1%), or repeat thrombolysis (68.7%, overall $p = 0.004$). Overall mortality among the three groups was similar. Revascularization-free survival at 6 months was statistically similar, but tended to favor the PCI group (86.2% for the rescue PCI group vs. 77.6% in the conservative therapy arm vs. 74.4% in the repeat thrombolysis group, overall $p = 0.05$).
Comment: The benefits of rescue PCI persisted for at least 1 year, as described in the long-term follow-up analysis of the REACT trial (see *J Am Coll Cardiol* 2009;54:118–126).

146. **Wijeysundera HC,** et al. Rescue angioplasty or repeat fibrinolysis after failed fibrinolytic therapy for ST-segment myocardial infarction: a meta-analysis of randomized trials. *J Am Coll Cardiol* 2007;49:422–430.

The authors compiled results from eight trials of 1,177 patients randomized to rescue PCI or conservative therapy, with follow-up data to 6 months. Though they found no difference in overall mortality with rescue PCI (RR, 0.69; 95% CI, 0.46 to 1.05), there were significant reductions in heart failure (RR, 0.73; 95% CI, 0.54 to 1.00) and reinfarction (0.58; 95% CI, 0.35 to 0.97) when rescue PCI was compared to conservative therapy. However, there were increased rates of stroke (RR, 4.98; 95% CI, 1.10 to 22.5) and minor bleeding (RR, 4.58; 95% CI, 2.46 to 8.55). Repeat thrombolysis yielded only higher bleeding rates when compared to conservative therapy (RR, 1.84; 95% CI, 1.06 to 3.18), without any improvement in overall mortality (RR, 0.68; 95% CI, 0.41 to 1.14) or reinfarction (RR, 1.79; 95% CI, 0.92 to 3.48).

Cardiogenic Shock

147. **Berger PB,** et al. Impact of an aggressive invasive catheterization and revascularization strategy on mortality in patients with cardiogenic shock in the GUSTO I trial. *Circulation* 1997;96:122–127.

This analysis focused on 2,200 patients with SBP less than 90 mm Hg for 1 hour who survived 1 hour after onset of shock. The early angiography (24 hours or less) group had a lower 30-day mortality rate (38% vs. 62%; $p = 0.0001$). After multiple logistic regression analysis, the early angiography group was found to be younger (63 years vs. 68 years), to have had fewer prior MIs (19% vs. 27%), and to have been given thrombolysis earlier (2.9 hours vs. 3.2 hours). An aggressive strategy is still associated with a lower 30-day mortality rate (OR, 0.43; $p = 0.0001$). A subsequent GUSTO I analysis showed that most patients (88%) with cardiogenic shock who were alive at 30 days survived at least 1 year, and that those who underwent revascularization within 30 days had better 1-year survival than did patients not revascularized.

148. **Hochman JS,** et al. Should We Emergently Revascularize Occluded Coronaries for Cardiogenic Shock (**SHOCK**) Investigators. Early revascularization in acute MI complicated by cardiogenic shock. *N Engl J Med* 1999;341:625–634 (editorial, 686–688).

This prospective, randomized, multicenter trial was composed of 302 patients with STEMI (or new LBBB); pulmonary capillary wedge pressure, 15 mm Hg or more; cardiac index, 2.2 or less; SBP more than 90 mm Hg for 30 minutes before inotropes/vasopressors or IABP initiated; and HR, 60 beats/min. Patients underwent ERV within 6 hours (PTCA or CABG) or medical management [thrombolysis recommended (given in 64%), delayed revascularization allowed at 54 hours]. The ERV group had a 97% angiography rate and 87% revascularization rate [PTCA, 49% (at average 0.9 hours); CABG, 38% (average 2.7 hours)]. Among initial medical stabilization (IMS) patients, 4% had revascularization performed before 54 hours, and 22% underwent late revascularization. No significant difference was found in 30-day all-cause mortality (primary endpoint) between the two groups (ERV, 46.7%, vs. IMS, 56.0%; $p = 0.11$); however, at 6 months, a significant mortality benefit was associated with early revascularization strategy (50.3% vs. 63.1%; $p = 0.027$). In the subgroup of patients aged 75 years or younger, ERV was significantly better than IMS (at 30 days, 41% vs. 57%, $p < 0.01$; 6 months, 48% vs. 69%, $p < 0.01$). The PTCA success rate was 76%, and the mortality rate was 100% if PTCA did not achieve TIMI grade 2 or 3 flow.

Bare-Metal Stenting

149. **Antoniucci D,** et al. Florence Randomized Elective Stenting in Acute Coronary Occlusions (**FRESCO**). A clinical trial comparing primary stenting of the infarct-related artery with optimal primary angioplasty for acute MI. *J Am Coll Cardiol* 1998;31:1234–1239.

This prospective, randomized, multicenter study enrolled 150 patients seen within 6 hours of onset of symptoms with STEMI and who underwent successful primary PTCA. Patients were randomized to primary PTCA or primary PTCA followed by stenting. No PTCA was attempted if stenosis was less than 70% or the IRA could not be identified. No randomization to PTCA alone or stenting was performed if the reference diameter was less than 2.5 mm. Stenting success rate was 100%. At 6 months, the incidence of death, reinfarction, and repeated TVR due to recurrent ischemia at 6 months (primary endpoint) was only 9% in the stent group versus 28% in the PTCA group ($p = 0.003$). Repeated angiography was performed at 6 months, and the incidence of restenosis or reocclusion was 17% in the stent group and 43% in the PTCA group ($p = 0.001$).

150. **Suryapranata H,** et al. Randomized comparison of coronary stenting with balloon angioplasty in selected patients with acute MI. *Circulation* 1998;97:2502–2505.

This prospective, single-center study randomized 227 AMI patients seen within 6 hours of symptom onset (or after 6 to 24 hours if ongoing ischemia) to primary stenting (Palmaz–Schatz) or angioplasty (with bailout stenting only if prolonged inflation unsuccessful). Initial patients received warfarin for 3 months, but patients enrolled after January 1996 received ticlopidine, 250 mg/day for 2 weeks. Exclusion criteria were cardiogenic shock, prior bypass surgery or angioplasty, and prior MI. Angiographic exclusion criteria included unprotected left main, significant side branch jeopardy, excessive tortuosity, extensive thrombus, or inability to cross lesion with guide wire. Overall 6-month mortality rate was 2%. The stent group had fewer reinfarctions (1% vs. 7%; $p = 0.036$) and less need for subsequent TVR (4% vs. 17%; $p = 0.0016$). The stent group also had better cardiac event-free survival rate (95% vs. 80%; $p = 0.012$). The stent group had a larger reference vessel.

151. **Grines CL,** et al. for the **Stent PAMI** Study Group. Coronary angioplasty with or without stent implantation for acute myocardial infarction. *N Engl J Med* 1999;341: 1949–1956.

Design: Prospective, randomized, open, multicenter trial. The primary endpoint was the 6-month incidence of death, reinfarction, and disabling stroke, or ischemia-driven TVR.
Purpose: To compare stent implantation with primary angioplasty alone in AMI.
Population: 900 patients within 12 hours of symptom onset with ST elevation 1 mm or more in at least two contiguous leads or a nondiagnostic ECG with evidence of AMI in the catheterization laboratory and with lesions amenable to stenting.
Exclusion Criteria: Included prior administration of thrombolytic agents for index infarction, current use of warfarin, stroke in prior month, and cardiogenic shock.
Treatment: Angioplasty alone or stenting (heparin-coated Palmaz–Schatz).
Results: Acute procedural success rates were greater than 99% in both groups. The postprocedural TIMI grade 3 flow rates were 89.4% in the angioplasty group and 92.7% in the stent group ($p = 0.10$). At 6 months, the stent group had a larger mean luminal diameter (2.56 mm vs. 2.12 mm; $p < 0.001$) and lower restenosis rate (20.3% vs. 33.5%; $p < 0.001$). Stenting was associated with a significant reduction in the 6-month composite primary endpoint (12.6% vs. 20.1%; $p < 0.01$). This difference was driven entirely by a decreased need for TVR because of ischemia (7.7% vs. 17%; $p < 0.001$). The 6-month mortality rate was 4.2% in the stent group and 2.7% in the angioplasty group ($p = 0.27$). Bleeding rates were similar.
Comments: The use of glycoprotein IIb/IIIa inhibitors was infrequent (5%), rigid early generation stents were used (increased thrombus embolization), and high-pressure deployment and oversizing of the stent were common. Many of these practice patterns have now changed, and this finding should be reevaluated in future studies.

152. **Le May MR,** et al. Stenting versus thrombolysis in acute myocardial infarction trial **(STAT)**. *J Am Coll Cardiol* 2001;37:985–991.

A total of 123 patients with STEMI were randomized to primary stenting or accelerated tPA. Patients with cardiogenic shock, active bleeding, history of stroke, major surgery, severe hypertension, prolonged CPR, inadequate vascular access, PTCA within 6 months, prior stenting of culprit artery, and prior CABG were excluded. The primary endpoint was a 6-month composite of TVR. At 6-month follow-up, the primary endpoint (death, reinfarction, stroke, or repeated TVR) had occurred in 24.2% of stent patients and 55.7% of TPA patients ($p < 0.001$); this difference was due to a significant reduction in TVR in the stent group (14.5% vs. 49.2%; $p < 0.001$).

153. **Kastrati A,** et al. for the Stent versus Thrombolysis for Occluded Coronary Arteries in Patients with Acute Myocardial Infarction **(STOPAMI-2)** Study. Myocardial salvage after coronary stenting plus abciximab versus fibrinolysis plus abciximab in patients with acute myocardial infarction: a randomised trial. *Lancet* 2002;359:920–925.

Design: Prospective, randomized, open, multicenter trial. The primary endpoint was the salvage index (the ratio of the degree of myocardial salvage to the initial perfusion defect).
Purpose: To determine whether AMI patients benefit from the addition of glycoprotein IIb/IIIa inhibitors to fibrinolytic or mechanical reperfusion strategies.
Population: 162 patients with AMI seen within 12 hours of onset of symptoms.
Treatment: Stenting or alteplase. All received abciximab. Technetium-99m sestamibi scintigraphy was done at admission and at a median of 11 days in 141 (87%) patients.
Results: Stenting was associated with greater myocardial salvage than was alteplase (median, 13.6% vs. 8.0% of the left ventricle; $p = 0.007$). The salvage index was greater in the stent group than in the alteplase group [median, 0.60 (0.37 to 0.82) vs. 0.41 (0.13 to 0.58); $p = 0.001$]. Six-month mortality rate was 5% in the stent group and 9% in the alteplase group [RR, 0.56 (95% CI, 0.17 to 1.88); $p = 0.35$].

154. **Stone GW,** et al. for the Controlled Abciximab and Device Investigation to Lower Late Angioplasty Complications **(CADILLAC)** Investigators. Comparison of angioplasty with stenting, with or without abciximab, in acute myocardial infarction. *N Engl J Med* 2002;346:957–966 (see Ref. 54, full summary).

This 2,082-patient trial found a significantly lower incidence of major events with stenting compared with angioplasty, regardless of abciximab use (see Ref. 54 for full summary).

Drug-eluting Stents

155. **Valgimigli M,** et al. for the Multicentre Evaluation of Single High-dose Bolus Tirofiban vs Abciximab With Sirolimus-eluting Stent or Bare Metal Stent in Acute Myocardial Infarction Study (MULTISTRATEGY) Investigators. Comparison of angioplasty with infusion of tirofiban or abciximab and with implantation of sirolimus-eluting or uncoated stents for acute myocardial infarction: the multistrategy randomized trial. *JAMA* 2008;299(15):1788–1799.

Design: Prospective, randomized, open-label, 2×2 factorial design, multicenter, international trial. Primary endpoint for the stent comparison was a composite of death, reinfarction, or clinically driven TVR at 8 months. Primary endpoint for the drug comparison was at least 50% ST-segment resolution at 90 minutes, with a prespecified noninferiority margin.
Purpose: To evaluate alternative glycoprotein IIb/IIIa inhibitor strategies (using tirofiban), as well as the use of DES, in patients with STEMI.
Population: 745 patients with STEMI or new LBBB.
Treatment: Patients were first randomized to either high-dose bolus tirofiban or abciximab infusion; they were also randomized to receive a sirolimus-eluting stent (SES) or an uncoated BMS.
Results: For the drug comparison, 83.6% of patients had ST-segment resolution in the abciximab group, versus 85.3% in the tirofiban group ($p < 0.001$ for noninferiority). Each group had a similar rate of ischemic and bleeding adverse events. The primary endpoint in the stenting comparison was met in 14.5% of patients in the BMS group compared with 7.8% in the SES group ($p = 0.004$), which was significantly driven by a reduction in repeat

revascularization (10.2% vs. 3.2%). They reported a similar incidence of stent thromboses in the two groups.

156. **De Luca G,** et al. Efficacy and safety of drug-eluting stents in ST-segment elevation myocardial infarction: a meta-analysis of randomized trials. *Int J Cardiol* 2009;133: 213–222.

The reviewers compiled results from 11 trials, including 3,605 patients, comparing SES, paclitaxel-eluting stents (PES), and BMS in patients undergoing primary PCI for STEMI. Endpoints for SES and PES were combined into the DES group. At follow-up of 12 months, there were no differences in overall mortality (4.1% vs. 4.4%, $p = 0.59$), reinfarction (3.1% vs. 3.4%, $p = 0.38$), or stent thrombosis (1.6% vs. 2.2%, $p = 0.22$). However, the DES groups had lower rates of TVR (5.0% vs. 12.6%, $p < 0.0001$). In four trials of 1,178 patients, data at 18 and 24 months were similar.

157. **De Luca G,** et al. Short and long-term benefits of sirolimus-eluting stent in ST-segment elevation myocardial infarction: a meta-analysis of randomized trials. *J Thromb Thrombolysis* 2009 [Epub ahead of print]. DOI 10.1007/s11239-009-0305-7.

The authors repeated the previous meta-analysis, now limited to SES only, and including more contemporary trials. They combined data on 2,769 patients from nine randomized trials comparing BMS and SES in patients receiving primary PCI for STEMI. Follow-up at 12 months yielded significantly fewer incidents of TVR (4.9% vs. 13.6%; $p < 0.0001$) in the SES group, with a nonsignificant trend toward decreased mortality (2.9% vs. 4.2%; $p = 0.08$) and reinfarction (3.0% vs. 4.3%; $p = 0.06$). Rates of stent thrombosis appeared similar between the two groups (1.9% vs. 2.5%; $p = 0.36$). They report that long-term data at 2 to 3 years of follow-up from four of the trials (encompassing 569 patients) were similar.

158. **Chechi T,** et al. ST-segment elevation myocardial infarction due to early and late stent thrombosis: a new group of high-risk patients. *J Am Coll Cardiol* 2008;51:2396–2402.

The investigators explored a retrospective sample of patients with stent thrombosis who presented with STEMI (92, or 80% of thromboses), as compared with 98 patients with de novo STEMI. All received primary PCI therapy; however, those who presented with stent thrombosis were significantly less likely to achieve successful reperfusion ($p < 0.0001$), and had higher rates of distal embolization ($p = 0.01$). Patients with stent thrombosis had higher rates of major adverse cardiovascular and cerebrovascular events ($p = 0.03$), yet among hospital survivors mortality was similar ($p = 0.7$).

159. **Steg PG,** et al. for the Global Registry of Acute Coronary Events (GRACE) Investigators. Mortality following placement of drug-eluting and bare-metal stents for ST-segment elevation acute myocardial infarction in the Global Registry of Acute Coronary Events. *Eur Heart J* 2009;30:321–329.

In this multinational, observational registry of acute coronary syndromes, the investigators reviewed outcomes in 5,093 patients with STEMI receiving DES ($n = 1313$) compared with those receiving BMS ($n = 3780$). Baseline characteristics did differ significantly (with patients receiving BMS having higher risk characteristics); however, in risk-adjusted and propensity analyses, postdischarge mortality was not different at 6 months ($p = 0.21$) or 1 year ($p = 0.34$). Mortality at from 6 months to 2 years and from 1 to 2 years was significantly higher in the DES group (hazard ratio 4.90, $p = 0.01$ and hazard ratio 7.06, $p = 0.02$, respectively).

160. **Di Lorenzo E,** et al. The PASEO (PaclitAxel or Sirolimus-eluting Stent versus Bare Metal Stent in Primary Angioplasty) randomized trial. *J Am Coll Cardiol Intvervent* 2009;2:515–523.

Design: Prospective, randomized, open-label, trial. Primary endpoint was TLR at 1 year.
Purpose: To compare the two most common DES with each other, and with BMS for acute STEMI.

Population: 270 patients with STEMI within 12 hours of symptom onset.

Treatment: Primary angioplasty with implantation of either a BMS, SES, or PES.

Results: After 1 year, rates of TLR significantly favored the DES—BMS (14.4%), PES (4.4%, $p = 0.023$), and SES (3.3%, $p = 0.016$). There were no differences in the rates of death and/or reinfarction at 2 years.

161. **Brar SS**, et al. Use of drug-eluting stents in acute myocardial infarction a systematic review and meta-analysis. *J Am Coll Cardiol* 2009;53:1677–1689.

The authors combined results from 13 randomized trials encompassing 7,352 patients comparing BMS and DES in STEMI. Rates of TVR favored DES over BMS (RR, 0.44; 95% CI, 0.35 to 0.55), with no effect on death (RR, 0.89; 95% CI, 0.70 to 1.14), reinfarction (RR, 0.82; 95% CI, 0.64 to 1.05), or stent thrombosis (RR, 0.97; 95% CI, 0.73 to 1.28). These results remained consistent over 2 years of follow-up. They also reviewed results form 18 registry studies including 26,521 patients; similarly, DES significantly reduced TVR (RR, 0.54; 95% CI, 0.40 to 0.74). While mortality was significantly lower at 1 year, rates were similar between DES and BMS at 2 years.

ANGIOTENSIN-CONVERTING ENZYME INHIBITORS WITH OR WITHOUT NITRATES

General Reviews and Meta-analyses

162. **Latini R,** et al. for the Meeting Participants. ACE inhibitor use in patients with myocardial infarction: summary of evidence from clinical trials. *Circulation* 1995;92: 3132–3137.

This report is the result of a meeting of experts in Berlin in 1994, which included the investigators from the CONSENSUS, AIRE, SAVE, SOLVD, ISIS-4, GISSI-3, and V-HeFT trials, as well as additional experts. The resulting manuscript reviews the overall data on ACE inhibitors in CAD, with particular focus on acute MI. They support the aggressive use of ACE inhibitors, particularly in the early phase of acute MI and in patients with impaired LV function.

163. **ACE Inhibitor MI Collaborative Group.** Indications for ACE inhibitors in the early treatment of acute MI: systematic overview of individual data from 100,000 patients in randomized trials. *Circulation* 1998;97:2202–2212.

This meta-analysis was composed of four randomized trials (CONSENSUS II, GISSI-3, ISIS-4, and CCS-1), 98,496 total patients, in which ACE inhibitors were started within 36 hours of AMI. ACE inhibition was associated with a 7% reduction in 30-day mortality (7.1% vs. 7.6%; $p < 0.004$). Most of the benefit was observed within the first week of treatment. The greatest mortality benefit was seen in high-risk groups (e.g., anterior MI; Killip class 2 to 3; HR, 100 beats/min at entry). ACE inhibition also was associated with a reduction in nonfatal cardiac failure (14.6% vs. 15.2%; $p = 0.01$) but led to more frequent hypotension (17.6% vs. 9.3%; $p < 0.01$) and renal dysfunction (1.3% vs. 0.6%; $p < 0.01$).

164. **Domanski MJ,** et al. Effect of angiotensin converting enzyme inhibition on sudden cardiac death in patients following acute MI. *J Am Coll Cardiol* 1999;33:598–604.

The results of this meta-analysis of 15 trials with 15,134 patients suggest that part of the benefit of ACE inhibition in AMI is related to a reduction in risk of sudden cardiac death. The majority of deaths (87%) were cardiovascular, of which 38.2% were deemed sudden cardiac deaths. Overall, ACE-inhibitor therapy was associated with significant reductions in overall mortality [OR, 0.83 (95% CI, 0.71 to 0.97)], cardiovascular death [OR, 0.82 (95% CI, 0.69 to 0.97)], and sudden cardiac death [OR, 0.80 (95% CI, 0.70 to 0.92)].

Studies

165. **Pfeffer MA,** et al. on behalf of the Survival and Ventricular Enlargement **(SAVE)** Investigators. Effect of captopril on mortality and morbidity in patients with left ventricular dysfunction after MI. *N Engl J Med* 1992;327:669–677.

Design: Prospective, randomized, double-blind, placebo-controlled, multicenter study. Mean follow-up period was 42 months. Primary endpoint was all-cause mortality.

Purpose: To determine the effect of captopril on mortality and morbidity when started 3 to 16 days after MI in patients with LV dysfunction.

Population: 2,231 patients aged 21 to 80 years with an EF 40% or less but no overt heart failure.

Exclusion Criteria: Requirement or contraindication to ACE inhibition, creatinine greater than 2.5 mg/dL, and unstable post-MI course.

Treatment: Captopril initiated 3 to 16 days after MI and titrated from 12.5 mg, three times daily, to 25 mg, three times daily, by hospital discharge (and later 50 mg, three times daily if tolerated); or placebo.

Results: Captopril group had the following risk reductions—19% lower all-cause mortality (20% vs. 25%; $p = 0.019$), 21% lower cardiovascular mortality ($p = 0.014$), 25% fewer recurrent MIs (11.9% vs. 15.2%; $p = 0.015$), and 22% less severe heart failure requiring hospitalization ($p = 0.019$). No difference was observed in deterioration of 9% in EF as measured by repeated radionuclide ventriculography at mean 36 months (13% vs. 16%; $p = 0.17$). Overall, captopril was associated with a 14% reduction in composite ischemic index of recurrent MI, revascularization, and unstable angina ($p = 0.047$).

166. **Swedeberg K,** et al. on behalf of the Cooperative New Scandinavian Enalapril Survival Study **(CONSENSUS II)** Group. Effects of early administration of enalapril on mortality in patients with acute MI. *N Engl J Med* 1992;327:678–684.

Design: Prospective, randomized, double-blind, placebo-controlled, multicenter study. Average follow-up period was 188 days. Primary endpoint was all-cause mortality rate.

Purpose: To evaluate the effect on mortality of early i.v. administration of enalapril in AMI patients.

Population: 6,090 patients within 24 hours of symptom onset and one of the following—ST elevation in at least two contiguous leads, new Q waves, or elevated serum enzymes.

Exclusion Criteria: Included BP less than 105/65 mm Hg, history of adverse reaction to or requirement for ACE inhibition, and severe valvular stenosis.

Treatment: Intravenously enalaprilat, 1 mg, over a 2-hour period (stopped if BP decreased below 90/60 mm Hg). Oral enalapril was begun at 6 hours (initial dose, 2.5 mg, and increased up to 20 mg/day), or placebo.

Results: Trial was terminated early by the safety committee. No significant mortality difference was observed at 180 days: 10.2% (placebo) vs. 11.0% (enalapril). Enalapril was associated with more frequent hypotension (BP <90/50 mm Hg): 12% vs. 3% ($p < 0.001$).

167. **Acute Infarction Ramipril Efficacy (AIRE)** Study Investigators. Effect of ramipril on mortality and morbidity of survivors of AMI with clinical evidence of heart failure. *Lancet* 1993;342:821–828.

Design: Prospective, randomized, double-blind, parallel-group, placebo-controlled, multicenter study. Average follow-up period was 15 months. Primary endpoint was all-cause mortality.

Purpose: To evaluate whether ramipril started 3 to 10 days after MI reduces mortality in patients whose course is complicated by heart failure.

Population: 2,006 patients with a definite AMI and clinical evidence of heart failure at any point after MI.

Exclusion Criteria: Heart failure due to valvular disease, unstable angina, contraindications to ACE inhibition, and severe and resistant heart failure.

Treatment: Ramipril, 2.5 mg twice daily for 2 days, and then 5 mg twice daily if tolerated.

Results: All-cause mortality was significantly lower in the ramipril group—27% risk reduction (17% vs. 23%; $p = 0.002$). Ramipril patients also had a 30% lower risk of sudden death ($p = 0.011$) and a 19% risk reduction in combined endpoints consisting of death, severe heart failure, MI, and stroke ($p = 0.008$). No significant difference was observed in reinfarction or stroke rates.

168. **GISSI-3.** Effects of lisinopril and transdermal glyceryl trinitrate singly and together on 6-week mortality and ventricular function after acute MI. *Lancet* 1994;343:1115–1122.

Design: Prospective, randomized, open-label, 2×2 factorial, multicenter study. Primary outcomes were 6-week all-cause mortality and combination of death, heart failure at 5 days after MI, and EF 35% or less or 45% or more myocardial segments with abnormal motion.
Purpose: To evaluate the effect of lisinopril and nitrates, alone and in combination, on all-cause mortality and LV function after AMI.
Population: 18,895 patients seen within 24 hours with 1 mm or more ST elevation or depression in at least one limb lead or 2 mm or more in at least one precordial lead.
Exclusion Criteria: Severe heart failure, SBP less than 100 mm Hg, serum creatinine more than 177 μM, and severe comorbidity.
Treatment: (a) Lisinopril, 5 mg in the first 24 hours, and then 10 mg once daily for 6 weeks or open control; (b) glyceryl nitrate (GTN), 5 μg/min i.v., and increased by 5 to 20 μg/min or until SBP was lowered by 10%. At 24 hours, transdermal GTN was started (10 mg/day, 14 hours each day) for 6 weeks. If not tolerated, isosorbide mononitrate (50 mg once daily) or open control. Overall, 72% of patients received a thrombolytic agent, 31% were taking a β-blocker, and 84% aspirin.
Results: Overall, 6-week mortality rate was only 6.7%. Lisinopril was associated with significant mortality reduction (6.3% vs. 7.1%; OR, 0.88; $p = 0.03$), with survival curves beginning to diverge on the first day. Reduction also was seen in combined primary outcome (15.6% vs. 17.0%; OR, 0.90; $p = 0.009$). No difference between lisinopril and controls was observed in recurrent infarction, postinfarct angina, cardiogenic shock, and stroke. No difference in mortality was observed between patients with and without GTN (18.4% vs. 18.9%; $p = 0.39$). Of note, 13.3% of controls received nonstudy ACE inhibitors, and 57.1% received nonstudy nitrates.
Comments: At 6 months, the lisinopril group had fewer deaths and LV dysfunction (18.1% vs. 19.3%; $p = 0.03$). A subgroup analysis showed that lisinopril was more beneficial in diabetic patients (6-week mortality, 8.7% vs. 12.4%; OR, 0.68) than in nondiabetic patients ($p < 0.025$).

169. **Ambrosioni E,** et al. for the Survival of MI Long-term Evaluation **(SMILE)** Study Investigators. The effect of the angiotensin-converting-enzyme inhibitor zofenopril on mortality and morbidity after anterior MI. *N Engl J Med* 1995;332:80–85.

Design: Prospective, randomized, double-blind, placebo-controlled, multicenter study. Follow-up was 1 year. Primary endpoint was death or severe heart failure (three or more of following: S_3, bilateral pulmonary rales, radiologic evidence, peripheral edema).
Purpose: To determine whether short-term ACE inhibition after MI reduces mortality and severe heart failure.
Population: 1,556 patients (of 20,261 cardiac care unit patients) at less than 24 hours from symptom onset and not administered thrombolytic therapy.
Exclusion Criteria: Cardiogenic shock, SBP less than 100 mm Hg, creatinine greater than 2.5 mg/dL, and history of CHF or ACE inhibitor use.
Treatment: Zofenopril, 7.5 to 30 mg twice daily, or placebo.
Results: At 6 weeks, the zofenopril group had a significant 34% reduction in the incidence of death and severe heart failure (7.1% vs. 10.6%; $p = 0.018$). A significant 46% reduction in severe heart failure and a statistically nonsignificant 25% reduction in death was found (7.1% vs. 10.6%; $p = 0.19$). At 1 year, the zofenopril group had 29% lower mortality (10.0% vs. 14.1%; $p = 0.011$).

170. **ISIS-4** Collaborative Group. ISIS-4: a randomised factorial assessing early oral captopril, oral mononitrate and intravenous magnesium sulfate in 58,050 patients with suspected acute MI. *Lancet* 1995;345:669–685.

Design: Prospective, randomized, double-blind, partially placebo-controlled (including captopril arm), multicenter study. Primary endpoint was 5-week mortality rate.

Purpose: To assess the effects of early initiation of captopril, oral nitrate, and intravenously magnesium on mortality and morbidity in AMI patients.

Population: 58,050 patients with suspected AMI (confirmed in 92%) seen within 24 hours (median, 8 hours) of symptom onset.

Exclusion Criteria (recommended): Cardiogenic shock, persistent severe hypotension, severe fluid depletion, and negligibly low risk of cardiac death.

Treatment: Captopril arm received 6.25 mg, 12.5 mg 2 hours later, 25 mg at 10 to 12 hours, and then 50 mg twice daily for 28 days; or placebo. The isosorbide mononitrate (Imdur) arm received 30 mg, 30 mg 10 to 12 hours later, and 60 mg once daily for 28 days; 70% received thrombolytic therapy, and 94% antiplatelet therapy.

Results: Captopril was associated with a 7% reduction in mortality—7.19% versus 7.69% ($p^2 = 0.02$). The benefit doubled in high-risk groups (prior MI, CHF, anterior ST elevation). More hypotension was seen with captopril, but no increased deaths were seen among patients with low BP (90 to 100 mm Hg). Imdur administration did not have a significant effect on mortality (7.34% vs. 7.54%).

171. **Chinese Cardiac Study (CCS-1).** Oral captopril versus placebo among 13,634 patients with suspected acute MI: interim report from the Chinese Cardiac Study (CCS-1). *Lancet* 1995;345:686–687.

Design: Prospective, randomized, placebo-controlled, multicenter study. Primary endpoint was 4-week all-cause mortality.

Purpose: To assess the effect of ACE inhibition in a broad group of MI patients.

Population: 13,634 patients with or without ST elevation seen within 36 hours of symptom onset.

Exclusion Criteria: Persistent hypotension (SBP <90 mm Hg), long-term use of large doses of diuretics, and contraindications to ACE inhibitors.

Treatment: Captopril, 6.25 mg initial dose, 12.5 mg 2 hours later, and then 12.5 mg three times daily; or placebo.

Results: Captopril group had a nonsignificant mortality reduction at 4 weeks—9.05% vs. 9.59% ($p = 0.03$). Captopril was associated with a significant excess of hypotension, resulting in discontinuation of therapy (8.4% vs. 4.9%) and higher incidence of persistent hypotension (16.3% vs. 10.8%). In patients with an admission SBP less than 100 mm Hg, mortality was slightly higher in the captopril group (11.0% vs. 10.0%; $p = $ NS).

Comments: The additive results of CCS-1, ISIS-4, CONSENSUS-II, GISSI-3, and 11 smaller trials show a clear benefit of ACE inhibitors—6.5% odds reduction (7.27% vs. 7.73%; total of 100,963 patients).

172. **Dickstein K**, et al. the OPTIMAAL Steering Committee, for the OPTIMAAL Study Group. Effects of losartan and captopril on mortality and morbidity in high-risk patients after acute myocardial infarction: the OPTIMAAL randomised trial. *Lancet* 2002; 360:752–760.

Design: Prospective, randomized, double-blind, parallel, multicenter study. Primary endpoint: all-cause mortality. Mean follow-up, 2.7 years.

Purpose: To determine whether losartan is superior or noninferior to captopril at decreasing all-cause mortality in high-risk patients after AMI.

Population: 5,477 patients enrolled within 10 days of presentation AND with: (a) AMI and signs or symptoms of heart failure (rales, S_3, treatment with diuretics or vasodilators, persistent sinus tachycardia, or radiographic evidence of heart failure); (b) AMI and EF, less than

35%, or LV end-diastolic diameter (LVEDD) greater than 65 mm; (c) new Q-wave anterior wall MI; OR (d) reinfarction with previous pathologic Q waves in the anterior wall.

Exclusion Criteria: Included SBP less than 100 mm Hg, current ACE inhibitor or ARB therapy, unstable angina, stenotic valvular heart disease, and planned coronary revascularization.

Treatment: Losartan (target dose, 50 mg orally once daily) or captopril (target dose, 50 mg orally three times each day).

Results: At follow-up, no significant difference in all-cause mortality was found between the two groups (losartan, 18.2%; captopril, 16.4%; $p = 0.069$). The CI boundary (<1.10) showed that losartan did not fulfill criteria for noninferiority. No significant increase in mortality was found in either group when stratified by β-blocker use. The losartan group had a significantly lower CV mortality than did the captopril group (15.3% vs. 13.3%; $p = 0.032$). Losartan was better tolerated than captopril, with 17% discontinuing losartan for any reason compared with 23% with captopril ($p < 0.0001$).

Comments: Data from the RENAAL and LIFE trials suggest that higher doses of losartan may be more beneficial.

173. **Pfeffer MA**, et al. for the Valsartan in Acute Myocardial Infarction Trail (VALIANT) Investigators. Valsartan, captopril, or both in myocardial infarction complicated by heart failure, left ventricular dysfunction, or both. *N Engl J Med* 2003;349:1893–1906.

Design: Prospective, randomized, double-blind, multicenter, international trial. Primary endpoint was death from any cause at median follow-up of 24.7 months.

Purpose: To compare the efficacy of angiotensin-II receptor blockade (with valsartan) versus ACE inhibitor (captopril) or both in patients with acute MI.

Population: 14,703 patients aged 18 or older, with recent MI (0.5 to 10 days prior), and evidence of heart failure clinically or LV systolic dysfunction (EF $\leq35\%$ on echo or angiography, $\leq40\%$ on radionucleotide scan).

Exclusion Criteria: Previous intolerance to ACE inhibitors or ARBs.

Treatment: Valsartan, valsartan plus captopril (combination), or captopril alone.

Results: Overall mortality at follow-up was similar among the three groups (hazard ratio for valsartan compared to captopril 1.00, 97.5% CI, 0.90 to 1.11; $p = 0.98$; hazard ratio for combination group compared to captopril 0.98, 97.5% CI, 0.89 to 1.09; $p = 0.73$). These comparisons met the prespecified test for noninferiority ($p = 0.004$). The highest rate of drug-related adverse events occurred in the combination-therapy group.

NITRATES

General Reviews

174. **Yusuf S,** et al. Effect of intravenous nitrates on mortality in acute MI: an overview of the randomized trials. *Lancet* 1988;1:1088–1092.

Analysis of data from seven small i.v. NTG trials enrolling 851 patients found that use of i.v. NTG was associated with a significant 41% mortality reduction (12.0% vs. 20.5%; $p < 0.001$). Analysis of three trials studying i.v. nitroprusside found that its use was associated with a nonsignificant mortality reduction (14.3% vs. 17.8%).

Studies

175. **ISIS-4 Collaborative Group.** ISIS-4: a randomised factorial assessing early oral captopril, oral mononitrate and intravenous magnesium sulfate in 58,050 patients with suspected acute MI. *Lancet* 1995;345:669–685.

This megatrial that enrolled 58,050 patients with suspected AMI admitted within 24 hours of symptom onset included a randomization to oral mononitrate (30 mg, 30 mg 10 to 12 hours later, and then 60 mg/day for 28 days), or placebo. In the nitrate arm, a nonsignificant reduction was seen in 35-day mortality (7.34% vs. 7.54%). Nearly half the placebo group received i.v. nitrate therapy, which could have diluted the results. See Ref. (171) for a full summary.

CALCIUM-CHANNEL BLOCKERS

176. **The Danish Study Group on Verapamil in MI (DAVIT I).** Verapamil in acute MI. *Eur Heart J* 1984;5:516–528.

This randomized trial was composed of 3,498 patients younger than 75 years with suspected MI. Patients received verapamil, 0.1 mg/kg i.v., followed by 120 mg orally three times daily; or matched placebo. Treatment continued for 6 months in the 1,436 (41%) patients with confirmed MI. Verapamil use was associated with a nonsignificant 9% mortality reduction at 6 months (12.8% vs. 13.9%; OR, 0.91; 95% CI, 0.67 to 1.24).

177. **Wilcox RG,** et al. Trial of Early Nifedipine in Acute MI (TRENT) study. *BMJ* 1986;293:1204–1208.

Design: Prospective, randomized, double-blind, placebo-controlled, multicenter study. Primary endpoint was all-cause mortality rate.
Purpose: To evaluate the effects of early nifedipine on mortality in acute MI patients.
Population: 4,491 patients 70 years or younger seen within 24 hours of onset of chest pain.
Exclusion Criteria: SBP less than 100 mm Hg or DBP less than 50 mm Hg; HR, more than 120 beats/min; and current treatment with calcium-channel blocker.
Treatment: Nifedipine, 10 mg four times daily, or placebo.
Results: Of the patients, 64% had confirmed MI. Nifedipine was associated with a nonsignificant 7% increase in mortality at 1 month (6.7% vs. 6.3%).

178. **The Multicenter Diltiazem Post-Infarction Trial (MDPIT)** Research Group. The effect of diltiazem on mortality and reinfarction after MI. *N Engl J Med* 1988;319:385–392.

Design: Prospective, randomized, double-blind, placebo-controlled, multicenter study. Mean follow-up period was 25 months. Primary endpoint was total mortality, cardiac death, and nonfatal MI.
Purpose: To evaluate the effects of long-term diltiazem on mortality or reinfarction rates after documented MI.
Population: 2,466 patients aged 25 to 75 years with a documented MI (enzyme confirmation required).
Exclusion Criteria: Included cardiogenic shock; second- or third-degree heart block; HR, less than 50 beats/min; and requirement for calcium antagonist.
Treatment: Diltiazem, 60 mg twice or four times daily, or placebo.
Results: No difference was observed in total mortality between the diltiazem and placebo groups (166 and 167 patients, respectively). However, among patients without pulmonary congestion (1,909 patients), diltiazem was associated with fewer cardiac events (hazard ratio, 0.77; 95% CI, 0.61 to 0.98), whereas diltiazem-treated patients with pulmonary congestion had more cardiac events (hazard ratio, 1.41; 95% CI, 1.01 to 1.96).

179. **The Danish Study Group on Verapamil in MI (DAVIT II).** Effect of verapamil on mortality and major events after acute MI (DAVIT II). *Am J Cardiol* 1990;66:779–785.

Design: Prospective, randomized, double-blind, placebo-controlled, multicenter study. Average follow-up period was 16 months. Primary endpoint was death and reinfarction.
Purpose: To evaluate the effect on total mortality and major cardiac events of verapamil started in the second week after MI.
Population: 1,975 patients younger than 75 years enrolled 7 to 15 days after proven MI.
Exclusion Criteria: Included BP less than 90 mm Hg and second- or third-degree heart block at 3 days.

Treatment: Verapamil, 120 mg three times daily (once- or twice-daily dosing allowed in cases of adverse drug reactions), or placebo.

Results: Verapamil group had 17% fewer major events (18.0% vs. 21.6%; p = 0.03) and 20% lower mortality (11.1% vs. 13.8%; p = 0.11). A significant mortality reduction was seen in patients with CHF (7.7% vs. 11.8%; p = 0.02), whereas no benefit was seen in those without CHF (17.9% vs. 17.5%).

180. **Goldbourt U,** et al. Secondary Prevention Reinfarction Israel Nifedipine Trial **(SPRINT 2)**. Early administration of nifedipine in suspected acute MI. *Arch Intern Med* 1993;153:345–353.

Design: Prospective, randomized, double-blind, placebo-controlled study. Primary endpoint was 6-month all-cause mortality rate.

Purpose: To evaluate the effect on mortality of nifedipine started early after AMI in high-risk patients.

Population: 1,006 patients aged 50 to 79 years meeting at least one of the following criteria— prior MI, angina in preceding month, hypertension, NYHA class II or higher, anterior MI, and lactate dehydrogenase three times the upper limit of normal.

Treatment: Nifedipine, 20 mg three times daily (6-day titration period), or placebo.

Results: Trial was terminated early. The nifedipine group had a 20% higher 6-month mortality rate (18.7% vs. 15.6%; 95% CI, 0.94 to 1.84). The majority of the mortality difference was owing to excessive mortality during the first 6 days (7.8% vs. 5.5%; CI, 0.86 to 3.0). No differences were observed in reinfarction rates (5.1% vs. 4.2%) or in outcomes based on CHF status.

181. **Rengo F,** et al. Calcium Antagonist Reinfarction Italian Study **(CRIS)**. A controlled trial of verapamil in patients after acute MI: results of the CRIS. *Am J Cardiol* 1996;77:365–369 (editorial, 421–422).

Design: Prospective, randomized, double-blind, placebo-controlled study. Mean follow-up period was 2 years. Primary endpoint was all-cause mortality rate.

Purpose: To evaluate the effects of verapamil on mortality and major cardiac endpoints in AMI patients.

Population: 1,073 patients aged 30 to 75 years who survived 5 days after an AMI.

Exclusion Criteria: NYHA class III/IV heart failure; HR, less than 50 beats/min; SBP less than 90 mm Hg or greater than 190 mm Hg; DBP greater than 110 mm Hg; long-term therapy with calcium antagonists or β-blockers.

Treatment: Verapamil, 120 mg orally every 8 hours, or placebo started 7 to 21 days (mean, 13.8 days) after admission.

Results: No differences were observed between the verapamil and placebo groups in all-cause mortality (30 and 29 deaths, respectively). The verapamil group had 20% fewer reinfarctions and 20% less angina.

Comments: Editorial reports that pooled data from nine trials show that verapamil is associated with a favorable effect on reinfarction (OR, 0.81; 95% CI, 0.67 to 0.98) but no overall mortality benefit (OR, 0.93; 95% CI, 0.78 to 1.10).

182. **Boden WE,** et al. for the Incomplete Infarction Trial of European Research Collaborators Evaluating Prognosis Post-thrombolysis (INTERCEPT). Diltiazem in acute myocardial infarction treated with thrombolytic agents: a randomised placebo-controlled trial. *Lancet* 2000;355:1751–1756.

Design: Prospective, randomized, double-blind, multicenter, international, placebo-controlled study. Primary endpoint was a composite of cardiac death, reinfarction, or refractory ischemia.

Purpose: To evaluate the effects of diltiazem on clinical outcomes in patients with acute MI who receive thrombolytic agents.

Population: 874 patients with acute MI, without CHF, who received thrombolytic agents.

Treatment: Diltiazem 300 mg daily or placebo, started within 36 to 96 hours of symptom onset, for a duration of up to 6 months.

Results: At 6 months, the diltiazem group had a nonsignificant 21% hazard reduction in death, MI, and refractory ischemia (hazard ratio, 0.79; 95% CI, 0.61 to 1.02; $p = 0.07$). The diltiazem group had a significant reduction in the incidence of nonfatal reinfarction or refractory ischemia (hazard ratio, 0.76; 95% CI, 0.58 to 1.00). There was a significant reduction in the need for repeat revascularization in the diltiazem group (hazard ratio, 0.61; 95% CI, 0.39 to 0.96).

MAGNESIUM

183. **Woods KL,** et al. Second Leicester Intravenous Magnesium Intervention Trial **(LIMIT-2).** Intravenous magnesium sulfate in suspected acute MI: results of LIMIT-2. *Lancet* 1992;339:1553–1558.

   This prospective, randomized, double-blind, placebo-controlled, single-center study randomized 2,316 patients with suspected AMI (no ECG criteria specified) seen within 24 hours. Patients received magnesium sulfate, 8 mmol over a 5-minute period, followed by 65 mmol over a 24-hour period; or saline. AMI was confirmed in 65%. The magnesium group had a 24% lower 28-day mortality rate (7.8% vs. 10.3%; $p = 0.04$). Long-term follow-up (mean, 2.7 years) showed persistent significant mortality benefit (16%) associated with magnesium.

184. **ISIS-4** Collaborative Group. ISIS-4: a randomised factorial assessing early oral captopril, oral mononitrate and intravenous magnesium sulfate in 58,050 patients with suspected acute MI. *Lancet* 1995;345:669–685.

   This megatrial of 58,050 patients with suspected AMI included a randomization to magnesium (8-mmol bolus over a 15-minute period, and then 72 mmol over a 24-hour period) or no magnesium. Magnesium group had a nonsignificant 6% increase in mortality (7.64% vs. 7.24%) and a higher incidence of CHF (+12/1,000), hypotension (+11/1,000), and cardiogenic shock (+5/1,000). No benefit of magnesium was seen in any subgroup.

185. **The Magnesium in Coronaries (MAGIC)** Trial Investigators. Early administration of intravenous magnesium to high-risk patients with acute myocardial infarction in the Magnesium in Coronaries (MAGIC) trial: a randomized controlled trial. *Lancet* 2002;360:1189–1196.

   This prospective, randomized, placebo-controlled, multicenter trial enrolled 6,213 high-risk AMI patients aged 65 years or older seen within 6 hours of symptom onset who were ineligible for reperfusion or eligible for reperfusion. Exclusion criteria included high-grade AV block, cardiogenic shock, and renal failure. Patients received i.v. magnesium (2-g i.v. bolus over a 15-minute period, and then 17 g over a 24-hour period) or placebo. Of patients who underwent reperfusion (primarily thrombolysis), 96% received the magnesium at the time of reperfusion. At 30 days, no difference was found between the two groups in all-cause mortality (15% in both groups). No differences occurred when the patients were stratified by sex, geography, EF, concomitant medications, and other variables.

ANTIARRHYTHMICS

186. **Burkart F,** et al. Basel Antiarrhythmic Study of Infarct Survival **(BASIS).** Effect of antiarrhythmic therapy on mortality in survivors of MI with asymptomatic complex ventricular arrhythmias: BASIS. *J Am Coll Cardiol* 1990;16:1711–1718.

Design: Prospective, randomized, three-center study. Follow-up period was 1 year.
Purpose: To compare individualized antiarrhythmic therapy with low-dose amiodarone and no therapy.
Population: 312 of 1,220 consecutively screened MI survivors younger than 71 years with asymptomatic, complex ventricular arrhythmias (Lown class 3 or 4b) on 24-hour ECG before hospital discharge.

Treatment: (a) Individualized—initially quinidine or mexiletine (if both failed, others tried: ajmaline, disopyramide, flecainide, propafenone, sotalol); (b) amiodarone, 1 g/day for 5 days, and then 200 mg/day for 1 year; or (c) no therapy—drugs allowed if arrhythmias developed.

Results: Amiodarone group had a lower overall 1-year mortality rate compared with controls—5.1% vs. 13.2% ($p < 0.05$); mortality for individually treated patients was 10% ($p =$ NS vs. amiodarone).

Comments: Post hoc analysis showed that the benefit of amiodarone was restricted to those with an EF of 40% (1.5% vs. 8.9% 1-year mortality; $p < 0.03$). Late follow-up showed persistent benefit of amiodarone (after discontinuation at 1 year) compared with placebo: at 7 years, 30% versus 45% mortality ($p = 0.03$).

187. **The Cardiac Arrhythmia Suppression Trial (CAST) Investigators.** Preliminary report: effect of encainide and flecainide on mortality in a randomized trial of arrhythmia suppression after myocardial infarction. *N Engl J Med* 1989;321:406–412.

Design: Prospective, randomized, open-label (initial phase), double-blind (main phase), placebo-controlled, multicenter study. Follow-up period was 10 months.

Purpose: To evaluate whether suppression of asymptomatic or mildly asymptomatic ventricular arrhythmias after MI reduces death due to arrhythmia.

Population: 1,727 patients with MI in prior 6 days to 2 years, at least six ventricular premature contractions per hour on 24-hour Holter monitoring, EF 0.55 or less if 90 days or less after MI or 0.40 or less if more than 90 days after MI (if EF 30%, patients not eligible to receive flecainide), and suppressibility during open-label phase (at 4 to 10 days, 80% reduction of ventricular premature contractions and 90% reduction of unsustained runs of VT).

Exclusion Criteria: Ventricular arrhythmias associated with severe symptoms; unsustained VT with 15 beats at 120 beats/min; contraindications to drugs; and ECG abnormalities making rhythm interpretation difficult.

Treatment: Encainide, 35 or 50 mg orally three times daily; flecainide, 100 or 150 mg twice daily; or moricizine, 200 or 250 mg three times daily.

Results: Encainide and flecainide arms were discontinued early. Encainide and flecainide patients had more arrhythmic deaths [4.5% vs. 1.2% (placebo); RR, 3.6; 95% CI, 1.7 to 8.5], as well as higher overall mortality (7.7% vs. 3.0%; RR, 2.5; 95% CI, 1.6 to 4.5).

Comments: The moricizine arm of the trial continued. Later analysis showed that those patients with easily suppressible arrhythmias ($n = 1,778$) had fewer arrhythmic deaths than the 1,173 patients with difficult-to-suppress arrhythmias (RR, 0.59; $p = 0.003$). This likely explains the low placebo mortality rate (1.2%).

188. **Waldo AL,** et al. for the Survival with Oral D-sotalol **(SWORD) Investigators.** Effect of D-sotalol on mortality in patients with left ventricular dysfunction after recent and remote MI. *Lancet* 1996;348:7–12.

Design: Prospective, randomized, double-blind, placebo-controlled, multicenter study. Mean follow-up period was 148 days. Primary endpoint was all-cause mortality rate.

Purpose: To determine if the NYHA class III antiarrhythmic agent D-sotalol can decrease all-cause mortality in high-risk MI survivors.

Population: 3,121 patients with EF 40% or less and recent MI (6 to 42 days) or symptomatic heart failure (class II or III) with remote (longer than 42 days) MI.

Exclusion Criteria: Unstable angina, class IV heart failure, history of life-threatening arrhythmia, PTCA, or CABG in previous 14 days, and creatinine clearance 50 mL/min or less.

Treatment: D-Sotalol, 200 mg orally twice daily, or placebo.

Results: Trial was terminated early because of 65% higher overall mortality in the sotalol group: 5.0% vs. 3.1% ($p = 0.006$). Increased arrhythmic deaths (RR, 1.77; $p = 0.008$) accounted for the excess mortality. The effect was greatest in those with EF 30% or less (RR, 4.0 vs. 1.2; EF, 31% to 40%; $p = 0.007$).

189. **Julian DG,** et al. for the European MI Amiodarone Trial **(EMIAT)** Investigators. Randomised trial of effect of amiodarone on mortality in patients with left-ventricular dysfunction after recent MI: EMIAT. *Lancet* 1997;349:667–674.

Design: Prospective, randomized, double-blind, placebo-controlled, multicenter study. Mean follow-up period was 21 months. Primary endpoint was all-cause mortality rate.

Purpose: To evaluate the effect of amiodarone on mortality in post-MI patients with LV dysfunction.

Population: 1,486 patients aged 18 to 75 years with MI in the prior 5 to 21 days and EF of 40% or less by multiple-gated nuclear angiography (approximately 45% with EF 30% or less).

Exclusion Criteria: Amiodarone in previous 6 months; HR, less than 50 beats/min; second- or third-degree AV block; significant hepatic or thyroid dysfunction; need for antiarrhythmic(s) other than β-blockers or digoxin.

Treatment: Amiodarone, 800 mg/day for 14 days, 400 mg/day for 14 weeks, and then 200 mg/day; or placebo.

Results: Among all patients, total mortality was 13.4%, with no difference between amiodarone and placebo (RR, 0.99). No difference was observed in cardiac mortality (RR, 0.94; $p = 0.67$). The amiodarone group had fewer arrhythmic deaths (RR, 0.35; $p = 0.04$).

190. **Cairns JA,** et al. for the Canadian Amiodarone MI Arrhythmia Trial **(CAMIAT)** Investigators. Randomised trial of outcome after MI in patients with frequent or repetitive ventricular premature depolarisations: CAMIAT. *Lancet* 1997;349:675–682.

Design: Prospective, randomized, double-blind, placebo-controlled, multicenter study. Median follow-up period was 1.8 years. Primary endpoint was resuscitated VF or arrhythmic death.

Purpose: To determine the effect of amiodarone on overall mortality in post-MI patients with frequent or repetitive ventricular premature depolarizations.

Population: 1,202 patients with MI in the prior 6 to 45 days, EF 40% or less, and 24-hour ECG monitoring showing 10 ventricular premature depolarizations per hour or one run of three beats of VT at 100 to 120 beats/min.

Exclusion Criteria: Contraindications to amiodarone (prior intolerance); HR, <50 beats/ min; heart block (any degree); QT interval greater than 480 msec; VT at more than 120 beats/min.

Treatment: Amiodarone, 10 mg/kg/day for 2 weeks, 300 to 400 mg/day for 3 to 5 months, 200 to 300 mg/day for 4 months, and 200 mg for 5 to 7 days/week for 16 months; or placebo.

Results: Amiodarone group with nearly 50% fewer arrhythmic deaths plus resuscitated VF [3.3% vs. 6.0%; $p = 0.016$ (intention-to-treat analysis, $p = 0.029$)]. Total mortality was not different.

Comments: Primary analysis was not based on intention-to-treat analysis. The trial also had many dropouts (221 amiodarone and 152 placebo patients; >70% and >50%, respectively, stopped because of adverse effects).

191. **Teo KK,** et al. Effects of prophylactic antiarrhythmic drug therapy in acute MI. *JAMA* 1993;270:1589–1595.

This analysis focused on 138 randomized trials with approximately 98,000 enrolled patients. Lower mortality was seen with β-blockers (26,973 patients; OR, 0.81; $p = 0.00001$) and amiodarone (778 patients; OR, 0.71; $p = 0.03$). Higher mortality was seen with class I agents (11,712 patients; OR, 1.14; $p = 0.03$). A statistically nonsignificant impact of calcium-channel blockers was observed (10,154 patients; OR, 1.04; $p = 0.41$).

192. **Sadowski ZP,** et al. Multicenter randomized trial and a systematic overview of lidocaine in acute myocardial infarction. *Am Heart J* 1999;137:792–798.

A total of 903 patients seen within 6 hours of symptom onset with ST elevation were randomized to lidocaine (four boluses of 50 mg each every 2 minutes, and then 3 mg/min for

12 hours, and then 2 mg/min for 36 hours) or no lidocaine. The lidocaine group had significantly less VF (2.0% vs. 5.7%; $p = 0.004$) but tended toward increased mortality (9.7% vs. 7.0%; $p = 0.145$). A meta-analysis of these results and those from 20 other randomized studies with more than 11,000 patients revealed nonsignificant trends toward reduced VF (OR, 0.71; 95% CI, 0.47 to 1.09) and increased mortality rates (OR, 1.12; 95% CI, 0.91 to 1.36) with lidocaine.

193. **Amiodarone Trials Meta-Analysis Investigators**. Effect of prophylactic amiodarone on mortality after acute myocardial infarction and in congestive heart failure: meta-analysis of individual data from 6500 patients in randomised trials. *Lancet* 1997;350:1417–1424.

The investigators pooled data form 13 trials, 8 in post-MI patients and 5 in CHF, 9 of which were double-blind and placebo-controlled. The resulting cohort of 6,553 patients demonstrated a significant reduction in mortality by 13% (OR, 0.87; $p = 0.03$) for those taking amiodarone, with a particular reduction in sudden death (OR, 0.71; $p = 0.0003$). These results did not differ between the post-MI and CHF populations; however, the risk of sudden death was higher for those in the CHF group. They calculated an excess risk of pulmonary toxicity to be 1% per year.

INTRA-AORTIC BALLOON PUMP

194. **Ohman EM,** et al. **IABP** Trial. Use of aortic counterpulsation to improve sustained coronary artery patency during acute MI. *Circulation* 1994;90:792–799.

Design: Prospective, randomized, multicenter study. Primary endpoint was angiographically detected reocclusion of IRA during initial hospitalization.
Purpose: To determine whether 48 hours of aortic counterpulsation therapy after reperfusion established during emergency catheterization would reduce the rate of reocclusion of the IRA.
Population: 182 AMI patients who underwent catheterization within 24 hours with successful restoration of IRA patency.
Exclusion Criteria: Included cardiogenic shock, pulmonary edema requiring aortic counterpulsation, severe PVD, more than 75% restenosis in one or two major epicardial arteries and TIMI grade 2 or 3 flow achieved in IRA with thrombolytic therapy, and contraindication(s) to heparin.
Treatment: IABP for 48 hours or standard care.
Results: Primary angioplasty was performed in 106 patients, rescue angioplasty in 51 patients, and other methods (e.g., intracoronary thrombolysis) in the remaining 25 patients. Both groups had a similar incidence of severe bleeding complications and transfusions. Catheterization performed at a median of 5 days demonstrated that the aortic counterpulsation group had a lower IRA reocclusion rate (8% vs. 21%) and nearly 50% fewer clinical events (death, stroke, reinfarction, ERV, and recurrent ischemia; 13% vs. 24%; $p < 0.04$).

195. **Stone GW,** et al. A prospective, randomized evaluation of prophylactic intraaortic balloon pump (IABP) counterpulsation in high risk patients with acute MI treated with primary angioplasty. *J Am Coll Cardiol* 1997;29:1459–1467.

Design: Prospective, randomized, multicenter study. Primary endpoints were death, MI, IRA occlusion, stroke, new heart failure, and sustained hypotension.
Purpose: To determine whether AMI patients stratified as high risk benefit from a routine IABP strategy after PTCA.
Population: 437 PAMI II patients classified as high risk (meeting at least one of the following criteria: age older than 70 years, three-vessel disease, EF 45% or less, saphenous vein graft occlusion, persistent malignant ventricular arrhythmia, or suboptimal angioplasty result).
Exclusion Criteria: Cardiogenic shock, bleeding diathesis, and thrombolytic therapy before catheterization.
Treatment: IABP for 36 to 48 hours or standard care.

Results: The two groups had similar outcomes [composite endpoint incidence 28.9% (IABP) vs. 29.2%]. The IABP group had fewer unscheduled repeated catheterizations (7.6% vs. 13.3%; $p = 0.05$), but had more strokes (2.4% vs. 0%; $p = 0.03$). The authors suggest that the IABP effect may not have been detected because of low control group mortality (3.1%) and IRA occlusion rate (5.5%).

196. **Anderson RD,** et al. Use of intraaortic balloon bump counterpulsation in patients presenting with cardiogenic shock: observations from the GUSTO-I study. *J Am Coll Cardiol* 1997;30:708–715.

This analysis focused on 68 GUSTO I patients with cardiogenic shock who had an IABP placed (91% within 1 day). Early IABP use was associated with increased bleeding (moderate, 47% vs. 12%, $p = 0.0001$; severe, 10% vs. 5%, $p = 0.16$). IABP use also was associated with increased arrhythmias, procedures, and bypass surgery. However, these increases were owing longer time to death (2.8 days vs. 7.2 hours). However, in part, a trend toward lower 30-day mortality was seen with IABP use [57% vs. 67%; adjusted $p = 0.11$ (if revascularization patients were excluded, 47% vs. 64%; $p = 0.07$)].

197. **Thiele H,** et al. Percutaneous left ventricular assist devices in acute myocardial infarction complicated by cardiogenic shock. *Eur Heart J* 2007;28:2057–2063.

The authors introduce novel percutaneous left ventricular assist devices (LVADs), their design, implantation, advantages, and disadvantage. These include percutaneous cardiopulmonary bypass, axial flow pumps, and left atrial-to-femoral arterial LVADs. The authors compare these devices to the current standard, the IABP. Limitations of these therapies, as well as future directions of research, are also discussed.

198. **Seyfarth M,** et al. A randomized clinical trial to evaluate the safety and efficacy of a percutaneous left ventricular assist device versus intra-aortic balloon pumping for treatment of cardiogenic shock caused by myocardial infarction (Efficacy Study of LV Assist Device to Treat Patients with Cardiogenic Shock [ISAR-SHOCK]). *J Am Coll Cardiol* 2008;52:1584–1588.

Design: Prospective, randomized, open trial. Primary endpoint was change in cardiac index at 30 minutes. Secondary endpoints were lactic acidosis, hemolysis, and mortality at 30 days.
Purpose: To determine the benefit, if any, of the newer Impella LP2.5 LVAD over standard IABP for hemodynamic support in cardiogenic shock secondary to acute MI.
Population: 26 patients with acute MI complicated by cardiogenic shock (a device was implanted in 25; 1 died prior to implant).
Treatment: Implantation of the Impella LP2.5 percutaneous LVAD versus implantation of a standard IABP.
Results: Cardiac index was significantly higher in the LVAD group at 30 minutes (change in cardiac index 0.49 for LVAD vs. 0.11 for IABP; $p = 0.02$). Overall mortality was similar in both groups (46%).

199. **Sjauw KD,** et al. A systematic review and meta-analysis of intra-aortic balloon pump therapy in ST-elevation myocardial infarction: should we change the guidelines? *Eur Heart J* 2009;30:459–468.

The authors reviewed data from trials and observational cohorts of patients with STEMI complicated by cardiogenic shock. Their first analysis included seven randomized trials of 1,009 patients, demonstrating no change in 30-day survival between patients who did and did not receive an IABP, despite significantly higher bleeding and stroke rates in the IABP groups. In their second analysis of nine cohorts of 10,529 patients, use of IABP in patients receiving thrombolysis was associated with an 18% lower mortality at 30 days ($p < 0.0001$), at the expense of higher revascularization rates in this group. However, in those undergoing primary PCI, IABP was associated with a 6% higher 30-day mortality ($p < 0.0008$). While there were important methodologic caveats to the results of the cohort meta-analysis, these results challenge the current guideline recommendations.

OTHER TREATMENTS

200. **Malmberg K,** et al. Diabetic Insulin–Glucose Infusion in Acute MI **(DIGAMI)**. Randomized trial of insulin–glucose infusion followed by subcutaneous insulin treatment in diabetic patients with acute MI: effects on mortality at 1 year. *J Am Coll Cardiol* 1995;26:57–65.

Design: Prospective, randomized, open, multicenter study. Primary endpoint was all-cause mortality.

Purpose: To evaluate whether rapid improvement of metabolic control in diabetic patients with an insulin/glucose infusion decreases early mortality and subsequent morbidity.

Population: 620 patients with suspected MI and blood glucose 11 mM on admission (with or without prior diagnosis of diabetes).

Treatment: Continuous i.v. insulin infusion for 24 hours (started at 5 U/hr) or until normoglycemia was achieved (goal of 7 to 10 mM), and then s.c. insulin for 3 months; or conventional therapy.

Results: At 24 hours, the insulin/glucose-treated patients had lower glucose (9.6 mM vs. 11.7 mM) and 29% lower mortality at 1 year (18.6% vs. 26.1%; $p = 0.027$). Mortality reduction was most marked (52%) in patients with a low cardiovascular risk profile or no previous insulin therapy. Only 10% stopped insulin because of hypoglycemia with no associated morbidity.

Comments: Intense insulin may restore impaired platelet function, decrease plasminogen activator inhibitor (PAI)-1 activity, and possibly improve metabolism of noninfarcted areas. Long-term follow-up showed that lower mortality was maintained at a mean 3.4 years: 33% vs. 44% (RR, 0.72; $p = 0.011$), with the largest benefit seen in patients with no prior insulin therapy (RR, 0.49).

201. **Fath-Ordoubadi F,** et al. Glucose–insulin–potassium therapy for treatment of acute MI. *Circulation* 1997;96:1152–1156.

This analysis focused on nine well-designed randomized, placebo-controlled trials with 1,932 patients (all prethrombolytic era). GIK was associated with lower hospital mortality (16.1% vs. 21%; OR, 0.72; $p = 0.004$). A 48% reduction was seen in the four trials using high-dose GIK (to suppress free fatty acid levels maximally).

202. **Diaz R,** et al. on behalf of the Estudios Cardiologicos Latinoamerica **(ECLA)** Glucose–Insulin–Potassium Pilot Trial Collaborative Group. Metabolic modulation of acute MI. *Circulation* 1998;98:2227–2234.

Design: Prospective, randomized, open, multicenter study.

Purpose: To evaluate the feasibility of GIK administration in contemporary practice and to assess its effect on clinical endpoints in patients with AMI.

Population: 407 patients with suspected AMI seen within 24 hours of symptom onset.

Exclusion Criteria: Severe renal impairment or hyperkalemia.

Treatment: High-dose GIK (25% glucose, 50 IU insulin/L, and 80 mM KCl at 1.5 mL/kg/hr for 24 hours), low-dose GIK (10% glucose, 20 IU insulin/L, and 40 mM KCl at 1.0 mL/kg/hr for 24 hours), or control. GIK was started an average 10 to 11 hours after onset of symptoms.

Results: GIK-treated patients had nonsignificant reductions in several in-hospital events, including severe heart failure, cardiogenic shock, VF, and reinfarction. Among the 252 (61.9%) patients treated with reperfusion strategies (thrombolysis, 95%; PTCA, 5%), GIK-treated patients had a significant 66% reduction in in-hospital mortality (5.2% vs. 15.2%; RR, 0.34; $p = 0.008$). At 1-year follow-up, only the high-dose GIK patients undergoing reperfusion had a significant mortality benefit (RR, 0.37; log-rank test, 0.046). The GIK group had a higher frequency of phlebitis (severe in only 2%) and serum changes in plasma concentration of glucose or potassium.

Comments: High-dose regimen achieves maximal suppression of free fatty acid levels. A meta-analysis of 1,932 patients showed no interaction between GIK and reperfusion.

203. **Mahaffey KW,** et al. Adenosine as an adjunct to thrombolytic therapy for acute myocardial infarction: results of a multicenter, randomized, placebo-controlled trial: the Acute Myocardial Infarction STudy of ADenosine **(AMISTAD)** trial. *J Am Coll Cardiol* 1999;34:1711–1720.

Design: Prospective, randomized, placebo-controlled, multicenter study. Primary endpoint was infarct size.

Purpose: To assess whether adenosine as an adjunct to thrombolysis would reduce MI size.

Population: 236 patients seen within 6 hours of onset of chest pain lasting 20 minutes or longer and with ST elevation 0.1 mV or more in two contiguous leads. Clinical decision made to treat with thrombolytic therapy.

Exclusion Criteria: Included dipyridamole within past 24 hours, bronchospastic lung disease or prior bronchodilator therapy, advanced AV block, LBBB, and sustained bradycardia (<60 beats/min for >20 minutes).

Treatment: Adenosine (70 mg/kg/min i.v. for 3 hours) or placebo (normal saline) begun before thrombolytic therapy. Tc-99m sestamibi was injected before thrombolytic therapy began, and single-photon emission computed tomography (SPECT) imaging was performed within 6 hours.

Results: Infarct size was assessed in 83% of patients and was significantly reduced in adenosine-treated patients (adjusted $p = 0.03$). A 67% relative reduction in infarct size with adenosine was found in patients with anterior MI (15% in the adenosine group vs. 45.5% in the placebo group; $p = 0.014$) but no reduction in patients with nonanterior infarcts (11.5% for both groups; $p = 0.96$). A trend was seen toward more major clinical events in the adenosine group compared with placebo (22% vs. 16%; OR, 1.43; 95% CI, 0.71 to 2.89).

204. **Ross AM,** et al. for the AMISTAD II Investigators. A randomized, double-blinded, placebo-controlled multicenter trial of adenosine as an adjunct to reperfusion in the treatment of acute myocardial infarction (AMISTAD-II). *J Am Coll Cardiol* 2005;45:1775–1780.

This prospective, randomized, placebo-controlled trial enrolled 2,118 patients with anterior AMI seen within 6 hours of symptom onset. Patients were randomized to low-dose i.v. adenosine (50 μg/kg/min), high-dose adenosine (70 μg/kg/min), or placebo for 3 hours. Patients underwent reperfusion therapy (thrombolysis or mechanical reperfusion) within 15 minutes of initiation of study drug infusion. At 6 months, a nonsignificant reduction in the primary endpoint of death, new CHF, or first rehospitalization for CHF in the pooled adenosine groups (16.3%) versus placebo (17.9%). In the prespecified subgroup analysis of patients with reperfusion success, a significant reduction in death or CHF was seen in the pooled adenosine group versus placebo (11% vs. 15%; $p = 0.043$). Incidence of a primary endpoint event was significantly related to infarct size ($p < 0.001$).

205. **Van der Horst IC,** et al. on behalf of the Zwolle Infarct Study Group. Glucose–insulin–potassium infusion treated with primary angioplasty for acute myocardial infarction: the Glucose–Insulin–Potassium Study: a randomized trial (GIPS). *J Am Coll Cardiol* 2003;42:784–791.

This prospective, randomized, placebo-controlled, open trial enrolled 940 patients with AMI treated with primary angioplasty. Patients received potassium, 80 mmol in 500 mL, and 20% glucose at a rate of 3 mL/kg body weight/hr over 8 to 12 hours and continuous i.v. insulin titrated with dose adjustment every hour, or placebo. At 30 days, a nonsignificant trend was observed toward a reduction in overall mortality in the GIK group (RR, 0.82; 95% CI, 0.46 to 1.46). In a subgroup analysis, a significant reduction was found in overall mortality at 30 days among those without heart failure symptoms (Killip class 1) (RR, 0.28; 95% CI, 0.1 to 0.75).

The subsequent GIPS II study was halted early for futility, and thus failed to yield significant support to GIK therapy (see *J Am Coll Cardiol* 2006;47:1730–1731).

206. **The CREATE-ECLA Trial Group Investigators**. Effect of glucose–insulin–potassium infusion on mortality in patients with acute ST-segment elevation myocardial infarction: the CREATE-ECLA randomized controlled trial. JAMA 2005;293:437–446.

Design: Prospective, randomized, multicenter, international trial. Primary endpoint was death, cardiac arrest, cardiogenic shock, and reinfarction at 30 days.
Purpose: To evaluate the benefit, if any, of GIK infusion in patients with STEMI.
Population: 20,201 patients presenting with STEMI within 12 hours of symptom onset.
Treatment: High-dose GIK infusion for 24 hours or standard care.
Results: GIK infusion resulted in no significant changes in the rates of 30-day mortality (hazard ratio 1.03; $p = 0.45$), cardiac arrest (hazard ratio 0.93; $p = 0.51$), cardiogenic shock (hazard ratio 1.05; $p = 0.38$) or reinfarction (hazard ratio 0.98; $p = 0.81$). Rates of heart failure were similar at 7 days (hazard ratio 1.01; $p = 0.72$).
Comment: The subsequent OASIS 6-GIK trial of GIK infusion in STEMI was stopped early on publication of these results (see also *JAMA* 2007;298:2399–2405).

Specific Cases

ANTERIOR MYOCARDIAL INFARCTION

207. **Stone PH,** et al. Prognostic significance of location and type of MI: independent adverse outcome associated with anterior location. *J Am Coll Cardiol* 1988;11:453–463.

This retrospective analysis focused on 471 Multicenter Investigation of the Limitation of Infarct Size (MILIS) patients with a first MI showing an anterior location associated with poor outcome. Anterior versus inferior patients: larger infarcts (higher CK-MB fraction; $p < 0.001$), approximately three times more heart failure (40.7% vs. 14.7%), more than four times more in-hospital deaths (11.9% vs. 2.8%; $p < 0.001$), and higher cumulative cardiac mortality (27% vs. 11%; $p < 0.001$). Q wave versus non–Q wave: worse in-hospital course [higher CK-MB, lower EF, more heart failure and deaths (9.3% vs. 4.1%; $p < 0.05$)], but no significant difference in long-term cardiac mortality (21% vs. 16%). After adjustment for infarct size, anterior patients still had higher mortality rates. If location and type were considered, anterior patients still had worse outcomes (whether Q wave or non–Q wave).

INFERIOR MYOCARDIAL INFARCTION

208. **Berger PB,** et al. Incidence and prognostic implications of heart block complicating inferior MI treated with thrombolytic therapy: results from TIMI II. *J Am Coll Cardiol* 1992;20:533–540.

This retrospective analysis focused on 1,786 patients. Complete heart block occurred in 12% (6.3% at presentation). The complete heart block group had a higher unadjusted 21-day mortality rate (7.1% vs. 2.7%; $p = 0.007$), but adjusted RR was not statistically significant. Mortality was nearly five times higher in those with complete heart block after thrombolysis (9.9% vs. 2.2%; $p < 0.001$). Increased deaths were attributable to more severe cardiac dysfunction.

209. **Behar S,** et al. Complete atrioventricular block complicating inferior acute wall MI: short and long-term prognosis. *Am Heart J* 1993;125:1622–1627.

This analysis focused on 2,273 SPRINT Registry patients with inferior Q-wave MIs. An 11% incidence of complete heart block was observed (women, 14%; age 70 years, 15%). The complete heart block group had more than a threefold higher in-hospital mortality rate

(37% vs. 11%; $p < 0.0001$; adjusted OR, 2.0; 95% CI, 1.12 to 3.57). However, no difference in 5-year mortality was observed among hospital survivors (28% vs. 23%).

210. **Peterson ED,** et al. Prognostic significance of precordial ST segment depression during inferior MI in the thrombolytic era: results in 16,521 patients. *J Am Coll Cardiol* 1996;28:305–312.

This post hoc GUSTO I analysis focused on 6,422 patients without any precordial depression. The ST-depression group had a 47% higher 30-day mortality rate (4.7% vs. 3.2%; at 1 year, 5% vs. 3.4%; $p < 0.001$). Magnitude of depression (sum of V_1 through V_6) added significant prognostic information after risk factor adjustment: 36% higher mortality per 0.5 mm.

211. **Matetzky S,** et al. Significance of ST segment elevations in posterior chest leads (V_7 to V_9) in patients with acute inferior MI: application for thrombolytic therapy. *J Am Coll Cardiol* 1998;31:506–511.

This analysis showed that ST elevation in V_7 to V_9 correlates with posterolateral involvement, and such patients benefit more from thrombolysis. Eighty-seven patients who had a first inferior MI and were treated with rtPA were stratified according to the presence (46 patients) or absence (41 patients) of ST elevation in V_7 to V_9. The ST-elevation group had a higher incidence of posterolateral wall-motion abnormalities ($p < 0.001$) on radionuclide ventriculography, a larger infarct area (higher peak CK, $p < 0.02$), lower predischarge EF ($p < 0.008$), and higher incidence of death, reinfarction, or heart failure ($p < 0.05$). Patency of the IRA in the V_7 to V_9 elevation group resulted in an improved EF at discharge ($p < 0.012$), whereas EF in the nonelevation patients was unchanged, regardless of IRA patency.

RIGHT VENTRICULAR INFARCTION

212. **Zehender M,** et al. Right ventricular infarction as an independent predictor of prognosis after acute MI. *N Engl J Med* 1993;328:981–988.

This analysis of 200 consecutive patients showed that ST elevation in lead V_4R was highly predictive of RVI: sensitivity, 88%; specificity, 78%. ST elevation in V_4R also was associated with higher mortality (31% vs. 19% overall) and more in-hospital complications (64% vs. 28%).

213. **Kinch JW,** Ryan TJ. Right ventricular infarction. *N Engl J Med* 1994;330:1211–1217.

This excellent overview discusses the pathophysiology, diagnosis, complications, treatment, and prognosis of patients with RVI.

214. **Zehender M,** et al. Eligibility for and benefit of thrombolytic therapy in inferior MI: focus on the prognostic importance of right ventricular infarction. *J Am Coll Cardiol* 1994;24:362–369.

This prospective analysis focused on 200 patients with an inferior MI. Thrombolytic therapy (accelerated tPA regimen) was received by 36%; this group of patients had a lower mortality than did patients ineligible for tPA (8% vs. 25%; $p < 0.001$). However, benefit of tPA was restricted to patients with RVI complicating acute inferior MI: 76% lower mortality (10% vs. 42%; $p < 0.005$) and fewer overall complications (34% vs. 54%; $p < 0.05$). In the absence of RVI, no difference was observed in mortality (7% vs. 6%), whether or not patients received tPA.

215. **Bowers TR,** et al. Effect of reperfusion on biventricular function and survival after right ventricular infarction. *N Engl J Med* 1998;338:933–940.

This prospective study was composed of 53 inferior MI patients with echocardiographic evidence of RVI (RV free-wall dysfunction, dilatation, and depressed global performance). Complete reperfusion was achieved by balloon angioplasty in 77% of patients (i.e., normal flow in right coronary artery and its major RV branches) and led to recovery of RV function [mean score for free-wall motion, 1.4 (at 3 days) vs. 3.0 (baseline); $p < 0.001$]. In contrast, unsuccessful reperfusion (no RV branch flow) was associated with a lack of RV recovery, as well as persistent hypotension and low cardiac output (83% vs. 12%; $p = 0.002$) and markedly higher mortality (58% vs. 2%; $p = 0.001$).

216. **Zeymer U,** et al. Effects of thrombolytic therapy in acute inferior MI with or without right ventricular involvement. *J Am Coll Cardiol* 1998;32:876–881.

This analysis of 522 inferior MI patients from the HIT-4 trial showed that RV involvement is not an independent predictor of survival. RV involvement was associated with higher 30-day cardiac mortality rates (5.9% vs. 2.5%), but this was related to larger infarct size rather than to RVI. Among large inferior MI patients (sum ST elevation >0.8 mV or precordial depression), a proximal right coronary artery lesion was seen in 52% with and 23% without RVI. Among small-MI patients, lesions were mostly distal in location, and cardiac mortality was less than 1% irrespective of the presence of RVI.

217. **Shiraki H,** et al. Association between preinfarction angina and a lower risk of right ventricular infarction. *N Engl J Med* 1998;338:941–947.

This retrospective analysis focused on 113 patients with a first MI due to occlusion of the right coronary artery. Absence of preinfarction angina (defined as chest pain <30 minutes 7 or fewer days before MI) was a strong predictor of RVI (OR, 6.3; $p < 0.001$), complete AV block (OR, 3.6; $p = 0.01$), and combined hypotension and shock (OR, 12.4; $p < 0.001$). Angina in the preceding 24 to 72 hours was associated with a lower incidence of RVI (OR, 0.2; $p = 0.02$) and hypotension/shock (OR, 0.1; $p = 0.02$).

POSTERIOR MYOCARDIAL INFARCTION

218. **Boden WE,** et al. Electrocardiographic evolution of posterior acute MI: importance of early precordial ST-segment depression. *Am J Cardiol* 1987;59:782–787.

This analysis focused on 50 patients from the Diltiazem Reinfarction Study who had isolated precordial ST-segment elevation of 1 mm or more in at least two precordial leads (V_1 to V_4). Serial ECGs showed that 46% developed evidence of posterior MI, defined as R-wave 0.04 second or more in lead V_1 and R:S 1 or more in V_2. The posterior group had a higher peak CK than the anterior group (1,051 vs. 663 IU; $p < 0.009$). All 23 posterior MI patients had horizontal ST depression and upright precordial T waves versus downsloping ST depression and T-wave inversion in 27 patients with an anterior non–Q wave MI.

219. **Casas RE,** et al. Value of leads V_7–V_9 in diagnosing posterior wall acute MI and other causes of tall R waves in V_1–V_2. *Am J Cardiol* 1997;80:508–509. This large retrospective analysis found that 250 of approximately 17,000 hospital patients had leads V7 to V9 assessed because of a tall R in V1 and/or suspicion of posterior MI. Among this selected group, 110 patients had evidence of new or old posterior MI, and in 25% of cases, V7 to V9 were the only leads diagnostic of MI.

COCAINE-ASSOCIATED MYOCARDIAL INFARCTION

220. **Hollander JE,** et al. Prospective multicenter evaluation of cocaine-associated chest pain. *Acad Emerg Med* 1994;1:330–339.

This prospective cohort study was composed of 246 patients with cocaine-associated chest pain. Pain began at a median 60 minutes after cocaine use and persisted for 120 minutes. Fourteen (5.7%) patients had a confirmed MI (elevated CK-MB). ECG showed a low sensitivity (35.7%) and high specificity (89.9%). No clinical differences were seen between those with and without MI.

221. **Hollander JE.** The management of cocaine-associated myocardial ischemia. *N Engl J Med* 1995;333:1267–1272.

This review covers pathophysiology, initial evaluation, treatment, complications, diagnostic evaluation, long-term prognosis, and secondary prevention of cocaine-associated ischemia.

222. **Hollander JE,** et al. Predictors of coronary artery disease in patients with cocaine-associated MI. *Am J Med* 1997;102:158–163.

   This retrospective analysis of 70 patients from 29 centers found CAD, defined as 50% or more stenosis or positive stress test result, demonstrated in 70%. The patient with CAD was older (42 years vs. 31 years) and had more cardiac risk factors (2.3 vs. 1.5), hypertension (OR, 5.3), and bradyarrhythmias (OR, 8.0). A greater percentage also had inferior location ($p = 0.04$).

NON–Q WAVE/NON–ST ELEVATION MYOCARDIAL INFARCTION

See Chapter 3.

Assessment and Prognosis

GENERAL REVIEW ARTICLES/MISCELLANEOUS

223. **Shaw LJ,** et al. A meta-analysis of pre-discharge risk stratification after acute MI with stress electrocardiography myocardial perfusion and ventricular function imaging. *Am J Cardiol* 1996;78:1327–1337.

   This analysis of 54 studies (76% retrospective) with 19,874 patients shows the low positive predictive value of predischarge noninvasive testing.

224. **Morrow DA,** et al. TIMI risk score for ST-elevation myocardial infarction: a convenient, bedside, clinical score for risk assessment at presentation: an intravenous nPA for treatment of infarcting myocardium early II trial substudy. *Circulation* 2000;102:2031–2037.

   The TIMI risk score for STEMI was created as the arithmetic sum of independent mortality predictors based on a logistic regression analysis of the 14,114-patient Intravenously nPA for Treatment of Infarcting Myocardium Early II (InTIME II) trial. The 10 baseline variables constituting the TIMI risk score accounted for 97% of the predictive capacity of the multivariate model. These included age 65 to 74 years (2 points); age older than 75 years (3 points); diabetes, hypertension, or angina (1 point); SBP less than 100 mm Hg (3 points); HR more than 100 beats/min (2 points); Killip class II to IV (2 points); weight less than 67 kg (1 point); anterior STEMI or LBBB (1 point); and time to treatment more than 4 hours (1 point). The risk score showed a more than 40-fold graded increase in mortality (<1% with a score of 0 vs. 35.9% for a score >8). The prognostic capacity of the TIMI risk score was similar to the full multivariable model (c statistic, 0.779 vs. 0.784). External validation in the TIMI 9 trial showed similar prognostic capacity (c statistic, 0.746).

225. **Morrow DA,** et al. Application of the TIMI risk score for ST-elevation MI in the National Registry of Myocardial Infarction 3. *JAMA* 2001;286:1356–1359.

   The TIMI risk score was evaluated in 84,029 STEMI patients treated from 1998 to 2000 and data recorded in the NRMI 3 registry. Only 48% received reperfusion therapy. NRMI 3 patients were older and more often female and with a history of CAD than were those in the derivation set. A significant graded increase in mortality was found with increasing TIMI risk score (range, 1.1% to 30.0%; $p < 0.001$ for trend). The risk score showed strong prognostic capacity overall ($c = 0.74$ vs. 0.78 in derivation set). It was equally predictive in those treated with fibrinolysis ($c = 0.79$) and primary PCI ($c = 0.80$). Among patients not receiving fibrinolytic therapy, absolute mortality rates were much higher for a given risk score, but the same pattern (higher score, higher risk) was seen, although with lower discriminatory capacity ($c = 0.65$).

226. **Eagle KA,** et al. for the GRACE Investigators. A validated prediction model for all forms of acute coronary syndrome: estimating the risk of 6-month postdischarge death in an international registry. *JAMA* 2004;291:2727–2733.

The researchers used data from the GRACE multinational registry of patients with ACS, including 17,142 presentations, to develop a risk-prediction model for 6-month outcomes. A separate cohort of 7,638 was subsequently used to validate the model. In multivariable analyses, they identified significant predictors of 6-month mortality: older age, history of MI, history of CHF, increased pulse at presentation, lower SBP at presentation, elevated initial creatinine, elevated initial cardiac biomarkers, ST-segment depression on initial ECG, and not having PCI in-hospital (see also *Arch Int Med* 2003;163:2345–2353; *BMJ* 2006;333:1091 for additional risk-prediction analyses from GRACE).

ELECTROCARDIOGRAPHY, ARRHYTHMIAS, AND CONDUCTION SYSTEM

227. **Volpi A,** et al. In-hospital prognosis of patients with acute MI complicated by primary ventricular fibrillation. *N Engl J Med* 1987;317:257–261.

This analysis focused on 11,112 GISSI patients. Primary VF (defined as not due to shock or MI) occurred in 2.8% and was associated with a nearly twofold higher in-hospital mortality rate (10.8% vs. 5.9%; RR, 1.94; 95% CI, 1.35 to 2.78).

228. **Multicenter Investigation of the Limitation of Infarct Size (MILIS).** Prognosis after cardiac arrest due to ventricular tachycardia or ventricular fibrillation associated with acute MI. *Am J Cardiol* 1987;60:755–761.

This analysis focused on 849 MILIS study patients aged 75 years or younger with a confirmed MI. Mean follow-up period was 32 months. VT and VF patients had a fourfold higher in-hospital mortality rate (27% vs. 7%; $p < 0.001$). This difference was attributable to a sevenfold higher risk in patients with secondary causes of VT and VF (e.g., presence of heart failure, hypotension). A worse outcome was attained if the episode occurred after 72 hours (57% vs. 20%; $p < 0.05$). No cases of primary VT and VF occurred after 72 hours. No difference in mortality at follow-up was seen among hospital survivors.

229. **Berger PB,** et al. Incidence and significance of ventricular tachycardia and fibrillation in the absence of hypotension or heart failure in acute MI treated with recombinant tissuetype plasminogen activator: results from the Thrombolysis in Myocardial Infarction (TIMI) phase II trial. *J Am Coll Cardiol* 1993;22:1773–1779.

This analysis focused on 2,456 TIMI II patients without CHF or hypotension during the first 24 hours after study entry. Sustained VT or VF developed in 1.9% within 24 hours. Among patients undergoing angiography at 18 to 48 hours (per protocol), the VT and VF group had lower IRA patency (68% vs. 87%; $p = 0.01$). Mortality at 21 days was more than 10 times higher in the VT and VF patients (20.4% vs. 1.6%; $p < 0.001$). Survival from 21 days to 1 year was similar in both groups.

230. **Schroder R,** et al. Extent of early ST segment elevation resolution: a strong predictor of outcome in patients with acute MI and a sensitive measure to compare thrombolytic regimens. *J Am Coll Cardiol* 1995;26:1657–1664.

This prospective study was composed of 1,398 INJECT patients seen within 6 hours of symptom onset. ST resolution at 3 hours was classified into three groups: complete (>70%), partial (30% to 70%), and no (<30%) resolution. The 35-day mortality rates in these groups were 2.5%, 4.3%, and 17.5% ($p < 0.0001$). Even after baseline characteristics were included, ST resolution was the most powerful predictor of 35-day mortality.

231. **Mont L,** et al. Predisposing factors and prognostic value of sustained monomorphic ventricular tachycardia in early phase of acute MI. *J Am Coll Cardiol* 1996;28:1670–1676.

This retrospective analysis focused on 1,120 consecutive cardiac care unit patients. The incidence of monomorphic VT was 1.9%. This group had larger infarcts (peak CK-MB, 435 IU/L vs. 168 IU/L) and four times higher mortality (43% vs. 11%; $p < 0.001$). VT was an independent mortality predictor, whereas independent predictors of VT were CK-MB (OR, 11.8), Killip class (OR, 4.0), and bifascicular block (OR, 3.1).

232. **Hathaway WR,** et al. Prognostic significance of the initial electrocardiogram in patients with acute MI. *JAMA* 1998;279:387–391.

This retrospective analysis focused on 34,166 GUSTO I patients without paced or ventricular rhythms or LBBB. In multivariate analysis, 30-day mortality predictors were found to be the sum of ST deviation (depression and elevation; OR, 1.53), hazard ratio (OR, 1.49), and QRS duration.

233. **Volpi A,** et al. Incidence and prognosis of early primary ventricular fibrillation in acute MI: results of the GISSI-2 database. *Am J Cardiol* 1998;82:265–271.

This retrospective analysis focused on 9,720 patients with a first MI. Early (4 hours or less) and late (>4 to 48 hours) primary VF occurred in 3.1% and 0.6%, respectively. Recurrence rates were 11% and 15%. Early primary VF occurred more frequently if SBP was less than 120 mm Hg and in the presence of hypokalemia. In-hospital mortality was higher in patients with both early and late primary VF [ORs, 2.47 (95% CI, 1.48 to 4.13) and 3.97 (95% CI, 1.51 to 10.48)]. Mortality from hospital discharge to 6 months was similar for both primary VF subgroups and controls.

234. **Go AS,** et al. Bundle-branch block and in-hospital mortality in acute MI. *Ann Intern Med* 1998;129:690–697.

This large retrospective cohort study of 297,832 patients from 1,571 hospitals showed that the prevalences of RBBB and LBBB are similar (6.2% and 6.7%, respectively) and that RBBB is a stronger independent predictor of in-hospital death [adjusted OR, 1.64 vs. 1.34 (LBBB)].

235. **Cheema AN,** et al. Nonsustained ventricular tachycardia in the setting of acute MI. *Circulation* 1998;98:2030–2036.

This prospective database analysis showed that contrary to prevailing opinion, NSVT that occurs beyond several hours after AMI is associated with adverse outcomes. NSVT was identified in 118 patients within 72 hours of AMI. The control group was matched for age, sex, type of MI, and thrombolytic therapy. The NSVT group had more frequent in-hospital VF (9% vs. none; $p < 0.001$), but in-hospital mortality (10% vs. 4%) and follow-up mortality (10% vs. 17%) were not significantly different. However, a multivariate analysis showed that time from presentation to NSVT was the strongest mortality predictor (risk became significant at 13 hours and peaked at 24 hours; RR, 7.5).

236. **Savonitto S,** et al. Prognostic value of the admission electrocardiogram in acute coronary syndromes. *JAMA* 1999;281:707–713.

This retrospective analysis focused on 12,142 GUSTO-IIb patients. Presenting ECG characteristics included T-wave inversion in 22%, ST elevation in 28%, ST depression in 35%, and 15% with a combination of ST elevation and depression. The 30-day incidence of death or MI was 5.5% in patients with T-wave inversion, 9.4% in those with ST elevation, 10.5% in those with ST depression, and 12.4% in those with both ST elevation and depression. After adjusting for factors associated with increased death or MI at 30 days, compared with those with T-wave inversion only, patients with ST-segment changes were at significantly increased risk (ORs, 1.68, 1.62, and 2.27 for ST elevation, ST depression, and both, respectively). Admission CK levels were associated with increased risk of death (OR, 2.36) and death or MI (OR, 1.56). In a multivariate analysis, ECG category and CK levels at admission remained highly predictive of death and MI.

EXERCISE TESTING

237. **Hamm LF,** et al. Safety and efficacy of exercise testing early after acute MI. *Am J Cardiol* 1989;63:1193–1197.

This analysis focused on 151,949 tests performed at 570 institutions; 42% were symptom-limited tests. Overall, only 41 fatal (0.03%) and 141 major cardiac complications (0.09%) were noted. Symptom-limited testing was associated with a similar mortality rate, but with 1.9 times more major cardiac complications.

238. **Chaitman BR,** et al. Impact of treatment strategy on predischarge exercise test in TIMI-II. *Am J Cardiol* 1993;71:131–138.

This analysis focused on 3,339 patients showing a fourfold higher 1-year mortality rate if no predischarge exercise test was done (7.7% vs. 1.8%; $p < 0.001$). No predictive value of ST depression or chest pain was observed: conservative RR, 0.6 (95% CI, 0.1 to 2.9); invasive RR, 2.1 (95% CI, 0.5 to 9.4). However, catheterization and revascularization are recommended if ETT is positive.

239. **Jain A,** et al. Comparison of symptom-limited and low level exercise tolerance tests early after MI. *J Am Coll Cardiol* 1993;22:1816–1820.

This analysis focused on 150 consecutive patients [44 others were excluded (death, ischemia at rest or with minimal ambulation, complications, physician/patient preference)]. Bruce protocol was performed at 6.4 ± 3.1 days. Low-level test results were positive in only 23% versus 40% with symptom-limited tests ($p < 0.001$). At follow-up (15 ± 5 months), only 5 patients with a negative maximal test result versus 14 patients with a nondiagnostic symptom-limited test had cardiac events.

240. **Zaret BL,** et al. Value of radionuclide rest and exercise left ventricular ejection fraction in assessing survival of patients after thrombolytic therapy for acute MI: results of TIMI II Study. *J Am Coll Cardiol* 1995;26:73–79.

The 2,567 patients were studied at average 9 hours after onset of symptoms. Rest EF was strongly associated with 1-year mortality (overall, 9.9%). The RR for EF of 30% to 39% was 3.1; 40% to 49%, 2.2; and 50% to 59%, 1.2. The differential between rest and exercise EF was not helpful.

241. **Villella A,** et al. Prognostic significance of maximal exercise testing after MI treated with thrombolytic agents: the GISSI-2 data base. *Lancet* 1995;346:523–529.

This post hoc analysis focused on 6,295 GISSI-2 patients tested an average of 28 days after AMI. The same mortality rate (7.1%) was observed among those with a positive ETT result as in those who did not undergo testing; lower rates were associated with nondiagnostic and negative tests (1.3% and 0.9%, respectively). Independent predictors of mortality were symptomatic ischemia and low work capacity (RRs, 2.1 and 1.8).

ECHOCARDIOGRAPHY AND OTHER NONINVASIVE TESTS

242. **Sutton MSJ,** et al. Quantitative two-dimensional echocardiography measurements are major predictors of adverse cardiovascular events after acute MI. *Circulation* 1994;89: 68–75.

A total of 521 SAVE trial patients had echocardiograms at 11.1 ± 3.2 days. At 1 year, LVED and LV end-systolic areas were smaller in the captopril group ($p = 0.038, 0.015$). The captopril group had 35% fewer cardiovascular events. In these patients with cardiovascular events, a more than threefold increase in LV cavity areas was observed.

243. **Picano E,** et al. Stress echocardiography results predict risk of reinfarction early after uncomplicated acute MI: large-scale multicenter study. *J Am Coll Cardiol* 1995;26:908–913.

The 1,080 patients underwent a dipyridamole echocardiography study at 10 ± 5 days. Follow-up period was 14 months. A positive test result (44%) was associated with a higher reinfarction rate (6.3% vs. 3.3%; $p < 0.01$).

244. **Sicari R,** et al. ECHO Dobutamine International Cooperative (EDIC) Study. Prognostic value of dobutamine-atropine stress echocardiography early after acute MI. *J Am Coll Cardiol* 1997;29:254–260.

In this prospective, observational, multicenter trial, 778 patients with first MI were tested at an average of 12 days, with follow-up testing at 9 ± 7 months. Positive test results were attained in 56%. No difference in event rates (death, MI, unstable angina, angioplasty, bypass surgery) was observed regardless of positive or negative test results: 14% versus 12% ($p = 0.3$). However, when only spontaneously occurring events were considered, myocardial viability was the best predictor (hazard ratio, 2.0; $p < 0.002$). Wall-motion stroke index is a very strong predictor of cardiac deaths only (hazard ratio, 9.2; $p < 0.0001$).

245. **Migrino RQ,** et al. End-systolic volume index at 90 to 180 minutes into reperfusion therapy for acute MI is a strong predictor of early and late mortality. *Circulation* 1997;96:116–121.

The 1,300 patients underwent left ventriculography. End-systolic volume index of 40 mL/m^2 or less was independently associated with increased 30-day and 1-year mortality rates [adjusted ORs, 3.4 (95% CI, 2.0 to 5.9), 4.1 (95% CI, 2.6 to 6.2); $p < 0.001$]. Independent predictors of high end-systolic volume index of 40 or less were SBP less than 110 mm Hg, anterior MI, male, prior angina or MI, weight less than 70 kg, and HR 80 beats/min or less.

FLOW AND VESSEL PATENCY

246. **Dewood MA,** et al. Prevalence of total coronary occlusion during the early hours of transmural MI. *N Engl J Med* 1980;303:897–902.

This classic angiography study demonstrated the central role of thrombotic occlusion in the pathogenesis of transmural MI. A total of 322 patients underwent catheterization at less than 24 hours. Total occlusion of the IRA was seen in 87% at less than 4 hours versus 65% at 12 to 24 hours.

247. **Karagounis L,** et al. Does TIMI perfusion grade 2 represent a mostly patent artery or a mostly occluded artery? Enzymatic and electrocardiographic evidence from the TEAM-2 study (Trial of Eminase in Acute MI). *J Am Coll Cardiol* 1992;19:1–10.

This analysis focused on 359 TEAM II patients treated with APSAC or SK. Angiography was performed at 90 to 240 minutes. TIMI grade 3 flow was associated with earlier enzymatic peaks and better ECG indexes of MI than TIMI grade flows 0 to 2 ($p = 0.02$ to 0.0001). No differences were found between TIMI flow grades 0, 1, and 2.

248. **Gibson CM,** et al. Angiographic predictors of reocclusion after thrombolysis: results from TIMI-4. *J Am Coll Cardiol* 1995;25:582–589.

The 278 patients were randomized to APSAC, rtPA, or combination therapy. Higher reocclusion (at 18 to 36 hours) was associated with TIMI grade 2 versus 3 flow (10% vs. 2%; $p = 0.003$), ulcerated lesions (10% vs. 3%; $p = 0.009$), and positive collateral vessels (18% vs. 5.6%; $p = 0.03$). Similar trends were seen for eccentric (7% vs. 2%; $p = 0.06$) and thrombotic lesions (8% vs. 3%; $p = 0.06$). Reocclusion also was associated with more severe mean stenosis at 90 minutes (78% vs. 74%; $p = 0.04$).

249. **Simes RJ,** et al. Link between the angiographic substudy and mortality outcomes in a large randomized trial of myocardial reperfusion: importance of early and complete infarct artery reperfusion. *Circulation* 1995;91:1923–1928.

This GUSTO I substudy of 1,210 patients showed that TIMI grade 3 flow at 90 minutes was associated with decreased mortality. A model was developed that assumed any difference in treatment effects on 30-day mortality were mediated through differences in 90-minute IRA patency. The model showed a strong correlation ($r = 0.97$) between actual and predicted mortality rates. These data provide support for the idea that improved survival is due to achievement of early and complete reperfusion.

250. **Lenderink T,** et al. Benefit of thrombolytic therapy is sustained throughout 5 years and is related to TIMI perfusion grade 3 but not grade 2 flow at discharge. *Circulation* 1995;92:1110–1116.

This study showed the benefits of achieving TIMI grade 3 flow. Five-year follow-up data were analyzed on 923 hospital survivors enrolled in the ECSG studies. Patients with TIMI grade 3 flow had a 91% 5-year survival rate compared with 84% for the TIMI grade 0 to 1 and TIMI grade 2 groups ($p^2 = 0.01$).

251. **Anderson JL,** et al. Meta-analysis of five reported studies on the relation of early coronary patency grades with mortality and outcomes after acute MI. *Am J Cardiol* 1996;78:1–8.

This meta-analysis focused on five studies with 3,969 patients. The mortality rate was 8.8% for TIMI grade 0/1, 7% for grade 2, and only 3.7% for grade 2 patients (grade 3 vs. grade 2; $p = 0.001$). TIMI grade 3 flow also was associated with better EFs and less time to CK peak.

252. **Reiner JS,** et al. Evolution of early TIMI 2 flow after thrombolysis for acute MI. *Circulation* 1996;94:2441–2446.

This analysis of the GUSTO Angiography Study showed the benefit of progressing from early TIMI grade 2 flow to grade 3 at follow-up. Of 914 patients with TIMI grade 2 flow, 278 underwent angiography at both 90 minutes and 5 to 7 days. In the group that improved to grade 3 flow by the second catheterization (67%), a higher mean EF (57.5% vs. 52.8%; $p = 0.02$), better infarct zone wall motion ($p = 0.01$), and less visible thrombus (26% vs. 38%; $p = 0.04$) were found. However, TIMI grade 3 flow at 90 minutes remained the best, with less thrombus (42% vs. 58%; $p < 0.0001$) and highest 5- to 7-day EF (61.7% vs. 57.5%; $p = 0.002$).

253. **Pilote L,** et al. Determinants of the use of angiography and revascularization after thrombolysis for acute MI. *N Engl J Med* 1996;335:1198–1205.

This post hoc analysis focused on 21,772 GUSTO I patients; 71% had predischarge angiography, of whom 58% underwent revascularization (PTCA, 73%). Overall, the best predictor of angiography use was age [if younger than 73 years, 76% (vs. 53%)]. Among young patients, PTCA availability was the most important predictor [83% vs. 67% (no PTCA)]. The number two predictor was recurrent ischemia. Reassuringly, coronary anatomy was the top predictor of the use and type of revascularization. However, the study yielded several unexpected findings: (a) similar revascularization rate in those with three-vessel disease and LV dysfunction as those with an EF less than 50% and one- or two-vessel disease and LAD stenosis of 50% or less; (b) many without symptoms had revascularization for one- or two-vessel disease; and (c) patients younger than 80 years with CHF or cardiogenic shock had similar angiography rates to those without these findings.

254. **Selby JV,** et al. Variation among hospitals in coronary angiography practices and outcomes after MI in a large health maintenance organization. *N Engl J Med* 1996;335:1888–1896.

This retrospective cohort study was composed of 6,851 patients treated from 1990 to 1992 at 16 hospitals. By 3 months, 30% to 77% had undergone angiography. After multivariate analysis, angiography rates in all hospitals were found to be inversely related to the risk of death from heart disease and heart disease events ($p = 0.03$; $p < 0.001$). However, at higher-angiography-rate hospitals, angiography was associated with lower risks of death and any heart disease event (hazard ratios, 0.67 and 0.72). In patients without indications for angiography, less benefit was seen at high-volume centers (hazard ratios, 0.85 and 0.90).

255. **Barbagelata NA,** et al. TIMI grade 3 flow and reocclusion after intravenous thrombolytic therapy: a pooled analysis. *Am Heart J* 1997;133:273–282.

Analysis of 15 TIMI flow studies with 5,475 angiograms and 27 reocclusion studies with 3,147 angiograms. TIMI grade 3 flow rates at 60 and 90 minutes were as follows: with accelerated tPA, 57.1/63.2%; standard tPA, 39.5/50.2%; APSAC, 40.2/50.1%; and SK, 31.5% (90 minutes). Reocclusion rates were as follows: with accelerated tPA, 6.0%; standard tPA, 11.8%; APSAC, 3.0%; and SK, 4.2%.

256. **Puma JA,** et al. Support for the open-artery hypothesis in survivors of acute MI: analysis of 11,228 patients treated with thrombolytic therapy. *Am J Cardiol* 1999;83:482–487.

This analysis focused on 11,228 GUSTO I patients with available IRA patency data. Both univariate and multivariable analyses showed that an open artery was associated with a significantly lower 30-day mortality rate ($p < 0.001$). This benefit appears to extend beyond that provided by myocardial salvage because the effect remained after adjustment for LVEF.

257. **Gibson CM,** et al. Relationship between TIMI frame count and clinical outcomes after thrombolytic administration. *Circulation* 1999;99:1945–1950.

CTFC was measured in 1,248 patients in TIMI 4, 10A, and 10B trials. Patients who died in the hospital and by 30 to 42 days had higher CTFCs (69.6 vs. 49.5, $p = 0.0003$; 66.2 vs. 49.9, $p = 0.006$). In a multivariate model, CTFC was an independent predictor of in-hospital mortality (OR, 1.21 per 10-frame increase). The risk of in-hospital mortality increased in a graded fashion from none in patients with the fastest flow (0 to 13 frames, hyperemia, TIMI grade 4 flow) to 2.7% in patients with CTFC of 14 to 40 (CTFC 40 is the cutoff for TIMI grade 3 flow), to 6.4% in patients with CTFC greater than 40 ($p = 0.003$).

MICROVASCULAR PERFUSION

258. **Gibson CM,** et al. for the TIMI Study Group. Relationship of TIMI myocardial perfusion grade to mortality after administration of thrombolytic drugs. *Circulation* 2000;101:125–130.

The TMP grade system was developed to assess the filling and clearance of contrast in the myocardium. TMPG 0 was defined as no apparent tissue-level perfusion (no ground glass appearance of blush or opacification of the myocardium) in culprit artery distribution; TMPG 1 indicates presence of myocardial blush but no clearance from the microvasculature (blush or a stain was present on the next injection); TMPG 2 blush clears slowly (blush is strongly persistent and diminishes minimally or not at all during three cardiac cycles of the washout phase); and TMPG 3 indicates that blush begins to clear during washout (blush is minimally persistent after three cardiac cycles of washout). Among 762 patients enrolled in the TIMI 10B trial, a significant mortality gradient was found across TMPGs, with mortality lowest in those patients with TMPG 3 (2.0%), intermediate in TMPG 2 (4.4%), and highest in TMPGs 0 and 1 (6.0%; three-way $p = 0.05$). Even among patients with TIMI grade 3 flow in the epicardial artery, the TMPGs allowed further risk stratification of 30-day mortality: 0.73% for TMPG 3; 2.9% for TMPG 2; 5.0% for TMPG 0 or 1 ($p = 0.03$ for TMPG 3 vs. grades 0, 1, and 2; three-way $p = 0.066$). TMPG 3 flow was a multivariate correlate of 30-day mortality (OR, 0.35; 95% CI, 0.12 to 1.02; $p = 0.054$) in a multivariate model that adjusted for the presence of TIMI 3 flow ($p = NS$), the CTFC (OR, 1.02; $p = 0.06$), the presence of an anterior MI (OR, 2.3; $p = 0.03$), admission hazard ratio ($p = NS$), female sex ($p = NS$), and age (OR, 1.1, $p < 0.001$).

259. **Gibson CM,** et al. Relationship of the TIMI myocardial perfusion grades, flow grades, frame count, and percutaneous coronary intervention to long-term outcomes after thrombolytic administration in acute myocardial infarction. *Circulation* 2002;105:1909–1913.

This analysis examined 848 patients from the TIMI 10B trial (compared tPA with TNK) who had 2-year follow-up. Improved survival was associated with TIMI grade 2/3 flow (Cox hazard ratio, 0.41; $p = 0.001$), reduced CTFCs ($p = 0.02$), and an open microvasculature (TMPG, 2/3; hazard ratio, 0.51; $p = 0.038$). Rescue PCI of closed arteries (TFG, 0/1) at 90 minutes was associated with lower mortality ($p = 0.03$), and mortality trended lower with adjunctive PCI of open (TFG, 2/3) arteries ($p = 0.11$). In a multivariate model correcting for previously identified correlates of mortality (age, sex, pulse, LAD as culprit vessel, and any PCI during initial hospitalization), patency (TFG, 2/3; hazard ratio, 0.32; $p < 0.001$), CTFC ($p = 0.01$), and TMPG 2/3 remained associated with reduced mortality (hazard ratio, 0.46; $p = 0.02$).

260. **Gibson CM,** et al. for the TIMI Study Group. Association of duration of symptoms at presentation with angiographic and clinical outcomes after fibrinolytic therapy in patients with ST-segment elevation myocardial infarction. *J Am Coll Cardiol* 2004;44:980–987.

This analysis of 3,845 patients in various TIMI trials examined the relationship between TMPG and symptom duration in patients receiving thrombolysis for acute STEMI. Patients with impaired myocardial perfusion had longer median times from symptom onset to treatment (3 hours for TMPG 0/1 vs. 2.7 hours for TMPG 2/3, $p = 0.001$). This relationship remained robust in a multivariable model ($p = 0.007$). Furthermore, delayed time from onset of symptoms was also associated with increased 30-day mortality (6.6% for time >4 hours vs. 3.3%, $p < 0.001$). These findings highlight the potential pathophysiologic background for poorer clinical outcomes linked to delayed presentation.

261. **Cragg DR,** et al. Outcome of patients with acute MI who are ineligible for thrombolytic therapy. *Ann Intern Med* 1991;115:173–177.

This retrospective analysis focused on 1,471 patients; 16% were given thrombolysis on protocols (88% TIMI IIB), and 7% had nonprotocol lysis, primary balloon angioplasty, or both. The nonthrombolysed group was older, more likely to be female, and more frequently had hypertension and prior MIs. Ineligible patients had a fivefold higher mortality rate (19% vs. 4%; $p < 0.001$). Independent mortality predictors were age older than 76 years, stroke or other bleeding risk, ineligible ECG, or two exclusion criteria.

262. **Barbash GI,** et al. Significance of smoking in patients receiving thrombolytic therapy for acute MI: experience gleaned from the International tPA/Streptokinase Mortality Trial. *Circulation* 1993;87:53–58.

This analysis of 8,259 International tPA/SK Trial patients found a protective effect of smoking in patients with acute MI. Both nonsmokers (more diabetes, higher Killip class, and older) and ex-smokers had more in-hospital reinfarctions (4.7% and 5% vs. 2.7%; $p < 0.001$) and decreased in-hospital and 6-month mortality rates (13%/18%, 8%/12%, 5%/8%).

263. **Grines CL,** et al. Effect of cigarette smoking on outcome after thrombolytic therapy for MI. *Circulation* 1995;91:298–303.

This study showed that better outcomes in smokers with MI may be due to a low-risk profile. Analysis of 1,619 patients treated with tPA, urokinase, or both in six MI trials showed that smokers had similar 90-minute patency (but higher grade 3 flow: 41.1% vs. 34.6%; $p = 0.03$) but lower in-hospital mortality rates (4% vs. 8.9%; $p = 0.0001$). However, after adjustments [lower age (54 years vs. 60 years), more inferior MIs (60% vs. 53%), less three-vessel disease (16% vs. 22%), and higher baseline EF (53% vs. 50%)], no independent prognostic significance was associated with smoking.

264. **Lee KL,** et al. Predictors of 30-day mortality in the era of reperfusion for acute MI: results from an international trial of 41,021 patients. *Circulation* 1995;91:1659–1668.

Multivariate analysis showed the strong influence of age on mortality rate (only 1.1% if younger than 45 years, 20.5% if older than 75 years). Other factors associated with mortality included lower SBP, higher Killip class, elevated HR, and anterior infarct. These five factors contribute approximately 90% of prognostic information.

265. **Woodfield SL,** et al. Gender and acute MI: is there a different response to thrombolysis? *J Am Coll Cardiol* 1997;29:35–42.

This GUSTO Angiography Substudy analysis showed female gender to be an independent risk factor for mortality. The women had some high-risk features (e.g., older, more hypertension, diabetes, and heart failure) and some low-risk features (e.g., fewer prior MIs and bypass surgery, less smoking). The unadjusted 30-day mortality rate was nearly three times higher (13.1% vs. 4.8%; $p < 0.001$), and after multivariate analysis, female gender remained an independent mortality predictor.

OTHER

266. **Case RB,** et al. Living alone after MI. *JAMA* 1992;267:515–519.

This analysis of 1,234 MI patients with an average follow-up of 2.1 years showed that living alone was associated with 54% more endpoints (nonfatal MI plus cardiac death).

267. **Frasure-Smith N,** et al. Depression following MI. *JAMA* 1993;270:1819–1825.

This small study was composed of 222 MI patients who survived to hospital discharge. Patients were interviewed at average 7 days (major depression, 2 weeks). Depression was associated with a 4.3-fold higher mortality rate ($p = 0.013$). The impact was at least equivalent to that of LV dysfunction (Killip class) and prior MI. Editorial points out that typically 15% to 20% of post-MI patients have major depression.

268. **Kuhl EA,** et al. Relation of anxiety and adherence to risk-reducing recommendations following myocardial infarction. *Am J Cardiol* 2009;103:1629–1634.

Among 278 patients with acute MI, in multivariable analysis anxiety predicted poorer adherence to many risk-reducing therapies (pharmacologic and nonpharmacologic). It was the only predictor of poor adherence to smoking cessation.

269. **Jollis JG,** et al. Outcome of acute MI according to the specialty of the admitting physician. *N Engl J Med* 1996;335:1880–1887.

This retrospective analysis of 8,241 Medicare patients showed that cardiologists provide optimal care for MI patients. All-cause 1-year mortality HRs (based on admitting physician) were as follows: cardiologists, 0.88; family medicine, 0.98; general practitioner, 1.06; and other, 1.16. Cardiologist-treated patients were younger and healthier and had less diabetes, more Killip class I, lower predicted 30-day mortality rates (GUSTO I model; 18% vs. 20%), and longer hospital stay (9.3 days vs. 7.3 to 8.6 days). Cardiologists used thrombolysis about twice as often; used angiography, revascularization, treadmill tests, nuclear imaging, Holter monitoring, and echocardiography more frequently; and gave more patients aspirin, β-blockers, and heparin. In an analysis of all 1992 Medicare claims (approximately 220,000 patients), the same mortality pattern emerged: with cardiologists, 30%; internists, 37%; family medicine, 39%; and general practitioners, 40%. Although 82% of the attending physicians were the same as the admitting physician, the roles of consultants and transfers were not assessed.

270. **Bradley EH,** et al. Hospital quality for acute myocardial infarction correlation among process measures and relationship with short-term mortality. *JAMA* 2006;296:72–78.

The investigators sought to correlate quality-of-care measures, as determined by Centers for Medicare & Medicaid Services (CMS) and the Joint Commission on Accreditation of Healthcare Organizations (JCAHO), with 30-day clinical outcomes for acute MI in the

NRMI. Core measures, such as β-blocker use at admission/discharge, aspirin at admission/discharge, and ACE use, were significantly correlated with 30-day mortality rates of hospitals (correlation coefficients ≥ 0.40, $p < 0.001$ for pairwise comparisons). However, these measures captured only explained a small fraction of variability in hospitals' mortality rates (~6%).

271. **Williams SC,** et al. Performance of top-ranked heart care hospitals on evidence-based process measures. *Circulation* 2006;114:558–564.

Hospitals at the top of *US News & World Report's* "America's Best Hospitals" were assessed for compliance with measures from the American College of Cardiology and AHA's clinical treatment guidelines for heart failure and acute MI. They aggregated 10 rate-based, performance measures into a cardiovascular composite score. While on the whole, hospitals at the top of the list did better than the rest (86% of measures met vs. 83%, $p < 0.05$), only 23 of "America's Best Hospitals" met such standards more frequently than the overall average.

Complications of Myocardial Infarction

ARRHYTHMIAS, BUNDLE BRANCH BLOCK

272. **Antman EM,** Berlin JA Declining incidence of ventricular fibrillation in MI: implications for prophylactic use of lidocaine. *Circulation* 1992;86:764–773.

This analysis focused on 18 randomized trials with 4,754 patients. Earlier year of publication (range, 1969 to 1988) was a significant predictor of VF ($p = 0.002$), even after adjusting for other variables. The incidence of VF in controls decreased from 4.5% in 1970 to only 0.35% in 1990.

273. **Solomon SD,** et al. Ventricular arrhythmias in trials of thrombolytic therapy for acute MI: a meta-analysis. *Circulation* 1993;88:2575–2581.

This analysis focused on 15 randomized trials with 39,606 patients. Thrombolytic administration was associated with lower risk of VF during the entire hospitalization (OR, 0.83; 95% CI, 0.76 to 0.90; $p < 0.0001$) but not in the first 6 or 24 hours after thrombolysis (ORs, 0.98 and 1.00). Thrombolytic use also was associated with a higher incidence of VT during hospitalization (OR, 1.34; 95% CI, 1.15 to 1.55; $p < 0.0001$).

274. **Newby KH,** et al. Incidence and clinical relevance of the occurrence of bundle branch block in patients treated with thrombolytic therapy. *Circulation* 1996;94:2424–2428.

This study was composed of 681 TAMI-9 and GUSTO I patients who underwent continuous 12-lead ECG monitoring for 36 to 72 hours. BBB occurred in 23.6% (RBBB, 13%; LBBB, 7%; alternating, 3.5%). Mortality was 2.5 times higher in BBB patients compared with those without BBB (8.7% vs. 3.5%; $p = 0.007$). The highest mortality rate was observed in those with persistent BBB [19.4% vs. 5.6 (transient) and 3.5% (none); $p < 0.001$]. BBB patients also had decreased EF, increased peak CK, and more diseased vessels.

275. **Crenshaw BS,** et al. Atrial fibrillation in the setting of acute MI: the GUSTO I experience. *J Am Coll Cardiol* 1997;30:406–413.

AF on admission ECG in 2.5%, increasing to 7.9% after study enrollment. The group with early and late AF had more three-vessel disease, less TIMI grade 3 flow, more in-hospital strokes (3.1% vs. 1.3%; $p = 0.0001$), and more than twofold higher unadjusted 30-day and 1-year mortality rates (14.3% vs. 6.2%, $p = 0.0001$; 21.5% vs. 8.6%, $p < 0.0001$). In multivariate analysis, late AF predictors were age, peak CK, Killip class, and HR. Adjusted ORs of mortality were 1.1 for baseline AF (85% CI, 0.88 to 1.3) and 1.4 for late AF (95% CI, 1.3 to 1.5).

CARDIAC RUPTURE

276. **Becker RC,** et al. Cardiac rupture associated with thrombolytic therapy: impact of time to treatment in the LATE (Late Assessment of Thrombolytic Efficacy) study. *J Am Coll Cardiol* 1995;25:1063–1068.

This analysis of 5,711 LATE patients found that cardiac rupture was the listed cause of death in 53 (9.7%) of 547 patients who died in the first 35 days. No increased risk of rupture was found in the group receiving rtPA at 6 to 24 hours compared with the placebo group. However, rupture events did occur earlier in the thrombolytic group (treatment × time to death interaction; $p = 0.03$).

277. **Becker RC,** et al. A composite view of cardiac rupture in the U.S. National Registry of MI. *J Am Coll Cardiol* 1996;27:1321–1326.

In this analysis of 350,755 patients, thrombolytic administration (approximately 12,000 patients) was associated with 5.9% mortality (no thrombolytic therapy, 12.9%). Cardiac rupture was reported as the cause of death in 12% of patients who received thrombolysis [vs. 6% (no thrombolysis)] and occurred more frequently within the first 24 hours.

278. **Anzai T,** et al. C-reactive protein as a predictor of infarct expansion and cardiac rupture after a first Q-wave acute MI. *Circulation* 1997;96:778–784.

Elevated C-reactive protein (CRP) was shown to be a risk factor for cardiac rupture. CRP was measured every 24 hours in 220 patients. Among the rupture patients, CRP levels were twice as high (23.7 mg/dL vs. 12.2 mg/dL; $p = 0.001$). In a multivariate analysis, a CRP of 2 mg/L or more was an independent risk factor for rupture (RR, 4.72; $p = 0.004$), as well as LV aneurysm (RR, 2.11; $p = 0.03$), and 1-year cardiac death (RR, 3.44; $p < 0.0001$).

279. **Becker RC,** et al. Fatal cardiac rupture among patients treated with thrombolytic agents and adjunctive thrombin antagonists. *J Am Coll Cardiol* 1999;33:479–487.

This analysis of 3,759 patients enrolled in the TIMI 9A and 9B trials showed a 1.7% incidence of cardiac rupture. By multivariate analysis, independent predictors of rupture were age older than 70 years (OR, 3.77; 95% CI, 2.06 to 6.91), female gender (OR, 2.87; 95% CI, 1.44 to 5.73), and prior angina (OR, 1.82; 95% CI, 1.05 to 3.16). No association was found between the intensity of anticoagulation or type of thrombin inhibition (e.g., heparin or hirudin) and cardiac rupture.

280. **Moreno R,** et al. Primary angioplasty reduces the risk of left ventricular free wall rupture compared with thrombolysis in patients with acute myocardial infarction. *J Am Coll Cardiol* 2002;39:598–603.

This analysis consisted of 1,375 patients with AMI seen within 12 hours of symptom onset; 55.4% underwent primary angioplasty, and 44.6% were treated with thrombolytic therapy. FWR was diagnosed when sudden death occurred because of PEA with large pericardial effusion on an echocardiogram or when demonstrated postmortem or at surgery. The overall incidence of FWR was 2.5% (angioplasty, 1.8%; thrombolysis, 3.3%; $p = 0.69$). In the univariate analysis, the following were risk factors for FWR: age older than 70 years (5.2% vs. 1.2%; $p < 0.001$), female gender (5.1% vs. 1.8%; $p = 0.006$), anterior location (3.3% vs. 1.4%; $p = 0.02$), and treatment more than 2 hours after symptom onset (3.6% vs. 1.7%; $p = 0.043$). In the multivariate analysis, independent risk factors were age older than 70 (OR, 4.12; 95% CI, 2.04 to 8.62; $p < 0.001$) and anterior location (OR, 2.91; 95% CI, 1.36 to 6.63; $p = 0.008$), whereas treatment with primary angioplasty was an independent protective factor (OR, 0.46; 95% CI, 0.22 to 0.96; $p = 0.037$).

CARDIOGENIC SHOCK AND CONGESTIVE HEART FAILURE

281. **Goldberg RJ**, et al. Cardiogenic shock after acute MI: incidence and mortality from a community-wide perspective, 1975–88. *N Engl J Med* 1991;325:1117–1122.

This retrospective analysis focused on 4,762 AMI patients. Cardiogenic shock (incidence, 7.5%) patients had a high rate of mortality: 77% vs. 13.5%. No significant changes were noted between 1975 and 1988.

282. **Holmes DR Jr**, et al. Contemporary reperfusion therapy for cardiogenic shock: the GUSTO-I experience *J Am Coll Cardiol* 1995;26:668–674.

Cardiogenic shock occurred in 2,972 (7.2%) patients, with 89% of cases developing after hospital admission. These shock patients had a higher reinfarction rate (11% vs. 3%) and much higher mortality rate [57% (shock on presentation) and 55% (shock after admission) versus 3%; $p < 0.001$]. Shock developed less frequently in patients treated with rtPA (6.3% vs. 7.7% and 8.1% in SK groups). The 30-day mortality was lower among the 19% who underwent angioplasty (31% vs. 61%). An updated analysis of the GUSTO I trial demonstrated that, among 30-day survivors, mortality was similar between patients in the trial who experienced shock and those who did not, at 2% to 4% per year (see *J Am Coll Cardiol* 2007;50: 1752–1758.).

283. **Holmes DR Jr**, et al. Difference in countries' use of resources and clinical outcome for patients with cardiogenic shock after MI: results from the GUSTO trial. *Lancet* 1997;349:75–78.

Analysis of GUSTO data showed that the following features were evident among U.S. patients: younger ($p < 0.001$), more anterior MIs (49% vs. 53%), and treated earlier (3.1 hours vs. 3.3 hours; $p < 0.01$). They underwent procedures much more often: catheterization, 58% vs. 23%; PTCA, 26% vs. 8%; IABP, 35% vs. 7%; pulmonary artery use, 57% vs. 22%. Revascularization was associated with decreased mortality in all nations; however, the United States had a 24% lower 30-day mortality rate [50% vs. 66% (other nations); $p < 0.001$ (adjusted for revascularization rates)]. Authors suggest better U.S. outcomes are owing to earlier identification of patients as a result of closer monitoring.

284. **Goldberg RJ**, et al. Temporal trends in cardiogenic shock complicating acute MI. *N Engl J Med* 1999;340:1162–1168.

This observational study was composed of 9,076 patients admitted to all local hospitals of a metropolitan area (Worcester, MA) during eleven 1-year periods between 1975 and 1997. The incidence of cardiogenic shock was relatively stable during this period (average, 7.1%). Cardiogenic shock was associated with a 71.7% in-hospital mortality rate (vs. 12.0%; $p < 0.001$). A significant trend toward better in-hospital survival was seen among patients treated in the mid-to-late 1990s compared with mid-to-late 1970s [ORs, 0.49 (1993 and 1995) and 0.46 (1997)].

INTRACRANIAL HEMORRHAGE IN THROMBOLYSIS

285. **Maggioni AP**, et al. Risk of stroke in patients with acute MI after thrombolytic and antithrombotic therapy. *N Engl J Med* 1992;327:1–6.

This analysis focused on GISSI-2 and International Study patients; complete data were available on 20,768 patients. The in-hospital stroke rate was 1.14% (hemorrhagic, 0.36%; ischemic, 0.48%; undefined cause, 0.30%). Patients treated with tPA had a small but significant excess of stroke versus SK-treated patients (1.33% vs. 0.94%; adjusted OR, 1.42; 95% CI, 1.09 to 1.84). Factors associated with increased risk of stroke were older age, higher Killip class, and anterior infarction.

286. **Simoons ML,** et al. Individual risk assessment for intracranial hemorrhage during thrombolytic therapy. *Lancet* 1993;342:1523–1528.

This analysis focused on data from the Netherlands registry, ECSG, GISSI-2 and International Study Group trials, TIMI II trials, TAMI trials, and ISAM study. By multivariate analysis, independent predictors of intracranial hemorrhage were age older than 65 years (OR, 2.2; 95% CI, 1.4 to 3.5), body weight less than 70 kg (OR, 2.1; 95% CI, 1.3 to 3.2), hypertension on hospital admission (OR, 2.0; 95% CI, 1.2 to 3.2), and administration of alteplase (OR, 1.6; 95% CI, 1.0 to 2.5).

287. **Gurwitz JH,** et al. Risk for intracranial hemorrhage after tissue plasminogen activator for acute MI. *Ann Intern Med* 1998;129:597–604.

This analysis focused on 71,073 patients from the NRMI 2 treated with tPA between June 1994 and September 1996. The in-hospitalization intracranial hemorrhage rate was 0.95% [0.88% confirmed (CT or MRI)]. In multivariate models, the following were intracranial hemorrhage predictors: older age, female sex, black ethnicity, SBP more than 140 mm Hg, DBP greater than 100 mm Hg, history of stroke, tPA dose more than 1.5 mg/kg, and lower body weight.

REOCCLUSION, RECURRENT ISCHEMIA, AND REINFARCTION

288. **Benhorin J,** et al. Prognostic significance of nonfatal myocardial reinfarction. *J Am Coll Cardiol* 1990;15:253–258.

This analysis focused on 1,234 placebo patients in the Multicenter Diltiazem Trial. At follow-up (1 to 4 years), nonfatal MI had occurred in 9.4%, with a higher frequency in women and those with prior cardiac symptoms. Nonfatal MI was associated with a threefold higher risk of subsequent cardiac mortality (5.4 times higher if the index event was a first MI).

289. **Ohman EM,** et al. Consequences of reocclusion after successful reperfusion therapy in acute MI. *Circulation* 1990;82:781–791.

This analysis focused on 810 TAMI patients with repeated angiography at average 7 days that showed a reoccluded IRA in 12.4% (58% with symptoms). At follow-up, occluded patients had a similar EF, but worse infarct zone function and increased in-hospital mortality (11% vs. 4.5%; $p = 0.01$).

290. **Kornowski R,** et al. Predictors and long-term prognostic significance of recurrent infarction in the year after a first MI. *Am J Cardiol* 1993;72:883–888.

This retrospective analysis focused on 3,695 SPRINT patients, with a 1-year reinfarction rate of 6% (associated in-hospital mortality, 30%). Reinfarction predictors were peripheral vascular disease (adjusted RR, 2.12), anterior MI (RR, 1.62), angina before MI (RR, 1.53), CHF on admission (RR, 1.34), diabetes (RR, 1.33), hypertension (RR, 1.28), and age increment (RR, 1.13). Reinfarction rates were as follows: zero or one risk factor, 4.0%; five or six risk factors, 23.3%. Recurrent MI is the strongest long-term mortality predictor (adjusted RR, 4.76).

291. **Mueller HS,** et al. Prognostic significance of nonfatal reinfarction during 3 year follow-up of the TIMI II clinical trial. *J Am Coll Cardiol* 1995;26:900–907.

The incidence of reinfarction was 10.1% (43 of 339 died). Relative risks of death were 1.9 if reinfarction occurred at less than 42 days, 6.2 at 43 to 365 days, and 2.9 at 1 to 3 years.

292. **Verheught FWA,** et al. Reocclusion: the flip of coronary thrombolysis. *J Am Coll Cardiol* 1996;27:766–773.

This analysis focused on 61 studies with 6,061 patients undergoing angiography twice. Reocclusion usually occurs within weeks. Overall, an 11% reocclusion rate was observed, but a 16% incidence was seen in true occlusion studies; thus, initial occlusion is a risk factor.

Aspirin and heparin were not associated with benefit in prevention (APRICOT, HART trials). Hirudin and hirulog appear beneficial. Half of reocclusions are clinically silent. Revascularization is helpful, especially if symptoms are present.

293. **Bauters C,** et al. Angiographically documented late reocclusion after successful coronary angioplasty of an infarct-related lesion is a powerful predictor of long-term mortality. *Circulation* 1999;99:2243–2250.

Retrospective analysis of 528 patients who had a patent IRA after balloon angioplasty procedure 10 ± 6 days after MI. At 6-month follow-up angiography, IRA reocclusion occurred in 17% (TIMI flow grade 0 or 1). At long-term follow-up (median, 6.4 years), the reocclusion group had a 2.5-fold higher mortality rate (20% vs. 8%; $p = 0.002$). The actuarial 8-year total mortality rates were 28% and 10% ($p = 0.0003$), and the CV mortality rates were 25% and 7% ($p < 0.0001$). The mortality differences between reoccluded and patent IRA patients were greater in patients with an anterior MI.

294. **Ernst NM,** et al. on behalf of the Zwolle Myocardial Infarction Study Group. Impact of failed mechanical reperfusion in patients with acute myocardial infarction treated with primary angioplasty. *Am J Cardiol* 2005;96:332–334.

Among 1,683 patients undergoing primary PCI for acute MI at a single center, nearly 7% in this cohort did not achieve mechanical reperfusion—roughly half had failed primary angioplasty and the other half had late reocclusion. Predictors of failed PCI in univariate analysis were Killip class >1, LAD IRA, and TIMI flow grade 0/1 prior to PCI. In-hospital, 30-day, and 1-year mortality rates were all higher in the patients with failed reperfusion ($p < 0.001$ for each).

LEFT VENTRICULAR THROMBI

295. **Gueret P,** et al. Effects of full-dose heparin anticoagulation on the development of left ventricular thrombosis in acute transmural MI. *J Am Coll Cardiol* 1986;8:419–426.

This small prospective study showed that thrombi occur frequently in anterior MIs. Ninety patients (46 anterior, 44 inferior) seen an average 5.2 hours after onset of symptoms were randomized to heparin or no heparin. No thrombi were detected on first echocardiograms (done at 10.3 ± 8 hours). In the anterior MI group, 46% had thrombi at 4.3 ± 3.0 days [38% (heparin) vs. 52% (no heparin); $p = 0.76$]. No thrombi formed in the inferior group.

296. **Vecchio C,** et al. Left ventricular thrombus in anterior acute MI after thrombolysis. *Circulation* 1991;84:512–519.

This GISSI-2 ancillary echocardiography study was composed of 180 consecutive patients with first MI. Echocardiography was performed within 48 hours and before discharge. LV thrombi were found in 28% (no difference between the four treatment groups). Mural shape was more common, especially in heparinized patients. Only one in-hospital embolic event was documented.

297. **Vaitkus PT,** Barnathan ES. Embolic potential, prevention and management of mural thrombus complicating anterior MI: a meta-analysis. *J Am Coll Cardiol* 1993;22:1004–1009.

This analysis focused on 11 studies with 856 patients. Thrombus by echocardiography was associated with an OR of embolization of 5.45 (11% vs. 2%). In anterior MI patients, the OR was 8.0. Anticoagulation was associated with 86% less embolization. Primary anticoagulation led to 68% less embolization, whereas thrombolytic therapy was associated with 52% less embolization (16% vs. 32%).

298. **Greaves SC,** et al. Incidence and natural history of left ventricular thrombus following anterior wall acute MI. *Am J Cardiol* 1997;80:442–448.

This analysis focused on 309 Healing and Early Afterload Reducing Treatment (HEART) substudy patients, 78% with Q-wave anterior MIs. Echocardiography was performed on days 1, 14, and 90. LV thrombus rates were low: day 1, 0.6%; day 14, 3.7%; day 90, 2.5%. Only one thrombus was detected on two echocardiograms. Thrombus patients had a greater LV size increase and wall-motion abnormalities.

299. **Weinsaft JW,** et al. Detection of left ventricular thrombus by delayed-enhancement cardiovascular magnetic resonance: prevalence and markers in patients with systolic dysfunction. *J Am Coll Cardiol* 2008;52:148–157.

In 784 patients with impaired systolic function (EF < 50%), left ventricular thrombus was detected in 7% (both intracavitary and mural thrombi). In multivariable analyses, risk factors for thrombus included low EF, ischemic cardiomyopathy, and increased myocardial scarring on magnetic resonance.

VALVULAR DAMAGE AND SEPTAL DEFECTS

300. **Lehmann KG,** et al. Mitral regurgitation in early MI: incidence, clinical detection and prognostic implications. *Ann Intern Med* 1992;117:10–17.

This analysis focused on 206 TIMI I patients with contrast left ventriculography within 7 hours of symptom onset. Mitral regurgitation was present in 27 (13%) patients and associated with a markedly increased 1-year mortality rate (RRs, 12.2 and 7.5 by univariate and multivariate analyses, respectively).

301. **Lamas GA,** et al. Clinical significance of mitral regurgitation after acute MI. *Circulation* 1997;96:827–833.

This study was composed of 727 SAVE patients with catheterization and left ventriculography data (done within 16 days of MI). Mitral regurgitation (19.4%) patients were more likely to have a persistently occluded IRA (27.2% vs. 15.2%; $p = 0.001$). At follow-up (median, 3.5 years), mitral regurgitation patients had a more than twofold higher CV mortality rate (29% vs. 12%; $p < 0.001$), more severe CHF (24% vs. 16%; $p = 0.015$), and a higher rate of CV mortality, severe CHF, and reinfarction (47% vs. 29%; $p < 0.001$). In multivariate analysis, mitral regurgitation was an independent CV mortality predictor [RR, 2.0; 95% CI, 1.28 to 3.04].

302. **Crenshaw BS,** et al. for the GUSTO-I (Global Utilization of Streptokinase and TPA for Occluded Coronary Arteries) Trial Investigators. Risk factors, angiographic patterns, and outcomes in patients with ventricular septal defect complicating acute myocardial infarction. *Circulation* 2000;101:27–32.

Ventricular septal defect (VSD) complicated 0.2% of STEMIs in the GUSTO I trial (84 of 41,021). Predisposing factors included older age, anterior infarct, females, and no previous smoking; additionally, VSD more common when the IRA was the LAD and when it was totally occluded. Mortality was significantly higher at 30 days in patients with a VSD (73.8% vs. 6.8%; $p < 0.001$), and surgical therapy showed mortality benefit over medical management (30-day mortality, 47% vs. 94%; $p < 0.001$).

303. **Birnbaum Y,** et al. Ventricular septal rupture after acute myocardial infarction. *N Engl J Med* 2002;347:1426–1432.

This review article discusses numerous topics, including the incidence, risk factors, pathogenesis, hemodynamics, time course, clinical manifestations, angiographic findings, medical and surgical therapy, and prognosis of ventricular septal rupture after acute MI.

CHAPTER 5

Heart Failure

Christopher P. Cannon, Benjamin A. Steinberg, and
Justin M. Dunn

EPIDEMIOLOGY

Congestive heart failure (HF) is now responsible for more than 1 million hospital admissions each year in the United States, at a cost of nearly $40 billion (*Circulation* 2009;119;e21–e181).

The aging of the population and improved survival after myocardial infarction (MI) (*Circulation* 2008;118(20):2057–2062) has resulted in an increasing prevalence of HF, which now affects nearly 6 million Americans [National Health and Nutritional Examination Survey (NHANES) 2005 to 2006 National Center for Health Statistics (NCHS) and NHLBI]. Data from the Framingham Heart Study suggest that the incidence of HF over the past 50-year period has declined among women but not among men, whereas survival has continued to improve in both sexes (by 12% per decade), which accounts for the increasing prevalence (14). However, a large population-based study of Olmsted County, MN, residents showed no significant decline in incidence in either sex, and survival improved in both sexes but much more so in younger men than in women and older patients (12).

Most studies show women surviving longer than men (9,11,13,14), whereas the Studies of Left Ventricular Dysfunction (SOLVD) trial found the opposite. The explanation for this discrepancy may be that the SOLVD trial enrolled a higher percentage of women with coronary artery disease (CAD), and HF due to an ischemic etiology is associated with increased mortality. But analysis of the Candesartan in Heart Failure: Assessment of Reduction in Mortality and Morbidity (CHARM) trial data suggests that the gender difference cannot be fully explained by a difference in the prevalence of CAD between sexes (15).

Factors associated with an increased risk of HF are advanced age, male gender, black race, diabetes, obesity, smoking, CAD/previous MI, and hypertension (10,11). The Olmsted County data suggest the highest population attributable risk stems from CAD and hypertension (see *Am J Med* 2009;122:1023–1028). Among women, those with hypertension and diabetes are more likely than men to develop HF. Echocardiographic findings associated with increased risk include low left and/or right ventricular ejection fraction (EF), left ventricular (LV) dilatation, and valvular disease (34).

The 2005 American Heart Association (AHA)/American College of Cardiology (ACC) guideline update for heart failure (HF) introduced a new staging system for classifying HF. There are four stages involved in the development of HF, A to D. These are not intended to replace the New York Heart Association (NYHA) classification system, discussed below, but rather to complement it with a staging system that does not change with response to therapy. It also recognizes that there are established risk factors and structural prerequisites for the development of HF that may benefit from therapeutic intervention even before the development of symptoms.

Stage A: at high risk for HF but without structural heart disease or symptoms of HF.
Stage B: structural heart disease but without signs or symptoms of HF.
Stage C: structural heart disease with prior or current symptoms of HF.
Stage D: refractory HF requiring specialized interventions.

Among those diagnosed with HF, severity of signs and symptoms is predicted by functional class. Most of the NYHA classes are contained within Stage C (see above). The NYHA classification is as follows:

Class I: no limitation.
Class II: slight HF; comfortable at rest but ordinary activity causes fatigue, dyspnea, or angina.
Class III: marked failure; less than ordinary activity causes symptoms.
Class IV: severe failure; symptoms of HF at rest.

The mortality rate in NYHA class III patients with peak oxygen consumption of 10 to 15 mL/kg/min is 15% to 20% per year, and it increases to 50% per year or more in class IV patients with oxygen consumption of less than 10 mL/kg/min.

Also noteworthy is the Killip classification system, first developed in 1967. It stratifies post-MI patients based on their level of HF signs and symptoms. Patients with a lower Killip class have a lower 30-day mortality post-MI than patients with a higher Killip class:

Killip class I: no clinical signs of HF.
Killip class II: rales or crackles in the lungs, an S_3 gallop, and elevated jugular venous pressure (JVP).
Killip class III: frank acute pulmonary edema.
Killip class IV: cardiogenic shock or hypotension (measured as systolic blood pressure lower than 90 mm Hg), and evidence of peripheral vasoconstriction (oliguria, cyanosis, or sweating).

The acute HF syndrome is the presentation of symptomatic, decompensated HF (8). This is frequently triggered in the setting of other acute medical or surgical illness (commonly infectious), dietary or medication nonadherence, or acute coronary syndrome events. Such hospitalizations account for a significant morbidity in such patients, in addition to enormous healthcare resource expenditures.

Rehospitalization rates with 90 days are high, as are rates of postdischarge events. While outpatient management strategies have accumulated a significant evidence base, inpatient management has remained focused predominantly on fluid removal and symptomatic treatment with relatively less supporting data (as discussed herein).

HISTORY AND PHYSICAL EXAMINATION

Symptoms include dyspnea, fatigue, paroxysmal nocturnal dyspnea, orthopnea, and nocturia. Orthopnea appears to be the most sensitive symptom for predicting elevated pulmonary capillary wedge pressure (PCWP) (16). Impaired concentration may occur in individuals with decreased cardiac output at rest.

The physical examination may be notable for rales (often not present if chronic or gradual in onset), elevated JVP, presence of third heart sound, peripheral edema, cool extremities, narrowed pulse pressure, and tachycardia (see **Table 5.1**). Hepatomegaly and ascites are often seen with right HF. Most of these signs have limited sensitivity at predicting elevated PCWP. In one study, jugular venous distention, at rest or inducible by a hepatojugular test, had a sensitivity of 80% for predicting elevated PCWP (17). JVD and third heart sound have been shown to have prognostic significance (20). In another study, low pulse pressure was an excellent predictor of poor cardiac output, with a pulse pressure of less than 25% having a 91% sensitivity and 83% specificity for a cardiac index of 2.2 $L/min/m^2$ or less (16).

ETIOLOGY

Systolic dysfunction is due to pump failure, typically from ischemic cardiomyopathy, nonischemic dilated cardiomyopathy, hypertensive heart disease, or valvular disease. Alcohol and viral illnesses are responsible for some cases of nonischemic

TABLE 5.1 Findings of Physical Examination

	Systolic Dysfunction	Diastolic Dysfunction
Third heart sound	Frequent	Rare
Fourth heart sound	Rare	Frequent
Rales	Occasional	Occasional
Peripheral edema	Frequent	Rare
Jugular venous distention	Frequent	Rare
Cardiomegaly	Usual	Rare

(Modified from Braunwald E. *Heart Disease*. Philadelphia, PA: W.B. Saunders; 1997.)

dilated cardiomyopathy but many are idiopathic. High-output causes of HF are less common, and include anemia, hyperthyroidism, and pregnancy. Rare causes include Paget disease, arteriovenous fistula, pheochromocytoma, and beriberi.

Diastolic dysfunction is a component in approximately one half of HF cases [see *JAMA* 2003;289(2):194–202]. Most of these are classified as heart failure with preserved EF (HFpEF), though it should be noted that diastolic function is often abnormal in systolic HF. HFpEF is typically associated with hypertension, hypertrophic cardiomyopathy, and infiltrative disease. It is most prevalent among elderly women, most of whom have hypertension, diabetes, or both. Unlike systolic HF, there is a dearth of large clinical trials to guide the management of these patients. Current recommendations are to control hypertension, control ventricular rate to allow diastolic filling, and address the underlying etiology if possible (e.g., coronary revascularization for CAD) (7).

An important precipitating factor of HF is noncompliance with a prescribed drug regimen and poor diet (e.g., high salt). In one study of patients hospitalized for HF, more than 60% were found to be noncompliant with drugs and/or diet (1). Abrupt/acute precipitating causes of HF include acute MI, acute pulmonary embolism, acute mitral regurgitation and aortic insufficiency, acute ventricular septal defect, and infection. More chronic precipitating causes of HF include drugs [nonsteroidal anti-inflammatory drugs (vasoconstriction), potentially even aspirin in nonischemic HF (22, WATCH trial); verapamil, diltiazem, and procainamide (negative inotropy, though amlodipine and felodipine appear to be safe in HF); estrogens, androgens, minoxidil, and thiazolidinediones (see the RECORD trial, *Lancet* 2009;373:2125–3215) (water retention); doxorubicin (Adriamycin)], depression, and sleep apnea.

TESTS

1. Laboratory tests. The use of B-type natriuretic peptide (BNP) has been found to be beneficial in the evaluation and triage of patients with acute dyspnea in the emergency department (ED; also see *J Am Coll Cardiol* 2001;37:379). One of the largest such studies, the **BNP** multinational study, demonstrated the statistically significant impact of adding BNP levels to other clinical criteria, to make the diagnosis of HF as an explanation for patients presented with dyspnea (25,26). Moreover, BNP level was more predictive than any other single clinical criterion for making the diagnosis of acute HF. Data on BNP have expanded to include support for BNP-guided outpatient management, as demonstrated by the STARS-BNP study (29); however, these results could not be replicated in the TIME-HF study (31). Small studies of using BNP to aid in discharge planning and decrease length of stay have yielded mixed results (27,32).

    Additionally, BNP has been found to predict mortality in patients with ACS independent of HF (28,30).

Low serum sodium is common (neurohormonal activation) and linearly predictive of poor outcome (23); elevated creatinine and liver function tests also are predictors of poor outcome. Finally, inflammatory markers (e.g., c-reactive protein, TNF-alpha, IL-6) appear to be elevated in HF patients (see *Circulation* 2003;107:1486). Their prognostic role requires further study.

2. Chest radiograph. Findings of increased pulmonary capillary pressure are seen in approximately 50% of patients; bilateral pleural effusions and cardiomegaly also may be present.

3. Electrocardiography (ECG). Q waves and left bundle branch block are good predictors of systolic dysfunction. A wide QRS (more than 220 milliseconds) is predictive of increased mortality.

4. Echocardiogram. A simple and useful tool, echocardiography can help determine systolic versus diastolic dysfunction and left and/or right ventricular impairment.

5. Six-minute walk test. Short distance correlates with higher mortality and increased HF-related hospitalizations (34).

6. Metabolic stress testing. Used to measure oxygen consumption; a peak oxygen consumption of less than 12 to 14 mL/kg/min portends a poor prognosis (33).

7. Endomyocardial biopsy (EMB). Biopsy may be useful in selected cases, such as suspected amyloidosis, sarcoidosis, and giant cell myocarditis (24).

TREATMENT

Acute

1. Diuretics. Furosemide, 20 to 200 mg, is administered intravenously to alleviate lung edema due to volume overload, again by reducing preload. (Initial dose should be based on prior diuretic history.) Addition of a thiazide (e.g., metolazone or chlorothiazide) may help potentiate diuresis. In cases of massive fluid overload that respond poorly to diuretics, ultrafiltration may be effective (95). Additional, preliminary data from the DOSE trial failed to demonstrate the superiority of continuous-infusion diuresis (compared to bolus dosing), but did advocate for higher intensity dosing of bolus intravenous diuretics (up to 2.5 × the outpatient oral dose).

2. Nitrates. Nitroglycerin is given sublingually or intravenously in cases in which preload reduction is necessary to more rapidly reduce pulmonary congestion. IV nitroglycerin is ideal for patients with HF and hypertension, coronary ischemia, or significant mitral regurgitation. In the case of severe HF, nitroprusside administration should be considered if both PCWP and systemic vascular resistance (SVR) are elevated. Nitroprusside has a balanced arteriodilating/venodilating effect and also dilates the pulmonary vasculature.

3. Nesiritide. This form of human BNP causes vasodilation and has resulted in rapid symptomatic and hemodynamic improvement in patients with acutely decompensated HF (61). It is an attractive alternative to inotropes because it

causes rapid symptom relief without the risk of arrhythmias. In the Vasodilation in the Management of Acute HF (VMAC) study, nesiritide also was compared with nitroglycerin in the management of acutely decompensated HF. Although no significant difference was noted in outcomes at 24 hours, hemodynamic benefit was somewhat improved at 3 hours (62). No difference was found in length of stay between the groups, but a trend toward decreased readmissions in the nesiritide groups was noted (see *J Am Coll Cardiol* 2002;39:798). However, more recent studies have suggested that nesiritide may be associated with worsening renal function (see *Circulation* 2005;111:1487–1491) and monitoring of renal function is important. The effect of nesiritide on mortality is unclear, with some studies suggesting an increased risk of mortality with nesiritide (63). The mortality trend was never significant, but further study is ongoing.

4. Inotropic agents. No single agent has been found to be clinically superior, but adrenergic agents (such as dobutamine and dopamine and the phosphodiesterase inhibitor, milrinone) each may have a role in certain hemodynamic states such as relative hypotension with poor response to vasodilators and diuretics. Dopamine may be preferable in those with low blood pressure because dobutamine reduces SVR to a greater extent, but the gain in cardiac output added to the decrease in SVR with dobutamine typically leads to a slight *increase* in blood pressure. Milrinone has greater vasodilating-unloading properties, and works on both the systemic and pulmonary systems. This agent was evaluated for short-term use in acute exacerbations of HF in the OPTIME-HF trial and was not shown to be beneficial (86).

Data from small clinical trials and anecdotal case experience suggest that inotropic agents reduce hospitalization, lead to hemodynamic and clinical improvement, and may serve as a bridge to transplantation. Some reports have suggested that intermittent infusion therapy in outpatients also may be effective in attenuating HF symptoms in the long term (see *J Heart Lung Transplant* 2000;19:S49), but the safety of prolonged outpatient use of these agents has been questioned. Data from more than 1,000 patients with chronic HF randomized to milrinone or placebo showed an increase in mortality (30% vs. 24%) with more adverse reactions, including syncope and hypotension [Prospective Randomized Milrinone Survival Evaluation (PROMISE); (82)]. The increase in mortality has led some to suggest that inotropic drugs used in this fashion may exacerbate arrhythmias with subsequent sudden cardiac death. Intermittent outpatient infusion of either vasoactive drugs such as nesiritide or positive inotropic drugs has not been shown to improve symptoms or survival in patients with advanced HF.

Long-term Therapies
ANGIOTENSIN-CONVERTING ENZYME INHIBITORS

Clearly indicated if LV dysfunction is present (see **Table 5.2**), angiotensin-converting enzyme (ACE) inhibitors should be initiated before aggressively performing diuresis

TABLE 5.2 Differential Diagnosis

	Acute Heart Failure	Decompensated Chronic Heart Failure	Chronic Heart Failure
Severity of symptoms	Severe	Severe	Mild to moderate
Pulmonary edema	Rare	Common	Rare
Peripheral edema	Rare	Common	Common
Weight gain	None to minimal	Moderate to severe	Mild to moderate

(Modified from Braunwald E. *Heart Disease.* Philadelphia, PA: W.B. Saunders; 1997.)

in HF patients. They are first-line therapy in patients with systolic HF. The Cooperative North Scandinavian Enalapril Survival Study (CONSENSUS I) showed that enalapril reduced 1-year mortality by 31% in NYHA class IV patients (36), whereas the larger SOLVD trial enrolled NYHA class II and III patients and showed that enalapril reduced mortality by 16% (average follow-up, 41 months) (37). Subsequent trials have shown similar benefits with other ACE inhibitors [e.g., Veterans Administration Cooperative Vasodilator-Heart Failure Trial II (V-HEFT II), Acute Infarction Ramipril Efficacy Study (AIRE) (39)](**Table 5.3**). A meta-analysis of 32 studies found ACE-inhibitor therapy to be associated with significant reductions in total mortality and mortality or hospitalization for HF ($p < 0.001$ for both) (35).

The beneficial effect of administering larger doses of ACE inhibition has been demonstrated, though the benefit seems limited to reducing the risk of hospitalization. Effects on symptoms and mortality did not appear to differ (ATLAS; 41). The ATLAS trial randomized 3,164 patients with NYHA class II to IV HF and EF ≤30% to low-dose (2.5 to 5 mg/day) versus high-dose (32.5 to 35 mg/day) lisinopril. This trial demonstrated a nonsignificant 8% lower mortality and significant 24% fewer hospitalizations in patients treated with high-dose lisinopril.

The use of ACE inhibition in HFpEF has not shown a proven benefit in initial studies. The Perindopril in Elderly People with Chronic Heart Failure (PEP-HF) trial randomized 850 HF patients who were at least 70 years of age and had an LVEF of ≥45% and echocardiographic features suggesting possible diastolic dysfunction to receive perindopril at 4 mg/day or placebo. The primary endpoint was a composite of all-cause mortality and unplanned HF–related hospitalization with a minimum follow-up of 1 year. Though there was a trend toward benefit, the study was underpowered to make any treatment recommendations.

TABLE 5.3 Major ACE-inhibitor Trials

	Number of Patients	Patient Characteristics	Placebo Mortality	Hazard Ratio
V-HeFT II (57)	804	NYHA I–III	25% at 2 yr[a]	0.72
CONSENSUS I (36)	253	NYHA IV	52% at 1 yr	0.69
SOLVD (37)	2,569	NYHA II, III	40% at 3.4 yr	0.84
SOLVD Prevention (38)	4,228	NYHA I	16% at 3.1 yr	0.91
AIRE (39)	2,006	Post-MI, clinical HF	23% at 1.3 yr	0.73
SAVE (Chapter 4)	2,231	Post-MI, EF ≤40%	25% at 3.5 yr	0.81
ISIS-4 (Chapter 4)	58,050	24-hr post-MI[b]	7.7% at 5 wk	0.93

This table demonstrates that studies that enrolled higher risk patients showed a strong benefit (15% to 30% lower mortality) from ACE-inhibitor therapy, whereas a modest benefit was seen in the lower risk populations (SOLVD Prevention, ISIS-4). EF, ejection fraction; HF, heart failure; NYHA, New York Heart Association; MI, myocardial infarction; ACE, angiotensin-converting enzyme.

[a]Hydralazine and isosorbide.

[b]No HF required for enrollment.

ANGIOTENSIN II–RECEPTOR ANTAGONISTS

Current trial data comparing angiotensin II–receptor antagonists with ACE inhibitors confirm that ACE inhibitors should remain first-line therapy for patients with HF, and angiotensin II–receptor blockers should be reserved for those who are intolerant because of cough. In the ELITE trial, losartan was reported to have a lower mortality rate compared with captopril in patients with HF. Mortality was not the primary endpoint, and the trial enrolled only 722 patients (40).

Furthermore, these findings were not confirmed in the larger ELITE II study that again compared captopril with losartan in 3,152 patients. After a median follow-up of 1.5 years, losartan was not superior to captopril in reducing mortality, but was better tolerated (42).

Other angiotensin II blockers also have been evaluated in patients with HF. In the Val-HEFT trial, valsartan was compared with placebo in more than 5,000 HF patients with NYHA class II to IV symptoms (43). Whereas no difference in mortality was noted, patients had improved quality of life (QOL) and fewer hospitalizations. In addition, subgroup analysis showed a trend toward increased mortality in patients receiving valsartan, ACE inhibition, and β-blockers. In the Valsartan in Acute Myocardial Infarction (VALIANT) trial, 14,703 patients were recruited up to 10 days post-MI and randomized to one of the three treatment arms: captopril in a target dose of 50 mg t.i.d., valsartan target dose 160 mg b.i.d., or the combination of captopril 50 mg t.i.d. and valsartan 80 mg b.i.d. Valsartan was demonstrated to be as effective as a proven dose of captopril in reducing mortality as well as cardiovascular events including MI, but it was noninferior and did not show superiority over captopril alone (44).

In the Symptom, Tolerability, Response to Exercise Trial of Candesartan Cilexetil in Heart Failure (STRETCH) trial, candesartan was evaluated in a study of 844 patients with HF randomized to placebo or candesartan. Significant improvements in exercise tolerance, cardiothoracic ratio, and symptoms and signs of HF were noted (STRETCH). The CHARM trial evaluated the use of candesartan in various groups of patients in NYHA class II to IV (45). The trial compared candesartan to placebo and evaluated three groups of patients with (a) LVEF less than or equal to 40% treated with an ACE inhibitor (CHARM-added, $n = 2,300$); (b) LVEF of 40% or less, ACE-inhibitor intolerant (CHARM-alternative, $n = 1,700$); and (c) LVEF greater than 40%, not treated with ACE inhibitors (CHARM-preserved, $n = 2,500$). The results showed that candesartan reduced the composite outcomes, cardiovascular mortality, hospital admissions for HF, and all-cause mortality, particularly among patients with reduced LV systolic function.

A recently published trial, effects of high-dose versus low-dose losartan on clinical outcomes in patients with heart failure (HEAAL study), suggests that a higher dose of losartan provides mortality benefit over lower doses in patients with systolic HF intolerant of ACE inhibitors (47). This trial suggests that incremental inhibition of the RAS system is beneficial, and it does not necessarily require two different types of agents. At the time of this writing, losartan is not approved for HF in the United States, only for hypertension.

ARB therapy in HFpEF initially showed some promise with the results of the CHARM-preserved arm of the CHARM trial. In that arm of the trial, the addition of candesartan to the treatment regimen for patients with symptomatic HF and relatively preserved EF significantly reduced morbidity but did not reach the primary endpoint of CV death. The recent Irbesartan in Patients with Heart Failure and Preserved Ejection Fraction (I-PRESERVE) trial again did not show any difference in outcomes when irbesartan was compared to placebo in HFpEF patients (46).

DUAL RAS BLOCKADE (ACE/ARB)

The Randomized Evaluation of Strategies for Left Ventricular Dysfunction (RESOLVD) trial evaluated the effects of candesartan alone, enalapril alone, and their combination on exercise tolerance, ventricular function, QOL, neurohormone levels, and tolerability in HF (48). There were no differences among groups with regard to 6-minute walk distance (6MWD), NYHA functional class, or QOL.

However, there was a trend toward benefit on LV remodeling with the combination therapy.

The bulk of the data on dual RAS blockade in HF, however, come from CHARM-added, VALIANT, and Val-HeFT mentioned above (43–45). CHARM-added was the only trial that showed a reduction in cardiovascular deaths with dual therapy, and it also showed a lower rate of hospitalization for HF. However, all-cause mortality did not differ between groups. In post hoc analysis, Val-HeFT actually showed that dual therapy increased morbidity and mortality. Two recent meta-analyses suggest that dual RAS therapy is not beneficial (*Arch Intern Med* 2007;167:1930–1936; *J Card Fail* 2008;14(3):181–188), and there is a higher risk of discontinuation of therapy because of adverse effects such as hyperkalemia, renal dysfunction, and hypotension. Though there may be a subset of patients that benefit from dual RAS therapy, such as young patients with good renal function, the available data do not support the routine addition of an ARB to ACE-I therapy in HF patients.

DIURETICS

Optimal use of diuretics is the cornerstone of any successful approach to the symptomatic treatment of HF. Diuretics are used to control and reduce fluid retention. In most cases, they should be used in conjunction with an ACE inhibitor with or without a β-blocker. Smaller, older studies have demonstrated a reduction in JVPs, pulmonary congestion, peripheral edema, and body weight with diuretics. Some longer studies have shown improvement in cardiac function, symptoms, and exercise tolerance. However, there have been no long-term studies of diuretic therapy, and thus their effects on morbidity and mortality are not known. A few small studies have found that a continuous intravenous infusion of furosemide (compared with bolus therapy) in patients hospitalized with severe HF may provide improved diuresis and natriuresis (49); however, the most recent DOSE study found no benefit of continuous-infusion furosemide over bolus therapy.

ALDOSTERONE BLOCKERS

The Randomized Aldactone Evaluation Study (RALES), which evaluated the potassium-sparing diuretic spironolactone in patients receiving optimal therapy (including a loop diuretic), showed a significantly lower mortality rate among spironolactone-treated patients compared with those treated with a loop diuretic alone (50). When spironolactone therapy is initiated, hyperkalemia occurs frequently, so careful monitoring of serum potassium levels is necessary (see *N Engl J Med* 2004;351:543–551).

Eplerenone is a selective aldosterone blocker that has a favorable side-effect profile compared to aldosterone, especially a lower incidence of gynecomastia. The Eplerenone Post-acute MI Heart Failure Efficacy and Survival Study (EPHESUS) compared eplerenone with placebo in 6,632 MI patients with an EF ≤40%. The eplerenone group had a significant reduction in all-cause mortality compared to placebo (relative risk 0.85, $p = 0.008$).

Data regarding the use of aldosterone antagonists in HFpEF are limited. The ongoing Trial of Aldosterone Antagonist Therapy in Adults With Preserved Ejection Fraction Congestive Heart Failure (TOPCAT) will hopefully help clarify the role spironolactone in this patient population (see http://clinicaltrials.gov/ct2/show/NCT00094302).

DIGOXIN

Although the large Digoxin Investigation Group (DIG) mortality trial (55) found that digoxin had no significant effect on total mortality (positive or negative), it also found that digoxin-treated patients with HF and EF <45% had fewer hospitalizations than placebo patients. Physicians may consider adding digoxin in patients with persistent symptoms of HF despite therapy with diuretics, an ACE-I (or ARB), and a β-blocker (*Circulation* 2004;109:2942–2946, 2959–2964). If a patient is taking digoxin but not an ACE-I or β-blocker, treatment with digoxin should not be withdrawn, but appropriate therapy with the neurohormonal antagonists should be instituted. Two digoxin-withdrawal trials [the Randomized Assessment of Effect of Digoxin on Inhibitors of ACE (RADIANCE) and Prospective Randomized Study of Ventricular Failure and Efficacy of Digoxin (PROVED) (53,54)] showed that fewer hospitalizations for worsening HF occurred in those who continued taking digoxin.

Toxicity is a concern with digoxin, especially in patients over age 70, with impaired renal function, or with a low lean body mass. The DIG trial suggests that risk-adjusted mortality increased as the plasma concentrations exceeded 1.0 ng/mL, though overt toxicity is not often seen until levels are greater than 2 ng/mL. Toxicity at lower levels can be seen if hypokalemia, hypomagnesemia, or hypothyroidism coexist. One analysis suggests that women may not benefit from digoxin therapy and may be at increased risk for death (*N Engl J Med* 2002;347:1403–1411). Given the narrow therapeutic index and lack of mortality benefit of digoxin, the AHA/ACC writing committee recently changed their recommendation from class I to class IIa (5).

VASODILATORS

Hydralazine and Isosorbide Dinitrate

This combination was associated with a higher mortality rate than was enalapril in the Veterans Administration Cooperative Vasodilator-Heart Failure Trial (V-HeFT II; 25% vs. 18% at 2 years) (57), but yielded better results than placebo in V-HeFT I (56). Post hoc analysis of the V-HeFT trials suggested a significant benefit specifically in African Americans. This prompted the design of the African-American Heart Failure Trial (A-HeFT), which only enrolled self-identified black patients (58). The trial was stopped early due to the significant mortality benefit of the study drug combo (in addition to ACE-I and β-blocker). This trial led to the first FDA approval of a drug for a specific race (BiDil), a significant medical milestone. It is untested as to whether there would be added benefit of this combination in non-black patients when added to a background of ACE-I and/or β-blocker. Despite the lack of studies in ACE-I–intolerant patients, this combination may be considered as a therapeutic alternative in such patients.

Calcium-channel Blockers

Negative inotropic effects are not desirable in systolic dysfunction, and most calcium-channel blockers should generally be avoided in HF. However, in the Prospective Randomized Amlodipine Survival Evaluation (PRAISE) trial (59), amlodipine showed a trend toward lower mortality (-16%; $p = 0.07$), with a 46% lower mortality rate among patients with nonischemic cardiomyopathy. PRAISE-2 compared amlodipine with placebo in a group of patients without ischemic heart disease (60). Patients with HF with LVEF less than 30% were randomized to receive placebo or amlodipine. No significant difference was found in this cohort with regard to all-cause or cardiac mortality.

β-blockers

β-blockers are safe when given carefully in controlled fashion, but only three β-blockers—bisoprolol, metoprolol succinate (XL), and carvedilol—have been shown to be effective in reducing the risk of death in patients with chronic HF. Consensus recommendations advocate the use of these three β-blockers in patients with Stage C HF. However, they should not be used in those with severe, decompensated HF. All β-blocker trials of more than 1-month duration have shown improved LV function, and a meta-analysis of 17 randomized trials with approximately 3,000 patients showed an approximately 30% mortality reduction, mostly due to fewer sudden deaths.

The Cardiac Insufficiency Bisoprolol Study (CIBIS II) enrolled more than 2,600 NYHA class III or IV patients with an EF of less than 35% and found that bisoprolol-treated patients had a mortality rate approximately one third lower than that of placebo-treated patients, whereas the Metoprolol CR/XL Randomized Intervention Trial in HF (MERIT-HF) trial enrolled nearly 4,000 patients with an EF of less than 40% and found that metoprolol-XL reduced mortality by 35% compared with placebo (73).

The largest published experience to date of the nonselective β-blocker and α_1-antagonist carvedilol pooled data from different small studies (65,66) and found an impressive 65% mortality reduction at 6 months in carvedilol-treated patients (67). Carvedilol also was shown to be beneficial in improving EF and NYHA functional class, and reducing LV volumes (see *J Am Coll Cardiol* 2001;37:407). The Carvedilol Prospective Randomized Cumulative Survival (COPERNICUS) trial extended these results to a more advanced patient population with NYHA class IV symptoms (69). Patients with far advanced HF symptoms and those who could not reach compensation were not enrolled, nor were significant numbers of black patients. The Carvedilol or Metoprolol European Trial (COMET) directly compared these two agents in 3,029 patients. At a mean follow-up of more than 3 years, carvedilol was associated with a significantly lower mortality than metoprolol therapy (70). It should be noted, however, that this trial used the shorter acting metoprolol tartrate, not the extended-release metoprolol succinate. The MERIT-HF trial used metoprolol succinate (XL), and all trials directly comparing carvedilol to metoprolol used the shorter acting tartrate formulation.

Some trials suggest a benefit of β-blockers in asymptomatic HF patients, that is, those with Stage B HF. A post hoc analysis of the SOLVD-Prevention trial, looking at asymptomatic patients with an LVEF ≤35%, suggests a synergistic effect of β-blockers and ACE-I leading to significantly lower rates of mortality due to HF compared to ACE-I alone (75). The Carvedilol Post-infarct Survival Control in Left Ventricular Dysfunction (CAPRICORN) study evaluated the addition of carvedilol versus placebo in post-MI patients with LVEF ≤40% (76). Carvedilol reduced mortality risk by 23% and was equally effective in patients with or without HF symptoms. The Carvedilol ACE Inhibitor Remodeling Mild HF Evaluation (CARMEN) trial and Reversal of Ventricular Remodeling with Toprol-XL (REVERT) trial suggest the importance of high-dose β-blocker therapy in reducing cardiac remodeling in asymptomatic HF patients (77,78).

Not all trials of β-adrenergic blockade have shown positive results. The β-blocker Evaluation of Survival Trial (BEST) compared bucindolol with placebo in 2,708 patients with NYHA class III or IV symptoms and found no difference in overall mortality rates (71). These findings called into question the concept of beneficial class effects for β-blockade in HF. However, bucindolol did significantly reduce cardiovascular mortality by 14% versus placebo ($p = 0.04$). Additionally, subgroup analysis did suggest a significant mortality benefit in the non-black patient population but no benefit in black patients.

Again it is important to note that β-blockers should be continued in all HF patients unless they show signs of poor perfusion in the setting of decompensation.

AMIODARONE

One South American study of the Grupo de Estudio de la Sobrevida en la Insuficiencia Cardiaca en Argentina (GESICA) (79) showed a mortality benefit, whereas the more recent and better designed Survival Trial of Antiarrhythmic Therapy in HF (HF-STAT) (80) found no mortality advantage in the amiodarone group. In the HF-STAT, a trend was seen toward a lower mortality rate with amiodarone in the subgroup of patients with nonischemic cardiomyopathy. Analysis of the VALIANT study has shown that amiodarone should not be considered as part of the routine treatment of patients with HF, unless it is needed to prevent recurrent atrial fibrillation or symptomatic ventricular arrhythmias. Furthermore, a related, newly approved antiarrhythmic drug, dronedarone, was specifically found to be harmful in patients with HF, and is thus contraindicated in such patients (see Chapter 6 and *N Engl J Med* 2008;358:2678–2687).

SOME FAILED AGENTS

1. Oral milrinone (inotrope)—A higher mortality rate was found in the PROMISE trial, with more adverse reactions including syncope and hypotension (82).

2. Vesnarinone (inotrope)—Despite one study that suggested a benefit with 60 mg/day, a subsequent larger study showed increased mortality with 60 mg/daily compared with placebo (84).

3. Mibefradil (L-type calcium-channel blockade)—Mibefradil was compared with placebo in 2,590 NYHA class II to IV patients in the MACH-1 study (see *Circulation* 2000;101:758). A trend was noted toward increased mortality with mibefradil (14% higher at 3 months; $p = 0.09$). Patients comedicated with mibefradil and antiarrhythmics (class I or III), including amiodarone, had a significantly increased risk of death.

4. Omapatrilat (vasopeptidase inhibitor)—Omapatrilat was compared with enalapril in the OVERTURE study, but no mortality advantage was found (85). It was never approved by the FDA due to concerns that it was associated with a high incidence of angioedema.

5. Endothelin-receptor antagonism—Bosentan was compared with placebo in the Endothelin Antagonist Bosentan for Lowering Cardiac Events in Heart Failure (ENABLE) trial. No significant difference was seen in the primary endpoint of death or rehospitalization for HF in 1,613 patients with NYHA class IIIB or IV symptoms. Treatment with this drug led to fluid retention in some patients and further adverse cardiac events (see *J Am Coll Cardiol* 2002;40:1). The EARTH trial randomized 642 patients with NYHA class II to IV symptoms and LVEF 35% or less to darusentan or placebo for at least 1 month. At 6 months darusentan did not improve any variable of LV remodeling, and there was no change in LV end-systolic dimension (primary endpoint). Finally, tezosentan was compared with placebo in the Randomized Intravenous Tezosentan study (RITZ-4) (see *J Am Coll Cardiol* 2003;41:1452). No significant difference was seen in the primary composite endpoint of death, worsening HF, recent ischemia, and recurrent or new MI within 72 hours. Tezosentan was also compared to placebo for the treatment of acute decompensated HF in the large Value of Endothelin Receptor Inhibition with Tezosentan in Acute Heart Failure Studies (VERITAS), which enrolled 1,435 patients from three continents (see *JAMA* 2007;298:2009–2019). The study found no benefit of tezosentan versus placebo for the coprimary endpoints of change in dyspnea over 24 hours and a composite of death or worsening HF within 7 days.

INVESTIGATIONAL AGENTS

1. Levosimendan (calcium sensitizer, inotrope)—This agent has been around for several years, and results have been equivocal. The recent Survival of Patients With Acute Heart Failure in Need of Intravenous Inotropic Support (SURVIVE) trial (see *JAMA* 2007;297:1883–1891) randomized 1,327 patients with

acute decompensated HF and an EF <30% to either levosimendan or dobut-amine infusions. There was no difference in all-cause mortality at 180 days (primary endpoint) or in any of the secondary endpoints. A subgroup analysis of SURVIVE (see *Eur J Heart Fail* 2009;11:304–311) suggests that patients with chronic HF who are on β-blockers may have improved mortality in the setting of acute decompensated heart failure (ADHF) treated with levosimen-dan rather than dobutamine. A recent meta-analysis suggests a possible bene-fit of levosimendan pre- and postoperatively in cardiac surgery patients (see *J Cardiothorac Vasc Anesth* 2010;24:51–57).

2. Istaroxime (Na/K-ATPase, inotrope)—This novel inotrope may be a safe agent for short-term treatment of ADHF. The small phase II Hemodynamic, Echocardiographic, and Neurohormonal Effects of Istaroxime in Acute Heart Failure Syndromes (HORIZON-HF) trial suggests istaroxime increases sys-tolic BP, decreases HR, and has a lusitropic effect compared with other inotropes.

3. Myosin activators—These investigational drugs use a novel mechanism within the myocyte to directly activate myosin without increasing intracellular cal-cium. The effect is lengthening of systole without the unwanted increase in oxygen demand.

4. Vasopressin receptor antagonists—Conivaptan (V1a and V2 receptor antago-nist), tolvaptan (selective V2 antagonist, oral), and lixivaptan (V2 selective, oral) are all being studied. The largest study, Efficacy of Vasopressin Antagonist in Heart Failure Outcome Study with Tolvaptan (EVEREST) tri-als (see *JAMA* 2007;297:1319, 1332), failed to show improvement in outcomes but did improve symptoms with minimal adverse effects. The vaptans hold promise as a potential alternative to current diuretic agents as they cause free water loss without adverse effects often seen with loop diuretics such as hypotension, hyponatremia, and worsening renal failure.

BIVENTRICULAR PACING

Among those with chronic HF due to systolic dysfunction, 30% or more have elec-trical conduction defects (bundle branch block or intraventricular conduction delay) that cause delayed activation of portions of the ventricular myocardium. This dyssynchrony decreases efficiency of ventricular contraction and worsens sys-tolic function. Please see Chapter 6 for a discussion of biventricular (BiV) pacing, also known as cardiac "resynchronization" therapy (CRT).

SURGICAL OPTIONS

Left Ventricular Assist Device

Useful as a bridging device to transplantation, the left ventricular assist device (LVAD) significantly improves peak oxygen consumption (89). Failure of long-term therapy is predicted by several preoperative variables, including poor urine output, elevated central venous pressure, mechanical ventilation, prolonged prothrombin time, and reoperation (87). The use of the LVAD as destination therapy was evaluated in the REMATCH trial. A significant survival advantage was noted in patients with end-stage HF who received an LVAD, but this therapy was limited by device malfunction, the high incidence of infection, and the fact that only 25% of patients receiving LVAD were alive at 2 years (91).

The new HeartMate II trial compares a new continuous-flow device (HeartMate II) to the older pulsatile-flow HeartMate XVE (92). The devices were compared in 200 transplant-ineligible patients, thus using the devices as destination therapy. Patients with continuous-flow devices had improved survival rates at 2 years (58% vs. 24%; $p = 0.008$). As compared with patients with a pulsatile-flow LV device, there were significant reductions in the rates of major adverse events among patients with a continuous-flow LVAD—including hardware-related or nonhardware-related infection, arrhythmia, right HF, respiratory failure, and renal failure. The incidence of stroke did not differ significantly between the continuous-flow group and the pulsatile-flow group. There was a 38% relative reduction in the rate of rehospitalization among patients with a continuous-flow LVAD as compared with those with a pulsatile-flow device.

Coronary Artery Bypass Graft Surgery

In HF patients with CAD and moderate to severe LV dysfunction (EF <40%), coronary artery bypass graft (CABG) improves 3-year survival by 30% to 50%. It is not clear whether this magnitude of benefit is obtained in patients with primarily HF symptoms and little or no angina. There are no randomized trials of revascularization in patients with CAD, an LVEF <35% to 40%, and evidence of myocardial viability. Most observational studies have found that revascularization of hibernating myocardium in patients with ischemic cardiomyopathy improves both survival and LV function compared to medical therapy [see *J Am Coll Cardiol* 2005;46(4):567–574]. The Surgical Treatment for Ischemic Heart Failure (STICH) trial is a multicenter, international, randomized trial from the NHLBI that began enrolling patients in 2002 to determine whether a benefit over medical therapy can be found for coronary revascularization and whether this benefit can be enhanced by ventricular restoration surgery. The results, at least of the CABG versus medical therapy for ischemic cardiomyopathy arm, are expected around 2012 (see below for results of the ventricular restoration surgery arm).

Cardiac Transplantation

Heart transplantation should be considered if peak oxygen consumption is below 10 to 12 mL/kg/min on optimal therapy. Other eligibility criteria also must be met (typically, age 65 years or younger, no active infection, and no malignancy).

Experimental or Controversial Treatment

1. Ventricular remodeling operation: Batista procedure—A wedge of the LV muscle is removed from apex to base, and the mitral valve apparatus is often repaired or replaced. Various centers have reported perioperative mortality in

excess of 20%. The largest series reported a surgical mortality of 3.2%, but 16% required LVADs. Long-term results were disappointing, with an incidence of death, return to NYHA class IV symptoms, or need for transplant or LVAD of 50% at 1 year and 67% at 2 years. Mortality rates have ranged from 15% to 30%, and LVAD rescue is often necessary.

2. Surgical ventricular restoration: Dor procedure—This procedure was evaluated in the STICH trial (mentioned above) as an attempt to restore the LV's elliptical geometry at the time of CABG in ischemic cardiomyopathy patients (93). The procedure entails an anterior left ventriculotomy centered in the zone of anterior asynergy, a suture encircling the scar, and then a cinching of the suture to bring the healthy portions of the ventricular walls in contact with one another. In STICH, surgical ventricular reconstruction reduced the end-systolic volume (ESV) index by 19%, as compared with a reduction of 6% with CABG alone. Cardiac symptoms and exercise tolerance improved from baseline to a similar degree in the two study groups. However, no significant difference was observed in the primary outcome of death or cardiac rehospitalization at 48 months (59% in the CABG-alone group vs. 58% for CABG plus SVR, $p = 0.90$).

3. Mitral valve repair—This option has been used in patients with HF due to DCM, which is complicated by severe, refractory mitral regurgitation. In one study, mitral valve reconstruction resulted in significant NYHA class improvement and a 2-year survival rate of more than 70% (88). However, a more recent study evaluating MV repair at the time of CABG for ischemic MR showed no improvement in survival and no significant difference in NYHA functional class versus CABG alone [see *Ann Thorac Surg* 2004;78(3): 794–799].

4. Stem cells—Autologous stem cells have shown some promise in preliminary studies of ischemic cardiomyopathy patients [see *Circulation* 2003;107(18): 2294–2302]. Most studies of stem cells have been done in acute MI patients as an attempt to preserve myocardial function. Newer studies suggest that allogenic stem cells, peripherally infused, may present a more practical approach in MI patients (see *J Am Coll Cardiol* 2009;54:2277–2286).

MISCELLANEOUS

Tailored Therapy

Routine invasive hemodynamic monitoring with pulmonary artery catheters is *not* considered standard of care for most hospitalized patients with symptoms of worsening HF. This trend stems primarily from the Evaluation Study of Congestive Heart Failure and Pulmonary Artery Catheterization Effectiveness (ESCAPE) trial, a large randomized multicenter trial of tailored therapy with PA catheters versus clinical assessments in patients hospitalized with severe HF refractory to standard of care therapy (94). A meta-analysis of 13 randomized trials published at the time of the ESCAPE trial found similar results (see *JAMA* 2005;294:1664–1670).

The AHA/ACC guidelines recommend that invasive hemodynamic monitoring should be performed in patients with (1) presumed cardiogenic shock requiring escalating pressor therapy and consideration of mechanical support; (2) severe clinical decompensation in which therapy is limited by uncertainty regarding relative contributions of elevated filling pressures, hypoperfusion, and vascular tone; (3) apparent dependence on intravenous inotropic infusions after initial clinical improvement; (4) persistent severe symptoms despite adjustment of recommended therapies.

Continuous Positive Airway Pressure (CPAP)
In the Sleep Heart Health Study, the presence of sleep-disturbed breathing was associated with a 2.38 relative risk of HF independent of other known risk factors (see *Am J Respir Crit Care Med* 2001;163:19–25). In HF patients with depressed LV function and obstructive sleep apnea, treatment of the latter with CPAP has been shown to reduce SBP and improve LV systolic function (see *N Engl J Med* 2003;348:1233).

Exercise Training and Rehabilitation
Numerous studies have shown tolerability and benefits of exercise in most patients, and it is now recommended for most stable outpatients with chronic HF. Regular exercise typically results in increased peak oxygen uptake and increased peak workload. Patients with circulatory failure in addition to deconditioning may not respond to exercise training (90,91,96).

Multidisciplinary Approach
One study found that a comprehensive, nurse-directed management approach, consisting of patient and family education, prescribed diet, social service consult, medication review, and intensive follow-up, led to more than 50% fewer HF-related hospitalizations, improved QOL, and significant cost savings (2).

COMPLICATIONS

Sudden Cardiac Death

CAD is the major substrate of sudden cardiac death, and cardiomyopathies, valvular heart disease, and abnormalities of the conduction system also are implicated; the baseline EF is a significant predictor of sudden cardiac risk. Sudden cardiac death is responsible for 30% to 70% of deaths among those with HF. The incidence is 2% to 3% per year in those with asymptomatic LV dysfunction and up to 20% per year in those with severe HF. Patients with advanced HF who have a syncopal episode have a high incidence of subsequent sudden death [in one study, 45% at 1 year (100)]. The incidence of sudden cardiac death appears lower in patients receiving ACE inhibitors.

Whereas predictors of sudden cardiac death have been established in patients with prior MI and reduced EF (see Chapter 6, MADIT, MADIT II, and MUSTT), risk stratification is difficult because few clinical predictors are specific for sudden cardiac death in those with nonischemic HF. However, the Sudden Cardiac Death in Heart Failure Trial (SCD-HeFT) showed a significant decrease in mortality in patients with NYHA class II and III HF and EF <35% (see Chapter 6 for trial details), and ICD implantation is now recommended for these patients with ischemic or nonischemic cardiomyopathy.

Atrial Fibrillation

The prevalence of atrial fibrillation is approximately 20%, and it is associated with an increased risk of stroke (15% per year if LV dysfunction is present) and higher total mortality (99).

Embolism

Incidence is 1% to 2% per year in NYHA class II or III patients who are in normal sinus rhythm and 3% to 4% per year in patients awaiting transplantation. Oral anticoagulation should be considered if mural thrombus is present (embolic risk much higher).

REFERENCES

Guidelines, Miscellaneous

1. **Ghali JK,** et al. Precipitating factors leading to decompensation of heart failure: traits among urban blacks. *Arch Intern Med* 1988;148:2013.

   This study of 101 patients admitted to an inner city hospital with a diagnosis of HF established precipitating factor(s) in 93%. The most common causes were noncompliance with diet and/or drugs (63%), uncontrolled hypertension (44%), arrhythmias (29%; mostly atrial fibrillation), environmental factors (19%), inadequate therapy (17%), pulmonary infection (12%), emotional stress (7%), and MI (6%).

2. **Rich MW,** et al. A multidisciplinary intervention to prevent the readmission of elderly patients with congestive heart failure. *N Engl J Med* 1995;333:1190–1195.

   This prospective, randomized trial was composed of 282 high-risk patients aged 70 years or older hospitalized with HF. Patients were assigned to standard care (control group) or nurse-directed, multidisciplinary care, consisting of comprehensive education of the patient and family, a prescribed diet, social service consultation, medication review, and intensive follow-up. A trend was noted toward improved survival without readmission (primary endpoint) in the multidisciplinary intervention group (64.1% vs. 53.6%; $p = 0.09$). The total number of hospital admissions was significantly lower in the multidisciplinary intervention group (53 vs. 94; $p = 0.02$), including 56% fewer HF-related admissions (24 vs. 54; $p = 0.04$). The intervention group had an overall lower cost of care ($460 less per patient). Finally, in a subgroup of 126 patients, QOL scores at 90 days improved significantly more in the intervention patients ($p = 0.001$).

3. **Feenstra J,** et al. Drug-induced heart failure. *J Am Coll Cardiol* 1999;33:1152–1162.

This review discusses anthracyclines, cyclophosphamide, paclitaxel, mitoxantrone, other chemotherapeutic agents, nonsteroidal anti-inflammatory drugs, immunomodulating agents (e.g., interferons, interleukin-2), and antidepressants. The contributory roles of three major cardiac drug classes in causing HF also are reviewed: antiarrhythmics, β-blockers, and calcium-channel blockers.

4. **Hunt SA,** et al. ACC/AHA 2005 guideline update for the diagnosis and management of chronic heart failure in the adult: a report of the American College of Cardiology/American Heart Association Task Force on Practice Guidelines (Writing Committee to Update the 2001 Guidelines for the Evaluation and Management of Heart Failure). *J Am Coll Cardiol* 2005;46:1116–1143.

This consensus document outlines the assessment and therapy of patients with HF. The report outlines management of patients with symptomatic and asymptomatic LV dysfunction as well as patients with refractory end-stage HF. Interventions that are of proven value are discussed in detail, as are end-of-life issues and the treatment of special populations such as women, racial minorities, and elderly patients.

5. **Jessup M,** et al. 2009 focused update: ACCF/AHA guidelines for the diagnosis and management of heart failure in adults: a report of the American College of Cardiology Foundation/American Heart Association Task Force on Practice Guidelines, developed in collaboration with the International Society for Heart and Lung Transplantation. *Circulation* 2009;119:1977–2016.

This is the 2009 update to the published 2005 ACC/AHA guidelines on HF. Recent clinical trials were deemed important enough to warrant this focused updated, with a new section specifically focusing on treatment of hospitalized patients with HF (acute HF syndromes). The committee outlines multiple new recommendations for inpatients with HF, including diagnostic laboratory and imaging studies, medical management, and monitoring of progress in these patients. The update also addresses recommendations for patients with refractory, end-stage HF.

6. **Jessup M,** Brozena S. Heart failure. *N Engl J Med* 2003;348:2007–2018.

This article reviews the epidemiology, pathophysiology, and etiologies of HF. Treatment modalities are then discussed for patients in various stages (A to D) of HF. Two final sections briefly review nonpharmacologic therapies.

7. **Maeder MT,** et al. Heart failure with normal left ventricular ejection fraction. *J Am Coll Cardiol* 2009;53:905–918.

In this "State-of-the-Art" paper, the authors describe the population of patients with "heart failure with normal ejection fraction" (HFNEF), as well as pathophysiologic mechanisms. They detail a diagnostic criteria algorithm, echocardiographic measures, and biomarkers in support of future therapeutic options.

8. **Pang PS,** et al. The current and future management of acute heart failure syndromes. *Eur Heart J* 2010;31:784–793.

This review focuses on the enormous problem of acute, symptomatic, decompensated HF, termed "acute heart failure syndromes." The authors highlight the significance of the problem, its triggers, and outcomes. They also call to attention the disparity in evidence base in therapies for inpatient, versus outpatient, management of HF. Future therapeutic approaches are discussed, in an effort to emphasize the need for improved outcomes in these patients.

Epidemiology

9. **Schocken DD,** et al. Prevalence and mortality rate of congestive heart failure in the United States. *J Am Coll Cardiol* 1992;20:301–306.

This analysis focused on prevalence data obtained from the NHANES I (1971 to 1975) and mortality data from the NHANES-I Epidemiologic Follow-up Study (1982 to 1986). Prevalence based on clinical criteria was 2% for the noninstitutionalized U.S. population. Mortality increased with advancing age and was higher in men than in women (15-year rates in patients older than 55 years: men, 71.8%; women, 39.1%).

10. **Levy D,** et al. The progression from hypertension to congestive heart failure. *JAMA* 1996;275:1557–1562.

This analysis focused on 5,143 Framingham Study subjects with a mean follow-up period of 14.1 years. Hypertension antedated 91% of new HF cases. After risk-factor adjustment, hypertension was associated with relative risks of developing HF of approximately 2.0 (men) and 3.0 (women). Poor 5-year survival was observed among hypertensive HF subjects: 24% in men and 31% in women.

11. **Adams KF Jr,** et al. Relation between gender, etiology and survival in patients with symptomatic heart failure. *J Am Coll Cardiol* 1996;28:1781–1788.

This prospective, observational study was composed of 557 patients (177 women; nonischemic etiology in 68%). At a mean follow-up of 2.4 years, the all-cause mortality rate was 36%. Women with better survival ($p < 0.001$), primarily due to the lower mortality associated with a nonischemic etiology (men vs. women, relative risk 2.36; $p < 0.001$).

12. **Roger VL,** et al. Trends in heart failure incidence and survival in a community-based population. *JAMA* 2004;292:344–350.

To assess survival rates in patients with HF among various demographics, the investigators enrolled 4,537 patients with HF of Olmsted County, Minnesota, between 1979 and 2000. They found that men had a higher incidence of heart failure (378 per 100,000 for men vs. 289 per 100,000 for women), and survival was worse among men at mean follow-up of 4.2 years (RR, 1.33; 95% CI, 1.24 to 1.43). Five-year survival rates did improve from 1979–1984 to 1996–2000 (age-adjusted survival, 43% for 1979 to 1984 vs. 52% for 1996 to 2000; $p < 0.001$); however, these gains were predominantly limited to men and younger patients at the expense of little to no improvement among women and the elderly. The incidence of HF has not declined over two decades; however, overall survival has improved, at least in this community-based cohort.

13. **Adams KF,** et al. Gender differences in survival in advanced heart failure. *Circulation* 1999;99:1816–1821.

This analysis focused on 471 Flolan International Randomized Survival Trial (FIRST) patients, of whom 112 were women; 60% were NYHA class IV, and average EF was 18%. A Cox proportional-hazards model, which included adjustments for age, gender, and 6-minute walk results, showed a significant association between female gender and better survival. (Relative risk of death for men vs. women was 2.18; $p < 0.001$.)

14. **Levy D,** et al. Long-term trends in the incidence of and survival with heart failure. *N Engl J Med* 2002;347:1397–1402 (editorial, 1442–1444).

This analysis consisted of 1,075 Framingham Heart Study participants who developed HF from 1950 to 1999. As compared with the period from 1950 to 1969, the incidence of HF remained virtually unchanged among men in the three subsequent periods (1970 to 1979, 1980 to 1989, 1990 to 1999) but declined by 31% to 40% among women (rate ratio for 1990 to 1999, 0.69; 95% CI, 0.51 to 0.93). Survival after onset of HF improved in both sexes. The 30-day,

1-year, and 5-year age-adjusted mortality rates among men declined from 12%, 30%, and 70% in the period from 1950 to 1969 to 11%, 28%, and 59% from 1990 to 1999. Corresponding rates among women were 18%, 28%, and 57% (1950 to 1969) and 10%, 24%, and 45% (1990 to 1999). Overall, the survival after HF onset improved by 12% per decade ($p = 0.01$ for men, $p = 0.02$ for women).

15. **O'Meara E,** et al. Sex differences in clinical characteristics and prognosis in a broad spectrum of patients with heart failure: results of the Candesartan in Heart Failure: Assessment of Reduction in Mortality and Morbidity (CHARM) program. *Circulation* 2007;115:3111–3120.

   The CHARM trial consisted of three independent but related trials in which patients with NYHA class II to IV HF were randomized to placebo or candesartan based on EF and prior ACE experience—CHARM-Alternative (EF ≤40%, intolerant of ACE-I) with 2,028 patients, CHARM-Added (EF ≤40%, already taking an ACE-I) with 2,548 patients, and CHARM-Preserved (EF >40%) with 3,023 patients. The primary outcome for each of the trials was the composite of cardiovascular death or unplanned admission for HF; there was a primary endpoint for the overall program, as well: all-cause mortality.
   O'Meara et al. used the results of the CHARM trial to assess differences in outcome based on gender alone. They found that women had lower all-cause mortality (21.5% vs. 25.3% in men; adjusted HR, 0.77; $p < 0.001$), as well as cardiovascular death or HF admission (30.4% vs. 33.3% for men; adjusted HR, 0.83; $p < 0.001$). Risk of death in women was unrelated to cause of heart failure or EF (see below for additional description of the CHARM program).

Assessment and Prognosis

PHYSICAL EXAMINATION

16. **Stevenson LW,** Perloff JK. The limited reliability of physical signs for estimating hemodynamics in chronic heart failure. *JAMA* 1989;261:884–888.

   This prospective study was composed of 50 patients with known chronic HF. Orthopnea within the preceding week was the most sensitive (91%) symptom for predicting elevated PCWP (22 mm Hg or more). Physical signs were not sensitive at predicting elevated PCWP because rales, edema, and elevated mean JVP were absent in 18 (41.9%) of 43 patients. A measured pulse pressure of less than 25% had a 91% sensitivity and 83% specificity for a cardiac index less than 2.2 L/min/m^2.

17. **Butman SM,** et al. Bedside cardiovascular exam with severe chronic heart failure: importance of rest or inducible jugular venous distention. *J Am Coll Cardiol* 1993;22:968–974.

   This prospective study was composed of 52 patients with chronic HF who underwent right heart catheterization. The presence of jugular venous distention had a 57% sensitivity and 93% specificity for a PCWP of 18 mm Hg. The combination of jugular venous distention at rest or inducible by an hepatojugular test had a sensitivity of 81%, specificity of 80%, and 81% predictive accuracy.

18. **Badgett RG,** et al. Can the clinical examination diagnose left-sided heart failure in adults? *JAMA* 1997;277:1712–1719.

   This review of the literature asserts that the best findings for detecting increased filling pressure are jugular venous distention and radiographic redistribution. The best findings for detecting systolic dysfunction are abnormal apical impulse, cardiomegaly (by radiograph), and Q waves or left bundle branch block on ECG.

19. **Nohria A,** et al. Clinical assessment identifies hemodynamic profiles that predict outcomes in patients admitted with heart failure. *J Am Coll Cardiol* 2003;41:1797–1798.

In this seminal paper, the investigators identify clinical findings in inpatients with HF that help to categorize them into four different hemodynamic profiles: cold–wet, cold–dry, warm–wet, and warm–dry. The primary conclusion found that such a categorization could help predict outcomes in patients with HF (with the cold–wet patients fairing the worst). However, these profiles also provide a foundation on which to base decisions for clinical therapies and aggressiveness of interventions.

20. **Drazner MH,** et al. Prognostic importance of elevated jugular venous pressure and a third heart sound in patients with heart failure. *N Engl J Med* 2001;345:574–581.

This is a retrospective analysis of the SOLVD treatment trial, in which 2,569 patients with a history of symptomatic HF were randomly assigned to receive enalapril or placebo and followed for a mean of 32 months. Elevated JVP or a third heart sound was identified on physical examination at trial enrollment, and used to predict outcomes of hospitalization for HF and/or progression of HF. In multivariable analyses, the risk of all endpoints was increased in patients with an elevated JVP and/or third heart sound ($p < 0.05$ for hospitalization for HF, death or hospitalization for HF, and death from pump failure).

ETIOLOGY

21. **Luk A,** et al. Dilated cardiomyopathy: a review. *J Clin Pathol* 2009;62:219–225.

Causes of systolic HF, specifically those that lead to ventricular dilation, are broad and many. This review discusses the myriad causes, both genetic/heritable and acquired, highlighting the pathophysiology, pathology, and diagnostic criteria.

22. **Massie BM,** et al. Randomized trial of warfarin, aspirin, and clopidogrel in patients with chronic heart failure: the Warfarin and Antiplatelet Therapy in Chronic Heart Failure (WATCH) trial. *Circulation* 2009;119(12):1616–1624.

Design: Prospective, randomized, clinical trial. The primary outcome was the time to first occurrence of death, nonfatal MI, or nonfatal stroke.
Purpose: To determine the optimal antithrombotic agent for HF patients with reduced EFs who are in sinus rhythm.
Population: 1,587 men and women ≥18 years of age with symptomatic HF for at least 3 months who were in sinus rhythm and had left ventricular ejection fraction of ≤35%.
Treatment: Patients were assigned to one of the following three treatment arms—blinded aspirin 162 mg, blinded clopidogrel 75 mg daily, or open-label warfarin (target INR of 2.5 to 3.0 with a designated acceptable range of 2.0 to 3.5). There was no loading dose for either clopidogrel or aspirin.
Results: There was no difference between groups for the primary endpoint of death, nonfatal MI, or nonfatal stroke (HR 0.98 for warfarin vs. aspirin, 1.08 for clopidogrel vs. aspirin, and 0.89 for warfarin vs. clopidogrel; all p = NS). Rates of hospitalization for HF were significantly higher in the aspirin group than in the warfarin group ($p = 0.02$), and there were fewer strokes in the warfarin group, compared with either aspirin or clopidogrel. More bleeding occurred in the warfarin group, compared to clopidogrel [$p = 0.01$ ($p = 0.22$ for warfarin vs. aspirin)].

LABORATORY, OTHER

23. **Gheorghiade M,** et al. Relationship between admission serum sodium concentration and clinical outcomes in patients hospitalized for heart failure: an analysis from the OPTI-MIZE-HF registry. *Eur Heart J* 2007;28:980–988.

The investigators used the OPTIMIZE-HF registry, a cohort of patients hospitalized with HF, to measure 60- to 90-day outcomes based on serum sodium concentration at admission. In multivariable analyses of 48,612 patients from 259 hospitals, the risk of in-hospital death, follow-up mortality, and death or rehospitalization increased by 19.5%, 10%, and 8%, respectively, for each 3 mmol/L decrease in admission serum sodium below 140 mmol/L.

24. **Cooper LT,** et al. The role of endomyocardial biopsy in the management of cardiovascular disease: a scientific statement from the American Heart Association, American College of Cardiology, and the European Society of Cardiology. *Circulation* 2007;116:2216–2233.

This writing group provides 14 clinical scenarios in which EMB may be considered, with the strength of evidence supporting biopsy for each group. The writers intended to more specifically describe the evidence for and against EMB, balancing the procedural risk of potential clinical benefit, for each scenario.

25. **Maisel AS,** et al. for the Breathing Not Properly (BNP) Multinational Study Investigators. Rapid measurement of B-type natriuretic peptide in the emergency diagnosis of heart failure. *N Engl J Med* 2002;347:161–167.

Design: Prospective, blinded, multicenter study. Primary endpoint was diagnostic accuracy at the optimum cutoff of BNP and at 80% or more ED physician estimate of clinical probability of HF.
Purpose: To assess the correlation of serum BNP levels with the clinical diagnosis of HF.
Population: 1,538 patients with clinical suspicion for HF determined by the ED attending physician.
Exclusion Criteria: Advanced renal failure (creatinine clearance, <15 mL/min), acute MI, and overt cause of dyspnea (e.g., chest wall trauma).
Treatment: Standard evaluation and management for HF.
Results: The final diagnosis, as determined by two blinded independent cardiologists, was HF in 47% (744), with no findings of HF in 49% (770). BNP level, alone, was more diagnostic of HF than any other clinical marker. At a level of 100 pg/mL, diagnostic accuracy was 83.4%, with a negative predictive value of 96% at a cutoff of 50 pg/mL. In multivariable analyses, BNP added significantly to diagnostic certainty of HF.

26. **McCullough PA,** et al. B-type natriuretic peptide and clinical judgment in emergency diagnosis of heart failure: analysis from Breathing Not Properly **(BNP)** Multinational Study. *Circulation* 2002;106:416–422.

In this additional analysis of the BNP study, the investigators sought to quantify the additional diagnostic certainty provided by BNP in assessment of patients in the ED with possible HF (see above for further details of the BNP study). At an 80% cutoff level of certainty of HF, clinical judgment had a sensitivity of 49% and specificity of 96%. At 100 pg/mL, BNP had a sensitivity of 90% and specificity of 73%. In determining the correct diagnosis (HF vs. no HF), adding BNP to clinical judgment would have enhanced diagnostic accuracy from 74% to 81%. In those participants with an intermediate (21% to 79%) probability of HF, BNP at a cutoff of 100 pg/mL accurately classified 74% of the cases. The areas under the receiver operating characteristic curve were 0.86 (95% CI, 0.84 to 0.88), 0.90 (95% CI, 0.88 to 0.91), and 0.93 (95% CI, 0.92 to 0.94) for clinical judgment, for BNP at a cutoff of 100 pg/mL, and for the two in combination, respectively ($p < 0.0001$ for all pairwise comparisons).

27. **Mueller C,** et al. Use of B-type natriuretic peptide in the evaluation and management of acute dyspnea. *N Engl J Med* 2004;350:647–654.

To assess the impact of BNP-diagnosed HF on length of stay and cost of hospitalization, the investigators randomly assigned 452 patients with dyspnea to a diagnostic strategy involving BNP levels, or standard care. In those who had BNP levels measured, fewer required hospitalization and intensive care ($p = 0.008$ and $p = 0.01$, respectively), compared with the standard care group. Length of stay was lower in the BNP group (8 days vs. 11 days; $p = 0.001$), as was total cost of treatment ($p = 0.006$). Mortality at 30 days was similar ($p = 0.45$). The authors offer that improved, early diagnosis of HF in the ED, as aided by BNP measurement, can lead to more efficient treatment and hospitalization course. However, large-scale validation is required.

28. **Lindahl B,** et al. Serial analyses of N-terminal pro-B-type natriuretic peptide in patients with non-ST-segment elevation acute coronary syndromes: a Fragmin and Fast Revascularisation During Instability in Coronary Artery Disease (FRISC)-II Substudy. *J Am Coll Cardiol* 2005;45:533–541.

In patients with non-ST elevation ACS, the authors measured serial BNP levels at randomization, 48 hours, 6 weeks, 3 months, and 6 months. A minimum of three values were collected in 1,216 patients, in an effort to assess their prognostic value. Of note, values of BNP initially rose in the setting of ACS, but this appeared to be a transient phenomenon. However, at each time point, BNP level predicted mortality at 2 years. Predictability was better when measured during a chronic, stable period.

29. **Jourdain P,** et al. Plasma brain natriuretic peptide-guided therapy to improve outcome in heart failure: the STARS-BNP Multicenter Study. *J Am Coll Cardiol* 2007;49: 1733–1739.

The investigators sought to assess the utility of BNP-guided therapy in the management of outpatient HF. They enrolled 220 patients with NYHA II or III symptoms, and randomized them to conventional HF therapy, or therapy targeting a reduction in BNP to <100 pg/mL. The primary outcome was HF death or hospitalization for HF, and all patients were managed by a HF specialist. Overall, medication changes were more frequent in the BNP group (for all types of medications). This led to significantly higher mean doses of β-blockers and ACE-Is in the BNP group ($p < 0.05$). Subsequently, fewer patients experienced a primary endpoint event in the BNP group (24% vs. 52%; $p < 0.001$).

30. **Weber M,** et al. N-terminal B-type natriuretic peptide assessment provides incremental prognostic information in patients with acute coronary syndromes and normal troponin T values upon admission. *J Am Coll Cardiol* 2008;51:1188–1195.

The objective of this study was to assess the utility of BNP measurement in patients presenting with ACS and normal troponin T levels. From two independent registries, the investigators measured BNP in 2,614 patients—one cohort with confirmed ACS served as derivation for the other, with chest pain patients. Based on such analyses of patients with normal troponin T, they identified the best receiver operator curve result at a BNP cutoff of 474 pg/mL. At this level, BNP successfully discriminated high-risk ACS patients, significantly predicting mortality at 6 months in both datasets.

31. **Pfisterer M,** et al. BNP-guided vs. symptom-guided heart failure therapy: the Trial of Intensified vs Standard Medical Therapy in Elderly Patients With Congestive Heart Failure (**TIME-HF**) randomized trial. *JAMA* 2009;301:383–392.

In patients 60 years or older, with systolic HF, these investigators sought to demonstrate the superiority of BNP-guided management of outpatient HF, for the improvement of QOL and all-cause hospitalization rate. In all, 499 patients were randomized and stratified by age (60 to 74, 75 and older), and the patients, but not investigators, were blinded to their assignments. At 18 months of follow-up, there was no difference in the rates of rehospitalization (41% for BNP-guided vs. 40% for standard care; $p = 0.39$) and improvement in QOL was similar in the two groups. However, there was a significant interaction between outcome and age group—BNP-guided therapy appeared to improve outcomes only for younger patients (those aged 60 to 74 years).

32. **Singer AJ,** et al. Rapid Emergency Department Heart Failure Outpatients Trial (**RED-HOT II**): a randomized controlled trial of the effect of serial B-type natriuretic peptide testing on patient management. *Circ Heart Fail* 2009;2:287–293.

To determine the utility of BNP in discharging patients with HF, the investigators randomized 447 patients with acute HF exacerbations to care guided by serial BNP measurements, or to usual care. Notably, physicians were not given standardized management instructions in response to BNP measurements; they were only provided with the laboratory result. There were no differences in the primary endpoints of length of stay (6.5 days for each group), readmission within 30 days, or all-cause mortality. The small sample size and short follow-up, however, limit the conclusions from this study.

NONINVASIVE TESTING

33. **Mancini DM,** et al. Value of peak exercise oxygen consumption for optimal timing of cardiac transplantation in ambulatory patients with heart failure. *Circulation* 1991;83: 778–786.

   This study of 114 patients found a peak oxygen consumption of 14 mL/kg/min or less in 62 patients (35 were transplantation candidates, and 27 had noncardiac issues) and more than 14 mL/kg/min in 52 patients. All three groups had similar NYHA functional class, LVEF, and cardiac index. Patients with an oxygen consumption of more than 14 mL/kg/min had a lower PCWP and significantly better 1-year survival [94% vs. 70% (transplant candidates) and 47%]. A multivariate analysis found peak oxygen consumption to be the best survival predictor, whereas PCWP added further prognostic information.

34. **Bitner V,** et al. Prediction of mortality and morbidity with a 6-minute walk test in patients with left ventricular dysfunction. *JAMA* 1993;270:1702–1707.

   This analysis focused on 898 SOLVD patients with radiologic evidence of HF and/or EF less than 45%; mean follow-up period was 8 months. No significant test-related complications were found. Highest versus lowest performance level (distance walked, 450 m or more vs. <300 m): 71% lower mortality (3% vs. 10.2%), 51% fewer hospitalizations (19.9% vs. 40.9%), and 91% fewer HF hospitalizations (2% vs. 22.2%). Logistic regression analysis showed that EF and walk time were equally strong and independent predictors of mortality and hospitalization due to acute HF.

Treatment

ANGIOTENSIN-CONVERTING ENZYME INHIBITORS AND ANGIOTENSIN II INHIBITORS

Meta-analysis

35. **Garg R,** Yusuf S. Overview of randomized trials of angiotensin-converting enzyme inhibitors on mortality and morbidity in patients with heart failure. *JAMA* 1995;273: 1450–1456.

   This analysis focused on 32 studies with 7,105 patients. All studies were placebo controlled, 8 weeks in duration, and assessed all-cause mortality by intention to treat. ACE-inhibitor therapy was associated with significant reductions in total mortality (odds ratio, 0.77; 95% CI, 0.67 to 0.88; $p < 0.001$) and mortality or hospitalization for HF (odds ratio, 0.65; 95% CI, 0.57 to 0.74; $p < 0.001$). Patients with the lowest EF had the greatest benefit. The mortality reduction was mainly due to fewer deaths from progressive HF (odds ratio, 0.69; 95% CI, 0.58 to 0.83). Nonsignificant reductions were noted in the incidence of arrhythmic deaths (odds ratio, 0.91; 95% CI, 0.73 to 1.12) and fatal MI (odds ratio, 0.82; 95% CI, 0.60 to 1.12). No significant differences were found between several different agents (see **Tables 5.1 and 5.2**).

Studies

36. The Cooperative North Scandinavian Enalapril Survival Study **(CONSENSUS)** Group. Effects of enalapril on mortality in severe HF. *N Engl J Med* 1987;316:1429–1435.

Design: Prospective, randomized, double-blind, placebo-controlled, multicenter study. Average follow-up period was 6 months. Primary endpoint was all-cause mortality rate.

Purpose: To evaluate the effect of enalapril, in addition to conventional therapy, on mortality in patients with severe HF.

Population: 253 NYHA class IV patients with heart size larger than 600 mL/m^2 body surface area in men and more than 550 mL/m^2 in women.

Exclusion Criteria: Acute pulmonary edema, MI in prior 2 months, unstable angina, planned cardiac surgery, and serum creatinine more than 300 μM.

Treatment: Enalapril, 2.5 mg/day orally, up to 20 mg twice daily. All patients were taking diuretics, 94% taking digoxin, and 50% taking vasodilators (mostly isosorbide dinitrate).

Results: Trial was terminated early because of significant mortality benefit in the enalapril group—40% relative risk reduction (RRR) in mortality at 6 months (26% vs. 44%; $p = 0.0002$), 31% RRR at 1 year (36% vs. 52%; $p = 0.001$), and 27% RRR at end of the study (39% vs. 54%; $p = 0.003$). The entire mortality reduction was seen in patients with progressive HF (approximately 50% lower mortality). No difference in sudden death rates was observed. A significant mortality benefit was maintained at 2-year follow-up.

37. The Studies of Left Ventricular Dysfunction **(SOLVD)** Investigators. Effect of enalapril on survival in patients with reduced ventricular ejection fraction and congestive heart failure. *N Engl J Med* 1991;325:293–302.

Design: Prospective, randomized, double-blind, placebo-controlled, multicenter study. Average follow-up period was 41 months. Primary endpoint was all-cause mortality rate.

Purpose: To evaluate the effect of enalapril on mortality in patients with LV dysfunction and HF symptoms.

Population: 2,569 NYHA class II and III patients aged 21 to 80 years with an EF of 35% or less.

Exclusion Criteria: Active angina requiring surgery, unstable angina, or MI within the preceding month; renal failure; pulmonary disease; and current ACE-inhibitor therapy.

Treatment: Enalapril, 2.5 to 5 mg twice daily initially, and then increased at 2 weeks to 5 to 10 mg twice daily; or placebo. Other drugs were not restricted (e.g., diuretics, digoxin, vasodilators).

Results: Enalapril group had 16% lower mortality (35.2% vs. 39.7%, 16% risk reduction; $p = 0.0036$). The majority of this effect was owing to fewer deaths from progressive HF (16.3% vs. 19.5%; $p = 0.0045$). The enalapril group also had a lower rate of death and rehospitalization due to worsening HF (47.7% vs. 57.3%, 26% risk reduction; $p < 0.0001$). Sudden death rates were similar.

38. **The SOLVD Investigators**. Effect of enalapril on mortality and the development of heart failure in asymptomatic patients with reduced left ventricular ejection fractions. *N Engl J Med* 1992;327:685–691.

Design: Prospective, randomized, double-blind, placebo-controlled, multicenter study. Follow-up period was 37 months. Primary endpoint was all-cause mortality rate.

Purpose: To evaluate effect of enalapril on mortality in patients with LV dysfunction without overt HF.

Population: 4,228 patients aged 21 to 80 years with an EF of 35% or less and taking no medications for HF (diuretics allowed for hypertension, and digoxin for atrial fibrillation).

Exclusion Criteria: See SOLVD trial earlier.

Treatment: Enalapril, 2.5 to 20 mg orally per day, or placebo.

Results: Total mortality rates were 14.8% and 15.8% in the enalapril and placebo groups, respectively ($p = 0.30$). Most of this nonsignificant difference was due to 12% fewer cardiovascular deaths in the enalapril group (12.5% vs. 14.1%; $p = 0.12$). Fewer enalapril patients developed HF (20.7% vs. 30.2%; $p < 0.001$), and fewer required hospitalization due to HF (8.7% vs. 12.9%; $p < 0.001$).

39. The Acute Infarction Ramipril Efficacy Study **(AIRE)** Investigators. Effect of ramipril on mortality and morbidity of survivors of acute MI with clinical evidence of heart failure. *Lancet* 1993;342:821–828.

Design: Prospective, randomized, double-blind, placebo-controlled, multicenter study. Mean follow-up period was 15 months. Primary endpoint was all-cause mortality.

Purpose: To compare the effects of ramipril with placebo on overall mortality in acute MI survivors with early evidence of HF.

Population: 2,006 patients with an MI 2 to 9 days before study enrollment and clinical evidence of HF at any time since acute MI.

Exclusion Criteria: Severe HF (usually NYHA class IV), unstable angina, and HF of primary valvular or congenital etiology.

Treatment: Ramipril, 2.5 mg orally twice daily for 2 days, and then 5 mg twice daily; or placebo.

Results: Ramipril group had a 27% risk reduction in mortality (17% vs. 23%; $p = 0.002$). This benefit was already apparent at 30 days. Sudden cardiac deaths were reduced by 30% ($p = 0.011$).

Comments: AIREX follow-up study analyzed 603 patients at a mean 59 months, and the ramipril group still had a significantly lower mortality rate (RR, 0.64; 27.5% vs. 38.9%; $p = 0.002$).

40. Pitt B, et al. Evaluation of Losartan in the Elderly **(ELITE)**. Randomized trial of losartan vs. captopril in patients over 65 with heart failure. *Lancet* 1997;349:747–752.

Design: Prospective, randomized, double-blind, placebo-controlled, multicenter study. Primary endpoint was increase in creatinine clearance of 0.3 mg/dL.

Purpose: To compare the effects of angiotensin II–receptor inhibitor losartan with captopril on creatinine clearance and major cardiac events in elderly HF patients.

Population: 722 ACE inhibitor–naive patients in NYHA class II to IV and with EF of 40% or less.

Exclusion Criteria: Included SBP less than 90 mm Hg, acute MI or coronary angioplasty in the prior 72 hours, bypass surgery in the prior 2 weeks, unstable angina in the prior 3 months, and stroke or transient ischemic attack (TIA) in the prior 3 months.

Treatment: Losartan, 12.5 to 50 mg daily, or captopril, 6.25 to 50 mg three times daily for 48 weeks.

Results: Similar incidence of increased creatinine was observed in both groups (10.5%). Fewer losartan patients discontinued therapy: 12.2% vs. 20.8%; $p = 0.002$ (cough, 0 patient vs. 14 patients). The losartan group showed a trend toward lower rates of death and hospitalization (9.4% vs. 13.2%; $p = 0.075$) and a significant 45% lower overall mortality rate (4.8% vs. 8.7%; $p = 0.035$; sudden cardiac death: 5 patients vs. 14 patients). This mortality benefit was seen in all subgroups except women (240 patients, 7.6% vs. 6.6%).

Comments: Study was not designed to examine mortality.

41. **Packer M,** et al. Comparative effects of low and high doses of the angiotensin-converting enzyme inhibitor, lisinopril, on morbidity and mortality in chronic heart failure **(ATLAS)**. *Circulation* 1999;100:2312–2318.

Design: Prospective, randomized, double-blind, placebo-controlled, multicenter study. Primary endpoint was all-cause mortality. Follow-up period was 4 years.

Purpose: To evaluate the comparative efficacy of lisinopril on mortality in patients with LV dysfunction and HF symptoms.

Population: 3,164 patients with NYHA class II to IV HF and an EF of 30% or less.

Exclusion Criteria: Included acute coronary ischemic event or revascularization procedure in the prior 2 months, history of sustained or symptomatic ventricular tachycardia (VT), intolerance to ACE inhibitors, and serum creatinine greater than 2.5 mg/dL.

Treatment: Low-dose lisinopril (2.5 to 5.0 mg daily) or high-dose lisinopril (32.5 to 35 mg daily). Before randomization, all patients received lisinopril for 4 weeks to assess their ability to tolerate the drug. Digitalis, ACE inhibitors, or vasodilators were allowed but not mandated.

Results: Patients in the high-dose group had a nonsignificant 8% lower risk of death ($p = 0.13$) but a significant 12% lower risk of death or hospitalization for any reason ($p = 0.002$) and 24% fewer hospitalizations for HF ($p = 0.002$). Dizziness and renal insufficiency were observed more frequently in the high-dose group, but the two groups were similar in the number of patients requiring cessation of the study medication.

42. **Pitt B,** et al. Effect of losartan compared with captopril on mortality in patients with symptomatic heart failure: randomised trial—the Losartan Heart Failure Survival Study **(ELITE II).** *Lancet* 2000;355:1582–1587.

Design: Prospective, randomized, double-blind, placebo-controlled, multicenter study. Primary endpoint was all-cause mortality.

Purpose: To compare the mortality benefit of the angiotensin II–receptor inhibitor losartan with captopril in elderly HF patients.

Population: 3,152 ACE inhibitor–naive patients in NYHA class II through IV and with EF 40% or less.

Exclusion Criteria: Included ACE inhibitor or angiotensin II–receptor antagonist intolerance, SBP less than 90 mm Hg, diastolic blood pressure (DBP) greater than 95 mm Hg, hemodynamically important stenotic valvular heart disease, active myocarditis or pericarditis, ICD implantation, serum creatinine more than 220 mM, PTCA in previous week, and cerebrovascular accident (CVA) or TIA in previous 6 weeks; CABG surgery, acute MI, or unstable angina in previous 2 weeks.

Treatment: Losartan, 12.5 to 50 mg daily, or captopril, 6.25 to 50 mg three times daily.

Results: No significant differences were found between the two groups in all-cause mortality (11.7% vs. 10.4% average annual mortality rate) or sudden death or resuscitated arrests (9.0% vs. 7.3%; $p = 0.08$). Fewer losartan patients had adverse effects (9.7% vs. 14.7%; $p < 0.001$), especially cough (0.3% vs. 2.7%).

Comments: These results demonstrate the problem of drawing conclusions from trials enrolling small numbers of patients (i.e., ELITE I). The trial was not designed to address equivalence between the two treatments, so these findings do not provide evidence regarding the efficacy of losartan compared with placebo.

43. **Cohn JN,** et al. A randomized trial of the angiotensin-receptor blocker valsartan in chronic heart failure **(Val-HeFT).** *N Engl J Med* 2001;345:1667–1675.

Design: Prospective, randomized, double-blind, placebo-controlled, multicenter study. Primary endpoint was all-cause mortality.

Purpose: To determine the mortality benefit of adding valsartan to usual therapy for HF in patients with HF.

Population: 5,010 patients with NYHA class II to IV symptoms with EF 40% or less. Patients required to be on stable medical regimens, which could include diuretics, digoxin, ACE inhibition, and β-blockers.

Treatment: Valsartan, 40 to 50 mg daily, or captopril, 6.25 to 50 mg three times daily.

Results: No significant difference in overall mortality was found between the valsartan and captopril groups (19.7% vs. 19.4%). The incidence of the secondary combined endpoint of death or cardiac arrest with resuscitation, hospitalized for HF, or intravenous inotropic or vasodilator for 4 hours or more was significantly lower with valsartan (RR, 0.87; $p = 0.009$). This benefit was mainly owing to a lower incidence of hospitalization for HF (13.8% vs.

18.2%; $p < 0.001$). Treatment with valsartan also was associated with improvements in NYHA class, EF, signs and symptoms of HF, and QOL.

44. **Pfeffer MA,** et al. Valsartan, captopril, or both in myocardial infarction complicated by heart failure, left ventricular dysfunction, or both (**VALIANT**). *N Engl J Med* 2003; 349(20):1893–1906.

Design: Prospective, randomized, double-blind, multicenter (931 centers, 24 countries) noninferiority study.

Purpose: To compare valsartan, captopril, or both in a population of post-MI patients complicated by LV systolic dysfunction, HF, or both.

Population: 14,808 patients up to 10 days post-MI complicated by clinical or radiologic signs of HF, evidence of LV systolic dysfunction (an EF ≤0.35 on echocardiography or contrast angiography and ≤0.40 on radionuclide ventriculography), or both.

Treatment: Therapy was begun with either 20 mg of valsartan, 20 mg of valsartan plus 6.25 mg of captopril, or 6.25 mg of captopril alone. Doses were gradually increased in four steps, with the goal of reaching step 3 (80 mg of valsartan twice daily, 40 mg of valsartan twice daily, and 25 mg of captopril three times daily, or 25 mg of captopril three times daily) during the initial hospitalization and step 4 (160 mg of valsartan twice daily, 80 mg of valsartan twice daily, and 50 mg of captopril three times daily, or 50 mg of captopril three times daily), if clinically possible, by the 3-month visit.

Results: Mortality from any cause and cause-specific mortality were similar in the three treatment groups. The rate of the secondary endpoint of death from cardiovascular causes, recurrent MI, or hospitalization for HF was similar in the three groups.

45. **Pfeffer MA,** et al. Effects of candesartan on mortality and morbidity in patients with chronic heart failure: the **CHARM-overall** programme. *Lancet* 2003;362:759–766.

Design: Three parallel, randomized, double-blind, placebo-controlled clinical trials.

Purpose: To evaluate the effect of candesartan versus placebo on all-cause mortality in three different populations of HF patients.

Population: Overall, 7,601 patients (7,599 with data) were randomly assigned candesartan ($n = 3,803$, titrated to 32 mg once daily) or matching placebo ($n = 3,796$), and followed up for at least 2 years.

Treatment: Candesartan titrated to 32 mg daily versus placebo.

Results: Over median follow-up of 37.7 months, all-cause mortality trended to favor the candesartan group (23% vs. 25% in the placebo group, unadjusted HR 0.91, $p = 0.055$; adjusted HR 0.90, $p = 0.032$), and significantly favored cardiovascular death (18% vs. 20%, unadjusted HR 0.88, $p = 0.012$) and HF hospitalization (20% vs. 24%; $p < 0.0001$). Heterogeneity analyses were not significant across the component trials.

46. **Massie BM,** et al. Irbesartan in Patients with Heart Failure and Preserved Ejection Fraction (**I-PRESERVE**). *N Engl J Med* 2008;359:2456–2467.

Design: Prospective, randomized, placebo-controlled trial. Primary composite outcome was all-cause mortality or cardiovascular hospitalization (HF, MI, UA, arrhythmia, or stroke).

Purpose: To assess utility of irbesartan in HFpEF.

Population: 4,128 patients at least 60 years of age, with NYHA class II, III, or IV HF and an EF ≥45%.

Treatment: Irbesartan 300 mg daily or placebo.

Results: Irbesartan did not significantly reduce incidence of the primary endpoint (HR, 0.95; $p = 0.35$), all-cause mortality (HR, 1.00; $p = 0.98$), or rates of cardiovascular hospitalization (HR, 0.95; $p = 0.44$).

Comment: This trial added to the evidence that HFpEF is a unique clinical entity, not responsive (in terms of clinical endpoints) to classical HF therapies.

47. **Konstam MA,** et al. Effects of high-dose versus low-dose losartan on clinical outcomes in patients with heart failure **(HEAAL study)**: a randomised, double-blind trial. *Lancet* 2009;374:1840–1848.

Design: Prospective, randomized, double-blind, multicenter (255, 30 countries) trial. Primary endpoint was all-cause mortality or admission for HF over median 4.7 years of follow-up.
Purpose: To compare high-dose versus low-dose losartan in patients with HF.
Population: 3,846 patients with HF of NYHA class II, III, or IV, EF ≤40%, and intolerance to ACE inhibitors.
Treatment: Losartan 150 mg or losartan 50 mg daily.
Results: Incidence of a primary endpoint event was significantly lower in the high-dose losartan group (43% vs. 46%; $p = 0.027$); this was predominantly driven by significantly lower rates of HF admissions (HR, 0.87; $p = 0.025$). While expected adverse events were higher in the high-dose group (renal impairment, hypotension, and hyperkalemia), this did not yield significantly higher treatment cessation rates in this group.

48. **McKelvie RS,** et al. Comparison of candesartan, enalapril, and their combination in congestive heart failure: randomized evaluation of strategies for left ventricular dysfunction **(RESOLVD)** pilot study. The RESOLVD Pilot Study Investigators. *Circulation* 1999;100:1056–1064.

Design: Multicenter, double-blind, randomized, placebo-controlled trial.
Purpose: To compare candesartan alone, enalapril alone, and their combination for the endpoints of exercise tolerance, ventricular function, QOL, neurohormone levels, and tolerability over 43 weeks.
Population: 768 patients with NYHA class II, III, or IV HF, EF <0.40, and a 6MWD <500 m.
Treatment: Candesartan (4, 8, or 16 mg), candesartan (4 or 8 mg) plus 20 mg of enalapril, or 20 mg of enalapril.
Results: Over the 43-week study period, the groups did not differ with regard to 6MWD, NYHA class, or QOL ($p = $ NS). End-diastolic volume (EDV) and ESV increased less with combination (candesartan–enalapril) therapy than with candesartan or enalapril alone. The authors conclude that, while candesartan is as safe and effective as enalapril, the combination may have incremental benefit on ventricular remodeling.

DIURETICS

49. **Dormans TPJ,** et al. Diuretic efficacy of high dose furosemide in severe heart failure: bolus injection vs. continuous infusion. *J Am Coll Cardiol* 1996;28:376–382.

In this crossover study, 20 patients were randomized to an equal dosage by intravenous bolus or an 8-hour continuous infusion after a loading dose (20% total). Doses used ranged from 250 to 2,000 mg/24 hr. The continuous-infusion group had an increased urinary volume (2.9 vs. 2.3 L; $p < 0.001$) and better sodium excretion. Reversible hearing loss was seen in five intravenous-bolus patients (maximal plasma concentration, 95 μg/mL vs. 24 μg/mL; only nine patients, and the bolus plus 48-hour infusion yielded better results than intravenous boluses three times daily).

50. **Pitt B,** et al. Randomized Aldactone Evaluation Study **(RALES)** Investigators. The effect of spironolactone on morbidity and mortality in patients with severe heart failure. *N Engl J Med* 1999;341:709–719 (editorial, 753–755).

Design: Prospective, randomized, double-blind, placebo-controlled, multicenter study. Mean follow-up was 24 months. Primary endpoint was all-cause mortality.
Purpose: To evaluate whether spironolactone would significantly reduce mortality in patients with severe HF.
Population: 1,663 NYHA class III (69%) or IV (31%) patients with an EF of 35% or less. Ischemic etiology of HF in 54%.

Exclusion Criteria: Included valvular heart disease; unstable angina; hepatic failure; potassium, 5 mM or greater; creatinine, greater than 2.5 mg/dL.

Treatment: Spironolactone, 25 mg, or placebo once daily. Dose could be increased to 50 mg if worsening HF with normal potassium. All patients were taking loop diuretics, 95% were taking ACE inhibitors, and 74% were receiving digoxin.

Results: Spironolactone group had a significant (30%) reduction in mortality compared with placebo (35% vs. 46%; $p < 0.001$). This benefit was attributable to a lower risk of sudden death from cardiac causes (29% RRR) and death from progressive HF (36% RRR). Spironolactone was associated with a higher incidence of gynecomastia (10% vs. 1%; $p < 0.001$), whereas the incidence of serious hyperkalemia was similar (2% vs. 1%).

51. **Pitt B,** et al. for the EPHESUS (Eplerenone Post-acute MI Heart Failure Efficacy and Survival Study) Investigators. Eplerenone, a selective aldosterone blocker in patients with left ventricular dysfunction after myocardial infarction. *N Engl J Med* 2003;348:1309–1321 (editorial, 1380–1382).

Design: Prospective, randomized, placebo-controlled, double-blind, multicenter study. Primary endpoints were all-cause mortality and cardiovascular death or hospitalization for cardiovascular causes. Mean follow-up was 16 months.

Purpose: To evaluate the effect of eplerenone on morbidity and mortality among patients with acute MI complicated by LV dysfunction.

Population: 6,632 patients with an acute MI 3 to 14 days prior to randomization and LVEF = 40% by echocardiography.

Exclusion Criteria: Included use of potassium-sparing diuretics, creatinine >2.5 mg/dL, and potassium >5.0 mmol/L.

Treatment: Eplerenone, 25 to 50 mg twice daily, or placebo. Nearly all were on ACE inhibitors (94%) and 75% were on β-blockers.

Results: Eplerenone group had a significant reduction in all-cause mortality compared to placebo (14.4% vs. 16.7%; relative risk, 0.85; $p = 0.008$). It was also associated with a lower rate of cardiovascular death or CV-related hospitalization (RR, 0.87; $p = 0.002$). Eplerenone also had a 21% relative reduction in sudden cardiac death ($p = 0.03$). Serious hyperkalemia occurred more frequently with eplerenone (5.5% vs. 3.9%; $p = 0.002$), while hypokalemia was less common (8.4% vs. 13.1%; $p < 0.001$).

DIGOXIN

Review Article

52. **Hauptman PJ,** Kelly RA. Digitalis. *Circulation* 1999;99:1265–1270.

This review discusses the molecular and clinical pharmacology of cardiac glycosides, describes the clinical manifestations and treatment of digitalis toxicity, and examines recent trial data, with a focus on the DIG trial results.

Studies

53. **Packer M,** et al. Randomized Assessment of Effect of Digoxin on Inhibitors of ACE (RADIANCE) study. Withdrawal of digoxin from patients with chronic HF treated with ACE inhibitor. *N Engl J Med* 1993;329:1–7.

Design: Prospective, randomized, double-blind, placebo-controlled, multicenter study. Primary endpoint was study withdrawal due to worsening HF, time to withdrawal, and changes in exercise tolerance.

Purpose: To evaluate the effect of the withdrawal of digoxin from patients with chronic HF who were clinically stable while receiving digoxin, diuretics, and an ACE inhibitor.

Population: 178 NYHA class II or III patients taking digoxin, diuretics, and ACE inhibitors (captopril or enalapril).

Exclusion Criteria: SBP, 160 mm Hg or more or less than 90 mm Hg; DBP, greater than 95 mm Hg; history of supraventricular arrhythmias or sustained ventricular arrhythmias; MI in the prior 3 months; and stroke in the prior 12 months.

Treatment: Patients were randomized to continue digoxin or to placebo for 12 weeks.

Results: Cessation/placebo group had a markedly higher rate of worsening HF requiring withdrawal from the study (24.7% vs. 4.7; RR, 5.9; $p < 0.001$), lower EF ($p < 0.001$), decreased functional capacity (maximal exercise tolerance, $p = 0.033$; submaximal exercise endurance, $p = 0.01$; NYHA class, $p = 0.019$), and poorer QOL scores ($p = 0.04$).

54. **Uretsky BF,** et al. Prospective Randomized Study of Ventricular Failure and Efficacy of Digoxin **(PROVED).** Randomized study assessing effect of digoxin withdrawal in patients with mild–moderate chronic HF. *J Am Coll Cardiol* 1993;22:955–962.

Design: Prospective, randomized, double-blind, placebo-controlled, multicenter study. Primary endpoint was incidence of treatment failure, time to treatment failure, treadmill time, and 6MWD.

Purpose: To evaluate the effects of digoxin withdrawal in patients with mild to moderate HF.

Population: 88 NYHA class II or III patients in normal sinus rhythm and taking digoxin and diuretics.

Exclusion Criteria: SBP less than 90 mm Hg, acute MI or coronary angioplasty in the prior 72 hours, bypass surgery in the prior 2 weeks, unstable angina in the prior 3 months, and stroke or TIA in the prior 3 months.

Treatment: Patients were randomized to continue digoxin or to placebo for 12 weeks.

Results: Cessation/placebo group had lower exercise tolerance (–96 seconds vs. –4.5 seconds; $p = 0.003$), twice as many treatment failures (39% vs. 19%; $p = 0.039$), decreased time to treatment failure ($p = 0.037$), lower EF ($p = 0.016$), and higher heart rate ($p = 0.003$).

55. Digoxin Investigation Group **(DIG).** The effect of digoxin on mortality and morbidity in patients with heart failure. *N Engl J Med* 1997;336:525–533.

Design: Prospective, randomized, double-blind, placebo-controlled, multicenter study. Follow-up period was 37 months. Primary endpoint was all-cause mortality rate.

Purpose: To evaluate the effects of digoxin on mortality from any cause in HF patients.

Population: 6,800 patients with an EF of 45% or less and in normal sinus rhythm. Most patients were taking ACE inhibitors (94%) and diuretics (82%).

Treatment: Digoxin (average dose, 0.25 mg/day) or placebo.

Results: No significant difference in mortality rates (34.8% vs. 35.1%) was observed. The digoxin group had fewer HF hospitalizations (26.8% vs. 34.7%; RR, 0.72; $p < 0.001$) and showed a trend toward fewer HF deaths (RR, 0.88; $p = 0.06$), but this was offset by increased mortality due to other cardiac causes (not a prespecified outcome; 15% vs. 13%; $p = 0.04$). Subgroup analysis showed that greater reductions in death and hospitalization were due to worsening HF if EF less than 25% (–23% vs. –16%) or NYHA class III/IV (–22% vs. –18%). An overall decrease in hospital stays of only 9 per 1,000 patient years was observed. An ancillary trial of 988 patients with EF greater than 45% also showed no difference in mortality (both 23.4%).

Comments: Subsequent post hoc subgroup analysis (see *N Engl J Med* 2002;347:1403) showed that among women, a significantly higher mortality was seen in those assigned to digoxin therapy [33.1% vs. 28.9% (no digoxin)]; in contrast, mortality rates were similar in men. This finding among women persisted after a multivariate analysis was performed. Another post hoc analysis of 3,782 men with LVEF ≤45% found that the optimal serum digoxin concentration was 0.5 to 0.8 mg/mL (higher mortality if ≥0.9 mg/mL; see *JAMA* 2003;289:871).

VASODILATOR STUDIES

56. **Cohn JN,** et al. VA Cooperative Heart Failure Trial **(V-HeFT I).** Effect of vasodilator therapy on mortality in chronic congestive heart failure. *N Engl J Med* 1986;314:1547–1552.

Design: Prospective, randomized, double-blind, placebo-controlled, multicenter study. Mean follow-up period was 2.3 years. Primary endpoint was all-cause mortality rate.

Purpose: To determine whether two widely used vasodilator regimens could alter life expectancy in men with stable chronic HF.

Population: 642 men aged 18 to 75 years with chronic HF (defined as cardiac dilatation by chest radiography or echocardiography) or EF less than 45% in association with reduced exercise tolerance.

Exclusion Criteria: Exercise tolerance limited by chest pain, MI in prior 3 months, and requirement for long-acting nitrates, calcium-channel antagonists, and/or β-blockers.

Treatment: Prazosin, 20 mg once daily; hydralazine, 300 mg/day; and isosorbide dinitrate, 160 mg/day; or placebo. Digoxin and diuretics were permitted.

Results: Hydralazine–isosorbide dinitrate group had 38% lower mortality at 1 year [12.1% vs. 19.5% (placebo)], 25% reduction at 2 years [25.6% vs. 34.3% (placebo); $p < 0.028$], and 23% reduction at 3 years (36.2% vs. 46.9%). LVEF increased significantly at 8 weeks and at 1 year in the hydralazine–isosorbide dinitrate group (+2.9%, +4.2%; both $p < 0.001$). No significant benefits were seen with prazosin.

57. **Cohn JN,** et al. **V-HeFT II.** A comparison of enalapril with hydralazine–isosorbide dinitrate in the treatment of chronic HF. *N Engl J Med* 1991;325:303–310.

Design: Prospective, randomized, double-blind, placebo-controlled, multicenter study. Average follow-up period was 2.5 years. Primary endpoint was 2-year all-cause mortality rate.

Purpose: To compare the efficacy of enalapril with hydralazine plus isosorbide dinitrate in HF patients.

Population: 804 men aged 18 to 75 years in mostly NYHA class II/III and taking digoxin and diuretics.

Exclusion Criteria: MI or cardiac surgery in the prior 3 months and angina limiting exercise or requiring long-term medical therapy.

Treatment: Enalapril, 20 mg/day, or hydralazine, 300 mg/day, plus isosorbide dinitrate, 160 mg/day.

Results: Enalapril group had a 28% lower 2-year mortality rate (18% vs. 25%; $p = 0.016$) and a 14% lower overall mortality rate (32.8% vs. 38.2%; $p = 0.08$). This mortality difference was owing to fewer sudden cardiac deaths (57 patients vs. 92 patients), mostly in NYHA class I or II patients. At 13 weeks, the enalapril group had a greater reduction in BP, whereas the hydralazine–isosorbide dinitrate group had a greater increase in EF and exercise tolerance.

58. **Taylor AL,** et al. Combination of isosorbide dinitrate and hydralazine in blacks with heart failure (**A-HeFT**). *N Engl J Med* 2004;351:2049–2057.

Design: Prospective, randomized, double-blind, placebo-controlled multicenter trial. The primary endpoint was a weighted score composed of all-cause mortality, HF hospitalization, and QOL.

Purpose: To determine whether fixed-dose combination isosorbide dinitrate and hydralazine provides additional benefit in blacks with advanced HF.

Population: 1,050 black patients with NYHA class III or IV, dilated HF.

Treatment: Fixed-dose combination isosorbide dinitrate plus hydralazine or placebo.

Results: The study was terminated early due to significantly increased all-cause mortality in the placebo arm (10.2% vs. 6.2%; $p = 0.02$), which also had a lower mean primary composite score (–0.5 vs. –0.1; $p = 0.01$). All components of the composite score also significantly favored the isosorbide dinitrate plus hydralazine arm.

Comment: This trial led to the first FDA approval for a drug *for a specific racial group*.

59. **Packer M,** et al. Prospective Randomized Amlodipine Survival Evaluation **(PRAISE).** Effect of amlodipine on morbidity and mortality in severe chronic heart failure. *N Engl J Med* 1996;335:1107–1114.

Design: Prospective, randomized, double-blind, placebo-controlled, multicenter study. Average follow-up period was 14 months. Primary endpoint was mortality and CV morbidity [hospitalization for 24 hours for MI, pulmonary edema, severe hypoperfusion, VT, or ventricular fibrillation (VF)].

Purpose: To assess the safety and efficacy of the calcium-channel antagonist amlodipine in patients with severe chronic HF.

Population: 1,153 patients with an EF less than 30%. HF was associated with ischemic disease in 732 (63.5%) patients.

Exclusion Criteria: Unstable angina or MI in the prior month, cardiac arrest or sustained VT or VF in the prior year, stroke or cardiac revascularization in the prior 3 months, SBP less than 85 or 160 mm Hg or more, active myocarditis, constrictive pericarditis, and primary valvular disease.

Treatment: Amlodipine, 10 mg/day (5 mg/day for first 2 weeks), or placebo.

Results: Amlodipine group had a nonsignificant 9% lower incidence in the primary endpoint (39% vs. 42%; $p = 0.31$). It also had a nonsignificant 16% mortality reduction (33% vs. 38%; $p = 0.07$). Among nonischemic patients, amlodipine was associated with a 46% lower mortality rate ($p < 0.001$) and 31% fewer overall events ($p = 0.04$).

Comments: An interesting ancillary study of cytokines showed that high interleukin-6 levels correlated with increased HF and death ($p = 0.048$) and were reduced by amlodipine ($p = 0.006$) but to values still more than five times normal.

60. **PRAISE-2** (Prospective Randomized Amlodipine Survival Evaluation-2). Effect of amlodipine on morbidity and mortality in severe non ischemic chronic heart failure: preliminary results presented at the 49th Annual American College of Cardiology Scientific Sessions, Anaheim, CA, November 2000 [unpublished results].

Design: Prospective, randomized, double-blind, placebo-controlled, multicenter study. Primary endpoint was all-cause mortality and CV morbidity (hospitalization for 24 hours for MI, pulmonary edema, severe hypoperfusion, VT, or VF). Average follow-up was 4 years.

Purpose: To assess the safety and efficacy of the calcium-channel antagonist amlodipine in patients with severe nonischemic chronic HF.

Population: 1,652 patients with an EF less than 30% and NYHA class IIIb or IV symptoms despite therapy with diuretics, ACE inhibitors, and digoxin.

Exclusion Criteria: Included therapy with calcium-channel blockers, β-blockers, or cardiodepressant antiarrhythmic drugs; unstable angina or MI in the prior month; cardiac arrest or sustained VT or VF in the prior year; stroke or cardiac revascularization in the prior 3 months; SBP less than 85 or 160 mm Hg or greater; primary valvular disease.

Treatment: Amlodipine, 10 mg/day (5 mg/day for first 2 weeks), or placebo.

Results: No significant difference was found between the groups in all-cause mortality [31.7% (placebo), 33.7% (amlodipine); hazard ratio, 1.09; 95% CI, 0.92 to 1.29; $p = 0.32$]. No subgroup was found to receive a mortality benefit with amlodipine.

Comments: Further analysis using the combined population of PRAISE-1 and PRAISE-2 showed no significant differences in all-cause mortality.

61. **Colucci WS,** et al. for **Nesiritide Study Group.** Intravenous nesiritide, a natriuretic peptide, in the treatment of decompensated congestive heart failure. *N Engl J Med* 2000;343:246–253.

Design: Prospective, randomized, partially blinded, partially open, multicenter trial. Primary endpoint: change in pulmonary capillary pressure from baseline to 6 hours (efficacy trial); global clinical status and clinical symptoms (comparative trial).

Purpose: To evaluate an intravenous infusion of nesiritide, a BNP, in patients with decompensated HF.

Population: Efficacy study—127 patients with a PCWP of 18 mm Hg or more and cardiac index of 2.7 L/min/m^2; comparative trial, 305 patients.

Exclusion Criteria: Included dopamine, dobutamine, or intravenous vasodilator infusion for more than 4 hours; MI or unstable angina in the previous 48 hours; clinically significant valvular stenosis; hypertrophic or restrictive cardiomyopathy; constrictive pericarditis; or active myocarditis.

Treatment: Efficacy trial—Swan–Ganz catheter placed and randomization to double-blind treatment with intravenous placebo or nesiritide (0.015 or 0.030 μg/kg/min) for 6 hours. Comparative trial: hemodynamic monitoring not required and open-label therapy with standard agents or nesiritide for up to 7 days.

Results: In the efficacy trial, at 6 hours, nesiritide was associated with significant reductions in PCWP (6.0 and 9.6 mm Hg for 0.015 and 0.030 μg/kg/min, respectively, versus $+2.0$ mm Hg with placebo; $p < 0.001$). It was also associated with improved global clinical status in 60% and 67% of patients (vs. 14% in placebo group; $p < 0.001$), less dyspnea [57% and 53% vs. 12% (placebo); $p < 0.001$], and less fatigue [32% and 38% vs. 5% (placebo); $p < 0.001$]. In the comparative trial, the improvements in global clinical status, dyspnea, and fatigue were sustained with nesiritide therapy for up to 7 days and were similar to those seen with standard intravenous therapy for HF. The most common side effect was dose-related hypotension [symptomatic: 11% and 17% vs. 4%, $p = 0.008$ (comparative); 2% and 5% vs. none, $p = 0.55$ (efficacy)].

62. Publication Committee for the **VMAC** Investigators (Vasodilatation in the Management of Acute HF). Intravenous nesiritide vs nitroglycerin for treatment of decompensated congestive heart failure: a randomized controlled trial. *JAMA* 2002;287:1531–1540.

Design: Prospective, randomized, double-blind trial. Primary endpoints were change in PCWP in catheterized patients and self-evaluation of dyspnea at 3 hours after initiation of study drug.

Population: 489 inpatients with dyspnea at rest from decompensated HF, including 246 who received pulmonary artery catheterization (PAC).

Treatment: Intravenous nesiritide, intravenous nitroglycerin, or placebo added to standard medications for 3 hours, followed by nesiritide or nitroglycerin added to standard medication for 24 hours.

Results: At 3 hours, the mean decrease in PCWP from baseline was greater with nesiritide compared with placebo ($p < 0.001$) and nitroglycerin ($p = 0.03$). At 3 hours, nesiritide resulted in improvement in dyspnea compared with placebo ($p = 0.03$), but no significant difference was found between nesiritide and nitroglycerin in dyspnea or global clinical status. At 24 hours, the reduction in PCWP was greater in the nesiritide group (8.2 mm Hg) than in the nitroglycerin group (6.3 mm Hg), but no significant difference was noted in dyspnea and only modest improvement in global clinical status.

63. **Sackner-Bernstein JD**, et al. Short-term risk of death after treatment with nesiritide for decompensated heart failure: a pooled analysis of randomized controlled trials. *JAMA* 2005;293:1900–1905.

The authors reviewed the primary reports of completed clinical trials (as of December 2004), which predominantly compared nesiritide to diuretics or vasodilators. Data came from the sponsor (Scios Inc.), the FDA, PubMed, and scientific meetings manuals. The final study included 3 of 12 (862 patients total) randomized trials identified, as the remainder did not meet inclusion criteria of randomized, double-blinded trials in patients with acutely decompensated HF. Overall, all-cause mortality at 30 days trended to be higher in the nesiritide group (7.2% vs. 4.0%; RR, 1.74; $p = 0.059$). The meta-analysis signaled the possible harm caused by routine infusion of nesiritide for acutely decompensated HF.

β-BLOCKERS

Review Articles and Meta-analyses

64. **Lechat P**, et al. Clinical effects of β-adrenergic blockade in chronic heart failure. *Circulation* 1998;98:1184–1191.

This meta-analysis focused on 18 double-blind, placebo-controlled, parallel-group studies with a total of 3,023 patients. β-blocker use was associated with a 29% increase in EF ($p < 0.0001$) and 37% reduction in the risk of death or hospitalization for HF ($p < 0.001$). All-cause mortality was decreased by 32% ($p = 0.003$). A greater reduction for non-selective β-blockers compared with β_1-selective agents was seen (49% vs. 18%; $p = 0.049$). The effect of β-blocker use on NYHA functional class was of only borderline significance ($p = 0.04$).

Carvedilol Studies

65. **Packer M,** et al. Prospective Randomized Evaluation of Carvedilol on Symptoms and Exercise **(PRECISE).** Double-blind, placebo-controlled study of the effects of carvedilol in patients with moderate to severe heart failure. *Circulation* 1996;94:2793–2799.

Design: Prospective, randomized, double-blind, placebo-controlled, multicenter study. Primary endpoint was exercise tolerance.

Purpose: To evaluate the clinical effects of carvedilol in patients with moderate to severe HF.

Population: 278 patients with moderate to severe HF (dyspnea or fatigue at rest or on exertion for 3 months), an EF 35% or less, and receiving digoxin, diuretics, and an ACE inhibitor.

Exclusion Criteria: MI, unstable angina, CABG surgery, or stroke in the prior 3 months; uncorrected primary valvular disease; SBP less than 85 mm Hg or more than 160 mm Hg or DBP more than 100 mm Hg; heart rate, less than 68 beats/min; and use of calcium-channel blockers or antiarrhythmic drugs.

Treatment: During the open-label run-in period, carvedilol, 6.25 mg twice daily for 2 weeks. If tolerated, the patient was randomized to carvedilol, 12.5 twice daily initially, with titration over a 2- to 6-week period to 25 to 50 mg twice daily for 6 months, or placebo.

Results: Carvedilol patients had more frequent improvement in symptoms, as evaluated by changes in NYHA functional class ($p = 0.014$) and global assessments by the patient ($p = 0.002$) and the physician ($p < 0.001$). Carvedilol patients also had a significant increase in EF ($+8\%$ vs. $+3\%$; $p < 0.001$) and a significant decrease in morbidity and mortality (19.6% vs. 31.0%; $p = 0.029$). However, no significant effect was seen on exercise tolerance or QOL scores.

66. **Bristow MR,** et al. Multicenter Oral Carvedilol Heart Failure Assessment **(MOCHA).** Carvedilol produces dose-related improvements in left ventricular function and survival in subjects with chronic heart failure. *Circulation* 1996;94:2807–2816.

Design: Prospective, randomized, double-blind, placebo-controlled, multicenter study. Follow-up period was 6 months. Primary endpoint was change in walk test distances (6-minute corridor test and 9-minute self-powered treadmill test).

Purpose: To evaluate the effects of carvedilol in addition to standard therapy on clinical events and QOL in chronic HF patients.

Population: 345 patients aged 18 to 85 years with symptomatic, stable HF capable of walking 150 to 450 m in 6 minutes.

Exclusion Criteria: MI or stroke in the prior 3 months, uncorrected primary valvular disease, planned bypass surgery or balloon angioplasty, SBP less than 85 or more than 160 mm Hg, and use of calcium-channel blockers or antiarrhythmic drugs.

Treatment: Carvedilol, 6.25 to 25 mg/day, or placebo. Concomitant therapy included diuretics, digoxin, and ACE inhibitors.

Results: No differences were seen in submaximal exercise performance (as assessed by two walk tests) or HF symptoms. Carvedilol was associated with dose-dependent improvements in LV function ($+5\%$, $+6\%$, and $+8\%$ in low-, medium-, and high-dose groups vs. $+2\%$ with placebo; $p < 0.001$) and mortality (6.0%, 6.7%, and 1.1% vs. 15.5%; $p < 0.001$). When the three carvedilol groups were combined, the all-cause actuarial mortality risk was 73% lower ($p < 0.001$). Carvedilol patients also were hospitalized less frequently (by 58% to 64%; $p = 0.01$).

67. **Packer M,** et al. U.S. Carvedilol Heart Failure Study Group. The effect of carvedilol on morbidity and mortality in patients with chronic heart failure. *N Engl J Med* 1996;334: 1349–1355 (editorial, 1396–1397).

Design: Prospective, randomized, double-blind, placebo-controlled, multicenter study. Primary endpoint was mortality.

Purpose: To evaluate the safety and efficacy of carvedilol in patients with chronic HF.

Population: 1,094 chronic HF patients with an EF 35% or less and taking digoxin, diuretics, and an ACE inhibitor.

Exclusion Criteria: SBP less than 90 mm Hg, acute MI or coronary angioplasty in the prior 72 hours, bypass surgery in the prior 2 weeks, unstable angina in the prior 3 months, and stroke or TIA in the prior 3 months.

Treatment: After the 2-week open-label phase (5.6% failed to complete this period because of adverse events), patients were assigned to one of the four treatment groups based on exercise capacity [6-minute walk: mild, 426 to 550 m; moderate, 150 to 425 m; severe, <150 m (fourth group, dose-ranging protocol)] and randomized to carvedilol, 6.25 to 50 mg twice daily (titrated over a 2- to 10-week period), or placebo.

Results: At 6 months, carvedilol-treated patients had 65% lower mortality (3.2% vs. 7.8%; $p < 0.001$), 27% fewer CV-related hospitalizations (14.1% vs. 19.6%; $p = 0.036$), and a 38% reduction in death and hospitalization (15.8% vs. 24.6%; $p < 0.001$). Patients with an initial HR of more than 82 beats/min had the most benefit. More placebo patients had worsening HF.

Comments: Analysis combined patients from three different studies [PRECISE, MOCHA, Colucci WS, et al.]. This study had limited follow-up and only 53 total deaths; 7 carvedilol deaths occurred in the run-in period, and 17 (1.4%) patients were excluded because of worsening HF [more problematic in severe HF patients (only 3% of this study population)].

68. Heart Failure Research Collaborative Group, **ANZ** (Australia/New Zealand). Randomized, placebo-controlled trial of carvedilol in patients with congestive heart failure due to ischaemic heart disease. *Lancet* 1997;349:375–380.

Design: Prospective, randomized, double-blind, placebo-controlled, multicenter study. Average follow-up period was 19 months. Primary endpoint was changes in LVEF and treadmill exercise duration.

Purpose: To evaluate the longer term effects on death and other serious clinical events of carvedilol in patients with chronic stable HF.

Population: 415 NYHA class II or III patients with chronic stable HF.

Exclusion Criteria: Current NYHA class IV; primary valvular disease; SBP less than 90 mm Hg or more than 160 mm Hg or DBP more than 100 mm Hg; and MI, unstable angina, bypass surgery, or coronary angioplasty in the prior 4 weeks.

Treatment: Twenty-seven patients were withdrawn during the 2- to 3-week open-label phase of carvedilol therapy (3.125 mg daily to 6.25 mg twice daily). Carvedilol was then given at 6.25 to 25 mg twice daily, or placebo.

Results: At 1 year, the carvedilol group had an increased EF (+5.3%; $p < 0.0001$) and decreased end-diastolic and end-systolic dimensions [–1.7 mm ($p = 0.06$) and –3.2 mm ($p = 0.001$)]. However, no differences were noted in exercise treadmill time, 6MWD, NYHA class, or specific activity score. At 19 months, no difference was seen in the number of HF episodes, but the carvedilol group had a lower incidence of death and hospitalization (50% vs. 63%; RR, 0.74; 95% CI, 0.57 to 0.95).

Comments: ANZ echocardiographic substudy of 123 patients (echocardiograms at baseline and 6 and 12 months) showed that the carvedilol group had a LV end-diastolic volume index (LVEDVI) 14 mL/m^2 lower than placebo ($p = 0.0015$), LV end-systolic volume index (LVESVI) 15.3 mL/m^2 lower than placebo ($p = 0.0001$), and EF 5.8% higher ($p = 0.0015$).

69. **Packer M,** et al. for the Carvedilol Prospective Randomized Cumulative Survival Study **(COPERNICUS)** Group. Effect of carvedilol on survival in severe chronic heart failure. *N Engl J Med* 2001;344:1651–1658.

Design: Prospective, randomized, double-blind, placebo-controlled, multicenter study. Primary endpoint was changed in LVEF and treadmill exercise duration. Average follow-up period was 10 months.

Purpose: To evaluate the longer term effects on death and other serious clinical events of carvedilol in patients with chronic stable HF.

Population: 2,289 NYHA class III or IV patients with chronic stable HF.

Exclusion Criteria: Included HF due to uncorrected primary valvular disease or a reversible cardiomyopathy; eligibility for cardiac transplantation; contraindication to β-blocker therapy or use in the previous 2 months; coronary revascularization, acute myocardial or cerebral ischemic event in the previous 2 months; use of α-adrenergic blocker, calcium-channel blocker, or class I antiarrhythmic drug in the previous 4 weeks; SBP less than 85 mm Hg; creatinine more than 2.8 mg/dL.

Treatment: Patients received an initial dose of 3.125 mg of carvedilol or placebo twice daily for 2 weeks, which was then increased at 2-week intervals (if tolerated), first to 6.25 mg, and then to 12.5 mg, and finally to a target dose of 25 mg twice daily.

Results: A 35% decrease was seen in the risk of death with carvedilol (95% CI, 19% to 48%; $p = 0.0014$). A 24% decrease in the combined risk of death or hospitalization with carvedilol was found ($p < 0.001$). Fewer patients in the carvedilol group than in the placebo group withdrew because of adverse effects or for other reasons ($p = 0.02$). A subsequent report showed that more patients felt improved and fewer patients felt worse in the carvedilol group than in the placebo group after 6 months of maintenance therapy ($p = 0.0009$; see *Circulation* 2002;106:2194).

Comments: Patients not included were those with far-advanced HF symptoms and those who could not reach compensation. A small proportion of black patients was included.

70. **Poole-Wilson PA,** et al. Comparison of carvedilol and metoprolol on clinical outcomes in patients with chronic heart failure in the Carvedilol Or Metoprolol European Trial (COMET): randomised controlled trial. *Lancet* 2003;362:7–13.

Design: Prospective, randomized, double-blind, multicenter trial. Primary endpoints were all-cause mortality and the composite of all-cause mortality or all-cause hospital admission over a mean of 58 months.

Purpose: To compare carvedilol to metoprolol (both twice daily) in chronic HF.

Population: 3,029 patients with chronic HF (NYHA class II, III, or IV), previous cardiovascular hospitalization, EF <35%, and already on ACE inhibitors (as tolerated).

Treatment: Carvedilol (target dose 25 mg twice daily) or metoprolol (metoprolol tartrate, target dose 50 mg twice daily).

Results: The outcome of all-cause mortality heavily favored carvedilol (34% vs. 40%; $p = 0.0017$), and was consistent across predefined subgroups. However, the composite endpoint of mortality or all-cause admission was not significantly different between the two groups (74% for carvedilol vs. 76% for metoprolol; $p = 0.122$), perhaps owing to the high rates of incidence overall.

71. **Eichhorn E,** et al. A trial of the β-blocker bucindolol in patients with advanced chronic heart failure **(BEST)**. *N Engl J Med* 2001;344:1659–1667.

Design: Prospective, randomized, double-blind, placebo-controlled, multicenter trial. Primary endpoint was all-cause mortality. Average follow-up, 2.0 years.

Purpose: To evaluate the effect on survival of the β-blocker bucindolol in patients with advanced HF.

Population: 2,708 patients with NYHA III (92%) or IV (8%) HF and LVEF 35% or lower.

Exclusion Criteria: Included decompensated HF, eligibility for heart transplantation, reversible causes of HF, uncorrected primary valvular disease, hypertrophic cardiomyopathy, MI within the previous 6 months, PCI or CABG within 60 days, calcium-channel blocking or β-agonists within 1 week, β-blocking agents within 30 days, and amiodarone within 8 weeks.

Treatment: Bucindolol, 3 to 100 mg orally, or placebo.

Results: Trial terminated after seventh interim analysis. Mortality rates were similar between the two groups [411 deaths (bucindolol) vs. 449 deaths; unadjusted $p = 0.16$]. The bucindolol group had a significantly lower incidence of CV death and heart transplantation or death.

Comments: The neutral results of this study are surprising and challenge the concept of a beneficial class effect with β-adrenergic blockade.

Other Studies

72. **Waagstein F,** et al. Metoprolol in Dilated Cardiomyopathy **(MDC)**. Beneficial effects of metoprolol in idiopathic dilated cardiomyopathy (DCM). *Lancet* 1993;342:1441–1446.

Design: Prospective, randomized, double-blind, placebo-controlled, parallel-group, multicenter study. Follow-up period was 12 to 18 months. Primary endpoint was death and need for cardiac transplantation.

Purpose: To evaluate the effects of metoprolol versus placebo in patients with HF due to idiopathic DCM.

Population: 383 patients aged 16 to 75 years with LVEF less than 0.40; 94% were in NYHA functional class II or III.

Exclusion Criteria: Use of β-blockers or calcium-channel blockers, CAD (more than 50% stenosis), SBP less than 90 mm Hg, heart rate less than 45 beats/min, obstructive lung disease requiring β-agonists, and insulin-dependent diabetes.

Treatment: If the test dose was tolerated (metoprolol, 5 mg twice daily for 2 to 7 days), then patients were randomized to metoprolol [10 mg/day titrated up to 100 to 150 mg/day (mean, 108 mg/day)], or placebo.

Results: Metoprolol group had 34% risk reduction in death or need for heart transplantation (22.5% vs. 36.5%; $p = 0.058$). At follow-up, the metoprolol group had a significantly better improvement in LVEF (+0.12 vs. +0.06 at 12 months; $p < 0.0001$), increased exercise duration (+76 seconds vs. +15 seconds at 12 months; $p = 0.046$), and showed a trend toward lower PCWP (−5 mm Hg vs. −2 mm Hg; $p = 0.06$). The metoprolol group had better QOL (based on patient assessment at 12 and 18 months; $p = 0.01$), and a significant correlation was found between the NYHA classification made by the physician and the QOL assessment. A subsequent report showed that the metoprolol group had a significantly improved exercise oxygen consumption index ($p = 0.045$).

73. Cardiac Insufficiency Bisoprolol Study II **(CIBIS-II)** Investigators. The Cardiac Insufficiency Bisoprolol Study II (CIBIS II): a randomized trial. *Lancet* 1999;353:9–12.

Design: Prospective, randomized, double-blind, placebo-controlled, multicenter study. Mean follow-up period was 1.3 years. Primary endpoint was all-cause mortality rate.

Purpose: To evaluate the efficacy of bisoprolol in decreasing all-cause mortality in patients with symptomatic chronic HF.

Population: 2,647 NYHA class III or IV patients with LVEF less than 35%.

Exclusion Criteria: Uncontrolled hypertension, MI, or unstable angina in the prior 3 months, PTCA or CABG in the prior 6 months, heart rate less than 60 beats/min, or preexisting or planned therapy with β-blockers.

Treatment: Bisoprolol, 1.25 to 10.0 mg/day, or placebo. All patients were taking diuretics and ACE inhibitors.

Results: Study was terminated because bisoprolol showed a significant mortality benefit— 11.8% versus 17.3% (hazard ratio, 0.66; $p < 0.0001$). The bisoprolol group also had a lower incidence of sudden death (3.6% vs. 6.3%; hazard ratio, 0.56; $p = 0.0011$) and 20% fewer hospital admissions; treatment effects were independent of severity or cause of HF.

Comments: No run-in period provided a better estimate of clinical effectiveness of bisoprolol. The low mortality rates suggest that not all patients were NYHA class III and IV patients.

74. **MERIT-HF** Study Group. Effect of metoprolol CR/XL in chronic heart failure: metoprolol CR/XL randomized intervention trial in congestive heart failure (MERIT-HF). *Lancet* 1999;353:2001–2007.

Design: Prospective, randomized, double-blind, placebo-controlled multicenter study. Mean follow-up period was 1 year. Primary endpoint was all-cause mortality.

Purpose: To evaluate whether metoprolol CR/XL, once daily, in addition to standard therapy, could lower mortality in symptomatic HF patients with impaired EF.

Population: 3,991 NYHA class II to IV (II, 41%; III, 55%) patients with an EF of 40% or less. Two thirds of patients had an ischemic etiology of HF; 89% were taking an ACE inhibitor; 90% were taking a diuretic; and 63% were receiving digoxin.

Treatment: Metoprolol CR/XL, 12.5 mg (NYHA III or IV) or 25 mg (NYHA II) once daily; or placebo. Target dose was 200 mg/day with up-titration over an 8-week period. Randomization was preceded by a 2-week single-blind placebo run-in period.

Results: All-cause mortality was significantly lower in the metoprolol group (7.2% vs. 11.0%; RR, 0.66; $p < 0.001$). The metoprolol group also had a 38% reduction in CV mortality ($p < 0.001$), a 41% reduction in sudden death ($p < 0.001$), and a 49% reduction in death due to progressive HF ($p = 0.002$). The incidence of side effects was similar in both groups.

75. **Exner DV,** et al. Beta-adrenergic blocking agent use and mortality in patients with asymptomatic and symptomatic left ventricular systolic dysfunction: a post hoc analysis of the studies of left ventricular dysfunction. *J Am Coll Cardiol* 1999;33:916–923.

Design: Retrospective analysis of patients in the **SOLVD** trial, based on baseline β-blocker use.

Purpose: To determine if β-blocker use was associated with lower morality, and if the effect interacts with ACE-inhibitor use.

Population: 6,790 patients with HF (4,223 mostly asymptomatic, 2,567 symptomatic).

Results: In all, only 1,015 (24%) asymptomatic and 197 (8%) symptomatic patients were receiving β-blockers at baseline. However, these groups did have fewer symptoms and higher EFs than those not receiving β-blockers (in univariate analysis). β-blocker use was associated with significantly lower mortality in both cohorts, an effect that persisted in multivariable analysis for asymptomatic patients. Moreover, this effect was synergistic in patients who added enalapril to their β-blocker.

76. **Dargie HG.** Effect of carvedilol on outcome after myocardial infarction in patients with left-ventricular dysfunction: the **CAPRICORN** randomized trial. *Lancet* 2001;357: 1385–1390.

Design: Multicenter (163 centers, 17 countries), randomized, double-blind, placebo-controlled trial. Primary endpoint was all-cause mortality or cardiovascular hospitalization over a mean of 1.3 years.

Purpose: To assess the utility of adding carvedilol to standard medical therapy in post-MI patients with LV dysfunction.

Population: 1,959 post-MI patients with EF $\leq$40%.

Treatment: Carvedilol 6.25 mg (titrated to 25 mg twice daily, as tolerated), or placebo.

Results: The two groups did not differ significantly in their incidence of primary endpoint events (35% for carvedilol vs. 37% for placebo). However, all-cause mortality alone was significantly reduced in carvedilol (12% vs. 15%; HR, 0.77; $p = 0.03$). Additionally, cardiovascular death and nonfatal MI were also lower in carvedilol.

77. **Remme WJ,** et al. The benefits of early combination treatment of carvedilol and an ACE-inhibitor in mild heart failure and left ventricular systolic dysfunction: the carvedilol and ACE-inhibitor remodeling mild heart failure evaluation trial (CARMEN). *Cardiovasc Drugs Ther* 2004;18:57–66.

Design: Multicenter (63 centers, 13 countries), double-blind, randomized trial. Primary outcome was change in LVESVI at 18 months.

Purpose: To identify the benefit, if any, of combination ACE inhibitor plus β-blocker therapy, on ventricular remodeling in HF.

Population: 572 patients with mild, stable HF (NYHA class I, II, or III) with EF <40%.

Treatment: Carvedilol ($n = 191$), enalapril ($n = 190$), or their combination ($n = 191$). In the latter, carvedilol was up-titrated before enalapril.

Results: LVESVI was significantly reduced by 5.4 mL/m^2 ($p = 0.0015$) in the combination-therapy group, compared to enalapril alone. However, there was no significant difference between carvedilol alone and enalapril alone. Furthermore, carvedilol significantly reduced LVESVI by 2.8 mL/m^2 ($p = 0.018$) compared to baseline, whereas enalapril did not. LVESVI was reduced by 6.3 mL/m^2 ($p = 0.0001$) with combination therapy.

78. **Colucci WS,** et al. Metoprolol reverses left ventricular remodeling in patients with asymptomatic systolic dysfunction: the Reversal of Ventricular Remodeling with Toprol-XL **(REVERT)** trial. *Circulation* 2007;116:49–56.

Design: Randomized, double-blind, placebo-controlled trial. Primary endpoint was change in LVESVI from baseline to 12 months.

Purpose: To determine if β-blockers can attenuate LV remodeling in asymptomatic patients with LV systolic dysfunction.

Population: 149 patients with LVEF <40% and mild LV dilatation (LVEDVI >75 mL/m^2) due to idiopathic, ischemic, or hypertensive cardiomyopathy (without HF symptoms for at least 3 months).

Treatment: Extended-release metoprolol succinate 200 mg ($n = 48$) or 50 mg ($n = 48$) or placebo ($n = 53$).

Results: At 12 months, there was a 14 mL/m^2 decrease in LVESVI and a 6 $\pm$ 1% increase in EF in the 200-mg group ($p < 0.05$ vs. baseline and placebo for both). In the 50-mg group, LVESVI and LVEDVI decreased relative to baseline, but not significantly more than was seen with placebo.

AMIODARONE

79. **Doval HC,** et al. Grupo de Estudio de la Sobrevida en la Insuficiencia Cardiaca en Argentina **(GESICA).** Randomized trial of low-dose amiodarone in severe HF. *Lancet* 1994;344:493–498.

Design: Prospective, randomized, open, parallel-group, multicenter study. Follow-up period was 2 years. Primary endpoint was total mortality.

Purpose: To evaluate the effect of low-dose amiodarone on mortality in patients with severe HF without symptomatic ventricular arrhythmias.

Population: 516 NYHA class II to IV patients with stable functional capacity and not requiring antiarrhythmic therapy.

Exclusion Criteria: Amiodarone treatment during the prior 3 months; MI, HF onset, or syncope in the prior 3 months; and history of sustained VT or VF.

Treatment: Amiodarone, 500 mg/day for 14 days, and then 300 mg once daily for 2 years; or standard therapy (diuretics, digoxin, ACE inhibitors).

Results: Amiodarone group had 28% RR in mortality at 2 years (33.5% vs. 41.4%; $p = 0.024$) and 31% RR in hospitalization due to worsening HF (45.8% vs. 58.2%; $p = 0.0024$). Reductions were seen in both sudden death (27% RR; $p = 0.16$) and death due to progressive HF (23% risk reduction; $p = 0.16$). These benefits were present in all examined subgroups and were independent of the presence of nonsustained VT. Side effects were reported in 17 (6.1%) amiodarone patients, of whom 12 discontinued therapy.

Comments: The study was blinded only to coordination center personnel, had a unique population (10% with Chagas disease), and was terminated at the two-thirds point.

80. **Singh SN,** et al. Survival Trial of Antiarrhythmic Therapy in HF **(HF-STAT).** Amiodarone in patients with congestive heart failure and asymptomatic ventricular arrhythmia. *N Engl J Med* 1995;333:77–82 (editorial, 121–122).

Design: Prospective, randomized, double-blind, placebo-controlled, multicenter study. Primary endpoint was overall mortality and sudden death from cardiac causes. Follow-up period was 45 months.

Purpose: To evaluate the effect of antiarrhythmic therapy on mortality in patients with HF and asymptomatic ventricular arrhythmia.

Population: 674 patients with symptoms of HF, cardiac enlargement, fewer than 10 premature ventricular contractions, and EF of 40% or less.

Exclusion Criteria: MI in the prior 3 months, history of cardiac arrest or sustained VT, need for antiarrhythmic therapy, and SBP less than 90 mm Hg.

Treatment: Amiodarone, 800 mg/day for 14 days, 400 mg/day for 50 weeks, and then 300 mg/day; or placebo. Other therapy consisted of vasodilators (all patients), with or without digoxin or diuretics.

Results: No significant differences were found in mortality or sudden death [30.6% (amiodarone) vs. 29.2%; 15% vs. 19%; $p = 0.43$]. However, amiodarone was associated with a trend toward lower mortality in the subgroup of patients with nonischemic cardiomyopathy ($p = 0.07$). The amiodarone group also had better suppression of ventricular arrhythmias and a greater increase in EF at 2 years (+10.5% vs. +4.1%).

Comments: This VA-based trial had notable differences compared with GESICA—older patients (+6 years), more men (GESICA, 48% lower mortality in females vs. 26% in men), and healthier patients with higher EFs. However, subgroup analysis showed that the greatest benefits in HF-STAT occurred in NYHA class II patients.

INOTROPIC AND OTHER AGENTS

81. **DiBianco R,** et al. A comparison of oral milrinone, digoxin and their combination in the treatment of patients with chronic heart failure. *N Engl J Med* 1989;320:677–683.

This prospective, randomized trial was composed of 230 patients comparing 12 weeks of digoxin, milrinone, and their combination. Both agents alone improved exercise tolerance (+64 seconds vs. +82 seconds) and lowered frequency of decompensation [15% and 34% vs. 47% (placebo)]. Overall, no significant difference was found between the effects of the two drugs. Milrinone and digoxin were no better than digoxin alone.

82. **Packer M,** et al. Prospective Randomized Milrinone Survival Evaluation **(PROMISE).** Effect of oral milrinone on mortality in severe chronic heart failure. *N Engl J Med* 1991;325:1468–1475.

Design: Prospective, randomized, double-blind, placebo-controlled, multicenter study. Mean follow-up period was 6.1 months. Primary endpoint was all-cause mortality.

Purpose: To evaluate the effect of oral administration of the phosphodiesterase milrinone on mortality in patients with severe HF.

Population: 1,088 NYHA class III or IV patients and EF less than 35%.

Exclusion Criteria: Obstructive valvular disease; history of serious ventricular arrhythmia; MI in prior 3 months; SBP less than 85 mm Hg; and requirement for β-blockers, calcium-channel blockers, and antiarrhythmic drugs.

Treatment: Milrinone, 40 mg/day orally, or placebo. All patients were on digoxin, diuretics, and ACE inhibitors.

Results: Study was terminated early. Milrinone was associated with significantly higher all-cause mortality (30% vs. 24%; $p = 0.038$) and CV mortality rates (29.4% vs. 22.6%; $p = 0.016$). The milrinone group had a 69% increased risk of sudden cardiac deaths ($p = 0.005$), whereas no increased risk of death was found because of progressive HF. Adverse effects were worst among class IV patients (53% higher mortality; $p = 0.006$).

83. **Califf RM,** et al. Flolan International Randomized Survival Trial **(FIRST).** A randomized controlled trial of epoprostenol therapy. *Am Heart J* 1997;134:44–54.

This prospective, randomized trial was composed of 471 patients with an EF less than 25% (<30% if taking inotropes); NYHA class IIIB or IV symptoms for 1 month with digoxin, diuretic, and ACE inhibitor; cardiac index, 2.2 mL/kg/m^2 or less; and PCWP, 15 mm Hg. Patients were randomized to epoprostenol (initial dose, 2 ng/kg/min; median, 4.0) or standard care. The epoprostenol group had an increased cardiac index (1.81 to 2.61) and decreased PCWP (24.5 to 20.0 mm Hg), but showed a trend toward increased mortality ($p = 0.055$), prompting early termination of the trial.

84. **Cohn JN,** et al. for the Vesnarinone Trial Investigators. A dose-dependent increase in mortality with vesnarinone among patients with severe heart failure. *N Engl J Med* 1998;339:1801–1806.

This prospective, randomized, double-blind, placebo-controlled, multicenter study enrolled 3,833 patients with NYHA class III or IV HF and an LVEF 30% or less despite optimal treatment (any regimen of diuretics, vasodilators, ACE inhibitor, and digitalis). Patients received vesnarinone (30 or 60 mg) or placebo once daily. At follow-up (mean, 286 days), the placebo group had significantly fewer deaths than the 60-mg vesnarinone group (18.9% vs. 22.9%; $p = 0.02$). Increased mortality with vesnarinone was mostly owing to increased sudden death rate (12.3% vs. 9.1%). QOL (assessed by Minnesota Living with Heart Failure Questionnaire) improved significantly more in the 60-mg vesnarinone group than in the placebo group at 8 weeks ($p < 0.001$) and 16 weeks ($p = 0.003$), but by 26 weeks, the differences were no longer significant. Agranulocytosis occurred in 1.2% and 0.2% of those given vesnarinone, 60 and 30 mg/day, respectively.

85. **Packer M,** et al. Comparison of omapatrilat and enalapril in patients with chronic heart failure: the Omapatrilat Versus Enalapril Randomized Trial of Utility in Reducing Events **(OVERTURE).** *Circulation* 2002;106:920–926.

Design: Prospective, randomized, placebo-controlled, blinded, parallel-group, multicenter trial. Primary endpoint was all-cause mortality or hospitalization for HF. Average follow-up, 15 months.

Purpose: To prove superiority or noninferiority of the vasopeptidase inhibitor omapatrilat compared to enalapril in patients with HF.

Population: 5,770 patients with NYHA class II to IV HF for more than 2 months due to ischemic or nonischemic heart disease, EF less than 30%, hospitalized for HF in the past year, and receiving diuretics at the time of enrollment.

Exclusion Criteria: Included reversible cause(s) of HF, no HF admission in the previous 48 hours, probable cardiac transplant or LVAD candidate, acute coronary syndrome in the previous month, coronary revascularization or an acute cerebral ischemic event in the previous 3 months, and history of VT, VF, or sudden death (unless ICD had been placed and had not fired in the previous 2 months).

Treatment: Omapatrilat, 40 mg/day, or enalapril, 20 mg/day.

Results: A nonsignificant trend was found toward a lower incidence of death or hospitalization for HF in the omapatrilat group compared with the enalapril group (32% vs. 34%; $p = 0.19$). All-cause mortality rates were not significantly different (17% vs. 18%). The trend was strong enough to show that omapatrilat was not inferior to enalapril.

86. **Cuffe MS,** et al. for the Outcomes of a Prospective Trial of Intravenous Milrinone for Exacerbations of Chronic Heart Failure **(OPTIME-HF)** Investigators. Short-term intravenous milrinone for acute exacerbation of chronic heart failure: a randomized controlled trial. *JAMA* 2002;287:1541–1547.

This trial randomized 951 patients with exacerbation of chronic HF not requiring intravenous inotropic support to 48 hours of milrinone or placebo. A total of the median number of days hospitalized for CV causes within 60 days after randomization did not differ significantly between patients given milrinone (6 days) compared with placebo (7 days; $p = 0.71$). Sustained hypotension requiring intervention (10.7% vs. 3.2%; $p < 0.001$) and new atrial arrhythmias (4.6% vs. 1.5%; $p = 0.004$) occurred more frequently in patients who received milrinone. The milrinone and placebo groups did not differ significantly in in-hospital mortality (3.8% vs. 2.3%; $p = 0.19$) or 60-day mortality (10.3% vs. 8.9%).

MECHANICAL ASSIST DEVICES AND SURGICAL OPTIONS

87. **Oz MC,** et al. Screening scale predicts patients successfully receiving long-term implantable left ventricular assist devices. *Circulation* 1995;92(suppl II):169–173.

A risk-factor selection scale (range, 0 to 10) was developed based on an analysis of easily obtainable preoperative risk factors in 56 patients undergoing LVAD insertion. Points were assigned as follows: urine output less than 30 mL/hr (weight, 3), central venous pressure more than 16 mm Hg (weight, 2), mechanical ventilation (weight, 2), prothrombin time more than 16 seconds (weight, 2), and reoperation (weight, 1). The mortality rate among those with a score of 5 was 67%. The average score of nonsurvivors was 5.43 versus 2.45 among survivors ($p < 0.0001$).

88. **Bolling SF,** et al. Intermediate-term outcome of mitral construction in cardiomyopathy. *J Thorac Cardiovasc Surg* 1998;115:381–386.

The 48 NYHA class III or IV patients with severe DCM and 4+ mitral regurgitation underwent surgery; all had annuloplasty rings inserted, 7 had CABG for incidental disease, and 11 had tricuspid valve repair. Postoperative transesophageal echocardiography (TEE) showed no mitral regurgitation in 41 patients and mild mitral regurgitation in 7 patients. One- and 2-year actuarial survival rates were 82% and 71%. At a median follow-up of 22 months, NYHA class had improved significantly from 3.9 to 2.0.

89. **Mancini D,** et al. Comparison of exercise performance in patients with chronic severe heart failure versus left ventricular assist devices. *Circulation* 1998;98:1178–1183.

Metabolic exercise testing was performed in 65 HF and 20 LVAD patients. Peak oxygen consumption was significantly higher in the LVAD group (15.9 mL/kg/min vs. 12.0 mL/kg/min; $p < 0.001$). At peak exercise, the LVAD group also had a significantly higher HR, BP, and cardiac output, whereas PCWP was lower (14 mm Hg vs. 31 mm Hg; $p < 0.001$). LVAD patients also had better hemodynamic measurements at rest, including higher cardiac output and lower PCWP.

90. **Mancini DM,** et al. Low incidence of myocardial recovery after left ventricular assist device implantation in patients with chronic heart failure. *Circulation* 1998;98:2383–2389.

A retrospective chart review of 111 LVAD recipients identified only 5 successfully explanted patients. A prospective attempt to identify explantable patients by using exercise testing was then undertaken on 39 consecutive patients, of whom 15 were able to exercise with maximal device support. Peak average oxygen consumption was 14.5 mL/kg/min, and Fick cardiac output 11.4 L/min. Seven patients remained normotensive while exercising at 20 cycles/min, and their peak oxygen consumption decreased from 17.3 to 13.0 mL/kg/min. In one of these patients, the LVAD was successfully explanted.

91. **Rose EA,** et al. Randomized Evaluation of Mechanical Assistance for the Treatment of Congestive Heart Failure **(REMATCH)** Study Group. Long-term mechanical left ventricular assistance for end-stage heart failure. *N Engl J Med* 2001;345:1435–1443.

Design: Prospective, randomized, multicenter trial. Primary endpoint was all-cause mortality or hospitalization for HF. Average follow-up, 14.5 months.
Purpose: To prove superiority of the implantable LVAD compared with standard therapy in patients with end-stage HF.

Population: 129 patients with end-stage HF who were ineligible for cardiac transplantation.

Exclusion Criteria: Included eligibility for cardiac transplantation, absence of symptoms of NYHA class IV in the previous 90 days, EF 25% or less, or a peak oxygen consumption of more than 14 mL/kg/min.

Treatment: A vented electric LVAD or optimal medical therapy. Patients could continue β-blockers if they had been administered for at least 60 of the 90 days before randomization.

Results: The LVAD group had a 48% reduction in mortality compared with the medical-therapy group ($p = 0.001$). At 1 year, survival rates were 52% in the LVAD group and 25% in the medical-therapy group ($p = 0.002$), whereas the rates at 2 years were 23% and 8% ($p = 0.09$), respectively. The frequency of serious adverse events in the LVAD was 2.35 times that in the medical-therapy group (95% CI, 1.86 to 2.95), with a predominance of infection, bleeding, and malfunction of the device. The QOL was significantly improved at 1 year in the LVAD group.

Comment: Because fewer than 25% of LVAD patients were alive at 2 years, these results may not be of sufficient magnitude to convince the medical community and insurance companies that this technology (or at least this particular device) can be considered a good alternative to transplantation.

92. **Slaughter MS,** et al. Advanced heart failure treated with continuous-flow left ventricular assist device. *N Engl J Med* 2009;361:2241–2251.

Design: Randomized trial. Primary composite endpoint was survival free from disabling stroke and repair or replacement of the device at 2 years.

Purpose: To compare continuous-flow LVAD to older pulsatile-flow LVAD and the effect on long-term outcomes.

Population: A total of 200 patients were randomly assigned (in 2:1 ratio) to undergo implantation of a continuous-flow LVAD (134 patients) or a pulsatile-flow LVAD (66 patients). Previously, 60% had undergone CRT, and by the time of surgery, roughly 80% were receiving intravenous inotropes and 20% had an intra-aortic balloon pump.

Results: The continuous-flow device demonstrated better primary-endpoint achievement at 2 years, compared to the pulsatile-flow device (46% vs. 11%; $p < 0.001$), and patients with continuous-flow devices had better survival rates at 2 years (58% vs. 24%; $p = 0.008$). For secondary endpoints, the continuous-flow device proved superior in terms of reduced adverse events and device replacement, and improved QOL and functional capacity.

Comment: The 1-year survival of only 68% in the continuous-flow device group was attributed to early deaths in this patient population due to the advanced nature of their disease at the time of device implantation. Future studies will likely evaluate the benefit of implantation in patients with less-advanced disease.

93. **Jones RH,** et al. **STICH Hypothesis 2** Investigators. Coronary bypass surgery with or without surgical ventricular reconstruction. *N Engl J Med* 2009;360:1705–1717.

Design: A multicenter, nonblinded, randomized trial at 127 clinical sites in 26 countries. The primary outcome was the time to death from any cause or hospitalization for cardiac causes. Secondary outcomes included death from any cause at 30 days, hospitalization for any cause and for cardiovascular causes, MI, and stroke.

Purpose: The trial included two major components. Patients in the Hypothesis 1 component were randomly assigned to receive either medical therapy alone or medical therapy plus CABG. The Hypothesis 1 component of the trial is ongoing. Patients in the Hypothesis 2 component were randomly assigned to receive either medical therapy plus CABG or medical therapy plus CABG and SVR. The results of the Hypothesis 2 component are described herein.

Population: Patients were eligible for enrollment if they had surgically appropriate CAD and a LV EF of ≤35%.

Results: SVR reduced the ESV index by 19%, as compared with a reduction of 6% with CABG alone. Cardiac symptoms and exercise capacity improved similarly in the two groups. However, no significant difference was observed in the primary outcome, death, or cardiac rehospitalization (59% in the CABG-alone group vs. 58% for CABG plus SVR group, $p = 0.90$).

INVASIVE THERAPY

94. **Binanay C,** et al. Evaluation study of congestive heart failure and pulmonary artery catheterization effectiveness: the **ESCAPE** trial. *JAMA* 2005;294:1625–1633.

Design: Multicenter, randomized controlled trial. The primary endpoint was days alive out of the hospital during the first 6 months.

Purpose: To determine whether PAC is safe and effective for improving outcomes in hospitalized patients with severe HF.

Population: 433 patients hospitalized for HF, meeting one of the three severity criteria: (1) HF hospitalization within the previous year; (2) urgent visit to the ED; or (3) treatment during the previous month with more than 160 mg of furosemide daily (or equivalent). Additionally, patients had to have had at least 3 months of symptoms despite ACE inhibitors and diuretics, EF $\leq$30%, systolic BP $\leq$125 mm Hg, and at least one sign and one symptom of congestion.

Treatment: HF management guided by PAC placement or by clinical assessment. For both groups, target PCWP was 15 mm Hg and target right atrial pressure was 8 mm Hg.

Results: There was no significant difference in the primary outcome, between the two groups (133 days for the PAC group vs. 135 days for clinical assessment; $p = 0.99$). Mortality and days in the hospital were also not different. However, patients in the PAC group did have higher incidence of in-hospital complications (21.9% vs. 25; $p = 0.04$).

Comment: There was a trend toward improved outcomes at centers in the trial with higher enrollment and greater experience with PA catheters, suggesting that PA catheters may be beneficial if monitored closely by an experienced clinical team and if the data are acted upon quickly and appropriately.

95. **Constanza MR,** et al. for the UNLOAD Trial Investigators. Ultrafiltration versus intravenous diuretics for patients hospitalized for acute decompensated heart failure. *J Am Coll Cardiol* 2007;49:675–683.

The investigators randomized 200 patients with acute, hypervolemic, decompensated HF to either standard intravenous diuretic therapy or intravenous ultrafiltration for fluid and sodium removal. None of the patients was in cardiogenic shock, and all had baseline serum creatinine levels of less than 3.0 mg/dL. Patients in the ultrafiltration group had greater overall average weight loss at 48 hours, the primary endpoint (5.0 kg vs. 3.1 kg; $p = 0.001$). There were no differences in acute renal failure, hypotension, or adverse events between the groups. Additionally, while there were improvements in subjective dyspnea similarly in both groups, patients' report of improvement did *not* correlate with amount of fluid removed (in either group). Notably, patients in the ultrafiltration group had significantly lower rates of rehospitalization and rehospitalization days at 90 days. Additionally, those in the ultrafiltration group required lower doses of oral diuretic at discharge than those in the standard intravenous diuretic group, suggesting that ultrafiltration may have a "sparing" effect on the kidney.

EXERCISE/TRAINING

96. **Keteyiajn SJ,** et al. Exercise training in patients with heart failure. *Ann Intern Med* 1996;124:1051–1057.

This small randomized controlled trial was composed of 40 men with an EF of 35% or less. The treatment regimen was composed of three sets of three exercises, each performed for 11 minutes (target heart rate, 60% maximum) for 2 weeks, and then up to 80% as tolerated.

At 24 weeks, the exercise group had increased exercise duration (+2.8 minutes), 16% higher peak oxygen consumption, and increased power output (+20 W).

97. **Wilson JR,** et al. Circulatory status and response to cardiac rehabilitation in patients with heart failure. *Circulation* 1996;94:1567–1572.

This study showed that only some patients respond well to exercise and offered insights into the pathophysiology of nonresponders. Thirty-two patients underwent maximal exercise treadmill testing and then rehabilitation for 3 months. Twenty-one had a normal cardiac output response to exercise, of whom 43% responded to the rehabilitation regimen (more than 10% increase in peak oxygen consumption and anaerobic threshold). Of the other 11 patients, 3 stopped rehabilitation (because of exhaustion), and 1 responded (9%; $p < 0.04$). The former group was likely limited by deconditioning, whereas the latter group was impaired by circulatory failures.

98. **Hambrecht R,** et al. Regular physical exercise corrects endothelial dysfunction and improves exercise capacity in patients with chronic heart failure. *Circulation* 1998;98: 2709–2715.

This small prospective randomized study of 20 patients showed that exercise training resulted in increased peak oxygen uptake (+26% at 6 weeks; $p < 0.01$). This increase correlated with endothelium-dependent changes in peripheral blood flow ($r = 0.64$; $p < 0.005$), suggesting that improved endothelial function contributes modestly to increased exercise capacity.

Complications

99. **Middlekauff HR,** et al. Prognostic significance of atrial fibrillation in advanced heart failure: a study of 390 patients. *Circulation* 1991;84:40–48.

This retrospective analysis focused on 390 consecutive NYHA class III or IV patients with a mean EF of 19%. Actuarial survival and sudden death-free survival were significantly worse in the atrial fibrillation patients compared with those in normal sinus rhythm (52% vs. 71%; 69% vs. 82%; both $p = 0.0013$).

100. **Middlekauff HR,** et al. Syncope in advanced heart failure: high sudden death regardless of etiology. *J Am Coll Cardiol* 1993;21:110–116.

This retrospective analysis focused on 491 NYHA class III or IV HF patients with no history of cardiac arrest and a mean EF of 20%. Sixty (12%) patients had a history of syncope. At follow-up (mean, 1 year), sudden death had occurred in 14%, and 13% had died of progressive HF. The 1-year actuarial incidence of sudden death was more than threefold higher in patients with a history of syncope than in those without syncope (45% vs. 12%; $p < 0.00001$). The incidence of sudden death was similar in patients with either cardiac syncope or syncope from other causes (49% vs. 39%; $p =$ NS).

CHAPTER 6

Arrhythmias

Christopher P. Cannon, Benjamin A. Steinberg, and Jonathan
Walter Dukes

ATRIAL ARRHYTHMIAS

Epidemiology

Atrial fibrillation (AF) is the most common sustained arrhythmia in the US population with a lifetime risk for people over the age of 40 of approximately 25% (2) and leads to more hospitalizations than does any other arrhythmia. AF prevalence is highest in those with clinical cardiovascular disease and occurs most commonly among older age groups (2,4). The average age at onset is 70 to 74 years (age 65 years for lone AF); as with other cardiac illnesses, women tend to present at an older age than do men. AF is causally related to a substantial proportion of ischemic strokes, and AF patients appear to have higher adjusted mortality rates than do those without AF (3). Atrial flutter, a related but more organized rhythm, also is associated with a modestly higher stroke risk than that for individuals in normal sinus rhythm (8,10). The current consensus is that atrial flutter should be treated the same as AF, in terms of thromboembolic risk and prophylaxis.

Natural History

The clinical course of AF is heterogeneous: some patients have only self-terminating paroxysms that occur with variable frequency, whereas others always require intervention to terminate episodes. Spontaneous conversion rates are variable (<15% to as high as 78%) and depend on the population studied. Higher rates of spontaneous conversion are associated with shorter AF duration (<12 hours), younger age, and lack of associated heart disease. In general, patients who are older, have more structural heart disease, and have a longer history of symptoms tend to progress toward more persistent and chronic AF, sometimes despite aggressive management. Among patients with persistent (non self–terminating) AF, normal sustained release (SR) can be restored in most, but 50% or more will have recurrences within 1 year.

Etiologies and Risk Factors

Many new cases of AF do not have a single clear etiology. From 3% to 11% of AF patients have structurally normal hearts. Conversely, new-onset AF often occurs in the setting of acute cardiac or noncardiac illness. Common examples include pneumonia, pulmonary embolism, and other acute pulmonary conditions; sepsis; acute myocardial infarction (MI); and major surgery. In these cases, treatment of the underlying illness is of primary importance. Cardiac surgery is associated with a distinctly high risk of postoperative AF, which occurs in 30% to 40% of patients undergoing coronary artery bypass graft (CABG) or valve surgery. Other acute precipitants of AF include alcohol intoxication ("holiday heart syndrome"), pericarditis, myocarditis, and thyroid disease. AF also may be triggered by other primary arrhythmias that are curable by radio frequency (RF) catheter ablation.

A variety of chronic cardiac conditions are associated with the development of AF; most common among these are hypertension and congestive heart failure (CHF). In a multivariable model based on subjects followed up for 38 years in the Framingham Heart Study, odds ratios (ORs) for the development of AF were highest for CHF (men, 4.5; women, 5.9), followed by valve disease (1.8, 3.4), hypertension (1.5, 1.4), and diabetes mellitus (1.4, 1.6). Prior MI was an independent risk factor for men (OR, 1.4) but not women. Rheumatic heart disease has a strong association with AF, but because of its declining prevalence in developed nations, the valvular lesion now most frequently associated with AF is mitral regurgitation. AF is likely a sequela of these conditions as a result of atrial dilation inducing myocardial fibrosis and subsequent electrical remodeling. Other cardiopulmonary conditions associated with AF include hypertrophic, dilated, and restrictive cardiomyopathies; atrial septal defect and other congenital abnormalities; and the sleep apnea syndrome. In addition, many older patients with AF have concomitant sinus node dysfunction, known as the tachycardia–bradycardia syndrome. In those patients, both arrhythmias appear related to underlying degeneration and fibrosis of normal atrial tissue.

The following is a list of causes of AF classified by prevalence:

1. Major causes: hypertension, CHF, ischemic heart disease, and postcardiac surgery.
2. Common causes: alcohol intoxication, pulmonary disease, valvular heart disease, rheumatic heart disease, cardiomyopathy, and thyrotoxicosis.
3. Uncommon to rare causes: pericarditis, infiltrative disease, atrial myxoma, autonomic dysfunction, ventricular/atrial septal defect, and pulmonary embolism.

Stroke Risk Factors

Data from the Framingham Heart Study initially documented the roughly fivefold increased incidence of stroke among AF patients compared with age, sex, and hypertensive matched contemporaries without AF, and highlighted the remarkably high rates of stroke in patients with AF due to rheumatic heart disease (relative risk, 17.6). Predictors of stroke were further evaluated in a meta-analysis of pooled control-group patients from five major anticoagulation trials (6). Among clinical variables, independent risk factors for stroke (with associated ORs) included previous stroke or transient ischemic attack (TIA) (2.5), hypertension (1.6), CHF (1.4), age (1.4 per decade), and diabetes mellitus (1.7). One of the trials also assessed echocardiographic variables and found impaired left ventricular (LV) systolic function and increased left atrial (LA) size to be significant predictors, independent of clinical variables. In patients with nonvalvular AF, transesophageal echocardiography (TEE) has identified additional markers of stroke risk, including the presence of thrombus, spontaneous echo contrast or reduced flow velocity in the LA appendage, and complex atherosclerotic plaque in the aorta. The CHADS2 risk score, derived from a National Registry of Atrial Fibrillation cohort, is widely used to assess risk of stroke in patients with AF off anticoagulation (see *JAMA* 2001;285:2864–2870) (**Table 6.1**).

Treatment

The American College of Cardiology (ACC), American Heart Association (AHA), and European Society of Cardiology (ESC) published comprehensive guidelines in 2006, as a revision to their 2001 guidelines on the management of AF (1). The following will briefly cover key aspects of management; the reader is referred to the guidelines for a more detailed review of these topics.

RATE VERSUS RHYTHM CONTROL

Some patients are unstable or severely symptomatic with AF due to hypotension, CHF, and/or angina. In such cases, cardioversion must be performed promptly, and in some occasions as an emergency. Often, however, the symptoms due to AF can be eliminated or at least minimized by controlling the rate of ventricular response. When AF becomes persistent, practitioners and patients then face a choice between rate control and rhythm control as alternative long-term strategies. Beyond the elimination of AF-related symptoms, advocates of rhythm control have hypothesized (if not assumed) that maintenance of SR will reduce the rates of stroke and potentially death, compared with a rate-control approach. These hypotheses have been tested in the North American AFFIRM and European RACE randomized trials (11,12). In both trials, rhythm control failed to lower the incidence of stroke or death as compared to rate control with anticoagulation.

Despite these data, the debate continues as further studies, such as the "on-treatment" analysis of AFFIRM and substudies of the DIAMOND trial, suggested that SR is associated with a considerable reduction in the risk of death. But an AFFIRM subgroup analysis also confirmed that antiarrhythmic drugs are associated with an increased risk of death when controlling for the presence of SR. This means that in practice, the beneficial effects of maintaining SR with antiarrhythmics is negated by their underlying proarrhythmic and noncardiac toxicities (13–15). This has given further credence to the development of nonpharmacologic rhythm-control strategies such as RF cardiac ablation. As of now, these techniques

TABLE 6.1 Risk of Stroke in National Registry of Atrial Fibrillation (NRAF) Participants, Stratified by CHADS2 Score[a]

CHADS2 Score	NRAF Crude Stroke Rate per 100 Patient-years
0	1.2
1	2.8
2	3.6
3	6.4
4	8.0
5	7.7
6	44.0

[a]CHADS2 score is calculated by adding one point for each of the following conditions: recent congestive heart failure, hypertension, age at least 75 years, or diabetes mellitus, and adding two points for having had a prior stroke or transient ischemic attack. CI indicates confidence interval. (Data from Gage BF, Waterman AD, Shannon W, et al. Validation of clinical classification schemes for predicting stroke: results from the National Registry of Atrial Fibrillation. JAMA. 2001 Jun 13;285(22):2864-2870.)

are still considered second-line treatment and reserved for select groups, though their target population is broadening rapidly.

When deciding which management strategy to pursue, it is important to assess the severity of symptoms, exercise tolerance, and patient preference. Though further studies are needed, it appears that patients on a pharmacologic rhythm-control regimen continue to be at risk for thromboembolism (likely through asymptomatic recurrence of AF). Thus, it is imperative that chronic anticoagulation therapy be addressed to prevent thromboembolism in high-risk individuals regardless of the choice of rhythm versus rate control (1).

PHARMACOLOGIC AGENTS FOR CONTROL OF THE VENTRICULAR RATE

1. β-blockers: Multiple studies have been done comparing the efficacy of beta-blockers to placebo and these have shown their efficacy to be agent-specific. In the AFFIRM study they were also found to be more effective than calcium-channel blockers with 70% of patients on *beta-blocker*s reaching their target heart rate compared to 54% of patients on calcium-channel blockers (11). Atenolol (16), metoprolol (17), timolol, pindolol, and nadolol have all been showed to be more effective than placebo at both rest and with exercise. Studies looking at xamoterol (18) showed good exertional heart rate (HR) control, but were inconsistent at rest, while labetalol was shown to be ineffective at rest (19).

Carvedilol is often recommended for use in heart failure, but there are no trials that have compared its efficacy to placebo for use in rate control. For acute rate control, metoprolol 5 mg intravenous (i.v.) push every 5 minutes up to three doses, or an esmolol bolus of 500 μg/kg over a 1-minute period, followed by an infusion rate of 60 to 200 μg/kg/min are commonly prescribed. Commonly used once-daily oral beta-blockers include metoprolol and atenolol, 25 to 100 mg daily. Beta-blockers should not be used in patients with severe bronchospasm and should be used with caution in the presence of severe LV dysfunction.

2. Calcium-channel blockers: The nondihydropyridine calcium-channel blockers diltiazem and verapamil have been shown in several randomized trials to be more effective than either placebo or digoxin at reducing the ventricular rate both at rest and during exercise in patients with AF (17,20). When compared head-to-head, diltiazem and verapamil were shown to have equal efficacy. Usual doses include diltiazem (half-life, 1 to 2 hours), 0.25 mg/kg i.v. over a 2-minute period, and then 5 to 15 mg/hr; verapamil (half-life, <30 minutes), 0.075 to 0.15 mg/kg i.v. over a 2-minute period or 40 to 120 mg orally every 8 hours.

3. Digoxin (0.5 mg i.v., and then 0.25 mg i.v. every 4 hours for two to four doses, and then 0.125 to 0.375 mg orally once daily): Digoxin is felt to act by increasing vagal tone and not through direct myocardial effects. It is most effective for chronic AF, not paroxysmal AF, and it takes hours to achieve maximal effect, so it is not effective for acute rate control. It also works poorly if high sympathetic tone is present, and studies have shown it to be ineffective during exercise (10–12,19,42,92,93). For this reason, the guidelines recommend that its use should primarily be limited to those who are not physically active, such as the elderly or those with heart failure (1). In the case of heart failure, it has the additional benefit of treating the underlying symptoms of heart failure.

PHARMACOLOGIC AGENTS FOR THE ACUTE CONVERSION OF ATRIAL FIBRILLATION

Antiarrhythmic drugs have complex pharmacologic and physiologic actions, and all carry some potential for side effects, including both noncardiac toxicity and proarrhythmic activity (i.e., the induction of potentially dangerous rhythms other than the one being treated). These risks are modified by a number of factors, including renal function, gender, LV systolic function, LV hypertrophy, and the presence of coronary disease and/or prior infarction. Understanding of these risks is essential to maximize the therapeutic index of any treatment decision. When choosing to proceed with pharmacologic conversion, it is important to note that pharmacologic conversion is most effective when started within 7 days of the initiation of an episode of AF.

Intravenous Agents

1. Amiodarone (150 mg i.v. over a 10-minute period *or* 5 to 7 mg/kg over a 30- to 60-minute period, followed by 1.2 to 1.8 g/day continuously or in divided oral doses until 10 g total, and then 200 mg to 400 mg/day maintenance dosing):

Amiodarone is one of the most widely used antiarrhythmic medication, and it has class I, II, III, and VI antiarrhythmic properties. The data for amiodarone in the acute cardioversion of AF are mixed, but they overall favor the use of amiodarone for acute cardioversion (class IIa in the AHA guidelines) (1). In some trials, amiodarone showed little to no efficacy at acute cardioversion, while several meta-analyses have demonstrated that amiodarone has similar efficacy to other class 1C agents, though it is slower to convert patients to normal sinus rhythm (NSR) (21–24). It is generally more effective for AF of <7 days duration, but the SAFE-T trial as well as a recent meta-analysis showed that it has moderate efficacy compared to placebo when converting persistent AF as well (24,25). Overall, it is generally well tolerated in critically ill patients, and in those with structural heart disease and/or heart failure. In these patients it is considered first-line treatment for acute conversion. Adverse effects may include hypotension, sinus bradycardia, phlebitis, gastrointestinal upset, hepatic dysfunction, thyroid disorders (both hypo and hyper), pulmonary toxicity, and, very rarely, torsades de pointes.

2. Ibutilide (1 to 2 mg i.v. over a 10-minute period; can repeat once): Initial studies of this class III agent showed modest to high conversion rates with AF, particularly when administered with a few weeks of the onset of AF (26,31,44), but the data are insufficient to establish its efficacy for conversion of persistent AF of longer duration. These studies have also shown ibutilide to be slightly more effective at converting atrial flutter than AF, compared both to itself and to other antiarrhythmics (26,31). In one trial it was shown to have similar efficacy to amiodarone at converting new-onset AF, but superior efficacy at converting flutter (87% converted with ibutilide vs. 29% with amiodarone) (26). More recent studies have suggested that the addition of beta-blockade or magnesium to an ibutilide infusion will increase the conversion rate of both AF and flutter (32; see also *Pacing Clin Electrophysiol* 2007;30:1331–1335). Given ibutilide's propensity to prolong the QTc, there is an approximately 2% to 4% risk of sustained polymorphic ventricular tachycardia (VT) and torsades de points (highest incidence in women) (44). Administering 4 g of IV magnesium sulfate in concert with ibutilide was shown to decrease the QTc in one trial (33), though there are no studies showing that this decreases rate of torsades de points. In contrast, the coadministration of esmolol with ibutilide reduced the rate of torsades de points from 6.5% to zero (32). Overall, given this propensity for ventricular arrhythmia, it is recommended that ibutilide be avoided in patients with low ejections fractions in the recent AHA guidelines.

3. Procainamide (loading dose of 15 to 17 mg/kg at 20 mg/min, and then 2 to 6 mg/min i.v.): Hypotension occurs in 10% to 15% of patients, and QT prolongation and torsades de pointes are known risks. A few studies have shown procainamide to be more effective than placebo (34,35), but the studies of comparative effectiveness are mixed. One shows better effectiveness than propafenone, but most show poorer effectiveness compared to other antiarrhythmics in the conversion of acute-onset AF (<48 hours) (31,35). One study goes as far to suggest that it has no efficacy for persistent AF of greater than 48

hours, but this has not been adequately studied (34). Given these mixed data on its effectiveness, procainamide was classified as a IIb recommendation for acute conversion in the AHA/ACC/ESC (1).

4. Intravenous versions of flecainide and propafenone are available outside but not within the United States. Both are considered class I recommendations for conversion of AF 7 days or less in duration, and a class IIb recommendation for conversion of AF of more than 7 days in duration (1). Direct comparison of IV to oral flecainide showed similar efficacy, but shorter onset of action with IV flecainide (36). In comparative effectiveness studies, IV flecainide is similar in efficacy to IV ibutilide (37) and direct comparison of IV propafenone to IV ibutilide has suggested that ibutilide is more effective (38). When comparing IV and oral propafenone, IV propafenone was shown to have similar efficacy to oral propafenone, but a faster onset of action. Intravenous sotalol also is available outside the United States, but is not recommended for acute conversion of AF (see section below on Oral Agents).

Oral Agents

1. Amiodarone (600 to 1,200 mg daily in divided doses for 10 to 14 days, and then 200 to 400 mg orally once daily): Amiodarone is also available in an oral formulation, though most studies of acute cardioversion of AF were done using the IV form. Because of its large volume of distribution, oral amiodarone is much slower to take effect than other agents when used for acute conversion, though it has a very low incidence of proarrhythmia. One study found oral amiodarone to be more effective than placebo for the cardioversion of chronic AF (34% vs. 0%) (see *J Cardiovasc Pharmacol Ther* 2000;6:341–350). Because of the limited number of trials available, oral amiodarone has a class IIa recommendation for the cardioversion of AF both <7 and >7 days in duration (1).

2. Flecainide [200 to 300 mg orally (p.o.)]: A type Ic antiarrhythmic that has been shown to have similar efficacy at cardioversion in both the IV and oral forms and has a class I recommendation for the acute cardioversion of AF <7 days in duration, but has a class IIb recommendation for AF of >7 days in duration. A single oral loading dose of flecainide has been shown to be more effective than placebo at converting AF of <7 days duration. Those trials also showed flecainide has equal efficacy with oral propafenone, but it was more effective than oral amiodarone at both 3 and 8 hours postmedication administration. Direct comparison of IV to oral flecainide showed similar efficacy, but shorter onset of action with IV flecainide (36). Overall, the effectiveness of flecainide for AF of >7 days duration has not been adequately studied. For this reason it has a class IIb recommendation for AF of >7 days duration. However, it was studied as an outpatient regimen (along with propafenone), the "pill-in-the-pocket" approach, to good effect in selected patients (39). Side effects including transient hypotension, QRS widening, and conversion to atrial flutter with rapid ventricular response have occurred. This agent is contraindicated in patients with ischemia or LV dysfunction (1).

3. Propafenone (450 to 600 mg p.o.): This type Ic medication has been studied extensively in the literature and has a class I recommendation for the cardioversion of AF of <7 days in duration and a class IIb recommendation for AF >7 days in duration in the AHA guidelines (1). A meta-analysis looking at 11 studies of oral propafenone loading—usually 600 mg given in a single dose—for recent-onset AF (<7 to 14 days) estimated success rates between 56% and 83% (40). Its rate of conversion was also comparable to that of oral flecainide. Comparisons to placebo, oral amiodarone, and oral quinidine with AF of <7 days found superior rates of conversion with propafenone during the first 8 hours after drug administration. Most studies had <8 hours of follow-up, but those with longer follow-up times found little difference in the NSR rate between propafenone, amiodarone, or placebo at 24 hours postdrug administration (134). There are little data to support its use in AF of >7 days in duration. As with flecainide, transient arrhythmias around the time of cardioversion can occur, and the drug should be avoided in patients with impaired LV function or coronary disease. There are little data on its safety in those with structural heart disease.

4. Quinidine (0.75 to 1.5 g in divided doses over a 6- to 12-hour period): Considered moderately effective and has a class IIb recommendation for AF of both <7 and >7 days in duration (1). Most trials of quinidine were done with digoxin administered concurrently and in a quinidine load with repeated doses given every 2 to 3 hours until cardioversion or a total dose of 600 to 1,500 mg was achieved. Most studies compared quinidine plus digoxin to oral propafenone and placebo. They found that quinidine plus digoxin was less effective than propafenone until 24 hours postadministration, at which point the proportion of patient in normal SR is comparable between all three groups (41). The one study comparing quinidine/digoxin to oral sotalol found better efficacy with quinidine/digoxin. Quinidine can cause QT prolongation and torsades de pointes. Its vagolytic properties can increase the ventricular response; thus, coadministration of a rate-controlling agent is recommended (42).

5. Dofetilide (125 to 500 μg p.o., b.i.d.): This newer class III agent has a class I recommendation for the cardioversion of AF regardless of duration. Its efficacy in the conversion of AF/flutter to normal SR was established in two randomized, placebo-controlled trials: European and Australian Multicenter Evaluative Research on Atrial Fibrillation Dofetilide (EMERALD) and Symptomatic Atrial Fibrillation Investigation and Randomized Evaluation of Dofetilide (SAFIRE-D). Short-term conversion rates were approximately 10% for the 250-μg b.i.d. dose and approximately 30% for the 500-μg b.i.d. dose, compared with 1% for placebo (see *Physician's Desk Reference* package insert for details). The SAFIRE-D study specifically looked at chronic AF and showed that dofetilide is more effective at converting chronic AF at doses of 500 μg b.i.d. with most conversions occurring in the first 36 hours (47). QT prolongation and torsades de pointes can occur, and have led to requirements for inpatient drug initiation. Unlike that of most other agents, however, the

safety of dofetilide has been established in patients with LV dysfunction and coronary disease.

Given concerns over the use of antiarrhythmic drugs in patients with structural heart disease, additional safety studies were conducted. Dofetilide was compared with placebo in 1,518 subjects hospitalized with new or worsening CHF and LV dysfunction (DIAMOND-CHF) and 1,510 subjects with severe LV dysfunction after MI (DIAMOND-MI). In patients with AF at baseline, dofetilide was much more effective than placebo at restoring SR (44% vs. 13% at 1 year; $p < 0.001$) and maintaining SR (hazard ratio, 0.35; $p < 0.001$). Furthermore, patients in SR at baseline were less likely to develop new AF with dofetilide than with placebo (2.0% vs. 6.6%; $p < 0.001$). No difference in total mortality was found in either trial. Torsades de pointes was seen in 3.3% of dofetilide patients in DIAMOND-CHF, but after adjustments in the dosing algorithm, this was reduced to 0.9% in DIAMOND-MI. Dofetilide thus appears safe in the CHF/post-MI populations, but initiation of therapy must take place in hospital with careful dose calculation (based on creatinine clearance) and QT-interval monitoring (45,46).

6. Other: Sotalol and digoxin are not recommended for the acute conversion of AF (class III indication) (1). Both IV and oral digoxin have been shown to have no efficacy in converting AF to SR in several studies (48). Studies with sotalol have been mixed, with SAFE-T demonstrating similar efficacy to amiodarone with acute cardioversion (25). Calcium-channel blockers and disopyramide either have not been adequately studied or appear ineffective for the acute conversion of AF.

PHARMACOLOGIC AGENTS FOR LONG-TERM MAINTENANCE OF SINUS RHYTHM

With exceptions, the same oral agents reviewed earlier for immediate conversion also are used for maintenance of SR. Because of findings of increased mortality in specific clinical trials (CAST, SWORD), the class IA and IC drugs are generally recommended only for patients without structural heart disease. Brief additional comments follow.

1. Amiodarone (200 mg/day). In addition to its well-documented safety in the presence of coronary artery disease (CAD) and LV dysfunction, amiodarone appears to be the most effective agent for long-term maintenance of SR when compared to other 1C agents as shown in CTAF, AFFIRM, and SAFE-T (13,25,49). Despite its increased efficacy, the potential for noncardiac toxicity (liver, lung, thyroid) and other side effects (neurologic, skin discoloration) requires consideration, particularly in younger patients. For this reason the AHA/ACC/EHA guidelines recommend that amiodarone be reserved for first-line maintenance therapy only in those with heart failure, moderate to severe systolic dysfunction, and hypertension-associated severe LV hypertrophy. It may be used as second-line therapy for all other patients whose AF is refractory to other medications.

2. Dronedarone is a new multiclass antiarrhythmic with similar electrophysiologic properties to amiodarone, but without the iodine moiety that has been thought to cause amiodarone's thyroid, liver, and lung toxicities. Several randomized trials have shown dronedarone to have no proarrhythmic, thyroid, or pulmonary toxicities, and to be more effective than placebo at preventing recurrent AF (27). This safety profile was confirmed in the large ATHENA trial that also found dronedarone to be associated with a reduced risk of death and cardiovascular hospitalization compared to placebo in patients with AF or flutter (28). Dronedarone should be avoided in patients with class IV heart failure, as the ANDROMEDA trial found a doubling in the rate of death among patients with severe heart failure taking dronedarone (29). When comparing dronedarone directly to amiodarone, the DIONYSOS trial showed that amiodarone was associated with less AF recurrence, but had more side effects compared to dronedarone (30).

3. Dofetilide (125 to 500 μg p.o., b.i.d.). Dofetilide is the only antiarrhythmic drug other than amiodarone with good safety data in CHF and CAD (45,46). Both the DIAMOND and SAFIRE-D studies showed that dofetilide was more effective than placebo in the maintenance of SR and prevention of new AF (14,45–47). Dofetilide should be avoided in patients with renal impairment due to the increased risk of torsades de pointes. It also has a number of important drug-to-drug interactions. Initiation of this medicine should take place in an inpatient setting due to proarrhythmia.

4. Sotalol (80 to 160 mg p.o., b.i.d.). It is a type III antiarrhythmic with additional type II beta-blocker effects. In several studies, sotalol was shown to be better than placebo for the maintenance of NSR (25,50) and similar in efficacy to quinidine (51). Some studies comparing sotalol to propafenone demonstrated equal efficacy at less than 1 year (52), while other long-term studies showed propafenone to have better long-term efficacy after 6 months (53,54). In comparison to amiodarone, the CTAF and SAFE-T studies showed sotalol to be less effective than amiodarone at maintaining NSR (25,49,53). Sotalol is renally excreted and prolongs the QT interval. It is not recommended for use in heart failure, renal dysfunction, or in patients with marked LV hypertrophy.

5. Flecainide (100 to 150 mg p.o., b.i.d.). A type Ic antiarrhythmic that is better than placebo for maintenance of SR. In comparison to other antiarrhythmics, flecainide has similar efficacy to both quinidine and propafenone (55,56), but patients were less likely to have side effects and more likely to stay on flecainide. Its use should be targeted to patients with no structural heart disease.

6. Propafenone (150 to 300 mg p.o., b.i.d. to t.i.d.). A type Ic antiarrhythmic that is better than placebo for maintenance of normal SR (57). Higher doses result in increased efficacy, but were also shown to result in increased side effects (57). Propafenone is similar in efficacy to flecainide (55,56), but possibly better than quinidine. Some studies comparing sotalol to propafenone demonstrated equal efficacy at less than 1 year (52), while other long-term studies showed propafenone to have better long-term efficacy after 6 months (53,54). A few

studies have compared amiodarone to propafenone, with two showing superior efficacy (49,53) and one showing equal efficacy (58). It carries the same adverse effects and warnings as other class IC antiarrhythmics.

7. Class IA agents (disopyramide, quinidine, procainamide). As a group, the IA agents have less data supporting their efficacy than do either the IC or class III agents, although quinidine has been studied more than the others (42). Each of these agents is associated with QT prolongation and potentially important noncardiac adverse effects. Their use for maintenance of SR has been steadily declining, relative to other agents.

CATHETER AND SURGICAL ABLATION

Catheter Ablation

Promising early reports have led to growing enthusiasm for RF catheter-based ablation approaches targeting ectopic atrial foci that trigger AF, the great majority of which appear to arise in or near the ostia of the pulmonary veins. This approach has been studied mainly in relatively young patients with structurally normal hearts, and appears to improve or eliminate AF episodes in 50% to 70% of subjects, but is clearly more successful when AF is paroxysmal rather than persistent (see *Circulation* 2002;105:1077). The role of catheter ablation in the management of AF is an area of active research, but currently there are only a few small, randomized, controlled trials comparing catheter ablation to antiarrhythmic drug therapy. Of the available trials, most look at RF catheter ablation as second-line therapy for patients who failed antiarrhythmic drug therapy alone. Though follow-up is limited to 1 year, all found RF catheter ablation to be superior to antiarrhythmic drug therapy at maintaining NSR (59–63). Only one small, randomized, controlled trial has examined RF catheter ablation as first-line therapy for paroxysmal AF in patients not previously treated with antiarrhythmic medications, and this found RF catheter ablation to be superior to antiarrhythmic drug therapy at maintaining NSR (64).

Surgical Ablation

Cox and other investigators developed surgical approaches to compartmentalize the atria to alter the underlying substrate for AF. This procedure (the Cox maze) has undergone many revisions and a number of similar methods using ablative energy sources rather than incisions have been developed. These interventions are typically combined adjunctively with mitral valve or other cardiac surgery, though occasionally, they are used in patients with significant, symptomatic, persistent AF who have been refractory to all other interventions. Most studies of patients undergoing this procedure are of small sample size and without blinding, though several meta-analyses have confirmed that the maze procedures can result in the restoration of NSR in 60% to 90% of patients (65,66). Most recently, surgical pulmonary vein isolation (PVI) by RF ablation has been shown to be as effective as the modified Cox maze procedure at restoring NSR in patients with chronic AF and mitral valve (MV) disease (67,68).

ELECTRICAL CARDIOVERSION

Electrical cardioversion is favored for immediate management of unstable patients, and appears to have greater efficacy (approximately 70% to 90%) than drugs for the elective conversion of AF of short- to medium-term duration. Unfortunately, recurrence soon or late after cardioversion is common, with some studies showing a recurrence rate as high as 50%. Aside from minor skin irritation, adverse events are relatively rare and may include the unmasking of significant sinus bradycardia. The most significant potential risk related to cardioversion is thromboembolism, and specific guidelines regarding pericardioversion anticoagulation exist and are reviewed later.

Type and Amount of Energy

Although traditional teaching dictates starting cardioversion attempts at low energies (50 to 100 J), a randomized study using monophasic waveform devices found a significantly higher success rate at higher energies. Success rates were 14%, 39%, and 95%, respectively, with initial energies of 100, 200, and 360 J. Patients treated with higher initial energies received fewer shocks and lower cumulative energy, and no patient had detectable myocardial injury by troponin testing (see *Am J Cardiol* 2000;86:348–350). More recently, external defibrillators with biphasic waveforms have been introduced into clinical practice and have started to become standard of care. Studies using these defibrillators, compared with older monophasic devices, have shown equivalent to increased efficacy (69; see also *Am J Cardiol* 2004;93:1495–1499) at relatively lower energies and have been used successfully in patients for whom previous attempts with monophasic defibrillators failed [see *Am J Cardiol* 2002;90 (3):331–332]. Another study showed decreased cutaneous burns due to the lower energy used (see *Resuscitation.* 2006: Dec;71(3):293–300. Epub 2006 Sep 20.). Several studies have looked into how much energy should be applied to biphasic cardioversion. In two studies, longer duration of AF (70) and body mass index (BMI) of >25 (71) were both correlated with increased energy requirement to achieve cardioversion and both concluded that starting with higher doses results in fever shocks. Given this, the general recommendation is to start with 200 J for biphasic cardioversion.

Anticoagulation Before and After Cardioversion

It has been noted since the 1920s that cardioversion (either pharmacologic or electrical) is associated with a transient increase above the already elevated baseline risk of thromboembolism in AF. This is related in part to the release of already-formed clot in the left atria (72), as well as the delayed recovery of atrial mechanical function postcardioversion, resulting in de novo clots (also known as "stunning"). There is a lack of randomized, controlled trials on the use of anticoagulation during cardioversion, but given the long-observed risk in observation studies of thromboembolism with AF, specific recommendations regarding pericardioversion anticoagulation have been developed. The following summarizes the recommendations for antithrombotic therapy in patients undergoing cardioversion (see AHA/ACC/ESC guidelines for further details):

1. Patients with AF less than 48 hours in duration may be cardioverted without prior anticoagulation, but anticoagulation should be given for 4 weeks following cardioversion to prevent de novo clot (class IIa recommendation). There is a dearth of prospective data to support this empiric duration, but retrospective data suggest that embolic complications with this approach are rare (72; see also *J Am Coll Cardiol* 2002;40:934).

2. Patients with hemodynamically unstable AF of recent onset should be cardioverted as an emergency without preceding anticoagulation, but should be given heparin concurrently if possible, and treated afterward with warfarin [international normalized ratio (INR), 2 to 3] for 3 to 4 weeks.

3. Patients with AF of longer than 48 hours or unknown duration should be given anticoagulation with warfarin (target INR, 2 to 3) for at least 3 to 4 weeks before and after cardioversion.

4. Documenting the absence of thrombus in the LA appendage by TEE is an acceptable alternative to the 3 to 4 weeks of anticoagulation preceding cardioversion. The safety of this approach has been established through both nonrandomized and randomized studies (73,74).

The potential role of low-molecular-weight heparin compounds as a substitute for i.v. heparin or warfarin around the time of cardioversion is under investigation. One randomized study reported data suggesting the noninferiority of enoxaparin for this indication (86), but this is difficult to prove, given the generally low rate of embolic events during this short time.

LONG-TERM ANTICOAGULATION

Thromboembolic stroke is the most serious complication of AF, and many studies have been done to characterize this risk. In meta-analyses of AF studies (1,6,77,88,89), anticoagulation with warfarin reduced stroke risk by roughly 60% versus placebo, compared with approximately 20% reduction with aspirin. No difference in stroke rate was found between paroxysmal AF and chronic AF. When anticoagulation is used, a target INR of 2.0 to 3.0 should be targeted (77–87), as the SPAF III trial (86) showed an increased rate of ischemic stroke and embolic complications with lower INR (**Table 6.2**). Despite the clear benefit of anticoagulation with regards to the stroke risk, anticoagulation carries clear risks of hemorrhagic complications. In order to balance these risks, several guidelines have attempted to define risk-stratification schemes for patients with AF. The CHADS2 score is one of the most validated, and integrates aspects of the AFI and SPAF algorithms (**Table 6.2**).

Recommendations for long-term anticoagulation based on the AHA/ACC/ESC guidelines are listed as follows:

1. If the patient has lone AF (i.e., no stroke risk factors) or a CHADS2 score of 0, aspirin alone is considered by most experts to be adequate, as the baseline stroke risk of this cohort is low (approximately 0.5% per year) (5).

TABLE 6.2 Major Randomized Trials of Warfarin for Prevention of Thromboembolism in Nonvalvular Atrial Fibrillation

Annual Event Rate (%) Study	Primary Endpoint(s)	Target INR	Warfarin	Control	Value
AFASAK (78)	Stroke, TIA, embolic complications to viscera and extremities	2.8–4.2	2.0	5.5[a]	<0.05
BAATAF (79)	Ischemic stroke	1.5–2.7	0.4	3.0[b]	0.002
SPAF I (80)	Ischemic stroke, systemic emboli	2.0–3.5	2.3	7.4[a]	0.01
CAFA (81)	Nonlacunar stroke, non-CNS embolic event, ICH, other fatal hemorrhage	2.0–3.0	3.5	5.2[a]	NS
SPINAF (82)	Cerebral infarction	1.4–2.8	0.9	4.3	0.001
EAFT (83)	Vascular death, any stroke, MI, recent stroke/TIA, systemic embolism	2.5–4.0	8.0	15.0[a]	0.001
SPAF II (84)	Ischemic stroke, systemic emboli	2.0–4.5	1.9	2.7[c]	0.15
SPAF III (86)	Ischemic stroke, systemic emboli	2.0–3.0	1.9	7.9[d]	<0.0001
AFASAK II (87)	Stroke, systemic emboli	2.0–3.0	2.8	3.6[e]	NS

CAFA, Canadian atrial fibrillation anticoagulation; SPAF, stroke prevention in atrial fibrillation; INR, international normalized ratio; ICH, intracranial hemorrhage; MI, myocardial infarction; TIA, transient ischemic attack; CNS, central nervous system; NS, not significant.

[a]Placebo group.
[b]No treatment but aspirin allowed.
[c]Aspirin.
[d]Aspirin and fixed low-dose warfarin (mean INR, 1.3).
[e]Low-dose warfarin.

2. If the patient has CHADS2 score greater than 1, anticoagulation with warfarin is recommended (target INR, 2.0 to 3.0). Aspirin is an acceptable alternative to anticoagulation in patients with a CHADS2 score equal to 1.

3. The optimal duration of warfarin treatment after cardioversion is not known, although "at least" 3 to 4 weeks is recommended by the AHA/ACC/ESC criteria (1). Thus far, no study has clearly demonstrated that a strategy of SR maintenance reduces the risk of stroke if warfarin is discontinued.

INVESTIGATIONAL ANTICOAGULANTS

Several oral direct thrombin or factor Xa inhibitors are being tested as possible replacements for warfarin, as they do not require coagulation monitoring or dosage titrations. Dabigatran has shown excellent results in the recently published RE-LY trial where high- and low-dose dabigatran were compared to standard warfarin therapy for use in AF. Low-dose dabigatran (110 mg twice daily) was noninferior to warfarin at the prevention of thromboembolic events, but with a lower risk of bleeding events. High-dose dabigatran (150 mg twice daily) had decreased thromboembolic events compared to warfarin therapy and an equal risk of bleeding events (90). Another oral direct thrombin inhibitor, ximelagatran, was withdrawn prior to getting Food and Drug Administration (FDA) approval due to liver toxicity noted during testing (91). Three oral factor Xa inhibitors (rivaroxaban, apixaban, and edoxaban) are currently undergoing testing, but no outcomes data are available yet for their use in AF.

OTHER TREATMENT MEASURES

1. *Implantable atrial defibrillator.* Some patients with frequent, symptomatic episodes of AF for whom other modalities have failed may be candidates for sophisticated ICD devices that provide antitachycardia pacing as well as automated or patient-activated shocks to terminate atrial arrhythmias.

2. *Atrial pacemakers.* Pacing the right atrium from two sites and implanting pacemakers with automated atrial overdrive algorithms are two novel pacemaker-based interventions for reducing the "burden" of AF. These are reviewed separately (see the section "Cardiac Pacing Studies").

3. *Atrioventricular junction (AVJ) ablation with permanent pacemaker implantation.* In patients for whom maintenance of SR is no longer feasible or desired, but who still have significant symptoms with AF, benefits have been demonstrated with the combination of AVJ ablation and implantation of a ventricular pacemaker. This provides the ultimate form of rate control and eliminates the irregular ventricular response that in some patients contributes to symptoms, even at moderate rates. However, given that the atria remain in AF, the risk for clot and thromboembolism remains; thus, this strategy does not change the requirement for anticoagulation.

ATRIAL FIBRILLATION PREVENTION AFTER CARDIAC SURGERY

Postoperative AF is especially common after cardiac operations, occurring in approximately 25% of patients. Postoperative AF occurs most frequently on post-operative days 2 to 3. Several studies have shown that its occurrence is associated with higher morbidity. Among cardiac surgery patients, one study found that post-operative AF was associated with increased mortality at 1 and 6 months. Postoperative AF also results in an extended length of hospital stay.

The use of beta-blockers after surgery has been consistently shown to reduce the incidence of AF and has become standard practice (92). In one meta-analysis of 24 randomized studies, beta-blocker therapy reduced post-CABG AF by 77% (92). Preoperative initiation of beta-blockers also was found to be more effective than postoperative initiation.

Several randomized, controlled studies have evaluated the prophylactic use of i.v. or oral amiodarone (93). Although amiodarone typically reduced the incidence of in-hospital AF, these reductions translated into a significantly shorter hospital stay in only one trial, when oral amiodarone was started 7 days preoperatively (93). Only one randomized study has compared amiodarone with a beta-blocker (pro-pranolol; see *Am Heart J* 2001;142:811). Amiodarone was associated with a lower incidence of postoperative AF, but no difference in length of hospital stay was found. It has pulmonary toxicity, and an increased incidence of bradyarrhythmias has been seen in those receiving beta-blocker therapy; therefore, beta-blockers remain first-line therapy for AF prophylaxis, whereas amiodarone should be con-sidered in those who cannot take beta-blockers and who are at high risk (i.e., his-tory of AF, age older than 75 years, valve operations). Other trials have evaluated agents such as oral sotalol (no advantage over other beta-blockers with increased risk of torsades de pointes), dofetilide (more effective than placebo) (94), pro-cainamide (not effective), and verapamil (not effective).

VENTRICULAR ARRHYTHMIAS

Sudden cardiac death (SCD) accounts for more than 250,000 annual fatalities in the United States, and roughly half of all cardiac deaths are due to out-of-hospital car-diac arrest. The majority of these events are attributable to unstable ventricular arrhythmias.

Immediate Therapy: Automated External Defibrillators

Because most patients with witnessed cardiac arrest have "shockable" ventricular tachyarrhythmias just after collapse, and survival rates are critically related to the rapidity of defibrillation, substantial effort has been expended in developing and deploying automated external defibrillators (AEDs) in public areas. These devices, which require little to no training to operate, were originally shown to improve survival to hospital discharge among cardiac arrest victims when supplied to first-responder firefighters, as compared with waiting slightly longer for paramedics (95). Given both their ease of use and clear survival advantage, studies have been done to look at their effectiveness when deployed broadly in the community. Pilot studies of AED use in casinos (96) and commercial airplanes (97) demonstrated excellent performance of both AED rhythm diagnostics and shocking efficacy, leading to rates of survival to hospital discharge of 40% to 50% for victims of ventricular fibrillation (VF). These led to the large PAD study that looked at the use of AEDs by trained laypersons (19,000 volunteers) across multiple public venues in North America. The PAD study found a significant advantage in survival to hospital discharge when AEDs were used compared to cardiopulmonary resuscitation (CPR) alone (23.4% vs. 14%) (98). Though AEDs are now being placed in more and more locations, at the moment there is no evidence for the widespread deployment of AED in private homes, as a recent study found no survival advantage to home AED use compared to CPR alone (99).

Immediate Therapy: Intravenous Amiodarone

Two important trials, ARREST and ALIVE, have provided more robust data than smaller prior studies on the immediate resuscitation of cardiac arrest (100,101). These trials demonstrated that a bolus of i.v. amiodarone, when given to patients with pulseless VT or VF refractory to initial attempts at defibrillation, results in improved survival to hospital admission compared with either placebo or i.v. lidocaine. The ARREST and ALIVE studies were not large enough to demonstrate improvement in more pertinent endpoints, such as survival to hospital discharge, but nonetheless solidified the role of i.v. amiodarone as first-choice drug therapy for VT/VF in the year 2000 (and subsequent) Advanced Cardiac Life Support (ACLS) guidelines.

Secondary-prevention Trials: Drugs versus Implantable Cardioverter Defibrillators

Three important randomized trials comparing ICDs with antiarrhythmic drugs for survivors of cardiac arrest or hemodynamically significant ventricular arrhythmias were completed in the 1990s: CASH, CIDS, and AVID (**Table 6.3**). Subsequently, there was an explosion of data supporting the implantation of such devices in various populations. Device technology was in a phase of rapid evolution, and concurrent with execution of the trials, perspectives on drug therapy were changing as well.

The CASH study randomized cardiac arrest survivors to amiodarone, metoprolol, ICD, or propafenone (102). The propafenone group was terminated early because of excess mortality compared with the ICD group. At long-term follow-up, a nonsignificant trend toward lower all-cause mortality favored the ICD group versus the combined amiodarone and metoprolol groups. CIDS was a "purer" and more recent comparison of ICDs versus amiodarone for survivors of cardiac arrest and documented unstable VT (103). As with CASH, a trend emerged in favor of

TABLE 6.3 Survival Trials of ICD Therapy versus Conventional Medical Management

	AVID (104)	CASH (102)	CIDS (103)	MADIT I (113)	MADIT II (115)
Pt population/ entry criteria	Primary VF; or VT with syncope; or VT with EF ≤40% and significant symptoms	SCD survivors w/documented ventricular arrhythmias	VF; or cardiac arrest; sustained VT (poorly tolerated or EF ≤35%,) or syncope with spontaneous or inducible VT	Prior MI + EF ≤35%; NYHA class I–III + nonsustained VT on EPS	Prior MI, EF ≤30%, NYHA class I–III
Treatment	ICD vs. amiodarone or sotalol	ICD, amiodarone, metoprolol, or propafenone	ICD or amiodarone	ICD or conventional medical therapy	ICD or conventional medical therapy
Primary endpoint	All-cause mortality	All-cause mortality	All-cause mortality	All-cause mortality	All-cause mortality
Results	39% lower mortality for ICD patients (at 3 yr, 24.6% vs. 35.9%; $p < 0.02$)	38% lower mortality for ICD patients vs. amiodarone and metoprolol (36% vs. 44%; $p = 0.08$)a	20% lower mortality for ICD patients (8.2% per yr vs. 10.2% per yr; $p = 0.14$)	54% lower mortality for ICD patients (17% vs. 39%; $p = 0.009$)	28% lower mortality for ICD patients (at 20 months; 14.2% vs. 19.8%)

	DINAMIT (116)	SCD-HeFT (117)	IRIS (118)	AMIOVIRT (120)	DEFINITE (121)
Pt population/ entry criteria	6–40 days post-MI, EF <35%, weakened cardiac autonomic function	NYHA class II or III CHF and an EF of ≤35% recurrent VT	5–31 days post-MI, EF <35%, at least 1 predictor of NSVT	Stable, NIDCM, EF <35%, and asymptomatic complexes or NSVT	NIDCM, EF <36%, and premature ventricular
Treatment	ICD or conventional medical therapy	Amiodarone, ICD, or conventional medical therapy	ICD or conventional medical therapy	ICD or amiodarone	ICD or conventional medical therapy
Primary endpoint	All-cause mortality	All-cause mortality	All-cause mortality	All-cause mortality	All-cause mortality
Results	No benefit for mortality (reduced arrhythmia death offset by nonarrhythmia death)	23% lower mortality (hazard ratio for ICD patients offset by nonarrhythmia death)	No benefit for mortality (reduced arrhythmia death of follow-up)	Stopped early for futility (no effect at 1 or 3 years)	35% reduction in mortality hazard for ICD patients

EF, ejection fraction; ICD, implantable cardiac defibrillator; VF, ventricular fibrillation; VT, ventricular tachycardia; NYHA, New York Heart Association.

[a]Enrollment in the propafenone arm was stopped in 1992 because of a high mortality rate.

ICDs for the endpoints of total and arrhythmic mortality, but again did not reach statistical significance. The AVID trial was the largest and most definitive of the three trials, randomizing more than 1,000 patients to ICD or antiarrhythmic drug (96% amiodarone) (104). AVID showed significantly better 2-year survival in the ICD group (75% vs. 64%; $p < 0.02$), leading many observers to conclude that CASH and CIDS were simply underpowered. Thus, in aggregate, the trials indicate that ICDs are superior to drug therapy. As a result, ICDs are now generally used as first-line treatment in the secondary-prevention population.

Primary-prevention Trials: Antiarrhythmic Drugs

In the 1970s and early 1980s, various investigators observed a high incidence of sudden death in survivors of acute MI, and identified methods of predicting increased risk for future arrhythmic events, including depressed ejection fraction, complex ventricular ectopy/nonsustained VT (NSVT) on ambulatory ECG monitoring, the presence of late potentials on signal-averaged electrocardiogram (ECG), and the induction of sustained tachycardias with invasive electrophysiologic study (EPS). These insights led to primary-prevention trials in MI survivors, initially with antiarrhythmic drugs. Unfortunately, these trials demonstrated that with the exception of amiodarone, antiarrhythmic drugs actually appear to *increase* mortality in this patient population. In particular, Vaughan-Williams class I agents propafenone, encainide, flecainide (105), and moricizine (106) all demonstrated excess mortality compared with control groups in randomized studies of post-MI patients. In contrast, oral amiodarone appeared to reduce arrhythmic events and sudden death in several trials enrolling post-MI and CHF patients (108–111), although consistent improvements in all-cause mortality were not seen. This was confirmed in the amiodarone arm of the SCD-HEFT trial where all-cause mortality was not improved by amiodarone as compared to placebo (117). A meta-analysis of amiodarone trials (112) suggested a small advantage in overall survival compared with placebo or alternative antiarrhythmic drugs. The class III antiarrhythmic drug dofetilide had a neutral effect on mortality in post-MI and CHF patients, but is currently approved for use only in AF (see the section "Pharmacologic Agents for the Acute Conversion of Atrial Fibrillation").

Primary-prevention Trials: Drugs versus Implantable Cardioverter Defibrillators

After the disappointing results of antiarrhythmic drug trials, primary-prevention trials involving ICDs were completed. The ICD trials again focused on the post-MI population known to be at high risk for SCD, and the first two major trials—MADIT and MUSTT (113,114)—selected patients with low ejection fractions, NSVT, and inducible VT at EPS. As with the secondary-prevention trials, a clear advantage emerged in favor of ICDs compared with medical therapy with or without antiarrhythmic drugs.

Subsequently, the results of the MADIT II trial, which selected coronary patients >30 days post-MI on the basis of low ejection fraction alone (30% or less), demonstrated a statistically significant 28% relative reduction in mortality with prophylactic ICD implantation (115; see **Table 6.3**). These results were confirmed in the SCD-HeFT trial that found a 23% reduction in mortality with prophylactic ICD implantation when compared to both placebo and amiodarone in patients with a low ejection fraction (35% or less) and NYHA class II or III heart failure (117).

Given the impressive results of the primary-prevention ICD trials in ischemic cardiomyopathy, two trials looked into primary-prevention ICD placement in patients <30 to 40 days out from a MI. The DINAMIT and IRIS trials enrolled patients with decreased ejection fractions, elevated resting heart rates, and recent MIs (<40 and <30 days, respectively). Both found no decrease in all-cause mortality in the ICD arms compared to placebo, despite the fact that the IRIS study showed a decreased rate of SCD in the ICD arm (which was balanced by an increase in non-SCDs in that arm) (116,118). Based on the DINAMIT results (which were later confirmed in IRIS), the new 2008 ACC/AHA/Heart Rhythm Society (HRS) guidelines (122) consider as a class I recommendation ICD therapy for patients with LVEF less than 35%, NYHA class II or III heart failure (or left ventricular ejection fraction (LVEF) <30% for NYHA class I heart failure) at least 40 days post-MI and 3 months after coronary revascularization therapy.

Primary-prevention Trials: Nonischemic Cardiomyopathy Patients

In contrast to the progress in sudden death prevention in coronary disease patients outlined earlier, the question of whether antiarrhythmic drugs or ICDs provide additional mortality benefit for nonischemic cardiomyopathy patients beyond that provided by angiotensin-converting enzyme (ACE) inhibitors and beta-blockers has been more difficult to answer. Two small early studies showed no benefit of ICD in nonischemic dilated cardiomyopathy (NIDCM) compared to either placebo [Cardiomyopathy Trial (CAT)] or amiodarone (AMIOVIRT). The CAT compared ICD with control in only NIDCM patients (LVEF <30%) (119). The trial was terminated before completion of full enrollment because of a lower than expected mortality in the control group; as a result, the study was underpowered to detect a mortality difference between the two groups [26% (ICD) vs. 31.5%; p = NS]. AMIOVIRT compared amiodarone alone, to amiodarone plus ICD treatment in NIDCM (LEVF <35%) and found no difference in survival between treatment groups (120). These studies were followed up with the larger DEFINITE and SCD-HeFT trials. DEFINITE enrolled patients with dilated cardiomyopathy (DCM) (LVEF <35%), frequent premature ventricular contractions (PVCs), or NSVT and compared ICD to standard medical therapy with ACE inhibitors and beta-blockers. It found that the ICD arm was associated with a statistically significant reduction in the risk of SCD from arrhythmias, but there was only a trend to statistical significance in the reduction of all-cause mortality (the primary endpoint) in the ICD arm compared to standard treatment (121). This was likely due to a lower than expected mortality rate in the standard medical treatment arm leaving the study underpowered. The SCD-HeFT trial, which enrolled both ischemic and NIDCM patients, was the first trial to find a statistically significant reduction in all-cause mortality with ICD use in NIDCM (117). Based on this study, the 2008 AHA/ACC/HRS guidelines give prophylactic ICD placement a class I recommendation for patients with NIDCM and NYHA class II or III heart failure (122).

CARDIAC PACING STUDIES

Traditionally, permanent pacemakers have been used for the treatment of brady-arrhythmias. However, evolving pacemaker technologies have shown utility in the management of tachyarrhythmias, CHF, and, to a limited extent, vasovagal syncope.

Pacemaker Mode Selection Trials

In clinical practice, most cardiologists implant dual-chamber pacemakers in patients with bradyarrhythmias, except those with chronic AF. Despite the sound rationale for physiologic dual-chamber pacing—including maintenance of AV synchrony, avoidance of retrograde ventriculoatrial (VA) conduction, and preservation of normal heart rate response in patients with intact sinus node function—objective benefits of dual-chamber pacing have proved difficult to quantify prospectively. Confirming prior retrospective data, several clinical trials have shown that atrial or dual-chamber pacing, when compared with single-chamber ventricular (VVI) pacing, prevents pacemaker syndrome, and is associated with a lower incidence of new or permanent AF, particularly among patients with sinus node dysfunction. However, improvements in "harder" endpoints, such as stroke or death, were seen in one preliminary study but not confirmed in larger, later trials [CTOPP, MOST (124,125)]. Furthermore, in the Dual Chamber and VVI Implantable Defibrillator (DAVID) Trial Investigators, dual-chamber pacing was compared with ventricular backup pacing in 506 patients with an implantable defibrillator and EF of 40% or less, and the backup pacing group had a better 1-year survival free of death or hospitalization for CHF (83.9% vs. 73.3%; relative hazard, 1.61; 95% CI, 1.06 to 2.44) (126), suggesting unnecessary pacing, which might desynchronize the two ventricles, may be harmful. Most recently, investigators in the PACE trial demonstrated such detrimental effects that chronic right ventricle (RV) pacing can have on the LV (127).

Pacing for Vasovagal Syncope

Therapy for patients with frequent episodes of vasovagal syncope is generally unsatisfactory. Nonrandomized data previously suggested that a subset of vasovagal syncope patients with pronounced cardioinhibitory (bradycardia) physiology benefits from permanent pacing. To this end, pacemakers were developed that automatically pace at high rates when triggered by prespecified decreases in intrinsic heart rate (rate-drop response). Early randomized trials [such as the Vasovagal Pacemaker Study (VPS)] were unblinded, leaving suspect their results showing that implantation of pacemakers with rate-drop response resulted in a significant reduction in subsequent syncopal events (128–130). These were followed by the Second Vasovagal Pacemaker Study (VPS II) and SYNPACE, which were fully blinded studies of highly symptomatic patients with bradycardia during tilt-table testing. Contrary to the results of the unblinded studies, VPS II showed only a modest, nonstatistically significant benefit (131), while SYNPACE was terminated early due to the inability of pacing to show a statistically significant reduction in syncopal events at the interim analysis (132). It should be noted, especially given the VPS II results, that both studies were underpowered to see a modest effect with pacing, so larger trials will be needed to fully answer this question. At present, pacing for vasovagal syncope cannot be recommended as a first-line treatment.

Pacing for Prevention of Atrial Fibrillation

Based on the observed benefits of standard right atrial (RA) pacing in preventing AF in susceptible patients (reviewed earlier), investigators have explored whether the development of specialized pacing software to provide automated atrial overdrive pacing or the implantation of atrial leads at two separate sites can achieve even better suppression of AF than standard dual-chamber pacing. Overdrive RA pacing appears to reduce the "burden" of AF somewhat (133), but the superiority of dual-site versus single-site pacing has not been clearly established. Statistically significant findings for particular endpoints and/or in specific subgroups have been reported with these approaches, but the magnitude of benefit, the clinical relevance of the endpoints, and the future of these forms of therapy remain uncertain (134–136).

Resynchronization Therapy for Congestive Heart Failure

Of patients with chronic CHF due to systolic ventricular dysfunction, 30% or more have electrical conduction defects (bundle branch block or intraventricular conduction delay) that cause delayed activation of portions of the ventricular myocardium. The resulting electrical dyssynchrony within or between ventricles appears to impair further the mechanical efficiency of the heart, contributing to heart failure (HF) symptoms and possibly mortality. To address this, pacing systems incorporate leads delivered through the coronary sinus system that provide early stimulation to the epicardial surface of the posterolateral left ventricle, the site typically activated latest in these patients. These systems allow for LV or biventricular (BiV) pacing, known as cardiac "resynchronization" therapy (CRT).

After pilot studies demonstrated immediate hemodynamic benefits from LV or BiV pacing, a number of clinical trials were performed with several different pacing systems (see review: *J Am Coll Cardiol* 2002;39:194). Each of these studies had short- to intermediate-term follow-up and documented improvements with LV or BiV pacing in various subjective and objective measures of heart failure severity, including New York Heart Association functional class, 6-minute walk test, peak oxygen consumption, and quality of life (QOL) (137–140). In the MIRACLE study, 453 NYHA class III or IV patients with EF less than 35% who underwent BiV pacing system placement were randomized to active pacing (atrially synchronized BiV pacing) or no pacing for 6 months (140). The active-pacing group had significant improvement in all measured parameters, including EF and hospitalization for worsening HF.

More recent studies with longer follow-up have shown a significant survival advantage in addition to the symptom improvements seen with CRT treatment both with (CRT-D) and without ICD (CRT) compared to standard medical management (141). The COMPANION trial enrolled 1,520 patients with class III or IV CHF with QRS <120 msec and found death and hospitalization was significantly reduced with BiV pacing and BiV pacing plus ICD (CRT-D). In addition, the CRT-D group had a highly significant 36% mortality reduction compared to optimal drug therapy (142). This was further confirmed in the CARE-HF trial that looked at 813 patients with class II or IV heart failure and with a QRD >120 msec and an LVEF of <35%. Again, the CRT arm was associated with a decreased rate of the primary endpoint of death or hospitalization (39% CRT vs. 55% medical therapy; $p < 0.001$), but in this trial there was also a significant reduction in mortality in the CRT group (20% CRT vs. 30% medical therapy; $p < 0.002$) (144). These findings were in addition to the QOL and objective improvements that were also seen in the prior studies (141,144). The MADIT-CRT trial further broadened the potential impact of CRT to include patients with milder symptoms of CHF, NYHA class I or II, and demonstrated benefit of CRT-D therapy in this population (143). Given the high cost of these devices, criteria for optimal patient selection are extremely important.

These data, particularly the survival data, resulted in a class Ia recommendation in the updated 2008 ACC/AHA/HRS guidelines (122): "For patients who have LVEF less than or equal to 35%, a QRS duration greater than or equal to 0.12 seconds, and sinus rhythm, CRT with or without an ICD is indicated for the treatment of NYHA functional Class III or ambulatory Class IV heart failure symptoms with optimal recommended medical therapy." Such data also paved the way for FDA approval of dedicated BiV pacing systems (including ICDs with BiV pacing capability).

REFERENCES

Atrial Fibrillation

1. **Fuster V,** et al. ACC/AHA/ESC 2006 guidelines for the management of patients with atrial fibrillation: a report of the American College of Cardiology/American Heart Association Task Force on Practice Guidelines and the European Society of Cardiology Committee for Practice Guidelines (Writing Committee to Revise the 2001 Guidelines for the Management

of Patients with Atrial Fibrillation) developed in collaboration with the European Heart Rhythm Association and the Heart Rhythm Society. *J Am Coll Cardiol* 2006;48;e149–e246.

EPIDEMIOLOGY

2. **Lloyd-Jones DM,** et al. Lifetime risk for development of atrial fibrillation: the Framingham Heart Study. *Circulation* 2004;110(9):1042–1046.

A population-based study done in Framingham, MA, between 1968 and 1999 that included 3,999 men and 4,726 women. It found a lifetime risk for the development of AF in patients over the age of 40 to be 26% for men and 23% for women. Excluding patients with CHF and prior MI, the lifetime risk for AF was approximately 16%.

3. **Benjamin EJ**. Impact of atrial fibrillation on the risk of death: the Framingham Heart Study. *Circulation* 1998;98(10):946–952.

A population-based study done in Framingham, MA. After 40 years of follow-up, AF was associated with an OR for death of 1.5 (95% CI, 1.2 to 1.8) in men and 1.9 (95% CI, 1.5 to 2.2) in women after adjusting for age, hypertension, smoking, diabetes, LV hypertrophy, MI, CHF, valvular heart disease, and stroke. AF was also noted to diminish the female advantage in survival.

4. **Go AS**. Prevalence of diagnosed atrial fibrillation in adults: national implications for rhythm management and stroke prevention: the AnTicoagulation and Risk Factors in Atrial Fibrillation (ATRIA) Study. *JAMA* 2001;285(18):2370–2375.

A large cross-sectional study of adults aged 20 and older in an HMO population. The prevalence of AF was noted to be 0.95% (1.1% in men vs. 0.8% in women). In prevalence rate increased with age from 0.1% in adults less than 55 years of age to 9% in adults over the age of 80. Given this prevalence, they estimated that approximately 2.3 million US adults currently have AF, which is projected to increase 2.5-fold to more than 5.6 million by the year 2050, with more than 50% of affected individuals aged 80 years or older.

5. **Kopecky SL**, et al. The natural history of lone atrial fibrillation. *N Engl J Med* 1987;317: 669–674.

In this population-based study of Olmstead County, MN, residents between 1950 and 1980, 3,623 persons were found to have AF, of whom 97 (2.7%) were younger than 60 years (mean age, 44 years at diagnosis) and had no overt cardiovascular disease or precipitating illness. Among these lone AF patients, 21% had an isolated episode, 58% had recurrent AF, and 22% had chronic AF. At 15-year follow-up, only 1.3% of patients had had a stroke on a cumulative actuarial basis, and no difference was found in survival or stroke-free survival among patients with the three types of lone AF. Based on these findings, the authors suggest that routine anticoagulation may not be indicated in individuals with lone AF.

6. **Atrial Fibrillation Investigators.** Risk factors for stroke and efficacy of antithrombotic therapy in atrial fibrillation: an analysis of pooled data from 5 randomized controlled trials (AFASAK, SPAF, BAATAF, SPINAF, CAFA). *Arch Intern Med* 1994;154:1449–1457.

Pooled data from these five trials showed that warfarin use was associated with a 68% reduction in stroke risk (to 1.4% per year) and 33% lower all-cause mortality. This significant benefit of warfarin also was present in patients with paroxysmal/intermittent AF [1.7% per year (warfarin) vs. 5.7% per year (placebo)]. Risk factors for thromboembolism were history of hypertension, prior stroke or TIA, diabetes, and age older than 65 years. A nonsignificant increase was seen in the frequency of major bleeding. Two of these five trials randomized patients to an aspirin group; the pooled risk reduction versus placebo was 36%.

7. **Benjamin EJ,** et al. Left atrial size and the risk of stroke and death: the Framingham Heart Study. *Circulation* 1995;92:835–841.

   This analysis focused on 3,099 patients aged 50 years or older. For each 1-cm increase in LA size, the relative risk of stroke was 2.4 in men and 1.4 in women, and for death, 1.3 and 1.4 in men and women, respectively.

8. **Wood KA,** et al. Risk of thromboembolism in chronic atrial flutter. *Am J Cardiol* 1997;79:1043–1047.

   Retrospective analysis of 86 patients referred for RF ablation. The annual risk of embolic events was 3% (1.6% after exclusion of patients with TIA and pulmonary embolism). In a logistic regression model, no significant independent predictors of increased thromboembolic risk were found.

9. **Benjamin EJ,** et al. Impact of atrial fibrillation on the risk of death. *Circulation* 1998;98: 946–952.

   Of 5,209 Framingham Study participants, in 296 men and 325 women, AF developed during 40 years of follow-up. AF patients were more likely (at baseline) to smoke and have hypertension, LV hypertrophy on ECG, history of MI, CHF, valvular disease, and stroke or TIA. AF was associated with an adjusted OR for death of 1.5 (95% CI, 1.2 to 1.8) in men and 1.9 (95% CI, 1.5 to 2.2) in women. The presence of AF increased the risk of dying at all ages. Most of the excess mortality was seen in the first 30 days after AF developed.

10. **Seidl K,** et al. Risk of thromboembolic events in patients with atrial flutter. *Am J Cardiol* 1998;82:580–583.

    This retrospective analysis focused on 191 consecutive patients with atrial flutter. At an average follow-up of 26 months, embolic events had occurred in 11 (7%) patients. Acute (<48 hours) embolism occurred in four patients (three after DC cardioversion, one after catheter ablation). In multivariate analysis, the only independent predictor of embolic events was hypertension (OR, 6.5; 95% CI, 1.5 to 45).

RATE VERSUS RHYTHM CONTROL

11. **Wyse G,** for the Atrial Fibrillation Follow-up Investigation of Rhythm Management **(AFFIRM)** Investigators. A comparison of rate control and rhythm control in patients with atrial fibrillation. *N Engl J Med* 2002;347:1825–1833.

    This prospective, randomized, multicenter study enrolled 4,060 patients with AF more than 6 hours but less than 6 months in duration. Eligible patients were aged 65 years or older or had one or more risk factors for stroke, could not have failed cardioversion, and had to be willing to accept randomization to rate versus rhythm control. Patients were randomized to rhythm control with electrical cardioversion and antiarrhythmic drugs (initially 39% amiodarone, 33% sotalol, and 15% IC agents) or to rate control with standard agents. Amiodarone was ultimately given to 60% of patients. Warfarin was continued indefinitely in the rate-control arm but could be discontinued at the local physicians' discretion in the rhythm-control arm if SR was maintained for 1 month. At follow-up (average, 3.5 years), no significant differences were found between the two groups in all-cause mortality (primary endpoint) and other major secondary endpoints including stroke [7.3% (rhythm control) vs. 5.7%; *p* = NS].

12. **Van Gelder IC,** et al. A comparison of rate control and rhythm control in patients with recurrent persistent atrial fibrillation (**RACE**). *N Engl J Med* 2002;347:1834–1840.

    This smaller trial had a general structure similar to that of the AFFIRM, enrolling 256 patients in the rate-control group and 266 patients in the rhythm-control group. Discontinuation of warfarin after a period of SR was mandated by the study for the rhythm-control group. At 3 years, no statistically significant difference was seen between the groups in the primary composite endpoint of cardiovascular death, HF hospitalization, embolic events, severe bleeding, pacemaker implantation, or severe drug side effects [17.2% (rate control) vs. 22.0%]. Trends toward more embolic events, HF, and adverse drug events were seen in the rhythm-control arm. Event rates were higher in hypertensive patients.

13. **Corley SD,** et al. AFFIRM Investigators. Relationships between sinus rhythm, treatment, and survival in the Atrial Fibrillation Follow-up Investigation of Rhythm Management (AFFIRM) Study. *Circulation* 2004;109:1509–1513.

An "on-treatment" reanalysis of the AFFIRM study looking at the relationship to survival of cardiac rhythm status and antiarrhythmic drug use independently of each other. In this analysis both the presence of NSR and warfarin use were associated with a lower risk of death. After adjusting for NSR, antiarrhythmic drug use was associated with increased mortality. They concluded that NSR was either a determinate of survival or a marker of an unknown factor that was associated with survival. Increased mortality associated with antiarrhythmic drugs was likely negated by the survival benefit of NSR resulting in the similar mortality rate with rate control seen in the original AFFIRM analysis.

14. **Pederson OD,** et al. Efficacy of dofetilide in the treatment of atrial fibrillation–flutter in patients with reduced left ventricular function. A Danish Investigations of Arrhythmia and Mortality ON Dofetilide (DIAMOND) Substudy. *Circulation* 2001;104:292–296.

The subgroup analysis of the two DIAMOND studies (DIAMOND CHF, DIAMOND MI) that looked at the effect of NSR and dofetilide on the mortality and hospitalization rate of patients with AF and atrial flutter. Dofetilide was shown to be more effective than placebo at the maintenance of NSR (79% vs. 42%; $p < 0.001$), but dofetilide had no effect on all-cause mortality. When pooling patients from both treatment groups who achieved NSR and comparing them to those that did not, NSR was associated with a significantly lower mortality (see Ref. 46 for more details on the DIAMOND trial).

15. **Roy D,** et al. for the Atrial Fibrillation and Congestive Heart Failure (**AF-CHF**) Investigators. Rhythm control versus rate control for atrial fibrillation and heart failure. *N Engl J Med* 2008;358:2667–2677.

Design: Randomized, international, multicenter trial; the primary endpoint was time to cardiovascular death over mean follow-up of 37 months.
Purpose: To compare the strategy of rate control to that of rhythm control in patients with AF and concomitant CHF.
Population: 1,376 patients with AF and symptomatic CHF with EF ≤35%.
Treatment: Aggressive rhythm control with electrical cardioversion (repeat, if needed) if pharmacologic cardioversion failed, compared with pharmacologic rate control predominantly with beta-blockers and digitalis.
Results: Cardiovascular mortality was similar between the two groups at 37 months (27% of rhythm-control group vs. 25% in rate-control group; $p = 0.59$). Notably, secondary outcomes including worsening heart failure were similar between the two groups and subgroup analyses did not reveal any preferential effects.

ANTIARRHYTHMIC DRUG TRIALS FOR ATRIAL FIBRILLATION

16. **Farshi R,** et al. Ventricular rate control in chronic atrial fibrillation during daily activity and programmed exercise: a crossover open-label study of five drug regimens. *J Am Coll Cardiol* 1999;33:304–310.

The investigators compared five pharmacologic therapies for exercise-induced rapid ventricular rates in 12 patients with chronic AF. These included oral digoxin, diltiazem, atenolol, digoxin plus diltiazem, or digoxin plus atenolol; primary endpoint was variability in 24-hour ventricular rate monitoring. When compared to diltiazem alone and atenolol alone, the ventricular rate with the digoxin plus atenolol combination was significantly lower and proved to be the most effective therapy at suppressing diurnal fluctuations in rate.

17. **Ahuja RC,** et al. Digoxin or verapamil or metoprolol for heart rate control in patients with mitral stenosis—a randomised cross-over study. *Int J Cardiol* 1989;25:325–331.

An open-label, randomized, crossover study comparing digoxin (0.25 to 0.5 mg daily), metoprolol (50 to 100 mg twice daily), and verapamil (40 to 80 mg three times daily). In the AF arm (10 patients), 80% of patients on verapamil, 40% on metoprolol, and 30% on digoxin reported a >50% subjective improvement in heart rate control. When treadmill testing was performed, the total work done by the patients was 555 ± 232 kpm (no medications), $1,379 \pm 553$ kpm on verapamil, $1,251 \pm 575$ kpm on metoprolol, and 716 ± 340 kpm on digoxin.

18. **Lawson-Matthew PJ,** et al. Xamoterol improves the control of chronic atrial fibrillation in elderly patients. *Age Ageing* 1995;24:321–325.

A double-blind, crossover study comparing xamoterol (200 mg twice daily) plus placebo or digoxin. When xamoterol or digoxin were used alone, there was no difference in the daytime maximal heart rate (132 beats/min with xamoterol vs. 122 beat/min with digoxin; $p > 0.05$), while the nocturnal minimum heart rate was significantly higher with xamoterol (85 bpm compared to 62 beats/min; $p < 0.0001$). When xamoterol was combined with digoxin, the nocturnal minimum heart rate was significantly raised (68 beats/min; $p < 0.05$), and the daytime maximal heart rate was lowered (115 beats/min; $p < 0.05$). There were fewer pauses of >1.5 seconds with xamoterol alone.

19. **Wong CK,** et al. Usefulness of labetalol in chronic atrial fibrillation. *Am J Cardiol* 1990;66:1212–1215.

A randomized, crossover trial comparing labetalol to digoxin, digoxin plus labetalol, and placebo. There was no difference in the exercise tolerance between any groups. Digoxin showed no decrease in the maximal exercise heart rate compared to placebo (177 beats/min digoxin vs. 175 beats/min placebo; $p > 0.05$). Labetalol either with or without digoxin was shown to be more effective than placebo at reducing maximal exercise heart rate (156 beats/min labetalol alone, 154 beats/min labetalol plus digoxin, 177 beats/min placebo; $p < 0.01$).

20. **Botto GL,** et al. Modulation of ventricular rate in permanent atrial fibrillation: randomized, crossover study of the effects of slow-release formulations of gallopamil, diltiazem, or verapamil. *Clin Cardiol* 1998;21:837–840.

A randomized, crossover trial comparing gallopamil (100 mg twice daily), diltiazem (120 mg twice daily), and verapamil (120 mg twice daily) and digoxin alone. On digoxin, the peak exercise heart rate was 167 beats/min, which was significantly reduced to 149 beats/min with gallopamil ($p = 0.01$), 142 beats/min with diltiazem ($p < 0.001$), and 137 beats/min with verapamil ($p < 0.001$). There was no statistical difference between calcium-channel blockers.

21. **Hilleman DE,** et al. Conversion of recent-onset atrial fibrillation with intravenous amiodarone: a meta-analysis of randomized controlled trials. *Pharmacotherapy* 2002;22:66–74.

A meta-analysis of 18 randomized controlled trials looking at a total of 550 patients receiving IV amiodarone, 451 patients receiving other antiarrhythmic therapy, and 202 patients receiving placebo. The pooled unadjusted rate of conversion to NSR was 76% for IV amiodarone, 72% for other antiarrhythmics, and 60% for placebo. When looking just at the placebo-controlled trials, the conversion rates were 82.4% for IV amiodarone compared to 59.7% placebo ($p = 0.003$). There was no difference between IV amiodarone and the other antiarrhythmics in the antiarrhythmic controlled trials (72.1% vs. 71.9%; $p = 0.84$). Safety was similar in amiodarone and the other antiarrhythmics with 17% versus 14% adverse events including infusion phlebitis, bradycardia, and hypotension.

22. **Chevalier P,** et al. Amiodarone versus placebo and classic drugs for cardioversion of recent-onset atrial fibrillation: a meta-analysis. *J Am Coll Cardiol* 2003;41:255–262.

A meta-analysis of six studies with 595 patients comparing amiodarone to placebo and seven studies with 579 patients comparing amiodarone to class Ic antiarrhythmics. Statistical significance comparing amiodarone to placebo was not reached until 6 to 8 hours after infusion (RR, 1.23; $p = 0.022$) and continued through 24 hours (RR, 1.44; $p < 0.001$). Amiodarone was inferior to class Ic antiarrhythmics up to 8 hours postinfusion (RR, 0.67; $p < 0.00$) but no difference was seen after 24 hours (RR, 0.95, 0.50).

23. **Letelier LM,** et al. Effectiveness of amiodarone for conversion of atrial fibrillation to sinus rhythm: a meta-analysis. *Arch Intern Med* 2003;163:777–785.

A meta-analysis of 21 studies that compared amiodarone to placebo, digoxin, or calcium-channel blockers for the conversion of AF to SR. The relative risk for achieving SR with amiodarone compared to placebo digoxin or calcium-channel blocker was 1.4 in AF of <48 hours in duration (95% confidence interval of 1.25 to 1.57) compared to 4.33 in AF of >48 hours in duration (95% confidence interval of 2.76 to 6.77).

24. **Doyle JF,** et al. Benefits and risks of long-term amiodarone therapy for persistent atrial fibrillation: a meta-analysis. *Mayo Clin Proc* 2009;84:234–242.

A meta-analysis of 12 randomized controlled trials that involved 5,060 patients with persistent AF comparing amiodarone to either placebo or another rate-control drug. The rate of conversion was higher in amiodarone compared to placebo or rate-control drug (RR, 3.2; 95% CI, 1.9 to 5.5). No defense was seen in long-term mortality (RR, 0.95; 95% confidence interval, 0.8 to 1.1; $p = 0.51$). Discontinuation of therapy due to adverse effects was more common with amiodarone (RR, 3.0; 95% confidence interval, 1.4 to 6.2).

25. **Singh BN,** et al. for the Sotalol Amiodarone Atrial Fibrillation Efficacy Trial (SAFE-T) Investigators. Amiodarone versus sotalol for atrial fibrillation. *N Engl J Med* 2005;352: 1861–1872.

A double-blind, placebo-controlled trial of 665 patients with persistent AF comparing amiodarone, sotalol, and placebo. Patients were given oral preparations and were then followed for conversion to NSR. If no conversion was achieved by 28 days, the patients then underwent electrical cardioversion. The primary endpoint was time to recurrence of AF. Pharmacologic cardioversion in the first 28 days occurred in 27.1% of patients on amiodarone, 24.2% on sotalol, and 0.8% on placebo ($p = 0.45$ amiodarone vs. sotalol, $p < 0.001$ placebo vs. either sotalol or amiodarone). There was no statistical difference in the rate of conversion with electrical cardioversion for those who failed pharmacologic cardioversion at 28 days (72.3% on amiodarone, 73.5% on sotalol, and 67.9% on placebo; $p = 0.54$). The median time to recurrence of AF was 487 days with amiodarone, 74 days with sotalol, and 6 days with placebo in the intention-to-treat analysis, showing amiodarone to be superior to both sotalol and placebo ($p < 0.001$) and sotalol to be superior to placebo ($p < 0.001$). In a subgroup analysis looking at ischemic heart disease, there was no difference between sotalol or amiodarone and maintenance of NSR (median time to recurrence 428 days with sotalol, 569 days with amiodarone; $p = 0.53$).

26. **Kafkas NV,** et al. Conversion efficacy of intravenous ibutilide compared with intravenous amiodarone in patients with recent-onset atrial fibrillation and atrial flutter. *Int J Cardiol* 2007;118(3):321–325.

A prospective, randomized, controlled trial comparing IV ibutilide and amiodarone in 152 patients with AF and atrial flutter of 3 to 48 hours in duration. The rate of conversion for AF was not statistically different for ibutilide compared to amiodarone (77% vs. 69%; $p =$ NS). When looking at atrial flutter, ibutilide was more effective than amiodarone at cardioversion (87% vs. 29%; $p = 0.003$).

27. **Singh BN,** et al. Dronedarone for maintenance of sinus rhythm in atrial fibrillation or flutter. *N Engl J Med* 2007;357(10):987–999.

   A report of two double-blind, randomized, controlled trials enrolling 1,237 patients with paroxysmal AF to compare dronedarone (400 mg twice daily) to placebo in the maintenance of normal SR. In both trials the mean time to recurrence was shorter in the dronedarone arm than the placebo arm (41 and 39 days with dronedarone vs. 96 and 158 days with placebo; p 0.01 and 0.002 for dronedarone vs. placebo). There was no significant difference in the rate of pulmonary, thyroid, or liver toxicities between dronedarone and placebo.

28. **Hohnloser SH,** et al. Effect of dronedarone on cardiovascular events in atrial fibrillation. *N Engl J Med* 2009;360(7):668–678.

   The **ATHENA** trial. A double-blinded, randomized, controlled trial of 4,628 patients with paroxysmal or persistent AF/atrial flutter comparing dronedarone (400 g twice daily) to placebo. Dronedarone was associated with a reduced risk of both the primary combined endpoint of death or cardiovascular hospitalization compared to placebo (31.9% dronedarone vs. 39.4 placebo; $p < 0.001$) and the secondary endpoint of cardiovascular death alone (2.7% dronedarone vs. 3.9% placebo; $p = 0.03$). The principal side effects were gastrointestinal disturbances, bradycardia, QT prolongation, and serum creatinine increase.

29. **Kober L,** et al. Increased mortality after dronedarone therapy for severe heart failure. *N Engl J Med* 2008;358(25):2678–2687.

   The **ANDROMEDA** trial. A double-blind, randomized, placebo-controlled trial of 627 patients with severe LV systolic dysfunction (NYHA class III or IV) comparing dronedarone (400 mg twice daily) to placebo. The trial was stopped early due to safety reasons due to an increased risk of death in the dronedarone group (8.1% dronedarone vs. 3.8% placebo; $p = 0.03$). The deaths were principally due to worsening heart failure and not proarrhythmia.

30. **Le Heuzey, J.-Y., De Ferrari, G.M. Radzik D, Santini M, Zhu J, Davy J-M, A Short-Term, Randomized, Double-Blind, Parallel-Group Study to Evaluate the Efficacy and Safety of Dronedarone versus Amiodarone in Patients with Persistent Atrial Fibrillation: The DIONYSOS Study.** *J Cardiovasc Electrophysiol, 2010;21. 597–605.*

   DIONYSOS trial compared amiodarone 600 mg daily to dronedarone 400 mg wtice a day in the maintenance of normal SR postelectrical cardioversion done in 504 patients with persistent AF. There was a lower rate of AF recurrence in the amiodarone arm compared to the dronedarone arm (24.3% amiodarone vs. 36.5% dronedarone; $p < 0.001$). There were less thyroid toxicities, bradycardia, and premature study drug discontinuation in the dronedarone arm, but there were also more frequent gastrointestinal side effects in patients taking dronedarone.

31. **Stambler BS,** et al. Antiarrhythmic actions of intravenous ibutilide compared with procainamide during human atrial flutter and fibrillation: electrophysiological determinants of enhanced conversion efficacy. *Circulation* 1997;96:4298–4306.

   A randomized, partially blinded (ibutilide arm only), placebo-controlled study looking at ibutilide compared to procainamide in AF and atrial flutter. Ibutilide appeared to be more effective at cardioversion of AF than procainamide (32% vs. 5%; p value not stated) or placebo (0%). With atrial flutter, cardioversion occurred in 64% of patients on ibutilide, compared to 0% on procainamide or placebo (p value not stated). The difference in conversion rates between AF and atrial flutter with ibutilide did reach statistical significance at 32% versus 64% ($p < 0.05$).

32. **Fragakis N,** et al. Acute beta-adrenoceptor blockade improves efficacy of ibutilide in conversion of atrial fibrillation with a rapid ventricular rate. *Europace* 2009;11:70–74.

   An open-label, randomized, controlled trial in 90 patients comparing ibutilide alone to ibutilide plus esmolol infusion in the conversion of AF. When esmolol was combined with ibutilide, 67% converted to normal SR compared to 46% of patients given ibutilide alone (p 0.04).

It was also noted that the slower the heart rate was at the time of ibutilide administration, the higher the likelihood of cardioversion ($p = 0.015$). The addition of esmolol had the added effect of shortening the QTc (433 msec with esmolol, 501 msec without; $p = 0.003$). This may have attributed to the lower rates of proarrhythmia when comparing the esmolol infusion group (0%) to the ibutilide-alone group (6.5%, one case of sustained polymorphic VT, three of NSVT). Though there were no VT episodes in the esmolol group, there were two cases of severe bradycardia in that group.

33. **Caron MF,** et al. The effects of intravenous magnesium sulfate on the QT interval in patients receiving ibutilide. *Pharmacotherapy* 2003;23:296–300.

A double-blinded, randomized, placebo-controlled trial comparing adjunctive IV magnesium to placebo in 20 patients with AF and atrial flutter undergoing chemical cardioversion with ibutilide. A total of 4 g of magnesium sulfate was given to the patients in this study (2 g prior to ibutilide and 2 g after). In the placebo group, the QTc increased 18% from baseline 30 minutes after the administration of ibutilide (p 0.007) compared to 4.4% with magnesium (not statistically significant difference from baseline) (no magnesium vs. magnesium, $p = 0.04$). No torsades de pointes occurred in either group.

34. **Kochiadakis GE,** et al. Conversion of atrial fibrillation to sinus rhythm using acute intravenous procainamide infusion. *Cardiovasc Drugs Ther* 1998;12(1):75–81.

A double-blind, placebo-controlled trial in 114 patients with AF comparing IV procainamide plus digoxin to placebo plus digoxin. Conversion to normal SR within 1 hour of drug infusion occurred in 50.9% of patients receiving procainamide compared to 28.1% of patients receiving placebo (p 0.012). When stratifying by length of AF, the conversion rate in patients with AF of <48 hours in duration increased to 69% of patients on procainamide and 38.1% of patients on placebo (p 0.004). No patients with AF of >48 hours in duration converted to normal SR in either group. It was also noted that the rate of conversion was inversely proportional to LA size.

35. **Kochiadakis GE,** et al. A comparative study of the efficacy and safety of procainamide versus propafenone versus amiodarone for the conversion of recent-onset atrial fibrillation. *Am J Cardiol* 2007;99(12):1721–1725.

A single-blinded, placebo-controlled study in 362 patients with recent-onset AF comparing procainamide, propafenone, amiodarone, and placebo. Success was any conversion to normal SR within 24 hours of drug administration. The rates of conversion were 68.53% of patients on procainamide, 80.21% on propafenone, 89.13% on amiodarone, and 61.11% on placebo, with all medication groups being more effective than placebo ($p < 0.05$). Amiodarone and propafenone were also more effective than procainamide ($p < 0.05$). The time to cardioversion was faster for procainamide (median time 3 hours) and propafenone (medical time 1 hour) than amiodarone (median time 9 hours) or placebo (median time 17 hours) (log-rank $p < 0.001$).

36. **Alp NJ,** et al. Randomised double blind trial of oral versus intravenous flecainide for the cardioversion of acute atrial fibrillation. *Heart* 2000;84:37–40.

A randomized, double-blind, placebo-controlled trial of 79 patients comparing IV flecainide to liquid oral flecainide. There was no difference between the conversion rate of oral and IV flecainide. Two hours after drug administration, 64% of patients on IV flecainide and 68% of patients on oral flecainide converted to normal SR (p 0.74). This improved to 72% and 75%, respectively, at 8 hours (p 0.76). There was a difference in the mean time to cardioversion, with IV flecainide achieving cardioversion at a mean of 52 minutes postadministration compared to a mean of 110 minutes with oral flecainide (p 0.002).

37. **Reisinger J,** et al. Flecainide versus ibutilide for immediate cardioversion of atrial fibrillation of recent onset. *Eur Heart J* 2004;25(15):1318–1324.

A single-blinded, randomized, controlled trial compared IV flecainide to IV ibutilide in 207 patients with recent-onset AF (<48 hours). Success was any cardiovascular (CV) within 90 minutes of drug infusion. There was no difference between the conversion rate of IV flecainide (56.4%) and IV ibutilide (50.0%) (p 0.34).

38. **Zhang N,** et al. Comparison of intravenous ibutilide vs. propafenone for rapid termination of recent onset atrial fibrillation. *Int J Clin Pract* 2005;59(12):1395–1400.

A single-blinded, randomized, controlled trial of 82 patients with AF comparing IV ibutilide and IV propafenone. Success was any cardioversion within 90 minutes of drug infusion. Ibutilide was more effective at cardioversion than propafenone (70.73% with ibutilide vs. 48.78% with propafenone; $p = 0.043$).

39. **Alboni P,** et al. Outpatient treatment of recent-onset atrial fibrillation with the "pill-in-the-pocket" approach. *N Engl J Med* 2004;351:2384–2391.

In an effort to study the feasibility of outpatient self-administration of flecainide or propafenone for paroxysmal AF, the investigators enrolled 210 patients with recent, successful pharmacologic cardioversion with either agent (patients with adverse effects were excluded). They were given oral versions of either drug, to be self-administered with the onset of symptoms; in all, 165 patients had 618 episodes of arrhythmia over mean follow-up of 15 months. Attempted treatment of 569 episodes was successful in 534 (94%), with symptom resolution at mean 113 minutes. Health facility utilization (emergency room visits and hospitalizations) was significantly lower during the study period than the year prior to enrollment ($p < 0.001$ for both measures).

40. **Khan IA.** Single oral loading dose of propafenone for pharmacological cardioversion of recent-onset atrial fibrillation. *J Am Coll Cardiol* 2001;37(2):542–547.

A meta-analysis of 11 studies looking at a single oral loading dose of propafenone 600 mg for the conversion of AF. The published success rates ranged from 56% to 83% and depended on the duration of AF. The single oral loading dose regimen was significantly more effective than placebo only in the first 8 hours. After 24 hours it was no different than placebo. The conversion time varied from 110 to 287 minutes. Comparing IV to oral formulations, the IV form was more effective only in the first 2 hours, but after that both forms had equal effectiveness. Adverse effects were transient arrhythmia, transient QRS widening, and hypotension. The transient arrhythmias were principally at the time of conversion, and included bradycardia, atrial flutter, and junctional rhythms.

41. **Capucci A,** et al. Safety of oral propafenone in the conversion of recent onset atrial fibrillation to sinus rhythm: a prospective parallel placebo-controlled multicentre study. *Int J Cardiol* 1999;68:187–196.

A randomized placebo control trial in 246 patients with recent-onset AF (<48 hours) comparing oral quinidine (1,100 mg) plus digoxin (0.75 to 1 mg IV), oral propafenone (450 to 600 mg), oral propafenone (450 to 600 mg) plus digoxin (0.75 to 1 mg IV), and placebo. At 3 hours both propafenone groups (with and without digoxin) were more effective than quinidine plus digoxin and placebo ($p < 0.05$), but by 24 hours there was no statistical difference between treatment groups or placebo. The mean time to conversion was 4.0 ± 4.1 hours for the propafenone group, 5.0 ± 8.6 hours for propafenone plus digoxin, 5.4 ± 4.5 hours for quinidine plus digoxin, and 7.8 ± 7.2 hours for the placebo ($p < 0.01$ propafenone vs. placebo).

42. **Coplen SE,** et al. Efficacy and safety of quinidine therapy for maintenance of sinus rhythm after cardioversion: a meta-analysis of randomized controlled trials. *Circulation* 1990;82:1106–1116.

This analysis focused on six trials with 808 patients. Quinidine use was associated with less AF recurrence. At 3, 6, and 12 months, 69%, 58%, and 50% of quinidine-treated patients were in normal SR versus 45%, 33%, and 25% of controls. Despite the lower recurrence rates, the quinidine group had a higher all-cause mortality rate (2.9% vs. 0.8%; $p < 0.05$).

43. **Gosselink TM,** et al. Low-dose amiodarone for maintenance of sinus rhythm after cardioversion of atrial fibrillation or flutter. *JAMA* 1992;267:3289–3293.

This study was composed of 89 AF patients for whom previous therapy failed. A loading dose of amiodarone (600 mg over a 4-week period) was followed by an average daily dose of 204 mg. Fifteen (16%) patients converted to normal SR during loading; 90% were in SR after cardioversion, and 53% remained in normal SR at 3-year follow-up. No proarrhythmia was documented.

44. **Stambler BS,** et al. Efficacy and safety for repeated intravenous doses of ibutilide for rapid conversion of atrial flutter of fibrillation. *Circulation* 1996;94:1613–1621.

This randomized trial was composed of 266 patients with sustained (3 hours to 45 days) AF or flutter. Patients received one or two 10-minute infusions of ibutilide, separated by 10 minutes (1.0 mg plus 0.5 mg or 1 mg plus 1 mg) or placebo. Ibutilide converted 47% of patients overall (vs. 2% with placebo), with better success in atrial flutter than in AF (63% vs. 31%). The average time to termination was 27 minutes. No significant differences were seen between dosing regimens. Polymorphic VT occurred in 8.3%, but was sustained in 1.7%.

45. **Torp-Pedersen C,** et al. for the Danish Investigations of Arrhythmia and Mortality on Dofetilide **(DIAMOND-CHF)** Study Group. Dofetilide in patients with congestive heart failure and left ventricular dysfunction. *N Engl J Med* 1999;341:857–865.

Design: Multicenter, randomized, double-blinded, placebo-controlled trial. Primary endpoint was death from any cause at median follow-up of 18 months.
Purpose: To assess the safety of dofetilide, a novel antiarrhythmic, in patients with CHF, with severe LV dysfunction.
Population: 1,518 patients with symptomatic CHF and severe LV dysfunction.
Treatment: Dofetilide (500 μg for patients in AF, 250 μg for those in SR; doses were subsequently based on renal function) or placebo.
Results: As an assessment of safety, the primary endpoint of all-cause mortality was not different in the two groups (41% for dofetilide vs. 42% for placebo). Yet, there was a higher incidence of torsades de pointes in the dofetilide group (3.3% vs. 0%). However, patients in the dofetilide group were less likely to be hospitalized for worsening heart failure; for those in AF, they were more likely to be converted to SR (12% vs. 1%), and for those in the dofetilide group they were more likely to stay in SR.

46. **Kober L,** et al. for the Danish Investigations of Arrhythmia and Mortality on Dofetilide **(DIAMOND-MI)** Study Group. Effect of dofetilide in patients with recent myocardial infarction and left-ventricular dysfunction: a randomised trial. *Lancet* 2000;356:2052–2058.

Design: Multicenter, randomized, double-blinded, placebo-controlled trial. Primary endpoint was all-cause mortality, with secondary endpoints of cardiac and arrhythmic death.
Purpose: To assess the safety of dofetilide in patients with recent MI and severe LV dysfunction.
Population: 1,510 patients with severe LV dysfunction and recent MI within 7 days; at baseline 8% of patients had AF or atrial flutter.
Treatment: Dofetilide or placebo.
Results: There was no significant difference in outcomes between the two groups—all-cause mortality (31% for dofetilide vs. 32% for placebo), cardiac mortality (26% vs. 28%), and arrhythmic mortality (17% vs. 18%) were all similar. Patients in the dofetilide group with AF or flutter were more likely to convert to SR (42% vs. 13%; $p = 0.002$); however, all seven cases of torsades de pointes were in the dofetilide group.

47. **Singh S,** et al. Efficacy and safety of oral dofetilide in converting to and maintaining sinus rhythm in patients with chronic atrial fibrillation or atrial flutter: the symptomatic atrial

fibrillation investigative research on dofetilide (**SAFIRE-D**) study. *Circulation* 2000;102: 2385–2390.

A double-blind, placebo-controlled trial of 325 patients with AF and atrial flutter comparing dofetilide (125, 250, or 500 μg) to placebo. Conversion rates for dofetilide were 6.1% with 125 μg, 9.8% with 250 μg, and 29.9% with 500 μg compared to 1.2% with placebo [dofetilide vs. placebo was significant at 250 μg ($p = 0.015$) and 500 μg ($p < 0.001$)]. For those who were successfully cardioverted, the probability of remaining in normal SR at 1 year was 0.4 at 125 μg, 0.37 at 250 μg, and 0.58 at 500 μg compared to 0.25 with placebo (500 μg vs. placebo was significant at $p = 0.001$). Two patients (0.8%) on dofetilide experienced an episode of torsades de pointes between days 1 and 2 of treatment, and one patient (0.4%) experienced SCD on day 8.

48. The Digitalis in Acute Atrial Fibrillation (**DAAF**) Trial Group. Intravenous digoxin in acute atrial fibrillation. Results of a randomized, placebo-controlled multicentre trial in 239 patients. *Eur Heart J* 1997;18:649–654.

A double-blind, randomized, placebo-controlled trial of 239 patients with recent-onset AF (<7 days) comparing IV digoxin (variable weight-based dosing given at 3 to 4 time points) and placebo. At 16 hours, 51% of patients on digoxin and 46% of patients on placebo were converted to normal SR ($p = $ NS). Digoxin was associated with a lower heart rate at 2 hours compared to placebo (104.6 +/−20.9 beats per minute compared to 116.8 ± 22.5 beats per minute; $p = 0.0001$).

49. **Roy D,** et al. for the Canadian Trial of Atrial Fibrillation (**CTAF**) Investigators. Amiodarone to prevent recurrence of atrial fibrillation. *N Engl J Med* 2000;342:913–920.

Design: Prospective, randomized, multicenter trial. Mean follow-up of 16 months.
Purpose: To evaluate the efficacy of amiodarone in preventing recurrent AF.
Population: 403 patients with symptomatic AF.
Treatment: Amiodarone, sotalol, or propafenone (average daily doses at 1 year were 194, 231, and 554 mg, respectively).
Results: Only 35% of amiodarone patients had a documented recurrence of AF compared with 63% taking the other antiarrhythmics. Discontinuation of study drug due to adverse effects occurred in 18% of amiodarone patients and 11% of sotalol/propafenone patients ($p = 0.06$).

50. **Benditt DG,** et al. Maintenance of sinus rhythm with oral D,L-sotalol therapy in patients with symptomatic atrial fibrillation and/or atrial flutter. D,L-Sotalol Atrial Fibrillation/Flutter Study Group. *Am J Cardiol* 1999;84:270–277.

A double-blind, randomized, placebo-controlled trial of 253 patients with AF or atrial flutter comparing the SR maintenance efficacy of sotalol (at 80, 120, or 160 mg twice daily) to placebo. All patients were in SR at the initiation of treatment and they were followed for 12 months. The median time to recurrence on placebo was 27 days. With sotalol it was 106 days at 80 mg ($p = 0.066$ vs. placebo), 229 days at 120 mg (p 0.004 vs. placebo), and 175 days at 160 mg ($p = 0.102$). The 160-mg dose was associated with more side effects and dropouts. No cases of torsades de pointes, sustained VT, or VF were reported.

51. **de Paola AA,** et al. Efficacy and safety of sotalol versus quinidine for the maintenance of sinus rhythm after conversion of atrial fibrillation. **SOCESP** Investigators. *Am J Cardiol* 1999;84:1033–1037.

A randomized controlled trial of 121 patients postcardioversion for AF (<6 months) comparing sotalol (160 to 320 mg/day) and quinidine (600 to 800 mg/day). At 6 months, 74% of patients on sotalol and 68% on quinidine were still in normal SR ($p = $ NS). For those who had recurrences, the mean time to occurrence was longer in the sotalol group than with the quinidine group (69 days vs. 10 days; $p < 0.05$) and the average heart rate was lower in the sotalol group ($p < 0.05$). Interestingly, sotalol was more effective than quinidine for patients who had been in AF <72 hours prior to cardioversion (93% with sotalol vs. 64% with quinidine;

$p = 0.01$) while patients in AF >72 hours prior to cardioversion had better success on quinidine (68% on quinidine vs. 33% on sotalol; $p < 0.05$). 5% of patients in the sotalol group and 2% in the quinidine group experienced proarrhythmic events.

52. **Bellandi F,** et al. Long-term efficacy and safety of propafenone and sotalol for the maintenance of sinus rhythm after conversion of recurrent symptomatic atrial fibrillation. *Am J Cardiol* 2001;88(6):640–645.

A double-blind, placebo-controlled trial in 300 patients with AF comparing propafenone, sotalol, and placebo at the maintenance of normal SR postcardioversion. At 1-year postcardioversion, 63% of patients on propafenone and 73% on sotalol were in normal SR compared to 35% on placebo (placebo vs. either drug; $p = 0.001$). The dropout due to side effects was equal in the propafenone and sotalol groups (9% and 10%, respectively). The likelihood of remaining in SR was higher for younger patients with smaller LA size and without heart disease.

53. **Kochiadakis GE,** et al. Amiodarone, sotalol, or propafenone in atrial fibrillation: which is preferred to maintain normal sinus rhythm? *Pacing Clin Electrophysiol* 2000;23: 1883–1887.

An open-label, randomized, controlled trial of 214 patients with AF comparing amiodarone (200 mg daily), propafenone (450 mg daily), and sotalol (320 mg daily) in the maintenance of normal SR. In this study, 77% of patients on amiodarone, 32% on sotalol, and 62.5% on propafenone were in normal SR at 36 months ($p < 0.01$ for both amiodarone and propafenone vs. sotalol).

54. **Kochiadakis GE,** et al. Sotalol versus propafenone for long-term maintenance of normal sinus rhythm in patients with recurrent symptomatic atrial fibrillation. *Am J Cardiol* 2004;94(12):1563–1566.

A single-blind, prospective, randomized, controlled trial in 254 patients with AF comparing sotalol (480 mg/day) to propafenone (150 mg three time daily) in the maintenance of normal SR. 81% of patients on sotalol, 52% on propafenone, and 87% on placebo experienced recurrence of AF ($p < 0.001$ for propafenone vs. sotalol or placebo). The mean period to recurrence was also greater with propafenone at 26 months compared to 18 months with sotalol and 11 months with placebo.

55. **Chimienti M,** et al. Safety of long-term flecainide and propafenone in the management of patients with symptomatic paroxysmal atrial fibrillation: report from the Flecainide and Propafenone Italian Study (FAPIS) Investigators. *Am J Cardiol* 1996;77:60A–65A.

A randomized, open-label trial of 200 patients with paroxysmal AF comparing flecainide (200 to 300 mg daily) with propafenone (450 to 900 mg daily). Efficacy was measured indirectly by the number of patients who completed the study at 12 months. 77% of flecainide-treated patients completed the study compared to 75% of propafenone-treated patients (p 0.72). 11% and 13% of patients dropped out due to lack of efficacy, respectively. There was no significant difference in the number of adverse events between groups.

56. **Aliot E,** et al. Flecainide AF French Study Group. Comparison of the safety and efficacy of flecainide versus propafenone in hospital out-patients with symptomatic paroxysmal atrial fibrillation/flutter. *Am J Cardiol* 1996;77:66A–71A.

A randomized, open-label trial of 97 patients with paroxysmal AF or atrial flutter comparing flecainide (50 to 150 mg twice daily) to propafenone (300 to 600 mg twice daily). The probability of staying on treatment at 1 year was high, but not statistically different in the flecainide group (0.619) compared to propafenone (0.469) ($p = 0.079$). There was no difference in the number of attacks per month between flecainide and propafenone (no attacks 81.6% vs. 81.5%, 1 attack 8.5% vs. 6.4%, and >2 attacks 9.1% and 10.1%, respectively; p not stated).

57. **Pritchett EL,** et al. Rythmol Atrial Fibrillation Trial (**RAFT**) Investigators. Efficacy and safety of sustained-release propafenone (propafenone SR) for patients with atrial fibrillation. *Am J Cardiol* 2003;92:941–946.

A double-blind, randomized, controlled trial of 523 patients with paroxysmal AF comparing propafenone SR (225, 325, or 425 mg twice daily) to placebo in the maintenance of normal SR. The median time to recurrence with propafenone SR was 112 days with 225 mg, 291 days with 325 mg, and >300 days with 425 mg compared to 41 days with placebo (*p* < 0.001 for 325 and 425 mg vs. placebo, and *p* = 0.014 for 225 mg vs. placebo). There were more adverse events leading to withdrawal in the 425-mg group (25% with 425 mg vs. 12.7% and 14.1% with 225 and 325 mg, respectively; *p* not reported).

58. **Kochiadakis GE,** et al. Long-term maintenance of normal sinus rhythm in patients with current symptomatic atrial fibrillation: amiodarone vs. propafenone, both in low doses. *Chest* 2004;125:377–383.

In this trial, the investigators randomized 146 patients with refractory AF, in a prospective, single-blinded manner, to amiodarone (200 mg/day) or propafenone (450 mg/day) after cardioversion and followed them for AF recurrence or side effects over approximately 20 months of follow-up. AF recurred in 25 of the 72 patients in the amiodarone group at a mean of 9.8 months, versus 33 of 74 patients in the propafenone group at an average of 3.8 months. However, 12 patients in the amiodarone group, compared with 2 in the propafenone group, reported side effects necessitating the withdrawal of study drug (while still in SR).

Catheter and Surgical Ablation

CATHETER ABLATION

59. **Stabile G,** et al. Catheter ablation treatment in patients with drug-refractory atrial fibrillation: a prospective, multi-centre, randomized, controlled study (Catheter Ablation for the Cure Of Atrial Fibrillation Study). *Eur Heart J* 2006;27:216–221 [Epub October 7, 2005].

This multicenter, randomized, controlled trial studied ablation therapy for patients with paroxysmal AF, in whom antiarrhythmic therapy had failed. These 137 patients enrolled and received either antiarrhythmic therapy alone or antiarrhythmic therapy plus cavotricuspid, left inferior pulmonary vein–mitral isthmus, and circumferential pulmonary vein ablation (CPVA). The primary endpoint, recurrence of AF (for >30 seconds) at 1 year, occurred in 63 of 69 patients in the control group (91.3%), versus 30 of 68 patients (including 4 who had atrial flutter recur) in the ablation cohort (44.1%; *p* < 0.001 for the comparison).

60. **Pappone C,** et al. A randomized trial of circumferential pulmonary vein ablation versus antiarrhythmic drug therapy in paroxysmal atrial fibrillation: the **APAF** Study. *J Am Coll Cardiol* 2006;48:2340–2347.

198 patients with paroxysmal AF resistant to routine drug therapy were randomized to maximum antiarrhythmic drug therapy (with either flecainide, sotalol, or amiodarone), or to CPVA. At 1 year, 93% of patients in the ablation group were free of atrial tachyarrhythmias, compared with 35% in the drug therapy group. Adverse events in the ablation group included one TIA and one pericardial effusion.

61. **Oral H,** et al. Circumferential pulmonary-vein ablation for chronic atrial fibrillation. *N Engl J Med* 2006;354:934–941.

This randomized, controlled trial of CPVA included 146 patients with chronic AF and assigned them to amiodarone and two cardioversions alone or in addition to CVPA. Cardiac rhythm was followed daily by telephonic monitoring for 1 year. Intention-to-treat analysis showed 74% of patients in the CVPA group versus 58% in the control group were free from AF and without antiarrhythmic drug therapy ($p = 0.05$). However, there was significant crossover (77% of the control group), and 26% of patients initially assigned to CVPA required repeat ablation for AF. They did observe a beneficial effect of SR on LA diameter.

62. **Jaïs P,** et al. Catheter ablation versus antiarrhythmic drugs for atrial fibrillation: the **A4** study. *Circulation* 2008;118(24):2498–2505.

    This was a randomized, multicenter, prospective trial of CVPA in 112 patients with paroxysmal AF; they were assigned to either CVPA or "new" antiarrhythmic drug therapy (alone or a combination of agents). Freedom from recurrence of AF was observed in 13 of 55 (23%) patients in the drug group, versus 46 of 52 patients (89%) in the ablation group at 1 year. Crossover, once again, was significant in the drug, as 63% (37 of 55) went on to undergo ablation.

63. **Wilber DJ,** et al. for the **ThermoCool AF** Trial Investigators. Comparison of antiarrhythmic drug therapy and radiofrequency catheter ablation in patients with paroxysmal atrial fibrillation: a randomized controlled trial. *JAMA* 2010;303(4):333–340.

    167 patients with paroxysmal AF (who had failed one antiarrhythmic drug) were randomized in a 2:1, unblinded fashion to either PVI or antiarrhythmic drug therapy (dofetilide, flecainide, propafenone, sotalol, or quinidine). Over 9 months of follow-up, freedom from AF persisted in 66% of patients in the ablation group, versus 16% of those in the drug therapy group ($p < 0.001$ for hazard ratio of 0.30 for ablation). Adverse consequences of treatment were recorded in 8.8% of those in the drug therapy group and 4.9% of those in the ablation group.

64. **Wazni OM,** et al. Radiofrequency ablation vs. antiarrhythmic drugs as first-line treatment of symptomatic atrial fibrillation: a randomized trial. *JAMA* 2005;293:2634–2640.

    In order to assess the use of PVI as first-line therapy for symptomatic, paroxysmal AF, the investigators randomized 70 patients to either PVI with RF ablation or antiarrhythmic drug therapy and followed for 1 year for the recurrence of AF. Such treatment failures occurred in 22 of 35 patients (63%) who received drug therapy, versus 4 of 32 patients (13%) who underwent PVI. QOL at 6 months improved significantly more for patients in the PVI group, and patients in this group had significantly fewer hospitalizations during the 1-year follow-up period (9% vs. 54% for drug therapy; $p < 0.001$).

SURGICAL ABLATION

65. **Barnett SD,** et al. Surgical ablation as treatment for the elimination of atrial fibrillation: a meta-analysis. *J Thorac Cardiovasc Surg* 2006;131:1029–1035.

    The authors review the evidence for use of the modified maze procedure [to include biatrial (BA) ablation, compared with traditional LA modification, for the treatment of AF, through use of MEDLINE search]. In all, 69 studies were included and captured outcomes in 5,885 patients with survival data up to 3 years. While patients receiving BA procedures did not demonstrate a survival advantage, they did remain free from recurrence of AF longer and in greater numbers at each time point.

66. **Reston JT,** et al. Meta-analysis of clinical outcomes of maze-related surgical procedures for medically refractory atrial fibrillation. *Eur J Cardiothorac Surg* 2005;28:724–730.

    The authors pooled data from four randomized studies and six retrospective comparisons of mitral valve surgery patients with paroxysmal AF undergoing valve repair alone or with simultaneous maze procedure. However, the authors included different studies for the assessment of different endpoints, with the total population culminating in 905 patients. There was no significant difference in mortality between the two groups; however, restoration of SR favored the maze group (80.7% vs. 17.3%; $p < 0.000001$), as did the rate of stroke

(0% vs. 5.8%; $p = 0.008$). The study offers weak evidence in favor of the maze procedure, but also highlights the dearth of sound clinical data on which to evaluate it.

67. **Albrecht A,** et al. Randomized study of surgical isolation of the pulmonary veins for correction of permanent atrial fibrillation associated with mitral valve disease. *J Thorac Cardiovasc Surg* 2009;138:454–459.

The authors sought to evaluate the efficacy of surgical PVI, compared with maze procedure, for the treatment of chronic, permanent AF. In a total of 60 patients they randomized 20 to each procedure (as well as a control group, which received no AF procedure with their mitral valve correction); all had concomitant mitral valve disease that was also corrected. Relative risk for AF late postoperatively was 0.07 in the PVI group ($p < 0.001$ vs. control) and 1.195 in the maze group ($p = 0.002$ vs. control). There was no statistical difference between the two interventions (RR, 0.358; $p = 0.215$). The study provides support to these surgical techniques for the correction of AF in the setting of mitral valve disease.

68. **Srivastava V,** et al. Efficacy of three different ablative procedures to treat atrial fibrillation in patients with valvular heart disease: a randomised trial. *Heart Lung Circ* 2008;17(3):232–240.

In patients undergoing surgical correction of rheumatic heart disease, the authors randomized 160 patients with concomitant AF to one of the following four strategies: BA ablation (Cox maze), LA portion of the Cox maze, PVI, or a control group (no maze). Ablation was performed with RF microbipolar coagulation and cryoablation. SR was restored in 6.25% of patients in the BA maze group, 57.5% in the LA maze, 67.5% of the PVI group, and 20% of patients in the control group. This suggested that the long bypass and cross-clamp times of the traditional Cox maze procedure may not be required to achieve SR in patients undergoing surgery for concomitant rheumatic valve disease.

ELECTRICAL CARDIOVERSION AND PERICARDIOVERSION ANTICOAGULATION

69. **Kawabata VS,** et al. Monophasic versus biphasic waveform shocks for atrial fibrillation cardioversion in patients with concomitant amiodarone therapy. *Europace* 2007;9:143–146.

The investigators at one center randomized 154 patients with AF and receiving amiodarone to serial biphasic or serial monophasic (using twice as much energy as the biphasic group) shocks for DC cardioversion of AF. Patients converted to SR on the first shock in similar proportions between the two groups; success with serial shocks was also similar. Number of shocks required was similar in the two groups as well.

70. **Wozakowska-Kaplon B,** et al. Efficacy of biphasic shock for transthoracic cardioversion of persistent atrial fibrillation: can we predict energy requirements? *Pacing Clin Electrophysiol* 2004;27:764–768.

In 94 patients referred for biphasic cardioversion for AF, the authors achieved a success rate of 89% in a stepwise increase in energy, as required. However, a mean of 2.2 shocks was required, with energy of 217 J; by comparison, success of cardioversion using either 50 J or 50 J then 100 J was only a combined 51%. Duration of AF was the only predictor of lower energy requirement, and thus it is recommended to start at 200 J for the vast majority of patients.

71. **Glover BM,** et al. Biphasic energy selection for transthoracic cardioversion of atrial fibrillation. The **BEST AF** Trial. *Heart* 2008;94:884–887.

The investigators prospectively randomized 380 patients with AF to either escalating biphasic energy (100, 150, 200, 200 J) or nonescalating biphasic energy (200, 200, 200 J) for cardioversion. Success of first shock was significantly higher in the nonescalating group (71% vs. 48%; $p < 0.01$) and for patients with a higher BMI. In patients with normal BMI (≤ 25 kg/m^2), there were no significant differences in the rate of success on the first shock, for subsequent shocks, or overall.

72. **Gentile F,** et al. Safety of electrical cardioversion in patients with atrial fibrillation. *Mayo Clin Proc* 2002;77:897–904.

The authors examined retrospectively the results of 834 successful electrical cardioversions in 717 patients, to identify the rate of thromboembolic complications. At 1-month post-cardioversion, the rate of thromboembolism was 0.9%, and they were all limited to patients without therapeutic INRs. In addition to subtherapeutic anticoagulation, diabetes and hypertension were also independently correlated with such events.

73. **Manning WJ,** et al. Cardioversion from atrial fibrillation without prolonged anticoagulation with the use of transesophageal echocardiography to exclude the presence of atrial thrombi. *N Engl J Med* 1993;328:750–755.

This study was composed of 94 patients with AF of more than 2 days' duration (average, 4.5 weeks). Eighty patients received heparin before cardioversion; 14 thrombi were seen by TEE versus only 2 of 14 seen on transthoracic echocardiography (2 of these patients died suddenly, whereas the other 10 were cardioverted after prolonged oral anticoagulation). No embolic events occurred in the other patients [78 of 82 successfully cardioverted (47 by drugs)].

74. **Klein AL,** et al. for the Assessment of Cardioversion Using Transesophageal Echocardiography **(ACUTE)** Investigators. Use of transesophageal echocardiography to guide cardioversion in patients with atrial fibrillation. *N Engl J Med* 2001;344:1411–1420.

Design: Prospective, randomized, open, multicenter study. Primary endpoint: embolic events.
Purpose: To evaluate the safety and efficacy of TEE-guided cardioversion in patients with AF.
Population: 1,222 patients with AF of more than 48 hours' duration.
Exclusion Criteria: Included atrial flutter (and no history of AF), long-term warfarin therapy, hemodynamic instability, and contraindications to TEE.
Treatment: Cardioversion after 3 or more weeks of warfarin or TEE-guided cardioversion. All received a minimum of 4 weeks of warfarin after cardioversion.
Results: No difference between the groups was found in the incidence of embolic events [0.5% (TEE-guided) vs. 0.8%]. The TEE approach was associated with lower rates of hemorrhage, mostly minor (2.9% vs. 5.5%; $p = 0.03$). The TEE group had a higher initial successful cardioversion rate (71.1% vs. 65.2%; $p = 0.03$); however, SR rates were similar at 8 weeks.

75. **Page RL,** et al. Biphasic versus monophasic shock waveform for conversion of atrial fibrillation: the results of an international randomized, double-blind multicenter trial. *J Am Coll Cardiol* 2002;39:1956–1963.

This prospective, randomized, double-blind, multicenter trial compared the effectiveness of monophasic versus biphasic shocks for the cardioversion of AF. The 203 patients were randomized to monophasic or biphasic shocking waveforms, and received successive shocks, as needed, at three shared energies (100, 150, and 200 J), and then maximum output for the respective devices (200 J biphasic, 360 J monophasic) and, if necessary, a final crossover shock at maximum output of the alternate waveform. The success rate was higher for biphasic than for monophasic shocks at each of the three shared energy levels (100 J: 60% vs. 22%; 150 J: 77% vs. 44%; 200 J: 90% vs. 53%; $p < 0.0001$). On average, biphasic patients required fewer shocks (1.7 vs. 2.8; $p < 0.0001$) and lower total energy (217 J vs. 548 J; $p < 0.0001$) for successful conversion. The biphasic shock waveform also was associated with a lower frequency of dermal injury (17% vs. 41%; $p < 0.0001$).

76. **Stellbrink C,** et al. Safety and efficacy of enoxaparin compared with unfractionated heparin and oral anticoagulants for prevention of thromboembolic complications in cardioversion of nonvalvular atrial fibrillation: the Anticoagulation in Cardioversion using Enoxaparin **(ACE)** trial. *Circulation* 2004;109:997–1003.

This European study included 496 patients with nonvalvular AF scheduled to undergo elective cardioversion. Subjects were randomized to i.v. unfractionated heparin followed by phenprocoumon, or to enoxaparin, 1 mg/kg twice daily for 3 to 8 days followed by 40 or 60 mg b.i.d. Most (86%) of the cardioversions were TEE-guided. The primary composite endpoint of all-cause mortality, neurologic events, embolic events, and major bleeding occurred (in intention-to-treat analysis) in 4.8% of unfractionated heparin patients and 2.8% of enoxaparin patients ($p_{noninferiority} = 0.013$). Investigators concluded that enoxaparin was not inferior.

LONG-TERM ANTICOAGULATION STUDIES

77. **Albers GW.** Atrial fibrillation and stroke: 3 new studies, 3 new questions. *Arch Intern Med* 1994;154:1443–1448.

Analysis of the trials showed that anticoagulation therapy was associated with a reduction in stroke rates of approximately 50% compared with placebo, whereas aspirin reduced the risk by approximately 25%. No significant difference in stroke rates was noted between those with paroxysmal and those with chronic AF. Based on these data, the following recommendations were proposed: (a) in individuals younger than 60 years with no risk factors (history of previous stroke, TIA, diabetes, hypertension), no therapy is required (stroke risk is <0.5% per year); (b) in patients aged 60 to 75 years with lone AF, aspirin only is adequate (risk is 2% per year without therapy); and (c) patients older than 75 years or younger than 75 years with risk factors should be given anticoagulation with warfarin.

78. **Peterson P,** et al. Atrial Fibrillation, Aspirin, Anticoagulation **(AFASAK)** study. Placebo-controlled, randomized trial of warfarin and aspirin for prevention of thromboembolic complications in chronic atrial fibrillation. *Lancet* 1989;333:175–178.

Design: Prospective, randomized, partially open (warfarin), partially blinded (aspirin vs. placebo) study. Follow-up period was 2 years. Primary endpoint was thromboembolic complications (TIA, minor stroke, nondisabling stroke, fatal stroke, or embolism to viscera or extremities).
Purpose: To assess the efficacy of low-dose warfarin in preventing strokes in patients with nonrheumatic AF.
Population: 1,007 patients aged 18 years with chronic AF.
Exclusion Criteria: Prior anticoagulation for 6 months, cerebrovascular events in the prior 1 month, and blood pressure (BP) greater than 180/100 mm Hg.
Treatment: Low-dose warfarin [target prothrombin time (PT), 1.2 to 1.5 times control (approximate INR, 2.8 to 4.2)]; aspirin, 75 mg/day; or placebo.
Results: The warfarin group had significantly fewer thromboembolic complications [1.5% vs. 6.0% (aspirin) and 6.3% (placebo)]. Vascular death occurred in 0.9%, 3.6%, and 4.5% of the warfarin, aspirin, and placebo groups ($p < 0.02$). Warfarin patients had more frequent nonfatal bleeding (6.3% vs. 0.6% and none of aspirin and placebo patients).

79. Boston Area Anticoagulation Trial for Atrial Fibrillation **(BAATAF).** The effect of low-dose warfarin on the risk of stroke in patients with non-rheumatic atrial fibrillation. *N Engl J Med* 1990;323:1505–1511.

Design: Prospective, randomized, open, controlled, multicenter study. Mean follow-up period was 2.2 years. Primary endpoint was ischemic stroke.
Purpose: To assess the efficacy of low-dose warfarin in preventing strokes in patients with nonrheumatic AF.
Population: 420 patients (mean age, 63 years) with chronic or intermittent AF.
Exclusion Criteria: Prosthetic valves, severe HF, stroke in the prior 6 months, and contraindications to or requirement for aspirin or warfarin therapy.
Treatment: Warfarin [target PT, 1.2 to 1.5 times normal (achieved in 83%)]; aspirin was allowed in the control group.

Results: Trial was terminated early because of strong evidence in favor of warfarin. The warfarin group had 86% fewer strokes [0.41% per year vs. 2.98% per year (control group); *p* = 0.002] and a 62% lower death rate (2.25% per year vs. 5.97% per year; *p* = 0.005). The warfarin group had more minor hemorrhages (38 patients vs. 21 patients).

80. **SPAF** Investigators. Stroke Prevention in Atrial Fibrillation Study: final results. *Circulation* 1991;84:527–539.

Design: Prospective, randomized, partially open (warfarin), partially blind (aspirin vs. placebo), multicenter study. Primary events were ischemic stroke and systemic embolism. Mean follow-up was 1.3 years.
Purpose: To determine the efficacy and safety of warfarin and aspirin compared with placebo for the prevention of ischemic stroke and systemic embolism in patients with nonrheumatic AF.
Population: 1,330 patients with chronic or intermittent AF.
Exclusion Criteria: Prosthetic valves, mitral stenosis, MI in the prior 3 months, and stroke or TIA in the prior 2 years.
Treatment: Group 1 [627 patients (most 75 years or younger)—warfarin (target PT, 1.3 to 1.8 times normal (approximate INR, 2.0 to 4.5)]; aspirin, 325 mg/day; or placebo. Group 2 (703 nonanticoagulation candidates): aspirin or placebo.
Results: Aspirin-treated patients had 67% fewer primary events than did placebo patients (3.6% per year vs. 6.3% per year; *p* = 0.02). In the warfarin-eligible patients, warfarin reduced the risk of primary events by 67% compared with placebo (2.3% per year vs. 7.4% per year; *p* = 0.01). Primary events or death were reduced 58% by warfarin (*p* = 0.01) and 32% by aspirin (*p* = 0.02). Disabling stroke or vascular death was reduced 54% by warfarin and a nonsignificant 22% by aspirin (*p* = 0.33). Significant bleeding rates were similar in all three groups (1.4 to 1.6% per year). Significant risk factors for stroke were (a) prior cerebrovascular accident, (b) CHF within preceding 100 days, (c) hypertension, and among the echocardiographically assessed features, (d) left atrium more than 5 cm, and (e) LV dysfunction. If one clinical factor was present, the risk of stroke was 7% per year; if two or all three factors were present, the risk was 18% per year. The group without any risk factors (26%) had an event rate of only 1% per year.
Comments: Placebo arm of group 1 was discontinued in late 1989 because of the strong evidence of superiority of both warfarin and aspirin over placebo.

81. **Connolly SJ,** et al. Canadian Atrial Fibrillation Anticoagulation study **(CAFA).** *J Am Coll Cardiol* 1991;18:349–355 (editorial, 301–302).

Design: Prospective, randomized, double-blind, placebo-controlled, multicenter study. Primary endpoint was nonlacunar ischemic stroke, other systemic embolism, and intracranial or fatal hemorrhage.
Purpose: To evaluate the effectiveness and safety of warfarin in AF patients.
Population: 378 patients with recurrent paroxysmal or chronic AF.
Exclusion Criteria: Clear indications or contraindications to anticoagulation, stroke, or TIA in the prior year, MI in the prior month, use of antiplatelet drug(s), and uncontrolled hypertension.
Treatment: Warfarin (target INR, 2 to 3) or placebo.
Results: Target INR was achieved with only 44% frequency (subtherapeutic values in 39.6%). The warfarin group had a nonsignificant 37% risk reduction in primary outcome events (3.5% per year vs. 5.2% per year; *p* = 0.26). Major/fatal and minor bleeding events were common with warfarin use (2.5% per year vs. 0.5% per year and 16% per year vs. 9.4% per year).
Comments: Trial was terminated early because of the AFASAK and SPAF results.

82. **Ezekowitz MD,** et al. VA Stroke Prevention in Non-rheumatic Atrial Fibrillation **(SPINAF).** Warfarin in the prevention of stroke associated with non-rheumatic atrial fibrillation. *N Engl J Med* 1992;327:1406–1412.

Design: Prospective, randomized, double-blind, placebo-controlled, multicenter study. Average follow-up period was 1.8 years. Primary endpoint was cerebral infarction.

Purpose: To evaluate whether low-intensity anticoagulation will decrease the risk of stroke in patients with nonrheumatic AF.

Population: 571 men, 46 with prior stroke, without echocardiographic evidence of rheumatic heart disease and AF on two ECG tracings 4 weeks apart.

Exclusion Criteria: Contraindications to or requirement for anticoagulation, BP greater than 180/105 mm Hg, and use of nonsteroidal anti-inflammatory drugs.

Treatment: Warfarin (target INR, 1.4 to 2.8) or placebo.

Results: A 79% risk reduction was observed among patients without a history of stroke (0.9% per year vs. 4.3% per year; $p = 0.001$). Significant benefit also was seen in patients older than 70 years (0.9% per year vs. 4.8% per year; $p = 0.02$) and with a history of prior stroke (6.1% per year vs. 9.3% per year). Major hemorrhage rates were similar [1.3% per year (warfarin) vs. 0.9% per year]. Cerebral infarction occurred more frequently among patients with a history of cerebral infarction [9.3% per year (placebo group) and 6.1% per year (warfarin group)].

Comments: An analysis of 516 evaluable admission computed tomography (CT) scans showed that 14.7% had one silent infarct. Strokes during the study were not predicted by infarct on admission CT scan, but rather by active angina [placebo group, 15% (angina) vs. 5%].

83. European Atrial Fibrillation Trial **(EAFT).** Secondary prevention in non-rheumatic fibrillation after transient ischemic attack or minor stroke. *Lancet* 1993;342:1255–1262.

Design: Prospective, randomized, partially open (anticoagulant therapy), double-blind aspirin treatment, placebo-controlled, multicenter study. Primary endpoints were death from vascular disease, any stroke, MI, and systemic embolism. Mean follow-up period was 2.3 years.

Purpose: To evaluate and compare the effectiveness of oral anticoagulation and aspirin in AF patients with recent minor cerebrovascular events.

Population: 1,007 patients with nonrheumatic AF and minor stroke or TIA in the previous 3 months.

Exclusion Criteria: Use of nonsteroidal anti-inflammatory or other antiplatelet drugs, MI in the prior 3 months, and scheduled coronary surgery or carotid endarterectomy within next 3 months.

Treatment: Group 1 (669 patients)—warfarin (target INR, 2.5 to 4.0), or aspirin, 300 mg daily, or placebo. Group 2: Contraindications to anticoagulation; 338 patients.

Results: Anticoagulation was more effective than aspirin and placebo—8% versus 15% and 17% annual rates of primary outcome events; risk of stroke was especially lower in warfarin-treated patients [4% per year vs. 12% per year (placebo)]. Overall, warfarin use was associated with 90 fewer vascular events per 1,000 patient years (vs. 40 with aspirin). Bleeding events were common in warfarin-treated patients [2.8% per year vs. 0.9% per year (aspirin patients)]. Analysis of group 2 patients showed that the optimal INR range was 2.0 to 3.9, with most bleeding complications occurring when the INR was greater than 5.0, and no significant treatment effect was seen if INR was less than 2.0.

84. **SPAF II.** Warfarin versus aspirin for prevention of thromboembolism in atrial fibrillation. *Lancet* 1994;43:687–691.

Design: Prospective, randomized, open, parallel-group, multicenter study. Primary events were stroke and systemic embolism. Mean follow-up period was 2.3 years.

Purpose: To define the long-term benefits and risks associated with warfarin compared with aspirin, according to age and risk of thromboembolism.

Population: 1,100 patients, 715 patients aged 75 years or younger and 385 older than 75 years, with AF in the prior 12 months.

Exclusion Criteria: Lone AF if younger than 60 years, and stroke or TIA in the prior 2 years.

Treatment: Warfarin (target INR, 2.0 to 4.5), or aspirin 325 mg daily.

Results: No significant difference was observed between groups. However, 12 of 28 events in the warfarin group occurred while patients were not taking warfarin. Thus, a 50% difference in favor of warfarin is evident if these events are excluded. Event rates per year for patients aged 75 years or younger were 1.3% vs. 1.9% ($p = 0.24$); older than 75 years, 3.6% vs. 4.8% ($p = 0.39$). Low-risk younger patients (no hypertension, recent HF, or prior thromboembolism) had a low 0.5% per year primary event rate. Among older patients, stroke rates were similar in the two treatment groups (aspirin, 4.3% per year; warfarin, 4.6% per year). Among warfarin-treated patients, the intracranial hemorrhage was significantly higher in older versus younger patients (1.6% vs. 4.2%; $p = 0.04$).

Comments: Randomization was performed separately for the two age groups.

85. **Hylek EM**, et al. An analysis of the lowest effective intensity of prophylactic anticoagulation for patients with non-rheumatic atrial fibrillation. *N Engl J Med* 1996;335:540–546.

This retrospective, case–control analysis focused on 74 consecutive patients with ischemic strokes taking warfarin (INR measured at admission) and 222 controls (INR measured closest to admission day of case patient). The risk of stroke increased significantly at INRs less than 2.0; the adjusted OR for stroke was 2.0 if the INR was 1.7 to 2.0, 3.3 if the INR was 1.5 to 2.0, and 6.0 if the INR was 1.3 to 2.0. Other independent risk factors were prior stroke (OR, 10.4), diabetes (OR, 2.9), hypertension (OR, 2.5), and smoking (OR, 5.7).

86. **SPAF III.** Adjusted-dose warfarin vs. low-intensity, fixed-dose warfarin and aspirin for high-risk patients with atrial fibrillation: SPAF III randomised clinical trial. *Lancet* 1996;348:633–638.

Design: Prospective, randomized, partially open, multicenter study. Primary events were ischemic stroke and systemic embolism. Mean follow-up period was 1.1 years.

Purpose: To compare the safety and effectiveness of a combination of low-intensity, fixed-dose warfarin plus aspirin with adjusted-dose warfarin in AF patients at high risk of stroke.

Population: 1,044 AF patients with one of the following—CHF or EF 25% or less, prior thromboembolism, systolic blood pressure (SBP) greater than 160 mm Hg, or woman older than 75 years.

Exclusion Criteria: Conditions requiring standard anticoagulation therapy and contraindications to aspirin or warfarin.

Treatment: Fixed-dose warfarin [initial INR, 1.2 to 1.5 (mean, 1.3)] and aspirin (325 mg/day) or adjusted-dose warfarin [INR, 2 to 3 (mean, 2.4)].

Results: Trial was terminated early. The low-INR group had four times more ischemic strokes and systemic emboli (7.9% per year vs. 1.9% per year; $p < 0.0001$). Rates of disabling stroke (5.6% per year vs. 1.7% per year; $p = 0.0007$) and of primary or vascular death (11.8% per year vs. 6.4% per year; $p = 0.002$) also were higher with combination therapy. Bleeding rates were similar. The greatest benefits of standard adjusted-dose warfarin were seen in patients with prior thromboembolism.

87. **Gullov AL**, et al. **AFASAK II.** Fixed minidose warfarin, aspirin alone and in combination, versus adjusted-dose warfarin for stroke prevention in atrial fibrillation. *Arch Intern Med* 1998;158:1513–1521 (editorial, 1487–1491).

Design: Prospective, randomized, controlled, single-center study. Primary endpoint was stroke and systemic thromboembolic events.

Purpose: To investigate the effects of minidose warfarin alone and in combination with aspirin in chronic AF patients.

Population: 677 patients (median age, 74 years) with chronic AF documented by ECG tracings at least 1 month apart.

Exclusion Criteria: Lone AF in patients 60 years or younger, SBP more than 180 mm Hg, diastolic BP more than 100 mm Hg, and stroke or TIA in the prior 6 months.

Treatment: Warfarin, 1.25 mg/day; warfarin, 1.25 mg/day; and aspirin, 300 mg/day; aspirin alone; or warfarin alone (target INR, 2 to 3).

Results: Trial was terminated early because of SPAF III results. One-year cumulative primary event rates were as follows: minidose warfarin, 5.8%; warfarin plus aspirin, 7.2%; aspirin alone, 3.6%; and adjusted-dose warfarin, 2.8% (*p* = 0.67). No significant differences were seen at 3 years. Major bleeding events were rare.

88. **Hart RG,** et al. Antithrombotic therapy to prevent stroke in patients with atrial fibrillation: a meta-analysis. *Ann Intern Med* 1999;131:492–501.

    The investigators combined data from 16 randomized trials of warfarin or aspirin in 9,874 patients with AF, for the prevention of stroke. Compared to placebo, warfarin reduced stroke by 62% (2.7% per year for primary prevention, 8.4% per year for secondary prevention), whereas aspirin reduced stroke by 22% (1.5% per year for primary prevention, 2.5% per year for secondary prevention). In head-to-head comparison, warfarin was better than aspirin at stroke prevention (RRR, 36%; 95% CI, 14% to 52%).

89. **Singer DE,** et al. The net clinical benefit of warfarin anticoagulation in atrial fibrillation. *Ann Intern Med* 2009;151:297–305.

    In an effort to assess the net clinical benefit of warfarin anticoagulation in AF, the authors pooled data on 13,559 adults, over 66,000 person-years of follow-up in an integrated health care delivery system. They balanced ischemic (presumed thromboembolic) stroke events against hemorrhagic events with an impact weight factor applied (hemorrhagic events counted 1.5× more than ischemic ones). After stratifying patients by CHADS2 score, investigators found an overall 0.68% net clinical benefit in favor of warfarin; however, this varied greatly across the spectrum of CHADS2 score. Those with a CHADS2 of 0 or 1 had essentially no clinical benefit, while those with a score of 4 to 6 derived a 2.22% yearly net clinical benefit. Notably, there was a significant net clinical benefit in older patients (those over 84 years) of 2.34%.

Investigational Anticoagulants

90. **Connolly SJ,** et al. and the **RE-LY** Steering Committee and Investigators. Dabigatran versus warfarin in patients with atrial fibrillation. *N Engl J Med* 2009;361:1139–1151.

    The investigators evaluated a novel direct thrombin inhibitor, dabigatran, in 18,113 patients with AF and increased stroke risk. Patients were assigned, in a randomized, unblinded fashion, to either dabigatran (at one of the following two doses: 110 or 150 mg both twice daily) or adjusted-dosing warfarin. Over a mean follow-up of 2 years, the primary endpoint of stroke or systemic embolism was followed. Rates of such an endpoint were 1.69% per year in the warfarin group versus 1.53% per year in the dabigatran 110-mg group and 1.11% in the 150-mg dabigatran group. Major bleeding occurred at 3.36% per year in the warfarin group, versus 2.71% per year in the dabigatran 110-mg group, and 3.11% per year in the dabigatran 150-mg group. Hemorrhagic stroke rates also favored dabigatran: 0.38% per year for warfarin, versus 0.12% and 0.10% for the 110- and 150-mg dabigatran groups, respectively. All of these margins met the statistical test for noninferiority except the bleeding comparison of warfarin and dabigatran 150 mg. There were no differences in the mortality rates among the groups.

91. **Olsson SB,** et al. for the Executive Steering Committee of the **SPORTIF III** Investigators. Stroke prevention with the oral direct thrombin inhibitor ximelagatran compared with warfarin in patients with non-valvular atrial fibrillation (**SPORTIF III**): randomised controlled trial. *Lancet* 2003;362:1691–1698.

    This open-label, randomized, multicenter trial enrolled 3,410 patients with nonvalvular AF and at least one other stroke factor. Patients received ximelagatran, 36 mg twice daily, or warfarin (goal INR 2-3; mean 2.5). At mean follow-up of 17.4 months, the ximelagatran group had a 1.6% annualized rate of stroke or systemic embolic events (vs. 2.3% with warfarin). An on-treatment analysis found a significant 41% relative risk reduction with ximelagatran (1.3% per year vs. 2.2% per year; $p = 0.018$). Ximelagatran was also associated with a significantly reduced risk of major or minor bleeding complications (25.8% vs. 29.8%; $p = 0.0065$), but also an increased incidence of liver enzyme elevations (6% vs. 1%; $p < 0.0001$). The latter typically occurred between 2 and 6 months, and enzyme normalized either spontaneously or after cessation of treatment.

ATRIAL FIBRILLATION PREVENTION AFTER SURGERY

92. **Andrews TC,** et al. Prevention of supraventricular arrhythmias after coronary artery bypass surgery: a meta-analysis of randomized controlled trials. *Circulation* 1991;84 (5 suppl):III236.

This meta-analysis included 1,549 patients from 24 randomized, controlled studies. Patients were excluded if they had an LVEF less than 30%, insulin-dependent diabetes, AV block, and sick sinus syndrome, and those undergoing noncardiac operations. The initiation of preoperative beta-blockers was found to be more effective than postoperative initiation, and beta-blocker therapy reduced post-CABG AF by 77%.

93. **Daoud EG,** et al. Preoperative amiodarone as prophylaxis against atrial fibrillation after heart surgery. *N Engl J Med* 1997;337:1785.

This prospective, randomized, double-blind study enrolled 124 patients scheduled to undergo elective cardiac surgery. Patients were randomized at least a week before surgery to oral amiodarone (600 mg/day for 7 days, and then 200 mg/day until hospital discharge), or placebo. Postoperative AF occurred significantly less in the amiodarone group (25% vs. 53%; $p = 0.003$). Amiodarone patients had a shorter and less costly hospital stay compared with placebo patients (6.5 days vs. 7.9 days, $p = 0.04$; $18,375 vs. $26,491, $p = 0.03$). No significant differences were seen between the groups in nonfatal and fatal postoperative complications.

94. **Serafimovski N,** et al. Usefulness of dofetilide for the prevention of atrial tachyarrhythmias (atrial fibrillation or flutter) after coronary artery bypass grafting. *Am J Cardiol* 2008;101:1574–1579.

In a randomized, double-blinded fashion, the investigators assigned 133 patients undergoing CABG, with or without valve surgery, to either dofetilide or placebo just prior to surgery. The primary endpoint of postoperative atrial tachyarrhythmias occurred in 36% of patients receiving placebo versus 18% of those receiving dofetilide (absolute RR, 18%; $p < 0.017$). In those patients on dofetilide who did develop an atrial tachyarrhythmia, their length of stay was still a day less than those in the placebo arm. There was no occurrence of torsades de pointes in either group.

Ventricular Arrhythmias

IMMEDIATE THERAPY: AUTOMATED EXTERNAL DEFIBRILLATORS

95. **Weaver WD,** et al. Use of the automatic external defibrillator in the management of out-of-hospital cardiac arrest. *N Engl J Med* 1988;319:661–666.

This prospective study of 1,287 consecutive cardiac arrest victims compared outcomes of defibrillation performed by first-responder firefighters using automatic external defibrillators with paramedics, who on average arrive on scene slightly later. Among patients for whom defibrillation was attempted, survival to hospital discharge was better when administered by firefighters (30%) than when waiting slightly longer for paramedics (19%; $p < 0.001$).

96. **Valenzuela TD,** et al. Outcomes of rapid defibrillation by security officers after cardiac arrest in casinos. *N Engl J Med* 2000;343:1206–1209.

This study tracked outcomes of treating cardiac arrest victims at a number of casinos with AEDs operated by (minimally) trained security officers. Of 105 subjects whose initial rhythm was VF, 53% survived to hospital discharge. Survival was better for witnessed than for unwitnessed arrests, and when defibrillation was performed in less than versus more than 3 minutes (74% vs. 49%). These results suggest that use of AEDs by nonmedical personnel is feasible and effective.

97. **Page RL,** et al. Automated external defibrillator use aboard a domestic airline. *N Engl J Med* 2000;343:1210–1216.

In this pilot study, AEDs were furnished aboard aircraft of one domestic US carrier. The 200 AED uses were reported, 99 of them for unconscious patients. Shocks were advised and delivered by the AEDs in 14 of 14 patients with VF, and in no patients with other rhythms (sensitivity and specificity of ECG diagnostics, both 100%). Survival to hospital discharge was 40% in the VF patients. Again, the use of AEDs by nonmedical personnel was supported.

98. **Hallstrom AP,** et al. for the Public Access Defibrillation (**PAD**) Trial Investigators. Public-access defibrillation and survival after out-of-hospital cardiac arrest. *N Engl J Med* 2004;351:637–646.

The investigators randomly assigned various community centers (malls, apartment complexes, etc.) to emergency response systems including layperson training of CPR or CPR plus use of AED. This included roughly 19,000 volunteers from across North America and the primary endpoint was survival to hospital discharge of out-of-hospital arrest victims. Among 128 arrests in the AED group, 30 survived to hospital discharge, compared to 15 of the 107 arrest victims in the CPR-only group ($p = 0.03$). There were no inappropriate shocks delivered, and functional status at discharge was not different between the two groups.

99. **Bardy GH,** et al. for the **HAT** Investigators. Home use of automated external defibrillators for sudden cardiac arrest. *N Engl J Med* 2008;358:1793–1804.

In 7,001 patients at high risk of SCD, namely those with recent anterior wall MI (but not candidates for internal defibrillator implants), investigators randomly assigned half to receive an AED for their home. For the primary endpoint of all-cause mortality over a median follow-up of 37.3 months, there was no difference in the two groups (6.4% in the AED group vs. 6.5% in the control; $p = 0.77$). However, only 35.6% of all deaths were considered to be of sudden, tachyarrhythmic etiology.

IMMEDIATE THERAPY: INTRAVENOUS AMIODARONE

100. **Kudenchuk PJ,** et al. Amiodarone for resuscitation after out-of hospital cardiac arrest due to ventricular fibrillation. *N Engl J Med* 1999;341:871–878.

Design: Prospective, randomized, placebo-controlled, double-blind, single-center trial. Primary endpoint was survival to hospital admission. Patients were followed up to hospital discharge.

Purpose: To determine whether i.v. amiodarone, compared with placebo, improved survival to hospital admission in shock-refractory VT/VF.

Population: 504 adult subjects with nontraumatic out-of-hospital cardiac arrest with ongoing pulseless VT or VF after three defibrillations.

Treatment: Epinephrine, 1 mg i.v., followed by amiodarone, 300 mg given as an i.v. push, or placebo, followed by standard ACLS-guided resuscitative measures.

Results: Amiodarone group had a significantly higher survival to admission compared with the placebo group (44% vs. 33%; $p = 0.03$). Amiodarone was associated with higher frequency of hypotension (59% vs. 48%; $p = 0.04$) and bradycardia (41% vs. 25%; $p = 0.004$) compared with placebo.

101. **Dorian P,** et al. Amiodarone as compared with lidocaine for shock-resistant ventricular fibrillation. *N Engl J Med* 2002;346:884–890 **(ALIVE)**.

Design: Prospective, randomized, double-blind, controlled, single-center study. Primary endpoint was survival to hospital admission.

Purpose: To compare i.v. amiodarone with lidocaine for shock-refractory VT/VF.

Population: 347 adult subjects with nontraumatic out-of-hospital cardiac arrest with ongoing pulseless VF after three defibrillations, i.v. epinephrine and a fourth defibrillation, or recurrent VF after initially successful defibrillation.

Treatment: Amiodarone, 5-mg/kg i.v. push plus lidocaine placebo, or lidocaine, 1.5-mg/kg i.v. push plus amiodarone placebo, followed by standard ACLS-guided resuscitative measures. A second dose of the same study drug (2.5 mg/kg amiodarone or 1.5 mg/kg lidocaine) could be given if VF persisted.

Results: Survival to hospital admission was better with i.v. amiodarone than with lidocaine (22.8% vs. 12.0%; $p = 0.009$). Patients treated early (less than the median of 24 minutes from ambulance dispatch to study drug administration) had better survival than those treated late, but within this subgroup, survival remained better with amiodarone (27.7% vs. 15.3%; $p = 0.05$).

SECONDARY-PREVENTION TRIALS: DRUGS VERSUS IMPLANTABLE CARDIOVERTER DEFIBRILLATORS

102. **Kuck KH,** et al. Randomized comparison of antiarrhythmic drug therapy with implantable defibrillators in patients resuscitated from cardiac arrest: the Cardiac Arrest Study Hamburg **(CASH)**. *Circulation* 2000;102:748–754 (also see *Am Heart J* 1994;127:1139).

This prospective study, initiated in 1987, initially randomized survivors of SCD in 3:1 fashion to treatment with oral propafenone, amiodarone, or metoprolol or to ICD implantation without concomitant antiarrhythmic drugs. The propafenone arm (56 patients) was terminated in 1992 after interim analysis revealed increased all-cause mortality and sudden death (12% vs. none; $p < 0.05$) with propafenone compared with ICD over an average follow-up of only 11 months. The remaining three arms of the study enrolled a total of 288 subjects: 99 ICD, 92 amiodarone, and 97 metoprolol. Final analysis at a mean follow-up of 57 months revealed a nonsignificant reduction in all-cause mortality favoring the ICD group over the combination of the amiodarone and metoprolol arms (36% vs. 44%; one-tailed p value 0.08). The relative improvement in survival with ICD compared with amiodarone/metoprolol was greatest at 1 year (42%), and progressively declined as the duration of follow-up lengthened.

103. **Connolly SJ,** et al. Canadian implantable defibrillator study **(CIDS):** a randomized trial of the implantable cardioverter defibrillator against amiodarone. *Circulation* 2000;101: 1297–1302.

This prospective, randomized study enrolled patients with documented VF or out-of-hospital cardiac arrest without a reversible cause, VT that was poorly tolerated or occurred in the presence of LVEF less than 35%, or syncope with spontaneous or inducible VT. Patients were randomized to oral amiodarone ($n = 331$; mean dose, 255 mg/day at 5 years) or ICD implantation ($n = 328$); 90% of ICD implants were transvenous. A moderate (21% to 28%) degree of crossover between groups occurred, and sotalol and β-blockers were more frequently used by ICD patients. Reductions in total mortality (8.2% vs. 10.2% per year; $p = 0.14$) and arrhythmic death (3.0% vs. 4.5% per year; $p = 0.09$) favored the ICD arm, but did not reach statistical significance. The trend toward improved survival with ICDs was viewed as consistent with the AVID trial, in which the survival benefit did reach statistical significance.

104. The Antiarrhythmics versus Implantable Defibrillators **(AVID)** Investigators. A comparison of antiarrhythmic-drug therapy with implantable defibrillators in patients resuscitated from near-fatal ventricular arrhythmias. *N Engl J Med* 1997;337:1576–1583.

Design: Prospective, randomized, open, multicenter study. Primary endpoint was all-cause mortality.

Purpose: To compare the efficacy of antiarrhythmic drugs (primarily amiodarone) with ICDs for secondary prevention of SCD.

Population: 1,016 subjects resuscitated from VF (45%) or hemodynamically unstable VT (55%) not due to a transient or correctable cause, with LVEF of 40% or less. Most (81%) had a clinical history of CAD.

Exclusion Criteria: Contraindication to amiodarone or ICD implantation.

Treatment: Patients were randomly assigned to antiarrhythmic drug treatment (96% amiodarone) or ICD implantation. Nearly all ICD implants were transvenous, with many pectoral. Crossover was approximately 10% in both groups. Beta-blocker use was three- to fourfold higher among ICD versus amiodarone patients.

Results: Mortality was significantly lower in the ICD group than in the antiarrhythmic drug arm at 1 year (10.7% vs. 17.7%), 2 years (18.4% vs. 25.3%), and 3 years (24.6% vs. 35.9%; $p < 0.02$).

Comments: The study was criticized for the imbalance in beta-blocker use, but the core conclusion of ICD superiority remains generally accepted.

PRIMARY-PREVENTION TRIALS: ANTIARRHYTHMIC DRUGS

105. The Cardiac Arrhythmia Suppression Trial **(CAST)** Investigators. Preliminary report: effect of encainide and flecainide on mortality in a randomized trial of arrhythmia suppression after myocardial infarction. *N Engl J Med* 1989;321:406–412 (see also Chapter 4).

In 1,727 post-MI patients, encainide and flecainide led to a significantly higher mortality rate through 10 months of follow-up (7.7% vs. 3.0% for placebo; relative risk, 2.5; 95% CI, 1.6 to 4.5). Arrhythmic death also was higher with the IC agents than with placebo (4.5% vs. 1.2%).

106. The Cardiac Arrhythmia Suppression Trial II **(CAST II)** Investigators. Effect of the antiarrhythmic agent moricizine on survival after myocardial infarction. *N Engl J Med* 1992;327:227–233.

CAST-II enrolled 2,699 subjects 6 to 90 days after MI with an EF of 40% or less and 6 or more PVCs/hour. Patients were randomized to placebo or the class I-C agent moricizine in the short-term (2 weeks; $n = 1,325$) and long-term (mean, 18 months; $n = 1,374$) protocols. The study was terminated early because of increased mortality associated with moricizine use in the 14-day protocol (2.6% vs. 0.5%; adjusted $p < 0.01$). Incidence of long-term deaths was similar (15% vs. 12%). The authors concluded that the use of moricizine after MI was not only ineffective, but also harmful.

107. **Waldo AL,** et al. Survival with oral D-sotalol **(SWORD)** investigators. Effect of D-sotalol on mortality in patients with left ventricular dysfunction after recent and remote myocardial infarction. *Lancet* 1996;348:7–12.

The 3,121 post-MI patients with an EF of 40% or less and NYHA class II to III HF were randomized to D-sotalol (100 to 200 mg, b.i.d.) or placebo. The D-sotalol arm exhibited higher all-cause mortality (5.0% vs. 3.1%), cardiac mortality (4.7% vs. 2.9%), and presumed arrhythmic deaths (3.6% vs. 2.0%) at a mean follow-up of 148 days (all p values <0.01).

108. **Doval HC,** et al. for the Grupo de Estudio de la Sobrevida en la Insuficiencia Cardiaca en Argentina **(GESICA)** Investigators. Randomised trial of low-dose amiodarone in severe congestive heart failure. *Lancet* 1994;344:493–498.

This trial randomized 516 Argentinean patients with CHF to amiodarone, 300 mg/day, or placebo. A significant proportion of patients had Chagas disease or alcoholism as the etiologies of their LV dysfunction. The trial found a nonsignificant 27% reduction in sudden death ($p = 0.16$) and a significant reduction in total mortality (33.5% vs. 41.4%; $p = 0.02$) in favor of amiodarone.

109. **Singh SN,** et al. for the Survival Trial of Antiarrhythmic Therapy in Congestive Heart Failure **(CHF-STAT)** Investigators. Amiodarone in patients with congestive heart failure and asymptomatic ventricular arrhythmia. *N Engl J Med* 1995;333:377–382.

Entry criteria for CHF-STAT were symptomatic CHF, EF less than 40%, more than 10 PVCs/hour, and cardiac enlargement. The majority (70%) of subjects had ischemic cardiomyopathy. The 674 subjects were randomized to amiodarone (maintenance dose, 300 mg/day) or placebo and followed up for a median of 45 months. Amiodarone showed no benefit in terms of overall mortality or SCD.

110. **Julian DG,** et al. Randomised trial of effect of amiodarone on mortality in patients with left ventricular dysfunction after recent myocardial infarction: **EMIAT.** *Lancet* 1997;349:667–674.

In 1,486 post-MI patients with an EF of 40% or less, all-cause mortality was similar for amiodarone versus placebo, but a 35% risk reduction ($p = 0.05$) occurred in arrhythmic deaths. The authors concluded that the systematic prophylactic use of amiodarone after MI (with low EF) was not indicated, but the lack of proarrhythmia supports the use of amiodarone in patients for whom antiarrhythmic therapy is indicated for other reasons.

111. **Cairns JA,** et al. Randomised trial of outcome after myocardial infarction in patients with frequent or repetitive ventricular premature depolarisations **CAMIAT.** *Lancet* 1997;349:675–682.

CAMIAT randomized 1,202 postinfarct patients with frequent ventricular ectopy (>10 premature ventricular depolarizations per hour) or NSVT to amiodarone or placebo. At a mean follow-up of 1.8 years, a reduction in combined resuscitated VF or arrhythmic death was found with amiodarone (4.5% vs. 6.9%; $p = 0.03$), but no significant difference was seen in all-cause mortality.

112. **Sim I,** et al. Quantitative overview of randomized trials of amiodarone to prevent sudden cardiac death. *Circulation* 1997;96:2823–2829.

This meta-analysis pooled the results of all trials randomizing subjects to amiodarone or alternative nondevice therapy (including placebo) for the prevention of sudden death, including a minority of subjects in secondary-prevention studies. Across trials, amiodarone reduced total mortality by 19% when compared with active control or "usual care" but only 10% when compared with placebo. The treatment effect of amiodarone, when pooled, appeared to be independent of the clinical population studied (post-MI, CHF, or SCD survivors).

PRIMARY-PREVENTION TRIALS: DRUGS VERSUS IMPLANTABLE CARDIOVERTER DEFIBRILLATORS

113. **Moss AJ,** et al. for the Multicenter Automated Defibrillator Implantation Trial **(MADIT)** Investigators. Improved survival with an implanted defibrillator in patients

with coronary disease at high risk for ventricular arrhythmia. *N Engl J Med* 1996;335:1933–1940.

Design: Prospective, randomized, open, multicenter trial. The primary endpoint was all-cause mortality. Average follow-up was 27 months.

Purpose: To compare the efficacy of ICDs with standard medical therapy (generally including antiarrhythmic drugs) for primary prevention of SCD in coronary patients at high risk for SCD.

Population: 196 adult patients with prior MI, documented NSVT, EF of 35% or less, and inducible VT or VF at EPS, not suppressible with i.v. procainamide.

Exclusion Criteria: Included previous cardiac arrest or VT with syncope, symptomatic hypotension, MI within 3 weeks, CABG surgery within 2 months, or PTCA within 3 months.

Treatment: Patients were randomly assigned to ICD implantation (50% transthoracic, 50% transvenous) or standard medical therapy. In the standard therapy group, 74% received amiodarone, 10% received type I antiarrhythmic drugs, and 7% received sotalol.

Results: Study enrollment was terminated prematurely when interim analysis passed prespecified stopping criteria. At follow-up, the mortality rate was 17% in the defibrillator group versus 39% in the conventional therapy group, a 54% reduction ($p = 0.009$).

114. **Buxton AE,** et al. for the Multicenter Unsustained Tachycardia Trial **(MUSTT)** Investigators. A randomized study of the prevention of sudden death in patients with coronary artery disease. *N Engl J Med* 1999;341:1882–1890.

Design: Prospective, randomized, open, multicenter trial. Primary endpoint was cardiac arrest or death from arrhythmia. Median follow-up duration was 39 months.

Purpose: To compare the efficacy of electrophysiologically guided therapy (antiarrhythmic drugs or ICDs if drugs failed) with standard medical therapy (not including antiarrhythmic drugs) for primary prevention of SCD in coronary patients at high risk for SCD.

Population: Adult patients with prior MI, documented NSVT, EF of 40% or less, and inducible VT or VF at EPS. Noninducible patients were followed up in a voluntary registry. The 704 inducible patients were randomized.

Exclusion Criteria: Syncope, sustained VT, or VF more than 48 hours after an acute MI; untreated exercise-induced ischemia.

Treatment: Standard medical therapy (not including antiarrhythmic drugs) or therapy based on serial electrophysiology (EP) testing, which consisted of an antiarrhythmic drug that suppressed VT inducibility, amiodarone (if two previous drug trials failed), or an ICD. Initially, ICDs were reserved for patients with three or more unsuccessful drug trials, but halfway through enrollment, this was relaxed to one or more. Ultimately, 46% of the EP-guided patients were discharged with ICDs, and 45% were treated with drugs: 26% class I, 10% amiodarone, and 9% sotalol.

Results: Overall, the EP group showed a lower rate of cardiac arrest or arrhythmic death ($p = 0.04$) and lower total mortality (hazard ratio, 0.80; $p = 0.06$). However, all the benefit was achieved among patients who had received an ICD (total mortality, 24% at 5 years), whereas patients treated with EP-guided antiarrhythmic drug therapy had a slightly higher mortality rate (55% at 5 years) compared with standard medical therapy without antiarrhythmic drugs (48%).

115. **Moss AJ,** et al. for The Multicenter Automatic Defibrillator Implantation Trial II **(MADIT II)** Investigators. Prophylactic implantation of a defibrillator in patients with myocardial infarction and reduced ejection fraction. *N Engl J Med* 2002;346:877–883.

Design: Prospective, randomized, open, multicenter trial. Primary endpoint was all-cause mortality. Average follow-up, 20 months.

Purpose: To compare the efficacy of ICDs with conventional medical therapy (primarily without antiarrhythmic drugs) for primary prevention of SCD in coronary patients at high risk for SCD.

Population: Adult patients with prior MI and EF of 30% or less.

Exclusion Criteria: FDA-approved indication for ICD implantation, NYHA class IV CHF, MI within 1 month, coronary revascularization procedure within 3 months, or other life-threatening condition.

Treatment: Patients were randomly assigned in 3:2 ratio to ICD implantation (all transvenous) or standard medical therapy. Amiodarone was used by 13% of ICD subjects and 10% of conventional therapy subjects at last study contact. Use of other cardiac medications, including beta-blockers and ACE inhibitors, was well balanced between groups.

Results: Total mortality was 19.8% in the conventional therapy group and 14.2% in the ICD group (hazard ratio, 0.69; $p = 0.016$). Benefits were consistent across all subgroups. A trend toward an increased rate of hospitalization for CHF was seen in the ICD group (19.9% vs. 14.9%; $p = 0.09$); this finding may be related to ventricular pacing worsening CHF by creating dyssynchrony in the heart (also see DAVID results; Ref. 125).

Comments: Based on these results, the updated ACC/AHA guidelines include ICD implantation in post-MI patients with LVEF 30% or less as a class IIa recommendation.

116. **Hohnloser SH,** et al. for the Defibrillator in Acute Myocardial Infarction (**DINAMIT**) Investigators. Prophylactic use of an implantable cardioverter-defibrillator after acute myocardial infarction. *N Engl J Med* 2004;351:2481–2488.

Design: Prospective, randomized trial; primary endpoint was all-cause mortality at mean follow-up of 30 months.

Purpose: To identify the benefit, if any, of ICD implantation early (6 to 40 days) after acute MI.

Population: 674 patients 6 to 40 days following acute MI; they also had reduced EF ($\leq35\%$) and weakened cardiac autonomic function (either depressed pulse variability or elevated 24-hour pulse rate).

Treatment: Placement of single-lead ICD programmed to shock for VT or VF, and for backup pacing at 40 bpm, as well as antitachycardia pacing for certain VT rates; or no device.

Results: Overall mortality did not differ between the two groups, as 62 of 322 patients in the ICD group died, versus 58 of 342 in the non-ICD group (hazard ratio for ICD group, 1.08; $p = 0.66$). Prespecified outcome of death from arrhythmia was significantly reduced, at 12 versus 29 in the ICD and non-ICD groups, respectively (hazard ratio for ICD group, 0.42; $p = 0.009$). This was offset by increased nonarrhythmia death in the ICD group.

117. **Bardy GH,** et al. for the Sudden Cardiac Death in Heart Failure Trial (**SCD-HeFT**) Investigators. Amiodarone or an implantable cardioverter-defibrillator for congestive heart failure. *N Engl J Med* 2005;352:225–237.

Design: Prospective, randomized trial; primary endpoint was all-cause mortality at median follow-up of 45.5 months.

Purpose: To identify best prevention of SCD for patients with CHF.

Population: 2,521 patients with NYHA class II or III CHF and an EF of $\leq35\%$.

Treatment: Standard CHF therapy plus placebo, standard therapy plus amiodarone, or standard therapy plus single-lead, shock-only ICD. The amiodarone versus placebo drug branches were double-blinded.

Results: Overall, 70% of patients enrolled for NYHA class II, with roughly half ischemic in etiology. In the placebo group, there were 244 deaths (29%), versus 240 (28%) in the amiodarone group (hazard ratio, 1.06 for amiodarone vs. placebo; $p = 0.53$), and 182 (22%) in the ICD group (hazard ratio, 0.77 for ICD vs. placebo; $p = 0.007$). Results did not differ based on etiology of CHF (ischemic vs. other). Of note, drug was discontinued in 22% and 32% of patients in the placebo and amiodarone groups, respectively; 14% of patients in the ICD group received open-label amiodarone at some point.

118. **Steinbeck G,** et al. for the **IRIS** Investigators. Defibrillator implantation early after myocardial infarction. *N Engl J Med* 2009;361:1427–1436.

Design: Prospective, randomized trial; primary endpoint was all-cause mortality at mean follow-up of 37 months.

Purpose: To test the hypothesis that patients at increased risk of ventricular arrhythmia would benefit from ICD placement early after MI.

Population: 898 patients within 5 to 31 days after acute MI with reduced EF (≤35%) and at least one of the following—heart rate ≥90 on the first available ECG (602 patients) or NSVT (≥150 bpm) on Holter (208 patients); 88 patients fulfilled both the heart rate and VT criteria.

Treatment: Single-chamber ICD placement or no device.

Results: There was no significant difference in mortality between those who received ICDs and those who did not (116 of 445 vs. 117 of 453, respectively; hazard ratio, 1.04; $p = 0.78$). However, incidence of SCD was lower in the ICD group (27 vs. 60; hazard ratio, 0.55; $p = 0.049$), with, once again, more nonsudden death events in the ICD group. There were no differences in outcomes among patients who fulfilled the different inclusion criteria.

PRIMARY-PREVENTION TRIALS: NONISCHEMIC CARDIOMYOPATHY PATIENTS

119. **Bansch D,** et al. for the Cardiomyopathy Trial (**CAT**) Investigators. Primary prevention of sudden cardiac death in idiopathic dilated cardiomyopathy. *Circulation* 2002;105:1453–1458.

    This prospective, randomized, multicenter trial enrolled 104 patients with recent onset of DCM (9 months or less), LVEF 30% or less, and in NYHA class II or III. CAD had to be excluded by angiography. Other exclusion criteria included history of MI, symptomatic bradycardia, VT, or VF. Patients were randomized to ICD or control. Trial was terminated early because 1-year mortality did not reach 30% in the control group. At mean follow-up of 5.5 years, no significant difference in mortality rates was found between the two groups (26.0% vs. 31.5%). The only predictor of mortality was impaired LVEF.

120. **Strickberger SA,** et al. Amiodarone versus implantable cardioverter-defibrillator: randomized trial in patients with non-ischemic dilated cardiomyopathy and asymptomatic nonsustained ventricular tachycardia—**AMIOVIRT**. *J Am Coll Cardiol* 2003;41: 1707–1712.

Design: Prospective, multicenter, randomized trial; primary endpoint was all-cause mortality at 3 years.

Purpose: To identify the benefit, if any, of ICD placement versus amiodarone in patients with NIDCM and a history of NSVT.

Population: 103 patients with NIDCM, EF ≤35%, and asymptomatic NSVT.

Treatment: Treatment with amiodarone or placement of an ICD.

Results: The study was stopped by the data safety and monitoring board (DSMB), as it met the prespecified stopping rule for futility. There were no differences in survival between the two groups at 1 or 3 years of follow-up (90% vs. 96% at 1 year, 88% vs. 87% at 3 years amiodarone and ICD, respectively; $p = 0.8$). Reported trends of improved arrhythmia-free survival and lower overall costs in the ICD group are difficult to interpret in the setting of stoppage for futility and a relatively small sample size.

121. **Kadish A,** et al. for the Defibrillators in Non-Ischemic Cardiomyopathy Treatment Evaluation (**DEFINITE**) Investigators. Prophylactic defibrillator implantation in patients with non-ischemic dilated cardiomyopathy. *N Engl J Med* 2004;350: 2151–2158.

Design: Prospective, randomized trial; primary endpoint was all-cause mortality at mean follow-up of 29 months.

Purpose: To identify the benefit, if any, of ICD placement in patients with NIDCM.

Population: 458 patients with NIDCM, EF <36%, and premature ventricular complexes or NSVT.

Treatment: Placement of a single-chamber ICD (with backup pacing rate of 40 bpm) with standard medical therapy or standard medical therapy alone. Standard medical therapy was a contemporary regimen including ACE inhibitors and beta-blockers.

Results: There were 28 deaths in the ICD group versus 40 in the medical therapy group (hazard ratio, 0.65; $p = 0.08$), and a significant reduction of sudden death from arrhythmia in the ICD group (3 vs. 17; hazard ratio, 0.20; $p = 0.006$). At 2 years, the mortality rate was 7.9% in the ICD group versus 14.1% in the medical therapy group.

Cardiac Pacing Studies

GUIDELINES

122. **Epstein AE,** et al. ACC/AHA/HRS 2008 guidelines for device-based therapy of cardiac rhythm abnormalities: a report of the American College of Cardiology/American Heart Association Task Force on Practice Guidelines (Writing Committee to Revise the ACC/AHA/NASPE 2002 Guideline Update for Implantation of Cardiac Pacemakers and Antiarrhythmic Devices). *J Am Coll Cardiol* 2008;51:e1–e62.

Two notable changes to these updated guidelines are that the following are now considered class Ia recommendations: BiV pacing in selected patients with HF, and ICD therapy for patients with a LVEF of 35% or less with class III or IV heart failure and at least 40 days post-MI.

MODE SELECTION TRIALS

123. **Lamas GA,** et al. for the Pacemaker Selection in the Elderly **(PASE)** Investigators. Quality of life and clinical outcomes in elderly patients treated with ventricular pacing as compared with dual-chamber pacing. *N Engl J Med* 1998;338:1097–1104.

This prospective, randomized, single-blinded, multicenter trial enrolled 407 patients older than 65 years who received dual-chamber pacemakers for bradycardia. Patients were then randomly assigned to a dual-chamber or ventricular-pacing mode. No significant differences between pacing modes were found for the primary endpoint of QOL or secondary endpoints of stroke or death. In patients with sinus node dysfunction, a trend toward less AF was seen with dual-chamber versus ventricular pacing (19% vs. 28%; $p = 0.06$). In addition, 26% of subjects assigned to ventricular pacing crossed over to dual-chamber pacing because of the symptoms of the pacemaker syndrome.

124. **Connolly SJ,** et al. for Canadian Trial of Physiologic Pacing **(CTOPP)** Investigators. Effects of physiologic pacing versus ventricular pacing on the risk of stroke and death due to cardiovascular causes. *N Engl J Med* 2000;342:1385–1391.

Design: Prospective, randomized, multicenter trial. Primary endpoint was stroke or cardiovascular death.

Purpose: To determine the benefits of physiologic (atrial or dual-chamber) pacing compared with ventricular pacing in patients with symptomatic bradycardia.

Population: 2,568 patients undergoing initial implantation of a permanent pacemaker for symptomatic bradycardia. Approximately 60% of patients had AV block, and 40% had sinus node dysfunction.

Exclusion Criteria: Chronic/persistent AF, prior AV junction ablation, and limited life expectancy.

Treatment: Implantation of physiologic (atrial or dual-chamber) or ventricular pacing system.

Results: At 3 years, no significant difference was found in the primary endpoint of stroke or cardiovascular death between physiologic and ventricular pacing groups (4.9% vs. 5.5%).

No significant differences in total mortality or CHF admission rates were seen. Physiologic pacing was associated with an 18% reduction in the incidence of AF (5.3% per year vs. 6.6% per year; $p = 0.05$).

125. **Lamas GA,** et al. for the Mode Selection Trial in Sinus-node Dysfunction **(MOST)** Investigators. Ventricular pacing or dual-chamber pacing for sinus-node dysfunction. *N Engl J Med* 2002;346:1854–1862.

Design: Prospective, randomized, multicenter study. Primary endpoint was death or nonfatal stroke.
Purpose: To determine the benefits of dual-chamber pacing compared with ventricular pacing in patients with sinus node dysfunction.
Population: 2,010 patients undergoing initial implantation of a dual-chamber pacemaker for sinus node dysfunction. Patients were required to be in SR at the time of randomization, but 45% had a history of AF.
Exclusion Criteria: Serious concurrent illness.
Treatment: All patients had dual-chamber pacemakers implanted, and then were randomized to dual-chamber (DDD) or ventricular (VVI) pacing modes.
Results: No difference was found between study groups in the incidence of death or nonfatal stroke. In adjusted analyses, small benefits favoring dual-chamber pacing were found for the secondary endpoints of hospitalization for HF (hazard ratio, 0.73; $p = 0.02$) and death, stroke, or hospitalization for HF (hazard ratio, 0.85; $p = 0.05$). Dual-chamber pacing was also associated with a lower incidence of any AF (hazard ratio, 0.79; $p = 0.008$) and progression to chronic AF (15% vs. 27% of those who had any AF; $p < 0.001$), and greater improvements in several QOL measures than with ventricular pacing. At the last follow-up, 31% of subjects originally assigned to ventricular pacing had crossed over to dual-chamber, about half of them for strictly defined pacemaker syndrome.
Comments: A subsequent secondary analysis revealed, as in MOST, a reduction not only in the incidence of AF with dual-chamber pacing, but also in the progression to chronic AF (2.8% per year vs. 3.8% per year with VVI pacing; $p = 0.016$) (see *J Am Coll Cardiol* 2001;38:167).

126. **Wilkoff BL,** et al. Dual Chamber and VVI Implantable Defibrillator **(DAVID)** Trial Investigators. Dual-chamber pacing or ventricular backup pacing in patients with an implantable defibrillator: the Dual Chamber and VVI Implantable Defibrillator (DAVID) Trial. *JAMA* 2002;288:3115–3123.

Design: Prospective, randomized, single-blind, parallel-group, multicenter trial. Primary endpoint was composite of death or first hospitalization for CHF.
Purpose: To determine the efficacy of dual-chamber pacing compared with backup ventricular pacing in patients with standard indications for ICD implantation but without indications for antibradycardia pacing.
Population: 506 patients with LVEF of 40% or less, no indication for antibradycardia pacemaker therapy, and no persistent atrial arrhythmias.
Treatment: All had an ICD with dual-chamber, rate-responsive pacing capability implanted. ICDs programmed to ventricular backup pacing at 40 per minute (VVI-40) or dual-chamber rate-responsive pacing at 70 per minute (DDDR-70).
Results: The VVI-40 group had a better 1-year survival free of composite endpoint [83.9% vs. 73.3% (for patients with DDDR-70); relative hazard, 1.61; 95% CI, 1.06 to 2.44]. A trend toward lower mortality in the VVI-40 group was noted (6.5% vs. 10.1%; relative hazard, 1.61; 95% CI, 0.84 to 3.09).

127. **Yu C-M,** et al., the Pacing to Avoid Cardiac Enlargement **(PACE)** Trial. Biventricular pacing in patients with bradycardia and normal ejection fraction. *N Engl J Med* 2009;361:2123–2134.

The investigators enrolled 177 patients with normal EF, bradycardia (due to either sinus node dysfunction or high-grade AV block), and an already-placed BiV pacemaker. They then randomized them to either BiV pacing or right ventricular apex pacing and followed EF and end-systolic volume at 12 months. At follow-up, EF was significantly lower in the RV pacing group (54% vs. 62%; $p < 0.001$), and LV end-systolic volume was higher in the RV pacing group (35.7 mL vs. 27.6 mL; $p < 0.001$). Average ventricular pacing was 98% in the BiV group and 97% in the RV pacing group ($p = 0.95$). Several issues were raised by this trial, particularly the persistent pacing of the RV in patients with sinus node dysfunction (as compared to dual-chamber pacing in an effort to spare the dyssynchrony induced by RV pacing). Investigators cite this as standard of care in China, where the trial was conducted; yet, the vast majority of such patients in the United States would receive dual-chamber devices, in an attempt to minimize dependence on RV pacing (for precisely the reasons demonstrated in the trial).

PACING FOR VASOVAGAL SYNCOPE

128. **Connolly SJ**, et al. for the North American Vasovagal Pacemaker Study **(VPS)** Investigators. A randomized trial of permanent cardiac pacing for the prevention of vasovagal syncope. *J Am Coll Cardiol* 1999;33:16–20.

Design: Prospective, randomized, open, multicenter study. Primary endpoint was time to first recurrence of syncope.

Purpose: To determine whether permanent pacemakers with rate-drop algorithms can reduce the frequency of vasovagal syncope.

Population: 54 patients with 6 or more prior syncopal episodes and a positive head-up tilt-table test, with syncope or presyncope and "relative bradycardia" (definition differed depending on whether test was performed with isoproterenol).

Treatment: Pacemaker implantation or continuation of medical therapy (not standardized).

Results: Study was terminated prematurely at first interim data analysis when a large treatment effect favoring pacemaker implantation was observed. Syncope had occurred in 19 (70%) of 27 no-pacemaker patients and only 6 (22%) of 27 pacemaker patients ($p < 0.001$). Time to first recurrence was 54 days in the no-pacemaker group and 112 days in the pacemaker group. Additional reductions in the rate of presyncopal events were seen in the pacemaker group, but were not statistically significant.

129. **Ammirati F**, et al. Syncope Diagnosis and Treatment Study Investigators. Permanent cardiac pacing versus medical treatment for the prevention of recurrent vasovagal syncope: a multicenter, randomized, controlled trial. *Circulation* 2001;104:52–57.

Design: Prospective, randomized, multicenter study. Primary endpoint was the first recurrence of syncope.

Purpose: To compare permanent dual-chamber pacemaker with pharmacologic therapy for recurrent vasovagal syncope.

Population: 93 patients with recurrent vasovagal syncope.

Treatment: Dual-chamber, permanent pacemaker implantation with setting of DDD (and a rate-drop response function), or pharmacologic therapy with the beta-blocker atenolol.

Results: Enrollment was terminated at the first interim analysis, as it demonstrated a significant effect favoring the pacemaker group (4.3% recurrence vs. 25.5%; $p = 0.004$) at a median of 135 days.

130. **Sutton R**, et al. Dual-chamber pacing in the treatment of neurally mediated tilt-positive cardioinhibitory syncope: pacemaker versus no therapy: a multicenter randomized study. The Vasovagal Syncope International Study (**VASIS**) Investigators. *Circulation* 2000;102:294–299.

Design: Prospective, randomized, multicenter study in Europe. Primary endpoint was the first recurrence of syncope, with mean follow-up of 3.7 years.

Purpose: To compare permanent dual-chamber pacemaker with standard therapy for recurrent neurally mediated syncope.

Population: 42 patients with severe cardioinhibitory tilt-positive neurally mediated syncope.

Treatment: Placement of permanent pacemaker set to DDI with rate hysteresis or no implant.

Results: Recurrent syncope was reduced to 1 patient with an event in the pacemaker group, versus 14 in the no-implant group (5% vs. 61%; $p = 0.0006$).

Comment: At repeat tilt-table testing 15 days after enrollment, there was no difference in responses between the two groups. This may highlight the potential confounding in this unblinded trial.

131. **Connelly SJ,** et al. for the Second North American Vasovagal Pacemaker Study Investigators **(VPS-II).** Pacemaker therapy for prevention of syncope in patients with recurrent severe vasovagal syncope. *JAMA* 2003;289:2224–2229.

Design: Prospective, randomized, double-blind, multicenter study. Primary endpoint was time to first recurrence of syncope.

Purpose: To determine if pacing therapy reduces the risk of syncope in patients with vasovagal syncope.

Population: 100 patients with 6 or more prior syncopal episodes or ≥ 3 in prior 2 years and a positive tilt-table test.

Treatment: Dual-chamber pacing (DDD) with rate-drop response or ODO.

Results: At 6 months, the cumulative risk of syncope was 40% for the ODO group and 31% for the DDD group. There was a nonsignificant 30% relative risk reduction in time to syncope with DDD pacing ($p = 0.14$). Lead dislodgement or repositioning occurred in seven patients.

132. **Raviele A,** et al. Vasovagal Syncope and Pacing Trial Investigators. A randomized, double-blind, placebo-controlled study of permanent cardiac pacing for the treatment of recurrent tilt-induced vasovagal syncope. The vasovagal syncope and pacing trial **(SYNPACE).** *Eur Heart J* 2004;25:1741–1748.

Design: Prospective, randomized, double-blind, placebo-controlled, multicenter study. Primary endpoint was time to first recurrence of syncope at median follow-up of 715 days.

Purpose: To determine if *blinded* pacing therapy reduces the risk of recurrent syncope in patients with vasovagal syncope.

Population: 29 patients with history of recurrent syncope and positive head-up tilt testing with asystolic or mixed response.

Treatment: All patients underwent permanent pacemaker implantation; they were then randomized to pacemaker ON or pacemaker OFF.

Results: At follow-up, recurrent syncope occurred in 50% patients with pacemaker ON and 38% of patients with pacemaker OFF ($p = $ NS); however, time to recurrence tended to be longer in the pacemaker ON group (median 97 days vs. 20 days; $p = 0.38$). These outcomes did not differ among patients with different responses to tilt testing.

Comment: The study highlights the importance of doing blinded, placebo-controlled trials to definitively resolve a hypothesis. While the study size is small, this trial very much put into question the results of earlier, unblinded trials of permanent pacemakers for syncope.

PACING FOR PREVENTION OF ATRIAL FIBRILLATION

133. **Carlson MD,** et al. A new pacemaker algorithm for the treatment of atrial fibrillation: results of the Atrial Dynamic Overdrive Pacing Trial **(ADOPT).** *J Am Coll Cardiol* 2003;42:627–633.

This study tested a specific pacing algorithm designed to pace the atrium above patients' intrinsic sinus rates to suppress AF, which is often triggered by atrial ectopic beats. Patients with sinus node dysfunction and two or more episodes of AF in the preceding month were randomized to dual-chamber pacing with or without this algorithm. Investigators reported an approximate 25% reduction in the "burden of AF."

134. **Fan K,** et al. Effects of biatrial pacing in prevention of postoperative atrial fibrillation after coronary artery bypass surgery. *Circulation* 2000;102:755–760.

In a cohort of 132 patients undergoing CABG surgery at a single center, patients were randomized to RA pacing, LA pacing, BA pacing, or no pacing after surgery. Overdrive pacing at 90 or 10 beats/min above the intrinsic rate up to 120 beats/min was performed for 5 days in the active-pacing arms. Rates of AF lasting 10 or more minutes or requiring intervention were 12.5% in the BA group and 36%, 33%, and 42% in the LA, RA, and no-pacing groups, respectively ($p < 0.05$ for all comparisons). Total length of stay was reduced about 2 days in the BA-pacing group, compared with the no-pacing group.

135. **Greenberg MD,** et al. Atrial pacing for the prevention of atrial fibrillation after cardiovascular surgery. *J Am Coll Cardiol* 2000;35:1416–1422.

Another single-center study randomized 154 cardiac surgery (CABG and valve replacement) patients to RA, LA, BA, or no pacing for 72 hours after surgery at rates of 100 to 110 beats/min. Beta-blocker use was strongly encouraged. AF lasting 1 hour or more and requiring urgent intervention occurred in 37.5% of subjects with no pacing, but in 8%, 20%, and 26% of subjects in the RA, LA, and BA groups, respectively. Thus, all pacing patients combined were significantly less likely to have AF than were no-pacing patients (17% vs. 37.5%; $p < 0.005$), but in contrast to the previously mentioned study by Fan et al., BA pacing was no better than RA pacing.

136. **Saksena S,** et al. Improved suppression of recurrent atrial fibrillation with dual-site right atrial pacing and antiarrhythmic drug therapy (Dual-site Atrial Pacing for Prevention of Atrial Fibrillation, **DAPPAF**). *J Am Coll Cardiol* 2002;40:1140–1150.

This prospective, randomized, single-blind, crossover study enrolled patients who had dual-chamber pacemakers implanted, with two atrial leads: one in the traditional high-RA position and one in the low RA, outside the ostium of the coronary sinus. Patients were then assigned to one of the following three pacing modes: high-RA overdrive, dual-site RA overdrive, or "support" (DDI or VDI at suggested rate of 50 beats/min) for 6 months, and then crossed over in random sequence to each of the other modes. Dislodgement of the "extra" low-RA lead was infrequent (1.7%). As expected, the "support" mode of pacing did the worst in terms of tolerability and rate of recurrent AF. Patients in the dual-site RA group were somewhat less likely to cross over because of mode intolerance than were patients in the high-RA group (time to crossover, 5.8 months vs. 4.7 months; $p < 0.01$) but had a similar proportion of mode-related adverse events. For the entire cohort, no significant difference was found between the dual-site and high-RA pacing groups for freedom from symptomatic AF or time to AF recurrence. Post hoc subgroup analysis did suggest the superiority of dual-site over high-RA pacing for AF suppression in patients with one or more AF episodes per week (hazard ratio, 0.62; $p = 0.006$), whereas a trend was seen only for patients taking antiarrhythmic drugs (hazard ratio, 0.67; $p = 0.06$).

RESYNCHRONIZATION THERAPY FOR CONGESTIVE HEART FAILURE

137. **Auricchio A,** et al. Effect of pacing chamber and atrioventricular delay on acute systolic function of paced patients with congestive heart failure: the Pacing Therapies for Congestive Heart Failure **(PATH-CHF).** Study Group. *Circulation* 1999;99: 2993–3001.

This single-blind study enrolled 42 patients with NYHA class III to IV CHF, EF less than 35%, and QRS durations greater than 120 msec, mostly due to left bundle branch block. All patients received BiV systems with the LV lead placed via limited thoracotomy. After implantation, the immediate hemodynamic performances of three different pacing modes (RV, LV, and BiV) were compared: LV pacing alone appeared most favorable. Patients then entered a 3-month crossover phase to select the optimal mode for the long-term phase, followed by a 12-month period of active pacing. At 12 months, BiV and LV pacing, compared with baseline, were associated with statistically significant improvements in 6-minute walk (446 m vs. 357 m; $p < 0.001$), peak oxygen consumption (1.19 L/min vs. 0.97 L/min; $p = 0.019$), anaerobic threshold (0.91 L/min vs. 0.76 L/min; $p = 0.018$), NYHA class (1.90 vs. 3.05; $p < 0.001$), and QOL (20 vs. 49; $p < 0.001$).

138. **Gras D,** et al. Cardiac resynchronization therapy in advanced heart failure: the multicenter InSync clinical study **(InSync).** *Eur J Heart Fail* 2002;4:311–320.

InSync was a nonrandomized study of BiV pacing, with all leads introduced transvenously. In the 103 subjects enrolled, on-treatment improvements (vs. baseline) were noted in NYHA class, QOL, and 6-minute walk. About half of the patients also had serial echocardiograms, and showed an increase in LVEF from 22% to 26% ($p = 0.006$). Only one procedure-related complication occurred.

139. **Cazeau S,** et al. for the Multisite Stimulation in Cardiomyopathies **(MUSTIC)** Study Investigators. Effects of multisite biventricular pacing in patients with heart failure and intraventricular conduction delay. *N Engl J Med* 2001;344:873–880.

Design: Prospective, randomized, single-blind, crossover, multicenter study. Primary endpoint was the 6-minute walk test.

Purpose: To assess the clinical benefits of BiV pacing (compared with no pacing) in HF patients with electrical conduction delays.

Population: 67 patients in SR with persistent NYHA class III symptoms despite optimal medical therapy, EF less than 35%, LVEDD more than 60 mm, QRS duration of >150 msec, and no other indication for pacemaker implantation. Nine patients withdrew before randomization, and 10 failed to complete both study phases.

Exclusion Criteria: Included hypertrophic or restrictive cardiomyopathy, treatable valve disease, acute myocarditis, recent acute coronary syndrome or revascularization procedure, and approved indication for ICD implantation.

Treatment: All patients had fully transvenous BiV pacing systems implanted, with RA and RV endocardial leads and LV leads introduced via coronary sinus branches. Two weeks after implant, patients were randomized to consecutive 3-month periods of "inactive" pacing (VVI at 40 beats/min) or "active" pacing in a crossover design. Optimal AV delay for active pacing was determined by echocardiographic evaluation at the time of implant.

Results: Initial implantation success rate was 92%. Early lead dislodgement occurred in eight patients and was corrected in all but three. Active pacing, as compared with "inactive," resulted in significant improvement in the average distance walked in 6 minutes (399 m vs. 325 m; $p < 0.001$). Active pacing also was associated with a 32% improvement in the QOL score ($p < 0.001$), and an 8% increase in maximal oxygen consumption ($p < 0.03$).

Comments: Similar benefits with BiV pacing were seen in 64 patients with chronic AF (see *Circulation* 2000;102:3349A).

140. **Abraham WT,** et al. for the Multicenter InSync Randomized Clinical Evaluation **(MIRACLE)** Study Group. Cardiac resynchronization in chronic heart failure. *N Engl J Med* 2002;346:1845–1853.

Design: Prospective, randomized, double-blind, controlled, multicenter trial. Primary endpoints were 6-minute walk, NYHA class, and QOL score.

Purpose: To assess the safety and efficacy of BiV pacing, compared with no pacing, in CHF patients with intraventricular conduction delay.

Population: 453 NYHA class III to IV patients with EF of 35% or less, LVEDD 55 mm or more, QRS duration of 130 msec or more, and 6-minute walking distance of 450 m or less.

Treatment: All received transvenous BiV pacing systems and then were randomized to active pacing (atrially synchronized BiV pacing) or no pacing for 6 months.

Results: Initial implantation success rate was approximately 92%; 30 patients required subsequent repositioning or replacement of the LV pacing lead. Compared with the control group, patients successfully treated with BiV pacing had significantly greater improvements in 6-minute walking distance (+39 m vs. +10 m; $p = 0.005$), peak oxygen consumption (+1.1 mL/kg/min vs. +0.2 mL/kg/min; $p = 0.009$), QOL (–18 points vs. –9 points; $p = 0.001$), time on treadmill (+81 seconds vs. +19 seconds; $p = 0.001$), and EF (+4.6% vs. –0.2%; $p < 0.001$). In addition, a significantly larger proportion of BiV patients improved one or more NYHA classes (68% vs. 38%; $p < 0.001$), and significantly fewer were hospitalized for worsening heart failure (hazard ratio, 0.50; $p = 0.02$).

141. **Young JB**, et al. Combined cardiac resynchronization and implantable cardioversion defibrillation in advanced chronic heart failure. The **MIRACLE ICD** trial. *JAMA* 2003;289:2685–2694.

Design: Prospective, randomized, double-blind, parallel-controlled, multicenter trial. Primary endpoints were changes between baseline and 6 months in QOL, functional class, and 6-minute walk distance.

Purpose: To examine the efficacy and safety of combined CRT and ICD therapy in patients with NYHA class III or IV CHF despite appropriate medical therapy.

Population: 369 patients with LVEF 35% or less, QRS duration of 130 msec, at high risk of life-threatening ventricular arrhythmias, and in NYHA class III or IV.

Treatment: All with ICD activated. Control group with CRT off.

Results: CRT group had a greater improvement in median QOL score ($p = 0.02$) and functional class ($p = 0.007$) compared to control group but there was no significant difference in change in 6-minute walk distance (55 m vs. 53 m; $p = 0.36$). CRT group did have a significant increase in peak oxygen consumption [+1.1 mL/kg/min vs. 0.1 (controls) mL/kg/min; $p = 0.04$].

142. **Bristow MR**, et al. for the Comparison of Medical Therapy, Pacing, and Defibrillation in Heart Failure (COMPANION) Investigators. Cardiac-resynchronization therapy with or without an implantable defibrillator in advanced chronic heart failure. *N Engl J Med* 2004;350:2140–2150.

This prospective, randomized, multicenter trial enrolled 1,520 patients with moderate or severe heart failure (HYHA class III or IV) due to ischemic or nonischemic causes with QRS >120 msec and PR interval >150 msec. Patients were assigned in 1:2:2 fashion to optimal medical therapy, optimal drugs plus CRT, or optimal drugs plus CRT with ICD (CRT-D). The primary endpoint was a reduction in death or hospitalization for any cause. At 1 year, the risk of the combined endpoint was reduced by 34% in the CRT group ($p < 0.002$) and 40% in the CRT-D group ($p < 0.001$). CRT-D significantly reduced the risk of death alone by 36% (p 0.003); CTR alone was not significant at 24% (p 0.059). The CRT-D mortality benefit was similar in those with ischemic and nonischemic etiologies.

143. **Moss AJ**, et al. for the **MADIT-CRT** Trial Investigators. Cardiac-resynchronization therapy for the prevention of heart-failure events. *N Engl J Med* 2009;361:1329–1338.

Design: Prospective, randomized, controlled trial. Primary endpoint was death from any cause or first nonfatal heart failure event over 2.4 years of follow-up.

Purpose: To identify the benefit, if any, of cardiac resynchronization on morbidity and mortality in patients with NYHA class I or II heart failure and ECG evidence of dyssynchrony.

Population: 1,820 patients with ischemic or nonischemic cardiomyopathy, EF ≤30%, QRS duration greater than 130 msec on ECG, and NYHA I or II symptoms.

Treatment: Conventional ICD placement or ICD placement with CRT, randomized in a 3:2 ratio favoring CRT.

Results: Treatment with CRT significantly reduced incidence of the primary endpoint when compared with ICD therapy alone (17.2% vs. 25.3%; $p = 0.001$). There was no difference between the ischemic or nonischemic groups; however, the composite primary endpoint was driven by a reduction in clinical heart failure events (13.9% for CRT-ICD vs. 22.8% for ICD-only; $p < 0.001$), without differences in mortality rates (3.3% for CRT-ICD vs. 2.5% in the ICD-only group). Total deaths, including those which occurred after a heart failure event, also were similar (6.8% for CRT-ICD vs. 7.3% for ICD-only; $p = 0.99$).

144. **Cleland JG,** et al. for the Cardiac Resynchronization—Heart Failure (**CARE-HF**) Study Investigators. The effect of cardiac resynchronization on morbidity and mortality in heart failure. *N Engl J Med* 2005;352:1539–1549.

Design: Prospective, randomized, controlled trial. Primary endpoint was death from any cause or unplanned hospitalization for cardiovascular event over a mean follow-up period of 29.4 months.

Purpose: To identify the effects of CRT on morbidity and mortality in patients with NYHA class III or IV heart failure.

Population: 813 patients with LV systolic dysfunction, NYHA III or IV symptoms, and cardiac dyssynchrony.

Treatment: Standard medical therapy alone, or with CRT.

Results: Primary endpoints were significantly reduced in the CRT group (39% vs. 55%; $p < 0.001$), and the effect was not just on morbidity, but mortality was significantly reduced in the CRT group as well (20% vs. 30%; $p < 0.002$). Additionally, CRT significantly improved several echocardiographic measures of LV function and efficiency.

TRIAL INDEX

SUBJECT INDEX

Page numbers followed by "*f*" indicate figures; and those followed by "*t*" indicate tables.